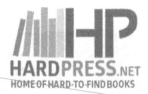

The Practice of Medicine
by Thomas Hawkes Tanner

Address:
HardPress
8345 NW 66TH ST #2561
MIAMI FL 33166-2626
USA
Email: info@hardpress.net

THE

PRACTICE OF MEDICINE.

—

VOL. I.

SIXTH EDITION.

THE

PRACTICE OF MEDICINE.

BY

THOMAS HAWKES TANNER, M.D., F.L.S.

MEMBER OF THE ROYAL COLLEGE OF PHYSICIANS,
FELLOW OF THE ROYAL SOCIETY OF LITERATURE, &c. &c.

IN TWO VOLUMES.

VOL. I.

THE SIXTH EDITION:

ENLARGED AND THOROUGHLY REVISED.

HENRY RENSHAW,

356, STRAND, LONDON.

1869.

[The right of Translation reserved.]

LONDON :
SAVILL, EDWARDS AND CO., PRINTERS, CHANDOS STREET,
COVENT GARDEN.

TO

WILLIAM FREDERICK DE LA RUE

THESE VOLUMES

ARE

INSCRIBED.

PREFACE.

A Sixth Edition of the Practice of Medicine having been demanded, all the time which could be spared from other onerous duties during the last two years has been devoted to rendering it more worthy of the great encouragement hitherto bestowed upon it. The fact of the book having been out of print for several months has been a subject of considerable regret, though it is hoped that the Reader will now reap the benefit of the unavoidable delay which has taken place in preparing the re-issue. For inasmuch as our knowledge of diseases and their treatment has been steadily advancing since the publication of the last edition in July 1865, I have been exceedingly unwilling to allow these volumes to pass out of my hands until such new matter as was necessary had been added, and until every page had been carefully and deliberately conned over. In this way the work has become much enlarged. Nevertheless, the original plan has been adhered to, of making its pages the medium of as much practical information as possible. Especially have I aimed at adopting a style which should be terse, without appearing obscure; while the endeavour has also been made to give particular prominence to those points which will aid the practitioner in the discharge of his responsible duties at the bedside.

Without attempting in any degree to deprecate criticism, it is still due to my readers to say how sincerely I trust it may not be thought that too dogmatic a tone has been adopted in the remarks upon the treatment of disease. But more than twenty years of daily observation have given me great confidence in the strength of the general principles which I have tried to inculcate in the following pages; and being thus zealously impressed, it is difficult (even were it advisable) to do otherwise than speak positively.

In conclusion, I cannot help expressing a hope that this work may still prove as useful, as its many friends have assured me it has hitherto been. While preparing each new edition I have felt my responsibility greatly increase; but the labour and anxiety have been lessened by bearing in mind Dr. Arnold's remark—" That so long as you humbly learn, so long you may hopefully teach."

HENRIETTA STREET, CAVENDISH SQUARE.

·17 *May* 1869.

GENERAL TABLE OF CONTENTS.

PART I.—GENERAL DISEASES.

PART IV.—DISEASES OF THE NERVOUS SYSTEM.

PART V.—DISEASES OF THE ORGANS OF RESPIRATION AND CIRCULATION.

GENERAL TABLE OF CONTENTS.

PART VI.—DISEASES OF THE THORACIC WALLS.

PART VII.—DISEASES OF THE ALIMENTARY CANAL.

PART VIII.—DISEASES OF THE LIVER.

CONTENTS

OF

THE FIRST VOLUME.

THE

PRACTICE OF MEDICINE.

PART I.
GENERAL DISEASES.

I. MORBID STATES OF THE BLOOD.

1. INTRODUCTION.—A nutritive fluid circulates through the tissues of all organised beings. This liquid, which is essential to life, is known as the sap in plants, and the blood in animals. The elaborated juice constituting the former is probably simply nutritive : the liquid flesh, as the latter has been termed, is a nutrient and something more, viz. the means by which used up materials are removed from the system.

In vain will the attempt be made to understand the nature of the various diseases to which the human body is liable, without a knowledge of the constitution and properties of the blood : that fluid which we have been emphatically taught "is the life of all flesh," through the instrumentality of which the various changes which attend the phenomena of life are accomplished, and by means of which the different organs and tissues of the body are directly nourished. The study of this subject, surrounded as it is with difficulty, is as interesting as it is important. And though it must be allowed that much has yet to be learnt, especially with regard to the chemical and microscopical characters of the blood in disease, yet not only are valuable observations gradually accumulating, but the improved methods of examination which can now be employed promise to yield very significant results.

The characteristics of the living organism are ceaseless change and ceaseless waste. Directly man begins to live, he begins to die. In the blood, as in the different tissues, the processes of decay and regeneration—of destruction and reconstruction, only terminate with the extinction of vitality. During action, the tissues waste ; during repose they are nourished, and the waste is repaired. That "the lamp of life" may burn brightly, the material for chemical action must be supplied in fitting proportions. Hence to breathe, to eat, to drink, to sleep—in other words, to maintain a due supply of the liquid by which nutrient matter is distributed to the various tissues—are the indispensable conditions of life. In the course of a single year an adult healthy man receives air and food and water amounting in the aggregate to more than 3000 lbs. (2240 lbs. = 1 ton); while in the same period of time he loses by urine and fæces, by transpired and expired matters, the same enormous amount of material. In infancy and youth the receipts are greater than the expenditure, and hence there is a gradual increase of weight. The bloodvessels, while they carry a certain amount of nutritive material to the tissues, only receive a smaller quantity of wasted material from them. But in old age this rule is reversed; and then as with the improvident, the means of repair become at length exhausted. The same thing happens in disease,—the general condition of equilibrium is upset; the balance being still further destroyed, owing to the useless or poisonous agents generated within the system not being removed as speedily or completely as is necessary.

Life is only to be maintained by the circulation of arterial blood; and whether no blood circulates through the arteries, or merely venous blood, the result is the same—death. When no blood circulates, death is said to take place from *syncope;* and this is of two kinds. Firstly, death by *anæmia,* in which there is a want of the due supply of blood to the heart, as is witnessed in fatal hæmorrhage, &c.; secondly, death by *asthenia,* where there is a failure in the contractile power of the heart—and this is seen to occur from the action of certain poisons, from intense grief or terror, from lightning, concussion, blows on the epigastrium, as well as from certain forms of apoplexy. It must be remembered that in some instances dissolution is due partly to anæmia and partly to asthenia; as may be particularly noticed in fatal cases of starvation, and in lingering disorders like phthisis, dysentery, &c.

When venous blood circulates through the arteries, life will be destroyed in one of two ways. In the first place we have death by *asphyxia,* or more correctly speaking by *apnœa* ['A = priv. + πνέω = to breathe], or *suffocation,* where the access of air to the lungs is prevented; as occurs in drowning, strangulation, choking, immobility of the respiratory muscles from tetanus, section of the phrenic and intercostal nerves, obstruction of the larynx by false membranes, many diseases of the lungs, and so on. Secondly, there is death by *coma,* in which the muscular movements required for respiration cease, owing to insensibility produced by some cerebral mischief; examples of which form are seen in many affections of the brain. Thus in death by apnœa we have successively impeded respiration, the circulation of venous blood, and insensibility; while in coma the order of the phenomena is reversed, and we find insensibility, cessation of the thoracic movements, and a stoppage of the chemical functions of the lungs.

The blood may be described as an albuminous fluid, charged with salts, holding fibrin in solution, and containing both coloured and colourless corpuscles. It is of high specific gravity, being on the average 1055, reckoning that of water as 1000 ; the extremes, compatible with health, varying from 1050 to 1059. The specific gravity is diminished by bleeding, anæmia, albuminuria, scurvy, gout, &c. ; while it is increased in cases of plethora, as well as in diseases attended with copious watery discharges—*e.g.* cholera, diabetes. The temperature is about 100° F.; being higher in the arteries than in the veins, with one or two exceptions. Bernard found the blood in the hepatic vein to range from 101° to 107° ; while in the aorta it varied from 99° to 105°. The reaction is constantly alkaline, the degree of alkalinity being greater during fasting than after food has been taken. The menstrual discharge, which consists of blood, offers no exception to this rule, in its pure state ; the acidity it sometimes manifests being merely due to the admixture of an acid mucus as the flow passes along the vagina. In fact, throughout the animal kingdom, the circulating fluid is always alkaline ; though it becomes spontaneously acid after death, owing—according to Bernard—to the sugar it contains being converted into lactic acid.

The statements made by physiologists as to the total quantity of blood present in the body vary greatly ; some observers estimating it at from one-fifth to one-eighth of the entire weight. Thus, Valentin says that from experiments on cats, dogs, rabbits, and a sheep, he was led to the conclusion that the blood has to the weight of the body a proportion of 1 to 4·08 to 1 to 6·32. Herbivorous animals had, on an average, less blood than carnivorous. Taking one-fifth as the mean value, he believes that a man of 30 to 40 years, whose average weight amounts to 140 lbs. would have 28 lbs. of blood. Wrisberg collected 21 lbs. 7¾ oz. from a very plethoric woman after decapitation ; while it is said that he saw 28 lbs. 11 oz. lost by uterine hæmorrhage ! On the other hand, Weber and Lehmann, from experiments on the bodies of two criminals who suffered death by decapitation, obtained results which seemed to show that the proportion was as 1 to 8 ; so that the body of a man weighing 140 lbs. would contain 17½ lbs. of blood. But again, the more recent and trustworthy investigations of Welcker tend to make it probable that even this proportion is too high ; and that in man and the mammalia generally the average relative weight of the blood to that of the body is only as 1 to 14. Hence the vessels of an adult healthy man will probably contain about ten pounds of blood ; the maximum being found as the digestion of a hearty meal is drawing to a close.

There is an immense difference—a difference of life and death —between the blood which enters, and that which issues from, the lungs. The former (venous blood) comes to the lungs charged with carbonic acid. The latter (arterial blood) is the fluid which maintains life, and which circulates between the lungs and the systemic capillaries. The course of the circulation is as follows :— The right auricle of the heart receives the blue venous blood of the whole body by the ascending and descending venæ cavæ and the coronary sinus.   From the auricular cavity it flows into the right ventricle, and so into the pulmonary artery to be distributed through the lungs.   Returning thence, the now crimson arterial blood is driven along the pulmonary veins into the left auricle, and then into the left ventricle.   From the latter it is urged into the aorta ; and by the ramifications of this vessel is distributed to all parts of the system, to be again returned by the capillaries and venous trunks and venæ cavæ.   The change of impure venous blood into pure arterial blood depends upon the exhalation of carbonic acid with the vapour of water, and the absorption of oxygen by the red blood-corpuscles ; so that a transudation of gases takes place as the blood in its flow through the pulmonary capillaries becomes exposed to the influence of the atmosphere in the cavities of the air cells.   The alteration from arterial to venous blood occurs in the systemic capillaries, and is due to the hæmatin yielding up the oxygen associated with it, and becoming charged with carbonic acid.   The theory, that in the act of respiration a combination or perfect oxidation took place in the lungs, owing to the oxygen from the air uniting with the carbon from the blood and forming carbonic acid, has been abandoned by some authorities. But since the experiments of Magnus, which led to the opinion that the oxygen and carbonic acid exist in the circulating fluid in solution or association and not in a state of intimate chemical combination, Liebig and others have adduced arguments tending to a revival of the first view.   Allowing that the question is undecided it seems to be generally thought that these gases are partly free in the blood, and partly in a state of loose chemical combination.   According to the researches of Pettenkofer on the elimination of carbonic acid and the absorption of oxygen by day and by night it appears, that large quantities of carbonic acid are formed during the day, while the absorption of oxygen at this time is comparatively small.   But at night, during repose, a considerable quantity of oxygen is absorbed ; which instead of being at once used up for oxidation, is, as it were, stored away in the system, ready for the wants of the ensuing day.   In other words, the process of oxidation has many intermediate stages ; and these occupy the oxygen for some hours within the system, before it is finally eliminated in the form of carbonic acid and water.

On minutely examining the blood as it exists while circulating in the vessels, we find it to consist of a transparent yellowish liquid called the liquor sanguinis or plasma ; which is formed of serum holding fibrin in solution, and in which are contained very numerous red discs termed blood corpuscles or blood cells, together with a few larger colourless corpuscles.   A red blood corpuscle, in the human subject, is a circular flattened cell without a nucleus; averaging $\frac{1}{3200}$ of an inch in diameter, and $\frac{1}{12000}$ in thickness, having an external structureless and elastic membrane, and red contents. The presence of an investing membrane is, however, denied by some physiologists. By such, these discs are regarded as homogeneous masses of a definite shape, rather than as bodies having a cell-wall with semi-fluid contents. In the first months of intra-uterine life, with all the mammalia, nuclei are present; while the same is the case during the whole existence of frogs, fishes, and birds. The corpuscles, as has been mentioned already, obtain oxygen in the pulmonary circulation, and transfer it to the most remote parts of the tissues they pervade,—being aptly termed carriers of oxygen; and then having given up this vivifying principle they return charged with carbonic acid to the pulmonary air cells, where they part with this impurity and receive a fresh supply of oxygen. The contents of the blood cells consist of a peculiar substance impregnated with red colouring matter, summarily called hæmatin. This latter contains a large amount of iron; and from it, under certain circumstances, three kinds of microscopic crystals can be obtained. The first variety of crystals has been named by Virchow *hæmatoidin*. They are formed spontaneously in the body, out of the hæmatin in coagula occurring in the Graafian vesicles, obliterated vessels, brain, &c. These crystals may be described as oblique rhombic columns of a yellowish-red or deep ruby tint, according to their thickness. Sometimes they resemble small crystals of uric acid or of the triple phosphates found in urine. And they are important because an effused mass of blood, as in apoplexy, cannot be removed, except by a large portion of it undergoing this form of crystallization. Moreover, hæmatoidin presents properties which show that it is allied to the colouring matter of the bile—biliverdin. The second kind of crystals has been called *hæmin*. Their pathological interest is small, inasmuch as they have to be produced artificially, by chemical tests; but they become of great significance to the medical jurist by affording a test of the presence of blood.* While the third class has received the name of *hæmatocrystallin*; crystals of this kind being very perishable, and only forming at a certain stage in the destruction of the blood cells. This crystalline substance was also formerly named globulin, owing to its erroneously supposed identity with the protein-body obtained from the crystalline lens.

The colourless or lymph corpuscles (termed *leucocytes* by Robin) have an average diameter of $\frac{1}{2500}$ of an inch. They are frequently circular and nearly spherical in shape, though they have the power of rapidly taking on various irregular forms. They are destitute of all colour, and very delicate in structure: whether they have

* The mode of obtaining these crystals as tests for the detection of bloodstains is shown in Virchow's work on *Cellular Pathology*, translated by Dr. Chance, p. 145. London, 1860.

any true cell-wall is uncertain. They possess soft and granular nuclei. The proportion of these white corpuscles to the red, in health, may be roughly stated as 1 to perhaps 370 or 400; although as they are immediately increased by food much will depend upon the time after a meal at which the examination is made. When first discovered they were mistaken for pus corpuscles, the result of pyæmia. The importance of these corpuscles in disease will be shown in the remarks subsequently to be made on leucocythemia. At present it need only be added, that many physiologists allow that they are identical with those bodies occurring in lymph, chyle, semen, colostrum, mucus, and pus, to which the general term *cytoid corpuscles* has been applied.

In addition to these red and white blood cells, the higher powers of the microscope reveal the presence of numerous minute molecules or granules, similar to those found in the lymph and chyle. During digestion especially, according to Gulliver, minute fatty particles may also be detected, exactly like those constituting the molecular base of chyle.

When the blood is fresh drawn from the body, it forms, in about ten minutes, a gelatinous mass; this singular alteration being caused by the tendency of the particles of fibrin dissolved in the plasma to agglutinate together. In some fifteen minutes, when the process of solidification is complete, the glutinous mass will be found to be shrinking and resolving itself into two distinct portions; which are known respectively as the *crassamentum* or *clot*, and *serum*. This shrinking is due to the further coagulation or contraction of the fibrin; and it continues for some thirty or forty hours, after which time no more serum is expressed. The *clot* consists, then, of the fibrin holding the red corpuscles entangled within the meshes it has formed. These corpuscles will either be equally diffused through the clot; or they may, by sinking from its surface, leave the upper part colourless. Where the latter happens, the colourless layer of fibrin, not being encumbered with corpuscles, contracts more than the lower part; and under these two circumstances the clot is said to be "buffed" and "cupped." The *serum* is the liquor sanguinis minus the fibrin; and consequently there is a most important distinction to be drawn between the plasma of living blood—so to speak, and the serum of blood removed from the vessels. This serum consists of a pale-coloured and watery solution of albumen; having a density of about 1029, being of alkaline reaction, and holding in solution many important substances. The albumen is probably associated or combined with soda; and it is the plastic material from which the tissues of all parts of the body are nourished, and by which the cells themselves grow. When deficient in quantity, indications of defective nutrition gradually become apparent. The fibrin probably arises from it, to be used up for the renovation and repair of the muscular tissues.

The attention of physiologists has long been directed to the discovery of the essential nature of this process of coagulation. But the question,—What is the cause of the solidification of the fibrin, in blood both in and out of the body? is still one that cannot be answered. There are objections to every theory which has been propounded :—to that of John Hunter, that " coagulation is an operation of life ;" to Hewson's, that the phenomenon is mainly due to the influence of atmospheric air ; to Scudamore's, that it is greatly promoted by the escape of carbonic acid ; to Draper's (a revived theory), that the fluidity of the blood during life is maintained by the muscular tissues picking out the fibrin, as it is solidified, for their nutrition ; and to Richardson's (now withdrawn), that the evolution of ammonia is the essential cause of the change We only know for certain that coagulation is favoured by rest, warmth, free access of air, and the multiplication of points of contact (Lister). Moreover, the subtraction of the influence of living vessels is, in all probability, largely instrumental in causing this phenomenon.

It is difficult to give the exact chemical composition of the blood ; since this fluid is not only altered in quantity and quality in different diseases, but it is also modified by the amount and variety of food taken. The following table, however, may be regarded as indicating the proportion of the constituents of healthy blood in 1000 parts :—

Water . . . . 784·

Oxygen . . ⎫
Carbonic acid ⎬ dissolved in the fluid.
Nitrogen . ⎭

Cell membrane ⎫ constituting the red corpuscles . . 131·
Hæmatin . . ⎭

Fibrin . . . . 2·5
Albumen . . . . 70·

Salts :—
Phosphate of soda, lime, magnesia, and iron . . ⎫
Sulphate of potash . . . . ⎬ 6·
Chlorides of sodium and potassium, silica, &c. . ⎭

Fats :—
Margarine . . . . . ⎫
Oleine . . . . . . ⎪
Seroline . . . . . ⎬ . . . . 1·2
Cholesterine . . . . ⎪
Phosphuretted fats, &c. ⎭

Extractive matters (creatine and creatinine among ⎫
the most important), with traces of urea, uric ⎬ 5·3
acid, biliary colouring matter, &c. . . . . . ⎭

The blood receives matter from three sources :—from the atmospheric air, through the lungs ; from the primary digestion, which takes place in the alimentary canal ; and from the secondary digestion, as that process is called by which the tissues which have served their purpose and become effete, are absorbed to be discharged from the economy. In return, it affords material for building up the tissues, for forming the secretions, and for producing the excretions ; while it also warms every part of the body. Hence, whatever interferes with the process of chylification, with respiration, with the excretory organs (as the bowels, liver, kidneys, and skin), and perhaps with the healthy condition of the nervous system, will affect the composition of the blood.   Mr. Paget adopts the proposition found in the writings of Treviranus,* to the effect that "each single part of the body, in respect of its nutrition, stands to the whole body in the relation of an excreted substance ;" and this certainly seems to be true.   Thus, to take only one example, it can readily be understood that the phosphates deposited in the bones are as effectually excreted from the blood as those which are discharged with the urine.   In health, then, when the sources of the blood are duly supplied, and when all the various organs and tissues abstract from this ever-circulating fluid the special materials they need, a general balance is maintained in the system ; but allow the rough materials for forming blood to be too large or too small in quantity, or let one organ act imperfectly, and every part of the body becomes necessarily more or less unfavourably affected.

The changes which take place in the blood under different circumstances will be noticed in treating of the various disordered states of the system.   It may, however, be useful to premise that as disease and death can arise from certain elements which are indispensable to the healthy nutrition of organs being deficient or absent in the food, so equally disastrous results will follow from injurious matters being retained or introduced in the blood.   To speak somewhat loosely, moreover, it can be noticed that inflammatory disorders remarkably modify the composition of the blood ; diminishing the albumen, doubling the amount of cholesterine, and increasing the quantity of fibrin to as much as even 10 parts in 1000.   During pregnancy the white corpuscles and the fibrin are increased, the red blood cells becoming rather deficient. Venesection, or hæmorrhage in any form, chiefly reduces the amount of the red particles, and to a slight degree lessens the quantity of the albumen and fatty matters ; while it also diminishes the density of the serum.   In Bright's disease and in cardiac dropsy the albumen is greatly diminished, owing to its escape in the urine or in the effused fluids ; whereas this element is probably increased in scrofula and cancer.   As regards starvation, scurvy, exhaustion from lingering disease, dipsomania, and fevers, the amount of fibrin is diminished.   A superalkaline condition of the blood may be produced

* *Die Erscheinungen und Gesetze des organischen Lebens*, Band i. p. 402. Bremen, 1831.   Mr. G. H. Lewes, in his work on the *Physiology of Common Life*, vol. i. p. 286, states that this conception is due to Caspar Friedrich Wolff, whose doctrine of epigenesis rests upon it.   See *Theorie von der Generation*, 1764.

by the use of alkalies, by abstinence from food, and by some forms of disease,—*e.g.*, typhoid and putrid fevers.

The chief source of the blood being the food, it follows that the careful selection and preparation of nutriment are among the most pressing necessities of our daily life. To expect to maintain healthy blood by scanty or improper food is as vain, as it is to hope that the healthy nutrition of the various tissues can be kept up by insufficient or morbid blood. There is, for example, no better established physiological axiom, than that the production of muscular activity depends on a free supply of pure arterial blood to the muscles; this supply being needed to facilitate that incessant transformation which is the necessary condition of muscular action, as well as to restore the waste. Of the various alimentary principles, not one of them taken singly is capable of maintaining the normal constitution of the blood. Albumen, fibrin, gelatine, gluten, sugar, starch, animal or vegetable fat, &c., consumed separately, cannot support life save for a very limited period. Moreover, in several experiments upon animals it has been found, that the attempt to maintain nutrition by any one of these substances alone, creates such disgust that the animal at length refuses to eat of it, even though dying of starvation. The value of every diet table, nay of every substance used as food, does not depend therefore upon the amount, however great, of any one alimentary principle that it may contain; but upon its possessing several such principles, blended in the proportions required for proper nutrition. Of the four organic elements (oxygen, hydrogen, nitrogen, and carbon) which principally compose the human body, nitrogen and carbon are those which have to be supplied most freely in the food; inasmuch as the phenomena of nutrition arise from the chemical interchanges of these elements, with the co-operating influences of oxygen and hydrogen, and certain salts. An average male adult in good health, performing an average amount of daily work, requires in the twenty-four hours from about 250 to 350 grains of nitrogen; from 3500 to 5000 grains of carbon; and perhaps 400 grains of salts. Or, if we speak of nitrogenous and carboniferous foods it appears, that three or four ounces of the former are needed to twelve or sixteen of the latter.

The *nitrogenous substances*, or albuminates, or plastic constituents of food, are those which are capable of being converted into the albumen or fibrin of the blood, and so of being assimilated subsequently by the tissues. The nitrogenous elements are in part heat-giving; but chiefly they are indispensable for the formation of muscular and nervous tissues, &c. The *fatty aliments,* including all animal and vegetable oils, are essential to nutrition. They are both plastic and calorifacient. To keep up mechanical force, the fats have to be furnished in due proportion just as the albuminates must be supplied. The *carbo-hydrates*, or starches and sugars and gums are believed to be simply combustible or heat-giving, and not plastic. In addition to these three great groups, it is necessary that certain *salts* and *water* be provided. Phosphate of lime, chloride of sodium, potash, magnesia, iron, and other saline matters are needed in the production of osseous and muscular and nervous substance; and as the body is constantly parting with these inorganic substances, so health cannot be maintained without their restoration. Fortunately, they are largely present in our drinking waters and meat and vegetables. Thus, the mineral elements in wheat, potatoes, watercresses, &c. are of great value. Then as water constitutes about four-fifths of the body, it can be understood how vitally significant the aqueous part of food must be. All important as solid food is, yet its loss is by no means so early appreciated by the system as is the deprivation of liquids. There still remains a group of substances which may be called *complemental foods*: that is to say, without acting as heat-givers, or muscle-makers, or bone-builders, these substances retard the destructive assimilation of tissue; while by their action on the nervous system they give rise to agreeable impressions, and render both mental and bodily labour less exhaustive than hard work proves to be without their aid. The chief articles in this class are tea and coffee, alcohol, and tobacco. They may all probably be regarded as compensating agents for a deficiency of food. Equally, where an excess of nourishment is consumed, the injurious consequences will be increased by these things—more especially by alcohol and tobacco.

An important question which remains to be noticed is, as to the quantity of food required for the maintenance of healthy nutrition? Now in answering this it is only possible to speak somewhat vaguely—to deal with generalities; so necessary is it that the amount should be modified according to age, climate, habits of life, custom, and so on. The healthy man who takes but little out of himself in the shape of work, will be called upon to restore less tissue-waste; and hence, his food ought to be less rich in flesh-formers than that of an active labourer—whether of mind or body. But granting this, there are still certain principles applicable to the average man, and these now claim a short notice. The daily loss of substance being great, an equivalent amount of liquid and solid aliment has to be introduced from without, if we would ward off disease and maintain life. Allow too much food to be consumed, and hyperæmia with other morbid conditions will result. Give too little, and inanition must be the consequence sooner or later. Too much work in proportion to the food can only lead to disease and death: it is impossible to obtain force without fuel. The daily discharge of water, as fluid or vapour, from the system being very large (it has been estimated at about 4 lbs. avoirdupois), it can be understood how urgent the demand for drink must be—as urgent almost as the need for oxygen. Of course, water is taken into the body in other ways than as a simple fluid, *e.g.*, abundantly in succulent meats and vegetables, &c. The amount of solid food required may be shown theoretically by estimating the solids in the various excretions. As actual observations are, however, more satisfactory, it suffices to refer to the experiments performed by Professor Dalton, of New York, on himself. This gentleman found that while living on an exclusive diet of bread, fresh meat, butter, and coffee with water for drink, the entire supply required during the twenty-four hours by a man in full health, taking free exercise in the open air, was as follows :—

Meat	16 ounces, or 1·00 lb. avoirdupois.	
Bread	19 ,, 1·19	,,
Butter or fat	3½ ,, 0·22	,,
Water	52 fl. oz., or 3·38	,,

That is to say, rather less than two and a half pounds of solid food, and rather over three pints of liquid. Had Professor Dalton been anxious to substitute other articles for the pound of meat, he might have secured the same amount of nitrogenous material (rather more than three and a half ounces) by taking four pints of milk, or fourteen eggs, or one pound and a half of oatmeal, or about two pounds of wheat flour or Indian meal, or five pounds of rice, or sixteen pounds of potatoes. None of these could, however, be taken continuously and solely without more or less detriment, except the milk and eggs. The latter must be nutritious, since they contain every principle required in the development of the chick. But of all the articles in daily use, there is not one which more perfectly illustrates what a model food should be than milk. This is shown very clearly in the following analysis of cow's milk by Payen :—

Water		86·40
Nitrogenised substances (casein, albumen, lacto- proteine, and matter soluble in alcohol) . . .		4·30
Lactose (sugar of milk or lactine)		5·20
Butter (or fatty matters)		3·70
A trace of colouring and aromatic matters.		
Salts, slightly soluble { Phosphate of lime . . ,, magnesia } ,, iron . .		0·25
Soluble salts { Chloride of sodium . . . ,, potassium . . . Phosphate and lactate of soda }		0·15
(Sp. Grav. 1032, at 60° Fahr.)		100·00

The foregoing table not only exhibits the value of milk as an article of ordinary diet, but it serves to illustrate the great importance which should be attached to this food as a restorative in disease. Believing that milk is less employed in the sick room than it deserves to be, the practitioner will find himself frequently reminded of its great utility in the ensuing pages.

It will now be convenient to notice in succession those disorders which in the present day are specially known as *blood diseases*.

2. HYPERÆMIA.—Plethora, or fulness of blood [*hyperæmia*, from Ὑπὲρ = in excess + αἷμα = blood; *polyæmia*, from Πολὺς = much;] consists of an increase in the whole mass of the blood, to an extent very variable in different cases. There is always a superabundance of the red corpuscles. The proportion of fibrin is probably unaltered, or it may be slightly increased [*hyperinosis*, from Ὑπὲρ = in excess + ἰς, ἰνὸς = the fibre of flesh]. The albumen of the serum is unchanged; the quantity of water being rather diminished.

When the blood merely exists in too great abundance in one or more particular organs or tissues we say that there is local hyperæmia, or partial plethora, or congestion, or determination of blood. There is no increase in the total amount of blood, nor in any of its constituents. Indeed partial plethora not uncommonly occurs in cases where the blood, taken as a whole, has been much diminished in quantity or quality by disease. Thus I have seen a woman lose a large quantity of blood by flooding directly after parturition, and yet the breasts have become greatly congested at the end of forty-eight hours, just prior to the secretion of milk. Again, if an organ be irritated mechanically, we cause an increased flow of blood to it through the arteries, thus giving rise to *active* congestion; a condition which, after a time, either decreases insensibly, or ends in hæmorrhage, or passes into inflammation. When the return of blood to the heart through the veins is impeded, as by the compression of one or more venous trunks, we have what is called *mechanical* congestion. Or again, the circulation of the blood through a part may be sluggish owing to want of tone in the walls of the veins and capillaries, as is often seen in persons debilitated by age or disease. We then have *passive* congestion.

The blood being directly fed by the chyle, it is evident that too free living must be one of the most common *causes* of hyperæmia. The normal waste of tissue, and consequent expenditure of blood, is also impeded by a sedentary mode of life. Sometimes this condition is hereditary; and not unfrequently I have found it occur in women after " the change of life." So again, plethora may result from the loss of an important part of the body. Thus, a spare man some months after amputation at the hip-joint became strong and robust and red-faced; for since he took as much food as he was accustomed to consume before the disease set in which rendered removal of his limb necessary, so of course he made as much blood as appeared needed for the nourishment of his body prior to nearly one-fourth part of it being removed.

The existence of general hyperæmia is marked by *symptoms* which cannot be overlooked. The face appears full and turgid, with a purplish tinge. The eyes seem rather small, and the conjunctivæ more moist than usual. There is distension of the capillaries, as can be observed on the lips and mucous surfaces. The pulse is large, somewhat hard, and resistent. There is also a turgid appearance of the veins. Obesity is sometimes an accompaniment, though by no means an infallible sign of plethora. Indeed, as will be mentioned in a subsequent section, many fat persons suffer from a deficiency, rather than from an excess, of blood ; and consequently they bear lowering measures during the progress of disease very badly.

Hyperæmia produces lassitude and indolence ; a desire for sleep, which is often accompanied with snoring and dreaming ; a liability to fits of vertigo and headache; and sometimes attacks of hæmorrhage, especially from the nose or from congested piles. In uncomplicated cases, there is not necessarily any special liability to dropsy, or fever, or inflammation. The blood, though present in excess, may yet be healthy, and will possibly be distributed equally to every part of the body. The chief fear is, that owing to the distension of the vessels the walls of one or more of them will give way ; a result of little moment if the blood escapes out of the body, though of vital consequence if it flow into the delicate structure of the brain from some ruptured capillaries.

The *treatment* of general plethora must consist in the adoption of a restricted diet, or the employment of non-nutritious substances ; in the avoidance of beer and all other alcoholic drinks ; in lessening the hours devoted to sleep ; and in the use of active exercise in pure air. Saline purgatives often do good (F. 165, 167, 169). The bromide of ammonium (F. 37) might be useful. So also, rather large doses of liquor potassæ (F. 73) have been recommended, especially where there is a rapidly-increasing tendency to grow fat ; although the efficacy of this medicine is very doubtful. In extreme cases the abstraction of blood ought to be had recourse to ; the quantity to be taken being measured by the immediate effects. Venesection judiciously employed will often afford sensible relief ; and provided the intervals between its employment be not too short, it is difficult to see what harm can arise. Of course I am supposing, that though the body is healthy in structure there exists more or less distress ; this being due to the blood-forming process going on too rapidly.

3. **ANÆMIA.**—Deficiency or poverty of blood [*anæmia*, from "Αναιμος = bloodless, the opposite condition to "Εναιμος = full blooded : *spanæmia*, from Σπανος = thin or poor + αἷμα = blood; *hydræmia*, from "Υδωρ = water; or *oligæmia*, from 'Ολίγος = little ;] arises generally in cases where there has been deprivation of the proper materials necessary for the formation of healthy blood ; such materials consisting of good food, pure air, light, sufficient clothing to afford protection from cold, &c. Anæmia is met with where

the digestive functions are imperfectly performed, as well as in the course of many serious chronic maladies. It occurs also in those diseases which are attended with a gradual draining of the circulating fluid,—as happens in persons suffering from bleeding piles, dysentery, women with menorrhagia or cancer uteri, &c. Profuse discharges of watery or albuminous fluids lead to it; while the same condition may of course be produced artificially by excessive venesection, the administration of mercury or antimony or active purgatives, and such like means. The anæmic state is not peculiar to any particular period of life: both males and females are equally affected by it. If the blood be analysed, it will be found that the red globules are deficient. Instead of existing in the proportion of about 130 per 1000 parts, as in health, they are reduced to 80 or 60, or even (in severe cases) to 30; while the hæmatin in those present seems paler than it should be. The number of the white cells is probably unaltered. The fibrin usually remains as in health, though it has sometimes been found diminished [*hypinosis*, from 'Υπὸ = under + ἰς, ἰνὸς = the fibre of flesh]. The liquor sanguinis is likewise poor in albumen; the quantity of water being more or less increased.

Those varieties of anæmia which are caused by tuberculosis, amyloid degeneration, fatty degeneration, albuminuria, carcinoma, scurvy, &c., will be treated of at length in succeeding pages.

Symptoms.—This disease proclaims both itself and its nature—impoverishment of the blood. The chief symptoms consist of a pale and waxy, or a sallow hue of the countenance and integuments generally; with a blanched appearance of the lips and tongue and inside of the mouth. The conjunctivæ are clear. The pulse is frequent, small, and quick—sometimes very quick. Attacks of frontal headache are often complained of; or there is an almost constant pain at the top of the head. Mental depression is generally a prominent symptom. And then we find more or less loss of appetite, with indigestion and flatulence and irregular action of the bowels; a free secretion of pale limpid urine; and great general debility with languor. There is often an enlargement of the thyroid gland; and with or without this an unnatural prominence of the eyeball (*exophthalmos, proptosis oculi*), producing a staring appearance as if the orbits were too small for their contents. The nervous sensibility is morbidly increased; and muscæ volitantes, with scintillations, are complained of. The temperature of the surface and extremities is below the normal standard. There may be œdema of the ankles, with or without albuminuria. While in women, the catamenial periods have either temporarily ceased; or they recur with regularity, but the fluid is pale and watery and usually scanty. Vaginal leucorrhœa is very common.

Then, in addition to the foregoing, the arteries in the neck are to be seen beating violently. The pulsations of the aorta can be readily felt just below the lower end of the sternum, by pressing on the stomach. It will likewise be observed that even moderate mental excitement or bodily exertion is attended by a sense of sinking, with fainting or syncope. There is also palpitation with hurried breathing. This panting dyspnœa is easily explained on the supposition that the blood cells are the carriers of oxygen; for allowing that these corpuscles are diminished, it necessarily follows that increased respiratory efforts must be established if the due oxygenation of the blood is to be maintained.

The suggestion has been made, that anæmia not only causes the respirations to be quickened, but that hurried breathing induces at length poverty of blood. The fact that housemaids in the lofty houses of large cities suffer thus, may perhaps be explained on this view. I have certainly found that steel alone fails to cure these cases. But when it is given during a rest of five or six weeks then speedy improvement takes place; the patient herself, in describing her progress towards recovery, often saying—" I seem to have more breath now."

On practising auscultation over different parts of the vascular system, certain inorganic murmurs can be heard. At the base of the heart, a soft systolic bruit or bellows-sound will frequently be detected; which may be traced distinctly up the aorta, and in the subclavian and carotid arteries. In some cases, an intermittent murmur, synchronous with the beat of the pulse, may be heard in all the large arteries. By placing the stethoscope over the large veins at the side of the neck, and especially in the right supraclavicular space, a continuous humming, or cooing, or even whistling sound—the *bruit de diable*—will be heard; a sound which is partly caused, as Dr. Ogier Ward first pointed out, by the descent of attenuated blood through the great cervical veins. Too much importance, however, must not be attached to this venous murmur. By making moderate pressure with the stethoscope it may be detected, though probably in a less degree than in anæmia, in the great majority of healthy individuals, and almost always in children and young women.

Where anæmia is of long continuance general atrophy sets in; together with dropsical effusions, great dyspnœa, diarrhœa, and profuse sweating. The pulse gets very frequent, irregular, and weak. The heart's action is rapid and palpitating. At times there are painful spasms or convulsions. Moreover, the low degree of vitality which exists, renders the system unable to resist the influence of any morbid poison to which it may be exposed. When death occurs it may take place gradually from exhaustion; or more suddenly from syncope, convulsions, or coma. The tissues will afterwards be found pallid and flabby: the heart and vessels will be comparatively bloodless. But no traces of structural disease can be detected, in cases of simple anæmia; with the exception, that the thyroid gland and possibly the spleen may be much enlarged.

Treatment.—Occasionally we meet with such serious cases, that we can for a time only trust to the most careful nursing, to the guarded exhibition of some preparation of cinchona, to the very frequent administration of wine or brandy, to the use of milk or cream or raw eggs or broth (F. 1, 2, 3, 17, &c.), to the application of warmth, and to the strict maintenance of the recumbent posture—possibly on a water bed. Nutrient enemata of cream and beef essence and wine may sometimes be needed, especially if the stomach cannot retain food. Otherwise, it is better not to attempt too much at first. These are instances, commonly, where there has been either gross neglect; or where the morbid state has arisen from some excessive loss of blood. Generally speaking, the patient is seen before matters have arrived at this very distressing stage. We then have the satisfaction of knowing that removal of the cause, the use of tonics and stimulants, the avoidance of all excesses, the due observance of mental and bodily repose, together with a suitable diet, will effect a cure. The remedies we particularly trust to are the various preparations of iron. If it be thought desirable to give metallic iron in a state of fine division, the practitioner will order the officinal ferrum redactum (F. 394); one grain of which is said to be equal to five grains of the citrate. This reduced iron is also valuable when combined with quinine (F. 380), or with aloes and nux vomica (F. 404). It ought only to be taken with the meals, as it otherwise is apt to cause disagreeable eructations of hydrogen. Then there is the citrate of iron and ammonia, which can often be borne when other preparations will not be tolerated. It may be prescribed with ammonia and citrate of potash (F. 403); or with cocoa-nut oil, brandy, strychnia, &c. (F. 391, 392, 394, and 408). Amongst other preparations also, it is well to remember the citrate of iron and quinia (F. 380); the phosphate of iron (F. 405); the tincture of perchloride of iron (F. 392, 402); the officinal pill of carbonate (saccharated) of iron; and the old officinal compound mixture of iron. The British Pharmacopœia, moreover, contains a formula for an "Aromatic Mixture of Iron," which is remarkable as forming about as inert a preparation as could well be concocted. It is only mentioned here that time may not be lost by prescribing it.

Attention should always be paid to the state of the bowels. If, as often happens, there is constipation, this condition will probably be aggravated by the use of steel. It becomes necessary, therefore, to avert this trouble by the combination of some aperient with the iron, or by the use of any mild cathartic, or by the employment of enemata. Steel and aloes (F. 154, 404); or this metal with Glauber's salts (F. 180, 181); or pepsine and aloes (F. 155); or either of the officinal extracts of aloes; or such remedies as magnesia, senna, sulphur, castor oil, &c., are sure to answer the purpose of the practitioner without proving too active for the patient.

The nervous system often requires to be calmed. This is done partly by the tonics already advised. But remedies such as ether, spirit of chloroform, Indian hemp, &c., are frequently needed in addition. As a rule, opium is best avoided ; but there are exceptional cases where it proves of great value. When there is much restlessness, soothing doses of henbane or hop are called for ; and when much palpitation, small doses of aconite do good (F. 325, 330, 342). Then plain nourishing food must be allowed as freely as it can be assimilated ; beginning with milk and raw eggs and beef tea, and port or Bordeaux or Hungarian wine, until we can advance to fish or poultry or mutton, cod liver oil, and unadulterated bitter ale or even good stout. Where the gastric juice is deficient in quantity, some preparation of pepsine will often work wonders (F. 420). A trial of one of the preparations of oxygen is also often advisable, particularly if there be much shortness of breath (F. 370). The only other curative agents to be remembered are out-door exercise, short of fatigue ; the respiration of pure air ; and cold bathing, particularly in sea water. Under the judicious use of such restoratives, the bloodlessness and all its resulting formidable symptoms entirely disappear ; though it must be remembered that as it takes a longer time to replace the red globules than the other constituents of the blood, so the remedies require to be persevered with for many weeks.

Transfusion of blood is said to have been successfully practised by some French physicians, during 1868, in two or three cases of severe anæmia. The only instance which I have found reported in the journals, ended unfavourably. The patient, who was dying from anæmia without any apparent organic disease, had blood from healthy subjects injected into his veins on four occasions by Professor Béhier. The quantity thus introduced within the space of a fortnight amounted to thirty-three ounces. At first the man seemed to rally ; but at a later period he was observed to exhibit symptoms of pulmonary and cerebral congestion. He died a few hours after the fourth operation. No morbid alterations of any importance were found on making the post-mortem examination ; only the organs were pale, flabby, and anæmic. It was remarked that the blood, which at first was quite watery and poor, had grown much thicker under the process of transfusion. The question naturally arises whether the injection of healthy blood can sufficiently excite the blood-forming organs to such a normal action as to keep up the supply of nutritive material. At present, the answer would seem to be in the negative.

In anæmia dependent on too severe mental occupation, the phosphate of iron or zinc, or the phosphoric acid in some tonic infusion (F. 376, 405, 414), together with cod liver oil, do much good. In such cases the blood gets poor and watery to a marked degree ; and hence requires to be enriched by rest from intellectual pursuits, a diet more than ordinarily rich in nitrogenous materials,

as well as by the employment of chalybeates. Coffee, wine or
bitter ale, and even tobacco in great moderation will prove useful.
Overwork of the brain produces undue destruction of the nervous
tissue, and consequent deterioration of the vital force, as certainly as too prolonged or too intense muscular action, or as
an insufficient supply of nourishment.

Invalids from tropical climates very often suffer from anæmia.
This will possibly be the result of long residence in malarious districts ; or it may be the sequel of hepatitis, fever, dysentery, and
cholera.   In the treatment of remittent and intermittent fevers,
&c., in India, bleeding and mercury and purgatives and low diet
often constitute the remedies.   Leeches appear to be employed
by dozens at a time; and of course they must usually produce
severe and protracted anæmia.   Sir James Ranald Martin mentions several cases where hundreds of these blood-suckers had
been used during an illness.   One gentleman, who was so unlucky
in 1855 as to fall from his horse, had twenty-two dozen applied at
once ; while another was invalided for life, after the employment
of at least three thousand leeches in six years.*   Necessarily, in
patients thus treated, the blood remains impoverished, and the
whole system enfeebled, for a very long time after the European
has returned home :—in fact, the disease, whatever its nature,
could hardly be more injurious than the remedy.   Amongst the
symptoms by which anæmia is especially characterized in tropical
invalids, we find repeated hæmorrhages, passive congestions of the
thoracic or abdominal viscera, and abdominal neuralgic pains.
Let the nature of these signals of debility be mistaken, or allow
depletion in any form to be resorted to, and very grave mischief
will result.   The only remedies of any avail are good food, ferruginous tonics, a complete holiday, and a residence in the country
air.   Sir Ranald Martin particularly recommends a visit to the
Highlands of Scotland, a suggestion not to be forgotten.

A peculiar form of anæmia, technically known as CHLOROSIS
[Χλωρὸς = green], frequently affects young women about the age of
puberty. According to some authorities this disease has its origin in
the nervous system; the disturbance of the digestive, circulatory, and
uterine functions being the effect of this morbid action.   Without
entirely denying this theory, I am sure that many cases which
have come under my notice have been dependent on, or at least
very intimately connected with, disordered menstruation, in combination probably with certain sexual causes.   The nervous system
has suffered equally with the circulating and the muscular, just as
all the tissues become affected when the blood is too poor to
nourish them properly.   But this suffering has appeared to me to

* *The Influence of Tropical Climates in producing the Acute Endemic
Diseases of Europeans.*   Second Edition, p. 652.   London, 1861.

stand in the relation of effect instead of cause. In chlorosis, the red corpuscles are pale and small, being also diminished in number, even to one-third of the normal standard; while the proportion of albumen in the liquor sanguinis is natural. The fibrin, in some instances, has been found to be increased, though no trace of any inflammatory action was to be discovered in the system. In chlorotic women the wax-like hue of the countenance is remarkable. Indeed, so peculiar is this pallor of the skin, that the disease is popularly spoken of as the *green sickness*. The subjects of it present certain prominent symptoms. Thus, they have a deficient or depraved appetite, gastric dyspepsia, inactivity of the liver, offensive breath, and constipation; the urine is abundant and pale and of low specific gravity, while the bladder is irritable so that it has to be frequently emptied; the integuments are puffy, perhaps œdematous; the mucous membranes have an exsanguine and flabby appearance; the tongue is flaccid and indented at the edges by the teeth, while the gums have a marked pallor and are inclined to be spongy; the pulse is frequent and small and quick; and the menstrual discharge is absent, or it appears at irregular times and is pale and scanty. There is an indisposition for all mental or bodily exertion; with vertigo, headache, intolerance of light and noise, palpitations, pain in the left side over the false ribs, backache, and various hysterical affections. The same cardiac and vascular murmurs are to be detected as in anæmia; and not unfrequently also the same enlargement of the thyroid gland, with the peculiar protrusion of the eyeballs.

These phenomena are developed gradually, and often after there have been symptoms of disordered menstruation for some little time. Dysmenorrhœa and leucorrhœa are very common precursors of chlorosis. In cases where the heart's action has become much enfeebled, there is a fear that syncope may occur suddenly and prove fatal. I have seen two or three instances also, in which all the symptoms have rapidly become aggravated, a condition of great drowsiness has followed, and the patients have died comatose at the end of a few hours.

The cure of this affection is not usually difficult. Perfect health may generally be restored by attention to the diet and mode of living, and by a course of chalybeates. I say " generally," because of those rare instances just alluded to, where severe symptoms set in suddenly, and death takes place as if from cerebral effusion. When we administer iron in cases of chlorosis and anæmia, it acts as a general tonic; while in all probability it becomes assimilated and enters directly into the formation of the blood globule, increasing the amount of hæmatin. The soluble preparations of steel are not so much more active than the insoluble, because the latter get oxidized in the alimentary canal. They must, however, be administered in a state of minute subdivision. According to some authorities, the more astringent the chalybeate, the greater its power; but this view is opposed to the results of my own observation.

4. **LEUCOCYTHEMIA.**—This remarkable affection may be best defined as a morbid state of the blood, in which the white corpuscles are greatly increased in number, while the red cells are much diminished. It is always connected with hypertrophy of one or more of the lymphatic glands, or of the spleen.

Leucocythemia has been particularly investigated—or, to speak more fairly, discovered—by Hughes Bennett and Virchow. The latter named it *Leukhemia*, or white blood; an objectionable term, inasmuch as the blood is not white, but of its usual colour. Dr. Bennett has therefore substituted the word *Leucocythemia*, from λευκὸς = white + κυτος = a cell + αἷμα = blood; literally white cell-blood. The first example of it was described by Dr. Bennett in October 1845, who regarded it as an instance of "suppuration of the blood without inflammation." It occurred in a case of hypertrophy of the liver, spleen, and lymphatic glands. Six weeks subsequently Virchow published the notes of a similar case; and gave what cannot but be deemed a more correct explanation of its nature. For he showed, that the bodies which Dr. Bennett regarded as pus globules resulting from some process of development in the blood itself, were really the colourless corpuscles of the blood very greatly increased in number.

Symptoms.—Very little is known of this disease or its causes at present. It occurs generally in adults; and decidedly is more frequent in advanced life than in the young. In cases where it has been found to exist, the majority of the patients have suffered from an unusual pallor, like that of anæmia; from great and progressive emaciation, with marked debility; from more or less swelling of the abdomen, owing to enlargement of the spleen, or liver, or both; from disordered respiration; as well as from increasing prostration and emaciation, gradually ending in death. In many cases, moreover, there has been obstinate diarrhœa; there have been repeated attacks of hæmorrhage in some form or other, but especially epistaxis; and there has been much suffering from nausea, jaundice, fever, and loss of appetite. Frequently, towards the close, there will be found œdema of the extremities; together with dropsical effusions into the pleuræ, pericardium, or peritoneum. Ascites is perhaps more common than other forms of dropsy; the fluid effused being especially abundant when there is great splenic enlargement.

The analyses which have been made of the urine in leucocythemia are few in number. But so far as those which have been published can teach us anything, they show that the uric acid is always augmented. This increase occurs absolutely as well as relatively to the urea. Thus in health, the proportion of uric acid to urea is about 1 : 60; while in the disease under consideration it has been found even higher than 1 : 20. The urea itself is present in greater proportion than in health, as is the sulphuric acid; while the chlorine is diminished. Leucine has also been detected, as it has in other morbid states of the system; though this substance is never present in healthy urine.

Diagnosis.—If we examine the blood of a patient affected with the symptoms just described, no mistake can be made with regard to the nature of the disease. On placing an ounce or two of leucocythemic blood, which has been freed from fibrin, in a narrow glass, the red corpuscles sink to the bottom, while the upper part of the mass looks like milk. This latter appearance is due to the colourless corpuscles; and it may be distinguished from that caused by fat, owing to the circumstance that it is not removed by ether. In extreme cases portions of the blood resemble pus.

On looking at the blood microscopically, under a magnifying power of 250 diameters, the yellow and colourless corpuscles are at first seen rolling together; the excess in the number of the latter being at once recognisable, and becoming more evident as the coloured bodies get aggregated together in rolls leaving clear spaces between them filled with the colourless ones. A drop of blood taken from a prick in the finger is sufficient for examination. The results of chemical analysis on nine occasions recorded by Dr. Hughes Bennett, show an excess of fibrin and a diminution of blood corpuscles.

Prognosis.—This is always unfavourable. The marasmus [Μαραίνω = to grow lean] generally increases steadily. All that can really be done is to try and put off the fatal termination : in this attempt we may sometimes be successful for one or two years.

Pathology.—In health the ratio of colourless to red corpuscles is about 1 : 373 (Donders and Moleschott); whereas in the disease under consideration they often stand to the red corpuscles in the high proportion of 1 : 3. According to many physiologists the red corpuscles are formed from the colourless ones by the direct transformation of the latter into the former. From numerous observations, however, Dr. Bennett believes with Wharton Jones that the coloured disc is merely the liberated nucleus of the colourless cell. The opinion, first promulgated by Hewson, that the blood corpuscles were derived from the lymphatic glands, has been generally rejected. But after a careful consideration of the subject, Dr. Hughes Bennett confirms this view. The conclusions this gentleman has drawn, after much laborious research, are these :— " 1. That the blood corpuscles of vertebrate animals are originally formed in the lymphatic glandular system, and that the great majority of them, on joining the circulation, become coloured in a manner that is as yet unexplained. Hence the blood corpuscles may be considered as a secretion from the lymphatic glands, although in the higher animals that secretion only becomes fully formed after it has received colour by exposure to oxygen in the lungs. 2. That in mammalia the lymphatic glandular system is composed of the spleen, thymus, thyroid, supra-renal, pituitary, pineal, and lymphatic glands. 3. That in fishes, reptiles, and birds, the coloured blood corpuscles are nucleated cells, originating in these glands; but that, in mammals they are free nuclei, sometimes derived as such from the glands, at others developed within colourless cells. 4. That in certain hypertrophies of the lymphatic glands in man their cell elements are multiplied to an unusual extent, and under such circumstances find their way into the blood, and constitute an increase in the number of its colourless cells. A corresponding diminution in the formation of free nuclei, and consequently of coloured corpuscles, must also occur. This is leucocythemia."*

From the foregoing it follows, that one or more of the blood-glands will be found enlarged in the disease under consideration. Most commonly this change is discovered in the spleen, liver, and lymphatics; less frequently the thyroid body and the supra-renal capsules are affected. Sometimes the spleen has weighed as much as nine pounds; but it must not be inferred that this organ cannot become greatly enlarged without the blood being leucocythemic. The liver has been found to be hypertrophied, or cirrhosed, or cancerous; though in some instances it has been perfectly healthy. The condition in which the increased proportion of colourless corpuscles appears to be dependent upon an affection of the lymphatic glands has been designated *Leucocytosis* by Virchow, in contradistinction to that due to splenic hypertrophy. But the foregoing remarks will show that this is a very unnecessary distinction; and one which, as it seems to me, can only lead to confusion.

Treatment.—The remedies which would appear to promise the most success, for a time, are certain tonics; especially perhaps, bark, iron in various forms, and quinine. Iodide of potassium and the chloride of potassium have been fruitlessly tried. As there is undoubtedly an increased metamorphosis of nitrogenous tissues in this disease, so plenty of good animal food will be indispensable; while cod liver oil may often no doubt prove beneficial. In the choice of subordinate restoratives and drugs, the practitioner must in a great measure be guided by the prominent symptoms in each case; always taking care to check any attacks of hæmorrhage or diarrhœa as soon as they arise.

5. **PIARHÆMIA.**—Healthy blood contains, on an average, somewhat less than two parts of fat in a thousand; and it probably exists in combination with potash or soda, as a kind of soap. Hence on a minute examination of normal blood no oil globules are to be seen. Milkiness of the serum or fatty blood [*piarhæmia*, from Πῖαρ = fat + αἷμα = blood; *pioræmia*, from Πίων = fat;

---

* *Clinical Lectures on the Principles and Practice of Medicine.* Fourth Edition, p. 891. Edinburgh, 1865.

or *lipæmia*, from Λίπα = fat;] is met with under certain circumstances in disease, and hence demands attention. Its physical causes are two—viz., free fat, and molecular albumen.

In the first place, piarhæmia is a *physiological* result of digestion, pregnancy, lactation, and hybernation. During the process of digestion, the lactescence of the serum is said by Becquerel and Rodier to begin about two hours after the ingestion of aliment, and to continue for two or three hours. The serum is found to be turbid and opalescent and semi-opaque; a transitory condition that is due to the absorption of the fatty matters of the food, which have been formed into an emulsion by the pancreatic juice and absorbed as such in the duodenum. Examined microscopically, this constitution of the serum is seen to be caused by the presence of a large number of fat globules and of molecular granules of albumen. According to Christison and Lecanu, the passage of the chyle into the blood renders the serum turbid; such turbidity lasting until the insoluble fatty matters—oleine, stearine, and margarine—enter into combination with the free soda of the blood, and become converted into the oleic, stearic, and margaric acids.

Secondly, lactescent serum is a *pathological* result of disease. The cases in which its occurrence has been noted are diabetes, chronic alcoholism, dropsy, jaundice, nephritis, hepatitis, pneumonia, and especially Bright's disease. In an interesting case of piarhæmia accompanying acute diabetes, recorded by Dr. Charles Coote, which ran its course very rapidly and was attended with great prostration, the blood after death was found fluid and homogeneous and of a dull-red colour like raspberry cream; while in a few seconds it separated into two distinct portions, the supernatant layer being of the colour and appearance of thick cream, while the subjacent portion presented the appearance of fluid venous blood. The creamy layer was certainly nothing but free fat, for it was wholly taken up by ether.

Various explanations have been given of the occurrence of fatty blood in disease. Formerly, pathologists attributed it to the passage of unaltered chyle into the circulation; an explanation which, though in some measure true, was shown by Hewson to be insufficient, since he observed this condition in many instances where the patients had taken little or no food for many days. Raspail maintained that the fat was set free in the blood for want of a free alkali to hold it in the form of a soap. Dr. Babington appeared to look upon piarhæmia as a fatty degeneration of the albumen of the blood. Rokitansky thinks it is often due to fatty degeneration of the colourless corpuscles, which are previously formed in excess, so that it is to be regarded as a modification of leucocythemia; but he also admits the direct introduction of fat into the blood, as well as the liberation of combined fat contained in it, to be possible causes. Virchow considers it as dependent upon the non-combustion of fat, and its consequent accumulation in the blood ; while he believes the presence of molecular albumen to be only a secondary phenomenon, the slow saponification of the excess of fat abstracting from the albumen of the blood the alkali required to keep the latter in solution. And lastly, Dr. C. Coote, from a comparison of all the facts which have been published upon this topic, concludes :*—1. That piarhæmia consists in an excess of saponifiable fat in the blood, and not in the mere liberation of fat from its combinations. 2. The excess of fat may be the result of two causes—viz. (a) the excessive ingestion of fat, as in piarhæmia during digestion; (b) the diminished elimination of the same, as in hybernation and pulmonary diseases. 3. Fat, if directly in-gested, may enter the blood with the chyle through the thoracic duct; though from the consideration of the case recorded by Dr. Coote, it seems that it may also be elaborated in and absorbed directly from the liver. 4. Piarhæmia is not a result of diabetes mellitus, for either may exist without the other. 5. The pathology of blood milky from molecular albumen must be considered as still almost wholly negative. Though probably never an independent affection, yet it is not a mere accidental occurrence of piarhæmia. Its apparent relation to albuminuria seems to point to some organic change in the constitution of the plasma of the blood itself.

6. **GLUCOHÆMIA.**—The excretion of sugar by the kidney, constituting a disease known as diabetes, or diabetes mellitus, or sac-charine diabetes [*diabetes*, from $\Delta\iota\dot{a}$ = through + $\beta a i \nu\omega$ = to move ; *melituria*, from $M\ell\lambda\iota$ = honey + $o\check{v}\rho o\nu$ = the urine ; *glucosuria*, from $\Gamma\lambda\nu\kappa\dot{\nu}\varsigma$ = sweet ; *glucohæmia*, from $\Gamma\lambda\nu\kappa\dot{\nu}\varsigma$ + $a\tilde{\iota}\mu a$ = blood ;] has at-tracted considerable attention since the time (about the year 1660) when Thomas Willis first observed the saccharine condition of the urine in this affection. More than a century later (1774) Matthew Dobson discovered, that the blood as well as the urine contains sugar in this disorder ; from which he inferred that the saccharine matter is not formed in the kidneys, but only eliminated by them. Four years afterwards (1778), Cowley succeeded in isolating the saccharine principle. John Rollo next taught (1796) that an animal diet lessens the amount of urine excreted, as well as the quantity of sugar. Then (1815) Chevreul learnt that the sugar differs from cane sugar, and resembles that of the grape; while ten years subsequently (1825) Tiedemann and Gmelin found that starch during its passage along the alimentary canal is transformed into sugar. Henceforth, the only justifiable opinion was to this effect :—viz. that the sugar formed in the stomach and alimentary canal, from the starchy and saccharine elements of the food, instead of being converted into other compounds, was absorbed and excreted by the kidneys. Dr. M'Gregor (1837) positively detected sugar in the serum of the blood, in the saliva, in the

* *The Lancet.* London, 8th and 15th September 1860.

stools, and also in the vomited matters of diabetic patients. It necessarily followed that the treatment of diabetes consisted in allowing a diet free from substances which could be converted into saccharine matter; and it is certain that thus the general symptoms were frequently alleviated, while the amount of sugar which could be detected in the urine was usually considerably diminished.

We now come to what may be appropriately called the physiological epoch in the history of diabetes. Just twenty-one years have elapsed since M. Claude Bernard asserted (in 1848) that animals, as well as vegetables, possess a sugar-forming power. Previously it had been the universal belief, that all the sugar found in the system was derived from the starchy and saccharine elements of the food. But Bernard's elaborate researches on what he has called the glycogenic function of the liver, were destined to direct attention to a new field. This eminent physiologist, while allowing that sugar could be formed during digestion, and that a certain portion might become absorbed, has yet further taught that this substance is a normal secretion of the liver. Thus, if a dog be fed for some time on a purely animal diet and then killed, the blood of the portal vein or that going to the liver will be found free from sugar; whereas the blood of the hepatic veins or that flowing from the gland, will be highly charged with it. He also proved that sugar may be formed in abnormal quantities by irritating the eighth pair of nerves at their origin in the fourth ventricle; while section of both these nerves suspends the sugar-forming function of the liver. In health the sugar produced by the liver passes into the hepatic veins, the inferior vena cava, the right cavities of the heart, and thence by the pulmonary artery to the lungs where it is consumed. When abnormally increased, the lungs cannot excrete all of it; and hence part passes off by the kidneys, producing diabetes. But although the division of the pneumogastric nerves has the effect just mentioned, yet the sugar-forming power of the liver is restored by irritating their upper cut ends; and diabetes can be produced just as if the origins of these nerves were excited. On the other hand, the application of an irritant to the lower ends of the divided nerves gives no result. Bernard therefore concludes that the nervous power which excites the liver to secrete the saccharine matter, does not originate in the brain, to be carried by the pneumogastrics to the hepatic organ; but rather that the stimulus proceeds along these nerves to the brain, and thence by reflex action is transmitted to the liver. Further consideration led to the opinion that in health the reflex action which excites the hepatic sugar-forming function originates in the stimulus given by the air we breathe to the pulmonary branches of the pneumogastrics. He believes, in short, that at each inspiration these branches receive a stimulus which is transported through the main trunks of the nerves to the brain, and is thence reflected by the spinal cord and the thoracic portion of the sympathetic to the liver. Experiments in proof of the foregoing showed, that when the function of respiration is stimulated—as by the exhibition of ether or chloroform—sugar temporarily appears in the urine. Again, it is supposed that just as the lungs act by reflex influence on the liver, so increased action of the liver acts upon the kidney; and hence that sugar produced in excess in one organ is excreted by the other.

Pursuing his investigations still further, Bernard was led to the conclusion (announced in March 1857) that the liver secretes a substance which is changed into sugar by some ferment, instead of forming the sugar directly. This glycogenic or sugar-forming substance, on being separated from the liver, presents the characters of hydrated starch; and when it comes into contact with the supposed ferment in the blood the transformation is effected. The sugar in the blood, when the latter reaches the lungs, is decomposed by the oxygen and disappears; so that the liver produces the glycogen which forms the sugar, whilst the lungs are the organs in which the latter is consumed. Of course during health, only the blood which circulates between the liver and the lungs contains saccharine matter; and, therefore, whenever this material is found in the circulation generally, it must be the consequence either of excess of hepatic power, or of diminished pulmonary action.

In July 1857, Dr. Harley published* his views on the pathology of diabetes, and showed that while agreeing in the main with Bernard, he yet doubted the conclusion of this physiologist that in the normal state respiration is the excitor of the glycogenic function of the liver. His experiments seem to indicate that if the pneumogastric carries the stimulus to the brain, to be thence transmitted by the spinal cord and splanchnic nerves to the liver, the point of departure of the stimulus is probably in the liver itself; and that the cause of the reflex action may originate in the stimulating effect of the portal blood upon the hepatic branches of the pneumogastric. Thus, if the stimulating effect of the blood of the portal vein be imitated by injecting into that vessel ether, chloroform, alcohol, or ammonia, the liver is excited to secrete an excess of sugar, and the animal operated upon is rendered for a time diabetic. This sugar belongs to that class of which grape sugar is the type. For just as in the vegetable kingdom there are two great types of sugar, cane and grape; so in the animal kingdom we find the representative of the first in milk sugar, and of the second in liver sugar. Dr. Harley also confirms the opinion of M. Chauveau that the sugar is not destroyed in any appreciable quantity during its passage through the lungs. On the contrary, he believes that this agent, formed by the liver, goes to the sup-

* *The British and Foreign Medico-Chirurgical Review*, vol. xx. p. 191. London, 1857.

free from admixture of azotized matters; whereas the substance found by Virchow is in more or less complete union with nitrogen. (2) The amyloid substance of Bernard is found in greatest abundance in the hepatic tissue about six hours after a full meal; from this time diminishing steadily and gradually if the animal be not fed. A diet containing much starch and sugar greatly increases the amount of amyloid substance formed in the liver (M'Donnell and Pavy). And (3) diabetes is the result of some defective action of the liver. What this defective action actually consists of, and what are the circumstances which give rise to it, still remain problems to be solved. It has long been known, as already mentioned, that a temporary diabetes is produced by pricking the floor of the fourth cerebral ventricle; by injuries to the base of the brain and cerebellum; by over mental work and anxiety; as well as by derangements of the stomach. Moreover, Dr. Pavy proved, in 1859, that a like condition ensues on injuring certain portions of the sympathetic—amongst other parts, the superior cervical ganglion. But how these various operations act can scarcely be surmised at present.

For the sake of convenience, as well as in accordance with custom, the symptoms and diagnosis and treatment of this affection will be considered in the section on renal disorders; though after the previous remarks it is hardly necessary to say, that the occurrence of saccharine urine is only a prominent symptom of one or more diseases.

7. **URÆMIA.**—The urine is one of the chief depurating secretions by which the normal condition of the blood is maintained. When, from any cause, the function of the kidneys becomes impaired or suppressed, urea (furnished, in great part at least, from the metamorphosis of the worn-out tissues, uric acid perhaps standing in the relation of an intermediate substance) and other substances which these organs ought to remove from the system are no longer eliminated, and they therefore accumulate in the blood, producing that morbid condition known as uræmia [from *urea*, + *aἷμα* = blood].

The important amount of work performed by the cells of the uriniferous tubes is very clearly shown in the following table by the Rev. Professor Haughton, of Trinity College, Dublin.* It exhibits the *natural daily constants of the urine of the average man;* the analysis giving results corresponding with those generally obtained, save that the uric acid is much below the average—scarcely one-half of the medium quantity discharged. From an examination of the table we cannot but infer that suppression of the renal excretion is one of the most dangerous events which can happen :—

* *The Dublin Quarterly Journal of Medical Science,* vol. xxxiv. p. 288. Dublin, 1862.

Excretion. Weight of Body 145 lbs.	Per day.	Per day per lb. of body-weight.
Urine.	52·62 oz., or 23021·25 grs.	2·84 drs., or 155·348 grs.
1. Urea	493·19 grs.	3·331 grs.
2. Uric acid	3·15 „	0·021 „
3. Phosphoric acid	32·36 „	0·218 „
4. Sulphuric acid	31·55 „	0·214 „
5. Chlorine.	106·56 „	0·673 „
6. Extractives	175·27 „	1·183 „
7. Balance (viz., inorganic bases) .	115·73 „	0·827 „
Total solids.	957·81 grs.	6·467 grs.

The quantity of urea excreted by the kidneys in the twenty-four hours is influenced by many circumstances. Thus it is increased by intellectual labour, by animal food, and by age—the young and old excreting less than individuals in the prime of life. There is also an increased amount in many diseases : e.g. the continued and eruptive fevers, inflammations of internal organs, ichorhæmia and diabetes. On the contrary, there is a decrease in chronic diseases accompanied by impaired nutrition, in convulsions, in some forms of paralysis, in cholera, in albuminuria, and in many fatal disorders towards their close. Of course this diminution may depend either on lessened production, as when the diet consists chiefly or exclusively of vegetable matter ; or it can be owing to arrested elimination—to lessened excretory activity of the kidneys, as happens in Bright's disease &c.

The term *uræmic intoxication* is employed to denote that peculiar kind of poisoning which results from the non-elimination of urea and other urinary constituents by the kidneys, and the consequent accumulation of these materials in the blood. As we shall presently see, considerable discussion has taken place as to whether the simple accumulation of urea is sufficient to account for the symptoms ; Frerichs asserting that the real poisonous agent is carbonate of ammonia resulting from the decomposition of the retained urea by some ferment in the blood. Moreover, the opinion entertained by most physiologists that the kidneys only separate already formed urea and uric acid from the blood seems about to be modified. If recent investigations prove to be correct, it will have to be granted that these organs manufacture as well as select. According to Oppler, a larger amount of urea is present in the blood after ligature of the ureters than after extirpation of the kidneys ; whilst, on the contrary, the quantity of creatine in the muscles is greater after the latter proceeding than after the former. And Zalesky, from numerous experiments upon animals, the results of which were published in 1865, has learnt that though urea and uric acid are found in the spleen and brain and other organs, still the largest proportion is formed in the kidneys themselves. Whatever conclusion, however, may be come to on either of these points, the significant clinical fact remains, that uræmic toxæmia is induced by whatever interferes with the excreting functions of the kidneys.

The direct effects of this poisoning are seen in a disturbed action of the two great nervous centres,—the brain and spinal cord. These centres will be affected either separately or together. Consequently we have three forms of uræmic poisoning :—(1) That in which a state of stupor supervenes rather abruptly, and from which the patient is aroused with difficulty. It is soon followed by complete coma, with stertorous breathing, as in ordinary poisoning from opium. (2) The variety in which convulsions of an epileptic character suddenly set in, often affecting the entire muscular system. There is complete insensibility throughout the attack, unless the convulsions are only partial. In this latter case, consciousness remains unimpaired. And (3) that kind in which coma and convulsions are combined.

Albuminuria with uræmia may arise from other conditions than structural disease of the kidney. The convulsions which occur during pregnancy and parturition are supposed by some to be caused by the pressure of the uterus, giving rise to active renal congestion ; while others regard them as due to a degradation of the maternal blood. Suppression of urine (*ischuria renalis*, or *anuria*) is a frequent and often fatal result of cholera, and of other morbid poisons in the blood. It now and then forms a very dangerous symptom during the progress of fever, and of the exanthemata— particularly scarlatina.

The *phenomena of uræmic poisoning* have usually been ascribed to the direct action of the urea retained in the blood. In 1851, however, Frerichs* advanced the opinion that the toxæmia is not due directly to this retention ; but to the conversion of the urea into carbonate of ammonia, through the influence of some particular ferment supposed to be present in the circulating fluid. At first, this view was almost universally accepted ; the experiments upon which it was based being regarded as convincing. Moreover, by its light an explanation was apparently given of those cases where individuals in the last stage of renal disease have their blood highly charged with urea, without any uræmic phenomena taking place ; simply, it was argued, because the unknown ferment, by means of which the urea is converted into carbonate of ammonia, is absent. But in a short time, when the nature of the ferment had been fruitlessly sought for, doubts began to be thrown on this hypothesis ; and more recently it would

* *Die Bright'sche Nierenkrankheit und deren Behandlung,* p. 111. Braunschweig, 1851.

appear to have been completely overthrown by the labours of Zimmerman,[*] Hammond,[†] Bernard,[‡] Richardson,[§] and others. Briefly it may be said that there are two highly important objections to the views of Frerichs : —(1) That ammonia is not an abnormal constituent of the blood. (2) There is no proof that urea, while retained in the blood, is converted into carbonate of ammonia. It is true that Frerichs detected ammonia in the breath of persons labouring under Bright's disease ; but Richardson, in conducting many examinations of persons in perfect health, failed to find it in only one.[||] The experiments which most strongly tend to support the views of Frerichs, are those performed by Dr. Alexander Petroff, of Dorpat. They were chiefly undertaken to disprove the validity of Dr. Oppler's explanations ; who, finding that the quantity of urea and extractives in the blood of dogs whose kidneys had been removed was much increased, and that the muscles contained more leucine and creatine than under ordinary circumstances, concluded that uræmic poisoning was caused by the accumulation of products of decomposition of nitrogenous matter within the centres of the nervous system. Very careful experiments appear to have been made by Dr. Petroff on the comparative effects of injections of ammonia into the blood, and the artificial production of uræmia. The following are the general conclusions at which he arrives : —(1) When the kidney function is interrupted, carbonate of ammonia is formed in the blood. (2) Injection of carbonate of ammonia into the blood produces symptoms strictly comparable to those of uræmia. (3) The degree in which these symptoms appear, and their character, depends on the proportion of ammonia in the blood, and the circumstances under which it exists there.

Nevertheless, as before mentioned, this attempted confirmation of Frerichs' theory has attracted but little attention. And it is certain, that authorities in this country now regard those views which were previously accepted as most probably correct. They have, in addition, been especially upheld by Dr. Hammond ; who,

---

[*] *The British and Foreign Medico-Chirurgical Review*, vol. xi. p. 289. London, 1853.

[†] *Physiological Memoirs*, p. 303. Philadelphia, 1863. Dr. Hammond's essay was first published in the *North American Medico-Chirurgical Review*, April 1858.

[‡] *Leçons sur les Propriétés Physiologiques et les Altérations Pathologiques des Liquides de l'Organisme*, tome ii. p. 36. Paris, 1859.

[§] *Clinical Essays*, vol. i. p. 133. London, 1862.

[||] The presence of ammonia in the expired air is roughly proved by holding a glass rod moistened with hydrochloric acid before the mouth, and obtaining the thick white fumes indicative of its presence. Or, more correctly, we may test for it by Richardson's process; which consists in moistening a slip of glass with hydrochloric acid, and exposing it to the suspected vapour. If ammonia be present, minute crystals of chloride of ammonium will be formed; and these are readily detected by a microscopic examination, with an object-glass of moderate power.

after much observation and numerous well-devised experiments, ascribes uræmic intoxication to the direct action of the elements of the urine retained in the blood upon the brain and nervous system, in a manner we do not yet understand. Of these excrementitious elements it is almost certain that urea is the most poisonous. The fact, that this substance in large quantity has been found in the blood of persons affected with renal disease in whom no symptoms of blood poisoning were present, at first sight appears to militate against this view. But then we must attribute some share of the mischief to the diminution of the corpuscles and albumen in the blood, as well as to the increase of the creatine and extractives, &c. And while allowing that these variations occur in different degrees in different subjects, so it may also be granted as Dr. Hammond suggests, that (as with most other poisons) all persons are not alike sensitive to the action of urea. Moreover, in kidney degeneration this salt generally accumulates very slowly; so that the system is thus enabled to tolerate a much greater quantity than when a large amount is suddenly thrown into the blood.

At the same time it is not denied, that after the urea has been secreted by the kidneys it can be readily decomposed into carbonate of ammonia when there is some impediment to the exit of the urine from the system. Thus, in examples of obstruction of the ureter, paralysis of the bladder, stricture of the urethra &c., the urea being acted upon by some animal matter as a ferment, will undergo decomposition; this change occurring more rapidly even than it does when the urine is out of the body, inasmuch as the secretion is maintained at a higher temperature, and is more supplied with mucus or pus. The decomposed product becoming absorbed, an excess of ammonia will soon collect in the blood; and then symptoms of ammoniacal poisoning (*ammonæmia*) result. The chief of these are a highly ammoniacal state of the breath and perspiration; a glazed appearance of the tongue and fauces; a sallow condition of the complexion; and attacks of rigors. In extreme cases, death may occur preceded by coma. The urine is offensive, it deposits amorphous phosphate of lime with crystals of ammoniaco-magnesian phosphate, and it is often purulent. The reaction is always alkaline, from the presence of the volatile alkali; so that if it be tested with reddened litmus paper a blue colour is produced, which can be removed by the application of gentle heat. When urine exhibits an alkaline reaction from the presence of a fixed alkali, the blue colour communicated by it to reddened litmus paper is permanent, instead of being destroyed by heat. This simple test is of great importance; for where there is alkalinity from the volatile alkali, the urine has been secreted acid, but has undergone decomposition afterwards. In the case of the fixed alkali, the kidneys have secreted sweet-smelling alkaline urine, in consequence of an increased alkalescence of the blood; this being due either to the consumption of a peculiar food or medicine, or to the existence of some morbid action in the system. In ammonæmia, medical interference often suffices to effect a rapid cure,— chiefly by taking care that the bladder is thoroughly emptied with a catheter, that this viscus is washed out every twelve hours with warm water, and that benzoic acid is freely administered.

If now we return from this digression and examine a typical case of uræmic poisoning, we shall find, on investigating the history, that there have been certain *premonitory symptoms*. Those particularly to be mentioned are œdema of the face and extremities, drowsiness, snoring during sleep, transitory attacks of mental confusion, partial paralysis of sensation, debility, biliousness, chilliness, nausea and vomiting, together with occasional sharp attacks of diarrhœa. Moreover, there is often a very fetid condition of the breath, owing to its being charged with ammonia. Then, the *acute symptoms* have been preceded by a chill or distinct rigor, and particularly by complete suppression of urine. Coma or convulsions, or both together, have set in unexpectedly; the coma perhaps being so profound that the patient cannot be roused. The skin is found cold, the complexion of a dusky tinge, the pupils insensible to light and dilated, the pulse slow and infrequent and intermittent, and the respiration obstructed. Frequently, however, the breath is no longer ammoniacal.

Now it is necessary to remember that it is not every case which presents all the symptoms just described. Thus, the practitioner will be occasionally puzzled by finding that there is merely coma without any convulsion; while the comatose condition will possibly be so slight that there is no difficulty in rousing the patient. The pupil may be natural; and neither dropsy, diarrhœa, nor vomiting shall have occurred. Nevertheless, there is either suppression of the functions of the kidneys; or if any urine can be obtained from the bladder it will be found highly albuminous, and proportionately deficient in urea.

The explanation of the ammoniacal state of the expired air is simple according to the views of Dr. Richardson. It has been already mentioned, that in all persons there is an exhalation of ammonia by the breath; while in healthy urine there is also a very small quantity of this volatile alkali present. In uræmia, prior to coma or convulsions, the amount of ammonia in the breath is increased, for the lungs are supplementing the kidneys. But when the acute symptoms have been developed, the alkali may be absent from the respired air; owing to the unfortunate circumstance that the compensating eliminating function of the lungs has become suppressed.

Under treatment the acute symptoms sometimes pass off, and recovery to a greater or less extent ensues. Even in those very unpromising cases where there is structural disease of the kidney, the patients will now and then rally for some little time.

The *diagnosis* of uræmic toxæmia is not unattended with difficulty. Without care it is not unlikely to be confounded with those other diseases of which coma and convulsions are the prominent symptoms. Thus uræmia simulates epileptic coma, apoplexy, hysteria, cerebral anæmia, acholia, cholæmia, and alcoholic or narcotic poisoning. But the diagnosis may generally be correctly made by inquiring into the functions of the kidneys. For, in all cases of renal coma or convulsions, we find either complete suppression of urine; or this excretion is scanty, of low specific gravity, deficient in urea, and highly albuminous. To distinguish suppression of urine from retention, it will possibly be necessary to use the catheter. Sometimes it happens that urea can be detected in the vomit, in the saliva, and in the sweat. When abundant in the latter, this salt has been found deposited on the skin in the form of a kind of scurf; which, on a minute examination, has been seen to consist of urea and scales of epithelium.

Moreover, urea is present in the blood in considerable quantity; as can be proved by the following method of analysis :—Take the serum procured after venesection or that which may be obtained from a good-sized blister, and add a few drops of acetic acid to it. Then evaporate to dryness over a water-bath; and extract the residue with boiling alcohol, which is a ready solvent of urea. This alcoholic extract is to be evaporated to dryness, treated with a few drops of distilled water, plunged into a freezing mixture, and then to have added to it a few drops of pure nitric acid. If urea be present, the characteristic crystals of nitrate of urea soon appear in the solution, and are positively recognised by the microscope.

From time to time it happens that a patient is not seen until he is comatose, and when (from the absence of friends) no account or previous history can be obtained. In a fatal case of epileptic coma which I saw some years ago under these circumstances, the symptoms so strongly resembled those due to uræmia, that no diagnosis could be made until the urine was drawn off and analysed. The attendants upon the patient concluded that some narcotic poison had been taken; and as there were certain incidental matters of a suspicious nature it was deemed necessary to hold a coroner's inquest. Not that there was any failure in the medical evidence, but unpleasant rumours began to be circulated, and publicity seemed necessary to remove them.*

The *treatment* of a case of uræmia must be considered under two heads :—1. Where there is an excessive excretion of urea, there is greater tissue waste than is desirable. It is probable that this may be checked by benzoic acid (F. 49); by citrate of iron and quinia (F. 380); as well as by digitalis, colchicum, acetate of potash, phosphate of soda, &c. Supposing that the occurrence of coma or convulsions is feared, the attempt should be made to purify the blood by means of those extensive excretory channels—

* *Medical Gazette.* New Series, vol. xiii. p. 578. London, 1851.

the skin and intestinal canal. Sweating can be induced by the
hot air bath, together with the copious administration of diluents,
such as tea and iced lemonade and cold water, &c. ; or by wrapping
the patient in the wet sheet (F. 136); or by sponging the body
with tepid vinegar—a proceeding which often produces copious
diaphoresis. The best purgatives, perhaps, are saline aperients
with colchicum (F. 141); or assafœtida and castor oil enemata
(F. 190); or elaterium, jalap, or podophyllin (F. 157, 151, 160).
Where there is debility, small doses of steel had better be given (particularly F. 392, 403). And I feel sure that I have done much
good in these cases by the prolonged exhibition of arsenic (F. 52,
399), though I am not prepared to state its mode of action. The
practitioner must carefully avoid the use of calomel ; for even one
or two moderate doses may develope mercurial ptyalism in cases of
renal disease. So also, opium is generally objectionable ; although,
on the principle of selecting the lesser of two evils, I have not
hesitated to resort to it where there has been great irritability or
sleeplessness. Blisters, nay even sinapisms, can be of no service,
while they have caused gangrene of the skin. Stimulants, such as
wine and brandy and whisky, are capable of causing much mischief, though used in moderate doses. Nevertheless, they are not
to be withheld if absolutely needed ; for given with caution, and
properly diluted, I have seen them do more good than harm. The
diet should be plain ; and while nourishing, ought not to contain
much animal food.

  2. As regards the management of those cases where the eclamp-
tic fits have set in, I know of no remedy so efficacious as chloroform
(F. 313). The inhalation of this agent, or of a mixture of chloroform and pure ether, may really be resorted to without fear;
though doubtless it requires some courage to administer it, particularly where the practitioner has not previously seen its value, and
where the patient is already insensible from the toxæmia. At the
same time, an antispasmodic mixture of ether, assafœtida &c., can
be used as an enema. Purgatives may be employed if the bowels
are loaded. If deemed advisable, sweating should be induced by one
of the means already mentioned. And lastly, venesection has been
advocated ; on the principle that in proportion as the cerebral and
renal congestions are relieved, consciousness will gradually be
restored. Without denying that opening a vein may sometimes be
useful where there is congestion of the brain, yet as I believe
there is an opposite state during all convulsions, the practice cannot
but be condemned. Moreover, it has happened to me to witness
examples of puerperal convulsions attended with flooding ; and in
some of these it was certain, that the more freely the blood came
away, the greater became the severity of the symptoms. Nevertheless, so far as I recollect none of the cases on which this
observation is founded, ended fatally ; so that they may be made
to tell both against and in favour of the abstraction of blood.

Finally, it appears certain that the formation and excretion of urea are much increased by a purely animal diet; and that the amount of this substance is greater under a rich or mixed, than under a spare or vegetable diet. Hence, when the kidneys act imperfectly it may not be unadvisable to attempt to limit the production of urea (or of creatine, if we incline to the views of Oppler and Zalesky) as far as possible. This is to be effected by the employment of starchy and fatty foods, as arrowroot and tapioca and sugar and cream &c.; all nitrogenous matters being allowed in diminished quantity. *Have seen Dr H's Sutton whief in uses of arsenic with such good little*

8. ACHOLIA.—The liver is the largest gland in the body; its weight, in the adult, varying from 2 to 4 lbs. During digestion it always becomes much congested; and consequently, while this function is in action, the organ is both larger and heavier than at other times. There are many reasons for believing that four different operations are conducted by the hepatic cells :—(1) The production of amyloid substance. (2) The manufacture of bile. (3) The final destruction of old blood corpuscles, probably after their partial disintegration in the spleen. While (4) they probably aid in the perfecting of the young corpuscles or blood cells.

Human bile is a complex fluid; being viscid, of a dark golden-brown tint, having a specific gravity of about 1018, and being neutral when perfectly fresh. The secretion of it is constantly going on; though this takes place most actively during digestion. The daily quantity of bile secreted in man is not positively determined; but if it bear any proportion to that in the carnivora we may estimate it, from the experiments of Bidder and Schmidt, at about 2½lbs. for an adult weighing 140lbs. The following, in addition to 88 per cent. of water, are the constituents of the bile :—(1) Biline or biliary matter; a compound of soda combined with two resinous acids—the glycocholic and taurocholic, forming glycocholate and taurocholate of soda. (2) Cholesterine, a crystalline fatty matter not peculiar to bile. (3) Biliverdin and bilifulvine, or colouring matter. (4) A resinous or waxy material. (5) Chloride of sodium. And (6) inorganic matter—chiefly soda, potash, magnesia, and lime.

Until very recently the physiologists of the present era have generally allowed (and the opinion is still maintained by many authorities) that none of the matters which constitute bile exist preformed in the blood; so that the constituents of this fluid have been supposed to arise not by a process of simple excretion, but by one of actual formation in the liver. The hepatic cells, it has been said, not only attract certain matters from the blood flowing through the capillary vessels, but they effect within their cavities a transmutation of these matters. Hence, disorganization of these cells—or, in other words, arrest of the functions of the liver—from any cause, must lead to acholia.

In order that the practitioner may become acquainted with the most recent opinions upon the formation of bile, attention will be fitly directed to some important researches on this matter. And, to begin, it must be confessed that our knowledge of the uses and pathological importance of *cholesterine* is not very precise. Dr. Austin Flint, junior, of New York, however, has made some observations, which if confirmed would go far to clear up many of the unsettled points relating to this substance. He has particularly examined cholesterine in its relations with seroline; the latter being a substance hitherto detected only in the serum of the blood (whence its name), but which Dr. Flint has found to exist normally in the fæces, and which therefore he has named stercorine. It is held that these two substances—cholesterine and seroline or stercorine—have a direct relation to each other; and that the knowledge of this relation, and of the function of cholesterine may explain those symptoms which attend the morbid condition termed acholia. For this latter term, Dr. Flint substitutes cholesteræmia. He believes that cholesterine is a product of the destructive assimilation of the nervous tissue, being absorbed from the substance of the brain and nerves by the blood, and eliminated by the liver. Hence in the bile there are two important elements having two separate functions:—" 1. It contains the glycocholate and taurocholate of soda; which are not found in the blood, are manufactured in the liver, are discharged mainly at a certain stage of the digestive process, are destined to assist in some of the nutritive processes, are not discharged from the body, and, in fine, are products of secretion. 2. It contains cholesterine; which is found in the blood, is merely separated from it by the liver and not manufactured in this organ, is not destined to assist in any of the nutritive processes but merely separated to be discharged from the body, and is a product of excretion."* As cholesterine is not found as such in the fæces (notwithstanding the contrary statement by several authors on physiological chemistry), Dr. Flint has made many experiments to determine what changes it undergoes; and the result of his investigations is, that it is converted into stercorine (or seroline). The retention then of cholesterine in the blood produces toxæmia, just in the same way as we have uræmic poisoning from the accumulation of urea. The difference in the gravity of the symptoms in the two varieties of jaundice (that from retention and that from suppression) is due to this circumstance :—viz., that in simple jaundice, dependent on the retention of the bile in the excretory passages, and the absorption of its colouring matter, the amount of cholesterine in the blood is not necessarily increased ; while in jaundice connected with structural change cholesterine is retained, and acts as a poison.

* *American Journal of the Medical Sciences.* New Series, vol. xliv. p. 337. Philadelphia, 1862.

Dr. Harley has likewise published* some valuable observations which tend to confirm the opinion that jaundice has a two-fold origin,—from *re-absorption*, owing to some obstruction to the escape of bile, and from *suppression* with retention in the blood of the matters which should be formed into bile by the liver. But he also believes that the liver is an excretive as well as a formative organ of the bile. The liver manufactures glycocholic and taurocholic acids. But it only separates from the blood the biliverdin† or colouring matter of the bile, and the cholesterine; which substances are not peculiar to the liver, but are always found in the blood independently of the presence or absence of the liver. In jaundice from suppression, the substances which the liver generates will be entirely wanting; while those which it merely excretes from the blood will collect in this fluid. Consequently, the biliverdin accumulates till the serum is saturated with this pigment; from which it exudes and stains the tissues, producing the colour we term jaundice. The elimination of this matter by the kidneys renders the urine of a saffron hue. Hence, Dr. Harley regards these symptoms as due to the imperfect excretion of biliverdin, quite independent of the presence or absence of the other constituents of the bile. The bile acids, not the bile pigment, induce the symptoms of poisoning. And from this it is argued, that when the colouring matter alone is found in the urine the jaundice is due to suppression; but when the biliary acids are present, it is clear that they must have been formed by the liver, and owing to some obstruction have been re-absorbed into the blood.

According to Dr. Lionel Beale, the view that in certain cases of jaundice there is suppressed action of the liver, that bile is not produced, and that no biliary acids are formed, is opposed to many facts. Entertaining the opinion that the colouring matters as well as the resinous acids are actually formed in the liver, he also thinks that in all cases of jaundice the bile has been formed by the hepatic cells; this fluid having been re-absorbed after its formation, and perhaps much of it again excreted in an altered form by the intestines. " It is easy to conceive," says Dr. Beale, " that the

---

* *Jaundice: its Pathology and Treatment.* London, 1863.

† There seems to be a repugnance on the part of chemists, in the present day, to work upon any subject without coining one or more new names. This extravagance only leads to confusion: for unfortunately, though two authorities write upon the same matter, at the same time, they will not adopt the same nomenclature. They only agree in discarding the terms which have been previously received. It is difficult to say by how many different denominations the bile-pigment is known. Dr. Thudichum (*A Treatise on Gall-stones*, p. 90. London, 1863) employs the word *cholochrome* to designate colouring matter of bile and all its varieties. For the brown colouring matter he retains the name *cholophæine*, for the green variety *cholochloine*. The older names of cholepyrrhine, biliphæine, and bilifulvine may be regarded as synonymous with cholophæine. Biliverdin and cholechlorine seem to be the synonyms of cholochloine.

relative proportion of the biliary acids and colouring matters produced, may be very different in different cases—that the quantity of the acids formed may vary greatly—that their composition may be affected, taurocholic acid being produced instead of glycocholic acid (Kühne)—that the quantity of blood corpuscles disintegrated by the presence of bile compounds in the blood varies—and that other chemical derangements may be caused although the action of the liver *cells* is not suspended even for a very short time."*

There are certain diseases of the liver—such as acute atrophy, impermeability of the bile ducts, cirrhosis, fatty degeneration, &c.—which lead to complete disorganization of this gland, and therefore to an arrest of its functions. Under these circumstances symptoms of blood-poisoning will arise, which very generally terminate fatally in a short time. Of course this toxæmia does not ensue in all cases, because sufficient healthy hepatic tissue may be left to do the necessary work.

Abnormal conditions of the nervous system are the essential *symptoms* in cases of acholia. Usually there is, first, a stage of excitement, characterized by noisy delirium and convulsions ; followed, secondly, by depression marked by somnolence and progressively increasing coma. Sometimes the first stage is absent, and the patients rapidly fall into a state of typhoid prostration, which passes into coma. Along with these symptoms we have hæmorrhage from the mucous membrane of the stomach and intestines, petechiæ with ecchymoses of the skin, and in a few cases jaundice.

The *treatment* must consist in the 'administration of active purgatives, particularly croton oil or podophyllin (F. 160, 168). Benzoic acid (F. 49), or the chloride of ammonium (F. 60), or the diluted nitro-hydrochloric acid (F. 378), can be tried, if there should be time for either of them to act. By these agents life will perhaps be prolonged for a brief period. Beyond this the cases are hopeless.

The term acholia [from 'A = privative + χολή = bile], signifying deficiency or absence of bile, has been here employed in the sense intended by Frerichs. Without therefore saying that this author's views are correct, we may, with our present imperfect knowledge, assume them to be so. Hence acholia must not be confounded with jaundice or cholæmia [from Χολή + αἷμα = blood], a morbid state in which bile exists in the blood owing to its re-absorption after having been formed by the liver. In the one case we have retained in the blood those substances by the metamorphosis of which bile is produced ; in the other, the blood contains the bile itself. The subject of jaundice has to be still further considered in the section on hepatic diseases.

9. PYÆMIA.—A very important morbid condition of the system, known frequently as ichorhæmia, or septicæmia, or

* *Kidney Diseases, Urinary Deposits, and Calculous Disorders.* Third Edition, p. 237. London, 1869.

pyæmia, [*ichorhæmia*, from ʻΙχὼρ = sanies, or any thin acrid matter discharged from wounds + αἷμα = blood ; *septicæmia*, from Σήπω = to putrefy ; *pyæmia*, or *pyohæmia*, from Πύον = pus ;] is caused by the introduction of ichorous or putrid matters into the blood.   This disease is generally known as pyæmia, or purulent absorption ; terms which are objectionable, inasmuch as they incorrectly lead to the inference that pus is present in the circulating fluid. Ichorhæmia is never a primary affection, but occurs subsequently to some injury or wound which takes on an unhealthy action. It may follow a boil or carbuncle, a diffused abscess, an attack of erysipelas, a burn, a compound fracture, a dissecting wound, a surgical operation, or the act of parturition—especially if any portion of placenta be left in the uterus to undergo decomposition. Suppurative inflammations of the joints, as well as acute inflammations and necroses of the shafts of the bones, especially seem to induce it.   But however brought about, ichorhæmia sets up a series of very grave symptoms, and often ends fatally.   The constitutional disturbance is so severe, that it sometimes seems at once to deprive the sufferer of all power of rallying ; while if he escape with life at the onset, he is not unlikely afterwards to succumb from the suppuration and other changes which occur in structures distant from the primary disease.   The chief of these changes consist of—extravasations of blood, especially in the lungs, the muscular substance of the heart, the spleen, the brain, and the areolar or connective tissue generally ; inflammatory consolidations of pulmonary, hepatic, and other structures ; and diffused or circumscribed, solitary or multiple, collections of pus.   These collections are most frequently met with in the liver, lungs, spleen, kidneys, brain, joints, &c.   In puerperal cases more especially, the eye is liable to suppurative inflammation, which ends in sloughing of the coats and extrusion of the humours.

On reviewing the *pathology* of ichorhæmia, the first question which requires an answer is this :—Do the symptoms depend upon the presence of pus cells in the blood ?   The attempt to solve this difficulty has given rise to a vast amount of controversy.   Until recently the question was always answered in the affirmative ; and consequently the name of pyæmia became current.   To explain how the pus cells passed into the blood and infected it, three hypotheses were regarded with more or less favour.   Thus it used to be said :—(1) The pus globules are absorbed (purulent absorption) from a suppurating cavity.   (2) The pus is the result of inflammation of the walls of the veins (phlebitis) ; this action leading to the production of pus in the venous channel, whence it is carried onwards into the general circulation.   (3) The pus is furnished by a suppuration of the blood itself.—How little dependence is to be placed on either of these theories will now be shown.

For the detection of pus in the blood the microscope has been almost exclusively depended on.   But since the publication of Dr.

Hughes Bennett's researches on Leucocythemia (in 1852) it has been generally allowed, that the so-called pus corpuscles which have been detected in the blood are identical with the colourless cells of that fluid; these bodies constituting, when in excess, the white cell blood.   Moreover, most pathologists agree that there is nothing peculiar in good and laudable pus which necessarily leads it to poison the blood.   The absorption of pus in its entirety is not possible; but there can be no doubt that the fluid portion of pus may be entirely absorbed, leaving behind merely the shrivelled cells deprived of their vitality.   This inspissation of pus occurs without producing any symptoms of the so-called purulent infection, unless indeed the fluid part be putrid.   Again, there is a second way in which the whole contents of an abscess can disappear—viz., by the pus cells undergoing fatty degeneration, becoming disintegrated, and reduced to a fluid condition in which absorption is rendered easy.   There is, of course, the possibility of an abscess bursting into a vein; but, in all probability, before this took place the canal of the vessel would be obliterated.   And so likewise, the peripheral lymphatic vessels may in the same manner become filled with pus; but before they reach a bloodvessel their course is interrupted by lymphatic glands, in which they break up into small branches, and through these no pus corpuscle could pass. Virchow well illustrates this occurrence by showing that in the process of tattooing, some of the cinnabar or gunpowder or the like finds its way into the lymphatic vessels, but is always separated by filtration in the nearest lymphatic glands.   Hence, while leucocythemia proves that corpuscles identical in form and size and structure and chemical composition with those of pus, may float in the blood and circulate innocuously, so the fact of the absorption of abscesses, either wholly or in part, demonstrates that healthy pus is not poisonous.   The truth, in short, seems to be, that what has been called pyæmia is not dependent upon pus cells mingling with the blood; but on contamination of the latter by some animal poison, or by any putrid or decomposing matter.   It is also certain that some decomposing fluids are more injurious than others, and hence the symptoms are of variable intensity.

Phlebitis and thrombosis have been regarded by many pathologists as sources of ichorhæmia, but it is rather doubtful if there be any connexion between these conditions so far as cause and effect are concerned.   A more reasonable view seems to be, that while the introduction of ichorous matter into the blood gives rise to a general poisoning of the system, so it may likewise produce a local inflammation in the coats of the veins, together with the formation of one or more clots.   It is not improbable, that among the first effects of phlebitis is an obstruction to the flow of blood through the vessel; this being produced either by the swelling of the coats of the vein, or by the formation of a clot.   But even if disintegration of this clot should afterwards occur, it is doubtful whether this process can lead by itself to any toxic effects. Severe mischief will arise mechanically, but there need be no blood-poisoning.

The *symptoms* of acute ichorhæmia are well-marked from the onset. The disease generally sets in with a severe rigor; followed by great heat of body, copious sweating, and increased frequency of pulse. The rise in temperature is remarkable; the thermometer in the axilla sometimes recording 104 or 105° Fahr. at the end of the first day. The rigors are occasionally repeated, perhaps periodically; or in their place various convulsive affections are substituted. In a lady who was long under my care with pelvic abscess, the re-formation of matter was sometimes preceded by a rigor and sometimes by an epileptiform seizure, but there was always one or the other to warn me of the mischief that had commenced. Then, if there is an open wound, it generally takes on an unhealthy appearance,—the surface quickly becomes pale and glassy; or instead of being bathed with laudable pus, its granulating surface looks indolent and the discharge from it ceases. Another symptom is a peculiar sweetish or fermentative odour of the breath and of the body generally. The aspect of the patient is peculiar, somewhat like that seen in typhus. At the same time, there is great prostration of both mind and body; together with extreme restlessness, sickness and frequent attacks of retching, diarrhœa with very offensive stools, dyspnœa and hiccough and cough, pains about the region of the heart, and perhaps low muttering delirium. The urine is scanty, high-coloured, and in exceptional cases albuminous: the chlorides have been found greatly diminished. The features become haggard; the face being alternately flushed and pallid. The pulse rises in frequency to 140 or upwards; while it is also small and quick. Auscultation will perhaps detect the signs of bronchitis or pneumonia: or a cardiac friction-sound and murmur may reveal the existence of pericarditis with endocarditis. The body wastes, the feebleness becomes extreme, the lips and tongue get brown and dry and covered with sordes, and the conjunctivæ and skin assume a sallow or even decided jaundiced hue. Not uncommonly, a sparse pustular eruption is observed on the chest or abdomen; or there will be spots or lines of congestion about the skin of the limbs or trunk; or small erysipelatous patches come out. Various parts of the body become excessively tender; while the suffering from diffuse suppuration in the tissues or joints may prove most severe. There is often subsultus tendinum. Profuse sweats, with perhaps effusion into the pleuræ or pericardium, or a low form of pneumonia or of hepatitis, increase the exhaustion; so that the patient dies worn out. When, on the other hand, the case terminates favourably, the fortunate escape has to be paid for by a wearying and tedious convalescence.

It follows from the foregoing, that there can scarcely be any mistake in the *diagnosis* except at the commencement of the disease.

Then it has sometimes been difficult to say exactly what the symptoms have been due to. Most frequently perhaps, when an error has been committed, the disturbance has been attributed to rheumatic fever, erysipelas, typhus, typhoid fever, scarlet fever, pneumonia, inflammation of the urinary organs, &c. The uncertainty can, however, generally be removed by remembering that ichorhæmia occurs in connexion with some wound, or injury, or attack of erysipelatous or other inflammation ; while the symptoms are more acute and increase more rapidly, and sooner give rise to alarming prostration than happens in the case of acute rheumatism or of any continued fever.

The *prognosis* in all forms of ichorhæmia is unfavourable ; but, it is especially so when the patient has been previously lowered by exhausting disease, by hæmorrhage, by a severe operation, or by insufficient food with residence in an unhealthy house. Taking all cases into consideration it is probable that 75 per cent. prove fatal. The mortality from this form of blood-poisoning amongst the wounded in the late American war was enormous. It formed one of the chief sources of death after amputation ; " and its victims are to be counted by thousands." There are said to be several valuable reports on this subject in the Surgeon-General's office at Washington, which will doubtless be published by and by.

The rate at which the symptoms may run on to a fatal termination varies, death frequently occurring within the week ; though with alternate remissions and relapses, it will possibly be deferred for some three months or more. If we were to tabulate the reports of a large number of fatal cases of ichorhæmia it would in all probability appear, that 40 per cent. had died by the end of the seventh day from the commencement of the attack ; 60 per cent. by the end of the fortnight ; 75 per cent. by the end of the fourth week ; 90 per cent. by the close of the second month ; 95 per cent. by the termination of the third month ; leaving five to struggle on for a longer but indeterminate period.*

* As a good example of the rapidity with which the symptoms will run on in an acute case, attention may be directed to the following instance recorded by Dr. William Addison :—On the 28th December, at 8 o'clock A.M., a physician pricked his finger while assisting to make the post-mortem examination of a lady who had died from puerperal peritonitis. In the evening he felt some pain and uneasiness at the part, and had it touched with nitrate of silver. During the night shiverings came on, and there was extreme restlessness. On the morning of the 29th the finger was much swollen, and red lines extended up the arm : leeches, fomentations, and poultices were applied. In the afternoon there was great prostration. On the 30th, the hand and arm were greatly swollen, the finger had put on a livid appearance, the glands in the axilla were affected, and the pain was very great. On the 31st the pulse was from 90 to 100, the breathing was irregular, and there was torpor with drowsiness. In the evening, the symptoms were found more alarming ; and there was an erysipelatous blush over the side of the chest, and in the axilla. During the night the breathing became more difficult, the drowsiness gradually passed into deep stupor, and death took place at 6 o'clock on the morning of the 1st January.—*Cell Therapeutics,* p. 36. London, 1856.

In contrast to the acute form there is a class of cases where the disease runs an essentially chronic course. The symptoms are of the same nature as are observed in acute ichorhæmia, save that they are much milder in character and are spread over a longer space of time. Moreover, there are sometimes intervals of apparent recovery, followed by relapses; each relapse, however, lessening in severity and peril. In this way, the disease has been known to extend over several months—possibly to last for a couple of years. The chief danger to be dreaded is that disease of the lungs will get developed. The risk of this is very greatly increased if there be a constitutional syphilitic taint in the system, or if there be any hereditary tendency to tuberculosis.

Ichorhæmia is particularly dreaded by obstetricians and surgeons, since it not unfrequently is the cause of highly dangerous symptoms after parturition (puerperal fever) and surgical operations. It may display itself in more ways than one. Thus, in some instances, the blood seems to be so immediately and deeply affected by the morbid matter, that the patient's death occurs before any local phenomena can be developed. In a second class, the intensity of the poison appears to be exerted upon the liver or the mucous membrane of the intestinal canal; in the one case there arising spontaneous efforts at elimination by the discharge of a large quantity of dark bile, in the other through a severe attack of diarrhœa or dysentery. Then there is a third set of cases where the serous membranes bear the brunt of the poison, and we have pleurisy, or pericarditis, or peritonitis; or the cutaneous surface is the part affected, and we find erysipelas, or a more or less copious eruption of boils. And again, there is a fourth class in which profuse suppuration ensues, giving rise to secondary abscesses in the lungs, liver, joints, eyes, &c.

Amongst the various forms of blood-poisoning is one to which the term *Cellulitis venenata* was formerly applied; meaning thereby a diffused form of inflammation of the connective tissue, arising from one or more punctures received in dissecting the dead body. Certain animal fluids are more dangerous than others, as the serum found in the abdomen after peritonitis, and that left after gangrenous inflammation. The bites of several venomous reptiles, as the cobra di capello, will also produce the same effects; and even the sting of the bee has proved fatal. The poison, whatever its nature, when thus absorbed gives rise to very severe constitutional disturbance; which, as in puerperal fever and erysipelas and the eruptive fevers, &c., may end fatally before sufficient time has elapsed for any appreciable local lesions to become produced. Where this does not happen, however, there sets in more or less severe inflammation of the connective tissue and absorbents, generally of the wounded limb, but sometimes of remote parts. The lymphatic glands are very often affected. The skin over the seat of inoculation and surrounding parts, becomes pale but tense and shining; while the swelling which occurs communicates a peculiar boggy feel to the touch. These inflammations are attended with rigors, restlessness, extreme pain, and great depression; while they either cause death in a few days, or they end in suppuration or gangrene. In fatal cases, death is preceded by delirium, offensive perspirations, a yellowness of the skin, dyspnœa, drowsiness, and deep stupor. When patients recover, it is often only to find the constitution permanently injured; or, at least, with the general powers of life so impaired that years elapse before perfect health is regained.

The effluvia given off from the dead body may be the cause of extensive toxæmia or blood-poisoning. These effluvia can, without injuring the party exposed to them, be carried by him to a third person placed under such circumstances as invite disease, and so provoke the most distressing results—a fact which demands the particular attention of obstetricians.* At the Lying-in hospitals of Vienna and Prague, a very large mortality was distinctly traced to a want of caution in admitting students from the dissecting-rooms to the wards. The surgeon also, who goes heedlessly from a case of erysipelas or any variety of unhealthy inflammation to the lying-in room, may set up most formidable mischief in the tenant of the apartment. The danger which arises from handling morbid preparations, unhealthy purulent secretions, &c., is equally great; and consequently the obstetric practitioner cannot exercise too much caution. If obliged to be present at any case of blood-poisoning or at a post-mortem examination, he should not visit any parturient woman until he has changed all his clothes, and has washed his hands thoroughly with some chlorine solution or other active disinfectant.

The *treatment* of ichorhæmia has to be conducted with considerable caution. Heroic remedies are out of the question. The painstaking and judicious practitioner may perhaps succeed in restoring his patient to health; but no brilliant cures are to be expected. For it must be remembered that this exhausting affection is most common during unhealthy seasons, when disorders of a low type are prevalent. Moreover, the sufferers from it are usually those whose constitutional powers are not of the first order. Hence, while endeavouring slowly to carry out the object of primary im-

* This statement as to the pernicious influence of these poisons is well illustrated by a case which occurred in the practice of Mr. Teale. This surgeon says:—"One evening, at the dissection of the body of a patient upon whom I had operated for strangulated hernia, several surgeons were present. Of these, two attended one case of midwifery each during the following night, and a third three cases. The two patients attended by the first two surgeons died of puerperal fever. Two of those attended by the third surgeon also died; and his third patient escaped death from this formidable malady with the greatest difficulty, after having been in extreme danger several days. It is an important fact, that no other cases occurred in the practice of these gentlemen."—*A Treatise on Abdominal Hernia*, p. 92. London, 1846.

portance—the purification of the blood, we must not fail to support the excessively depressed vital powers and to relieve pain.

Taking the latter indications first, it will suffice to say that stimulants are needed from the commencement; wine or beer appearing preferable in some instances, while in others brandy or gin or whisky have to be given.   In regulating the doses, and the intervals between them, there is scope for much judgment.   It is impossible to lay down any precise rules here.   I would, however, strongly insist upon the importance of ordering these remedies—so powerful for good or evil, as they are rightly or wrongly employed—in definite quantities.   All stimulants should be prescribed as drugs are ordered ; the exact dose, as well as the time for its administration, being distinctly stated at every visit.   Amongst other resuscitating agents the restorative soup (F. 2) will often be invaluable ; and so will the essence of beef (F. 3), or a mixture of brandy and eggs (F. 17).   Milk is of the greatest service, and should be given as freely as it can be digested.   Sometimes it happens that cream agrees better than milk.   Bark, with ether or ammonia (F. 371), is a good remedy ; while in some instances life would seem to have been preserved by the administration of three or four grains of quinine every four or six hours, until the head has become slightly affected.   Pain is to be relieved by opium, in doses sufficient to soothe and comfort the patient. Troublesome sickness can sometimes be controlled by the dilute hydrocyanic acid (F. 86, 362), by laurel water with citrate of soda (F. 348), by the citrate of potash in soda water (grs. 10 to 40, every three hours), by some preparation of bismuth (F. 65, 112), or by oxalate of cerium ; as well as by the application of linseed poultices, or sinapisms, or flying blisters to the epigastrium.   To check the thirst, iced drinks and cherry water ices are serviceable. Wenham Lake ice to suck can be allowed very freely.   Draughts of equal parts of iced soda water and milk, or of Seltzer water and champagne, are not only very refreshing, but will frequently be retained when the stomach rejects other drinks.   And then, in all cases, care must be taken that the patient's bed is placed in the centre of the apartment, that the hangings are removed, that a sufficient fire be maintained, and that the windows be opened. He must be kept in a pure cool atmosphere, night and day, even at the slight risk of catching cold.   In truth, however, this risk is merely a phantom.   Miss Florence Nightingale tells us that in the wooden huts before Sebastopol, with their pervious walls and open ridge ventilators, in which the sick and wounded soldiers sometimes said " they would get less snow if they were outside," such a thing as *catching cold* was never heard of.   The patients being well covered with blankets, were all the better for the cold air.*

To prevent the occurrence of ichorhæmia and erysipelas in our hospitals, the latter should be built in healthy localities ; plenty

* *Notes on Hospitals.*   Third Edition, p. 15.   London, 1863.

of light must be admitted into the wards ; while 2500 cubic feet
of space per bed ought to be allowed, with an interval of about 6
feet between each couch.   A good nurse—one who will quietly
but thoroughly carry out the physician's directions—is invaluable.
She will of course attend to the perfect cleanliness of the sufferer
and his bedding and his room.   To learn the cubical contents of a
room, multiply its length by the breadth and height.   The product
divided by the number of the beds, will give the amount for each bed.

To eliminate the poison from the system practitioners have
very commonly trusted to active purgatives, particularly to full
doses of calomel.   Even if there were no other remedies deserving
of trial, I should still discountenance the routine use of these
agents ; for I believe their mischievous effects to be second only
to those produced by bleeding.   At the same time, if at the commencement of the case there are indications that the intestines
are loaded, an aperient should be given—not a drastic purge. For
it has been shown previously, that foremost amongst the symptoms of ichorhæmia are sweating and vomiting and purging. Now
if we allow, as may fairly be done, that these evacuations are
critical or eliminative, yet it will be very wrong to push this view
to the illogical conclusion that more sweating and more intestinal action are to be encouraged. Without a doubt, if the skin be
inactive it will be frequently beneficial to induce perspiration.
With this object we may employ the vapour bath, or the wet-
sheet packing (F. 136), or even the acid sponging (F. 138) ; at
the same time administering diluents freely by the mouth.

After an elaborate series of experiments, Dr. Polli, of Milan,
has come to the conclusion that sulphurous acid, and various sulphites and hyposulphites, have the power of arresting all known
forms of fermentation, as well as of retarding putrefaction.* Many
diseases (typhus, pyæmia, puerperal fever, hospital gangrene, dissecting wounds, glanders, cholera, &c.), he asserts, arise from a
fermentation of some of the principles contained in the blood ;
and one grand object of his memoir is to prove the fallacy of
Bernard's view,—that the use of chemical agents capable of
arresting the fermentation would destroy the vital properties of
the blood.   Dr. Polli's experiments were of this nature :—A
certain number of dogs had putrid blood injected into their veins,
and all died but one.   An equal number had large and repeated
doses of the sulphites administered ; and subsequently the same
quantity of putrid blood was injected, as in the first cases.   All
recovered.   Then it was also found, that if the putrid blood were
mixed with a certain proportion of sulphite of soda before injecting
it, the dogs did not die as when putrid blood alone was employed.

* *Sulle Malattie da Fermento Morbifico, e sul loro Trattamento.* Milan,
1860.   See also, *British Medical Journal*, p. 339, 29 March 1862, and p. 441,
16 November 1867 : *Half-Yearly Abstract of Medical Sciences*, vol. xxxvii.
p. 245.   London, 1863 : and Mr. Henry Lee's Introductory Lecture at St.
George's Hospital, *On General Principles in Medicine*, p. 20.   London, 1863.

And again, an equal quantity of the discharge of glanders was injected into the femoral veins of two large dogs. One died, with the symptoms of glanders, in six days; the other, previously sulphited, quickly recovered. As to the mode of administration of the sulphites in man, Dr. Polli tells us that they may be fearlessly given in large doses. From 60 to 180 grains of the sulphite or hyposulphite of soda or magnesia can be given daily, in divided doses, for several days together. As the sulphite of magnesia (F. 48) is the richest in sulphurous acid, it is preferable to every other preparation. About twenty parts of water are needed for its solution.

Since becoming acquainted with Dr. Polli's views, I have had numerous opportunities of testing the efficacy of sulphurous acid and its combinations in various forms of blood-poisoning. And succinctly stated the result has appeared to me to be this,—that while on the one hand these agents certainly have done no harm, yet on the other side I find it difficult to persuade myself that they have proved of any service. On the whole, sulphurous acid with quinine has seemed to do more good than the acid alone. I have also tried various alkaline salts, such as the bicarbonate of potash, &c., but cannot bring forward the slightest evidence of their possessing valuable properties. And the same confession must be made with regard to the permanganate of potash; which, however beneficial as an antiseptic when applied externally, seems to have no value as an internal remedy in diseases like those under consideration.

As regards the local treatment of any ulceration or injury which may be present, it is necessary to insist upon the primary importance of cleanliness. Foul external wounds cannot be better managed than by the use of irrigation, so as to constantly remove all the unhealthy secretions. Continuous immersion of the part in tepid water is sometimes practicable and highly serviceable. If there be unhealthy discharges from internal organs—e.g. the ear, the nostril, the uterus—injections of warm water containing some antiseptic like the permanganate of potash ought to be employed several times in the twenty-four hours. Where abscesses have formed and are pointing it will be better to open them. If there be a reasonable fear that suppuration has occurred among the deeper tissues—beneath the fasciæ, free incision will be called for.

The remedies for chronic ichorhæmia are of the same description as the foregoing. Simply enumerated, they may be said essentially to consist of restoratives, nourishing food, pure air, tonics, and the removal of all sources of irritation from the system. Finally, in wounds from dissecting, or from the bites of reptiles, attempts are to be made by sucking or by the application of a cupping-glass to remove the poison from the puncture or bite. To prevent absorption, a ligature is at the same time to be tied between the wounded part and the trunk. It will also be advisable to apply lunar caustic freely to the wound. In other respects the treatment must be that just mentioned.

10. THROMBOSIS: EMBOLISM.—The fact has long since been proved by many independent observers, that when the blood contains—either absolutely or relatively—a great excess of fibrin (hyperinosis), or when this fluid gets contaminated by the introduction of foreign particles or other impurities, as well as when there exists any obstacle to the normal circulation, then fibrinous formations may take place during life in the heart, or in the arteries, or in the veins, or in the cerebral sinuses, or in the portal system. The symptoms which these solid substances (formerly known as polypi) give rise to are such, that their existence can with care be diagnosed. When a portion of fibrin coagulates in one of the arteries and is carried along by the blood-current, it will of course be arrested in the capillaries, if not before : when the solidification occurs in the veins, the clot need not necessarily be stopped till it reaches the lungs : when in the portal system, the liver capillaries will offer an obstacle to the further progress of the substance. And although it should be noticed that emboli may form in the lymphatics, yet the passage of these vessels through glands must prevent the transit of any body for any great distance along them.

Pathology.—Before entering upon this part of the subject, it is necessary to give an explanation of the terms employed. By *thrombosis* [Θρόμβος = a clot of blood] is generally understood the partial or complete closure of a vessel, by a morbid product developed at the site of the obstruction. The coagulum, which is usually fibrinous, is known as an *autochthonous clot* or *thrombus*. The term *embolism* ["Εμβολος = a plug] is used to designate an obstruction caused by any body detached and transported from the interior of the heart or of some vessel. The migratory substance is an *embolus.*

Thrombi or emboli vary in size—from a mass sufficient to obstruct the aorta, to a particle which can enter a capillary vessel. They consist not only of fibrin, but possibly of a fragment of gangrenous tissue, or perchance of a portion of tubercle or cancer which has got drawn into a vessel. The formation of a thrombus in a bloodvessel may act primarily by causing complete or partial obstruction. The secondary disturbances are twofold :—in the first place, larger or smaller fragments become detached from the end of the thrombus, and are carried along by the current of blood to remote vessels (embolism); or, secondly, the coagulum softens and becomes converted into a matter like pus,—constituting according to Virchow the process called " suppurative phlebitis."

These concretions are most frequently met with in diseases attended with great exhaustion or debility; and they have been especially found in cases of croup, diphtheria, scarlet fever, endocarditis, pneumonia, bronchitis, phthisis, typhus, purpura, erysipelas, hæmorrhage, and prostration from natural decay as well as from dissipation. With regard to croup, for example, my own experience would lead me to believe that death is much more frequently due to thrombi than to simple asphyxia. The formation of these substances seems also to be particularly favoured by the condition of the blood during pregnancy and the puerperal state. Thus in August 1863, I saw a lady whose general health was never good, who had advanced to the sixth month of her second pregnancy, and in whom the following series of events had occurred :—A sudden fright, apparently acting as the cause; succeeded by an attack of fainting, great rapidity of heart's action, agitation with nervous depression, and very severe pain in the left leg and ankle. When I visited her on the day following the occurrence of these symptoms there was much debility; while the foot and leg were very œdematous and cold, and no pulsations could be detected beyond the femoral artery. The symptoms, in short, were just those which would arise from the application of a ligature to the chief artery of the limb; and there was clearly the same necessity for establishing a collateral circulation to avoid gangrene.—Of another variety of these cases I met with an example in 1860 :—A delicate lady, twenty-five years of age, under my care, had such symptoms after the delivery of her first child, that I believe a small clot formed in the right side of the heart, though her labour had neither been difficult nor attended with more than ordinary hæmorrhage. For six weeks after her accouchement, the muscular prostration was so extreme that she literally could not turn over from one side to the other; and when the least attempt was made to raise her in bed, so as to change her linen, &c., the most severe attacks of dyspnœa set in.

The fibrinous masses either form suddenly, without the least warning, and at once cause death by obstructing the circulation; or else they arise gradually, and produce symptoms which creep on insidiously and last a long time. In the latter case, the masses (thrombi) become organized and attached to the walls of the heart, or they may soften and gradually deliquesce; while from these attachments, portions (emboli) can be carried away by the blood so as to block up the circulation at some extreme point. Perhaps the right auricle is the most common seat of these clots; but it can easily be understood that the edges of the valves, as well as the muscular and tendinous cords of the ventricles, are parts to which they readily become attached. Possibly, also, the small beadlike and warty exudations thrown out in endocarditis will sometimes form a foundation on which a concretion becomes deposited. The particles of solid fibrin carried away by the blood from the left side of the heart are usually arrested in the vessels of the brain, spleen, or kidney; while those from the right cavities pass by the pulmonary artery and its branches into the lungs.

Symptoms.—The indications presented when a coagulum has formed in the *heart* are always well-marked. They are likewise of the same general character, whatever may be the disease from

which the patient is suffering at the time of its formation.   Their
nature varies according as the concretion is deposited on the right
or on the left side of the heart.   When the obstruction is on the
right side, as is most commonly the case, the return of blood from
the systemic veins is prevented; and as the flow of blood to the
lungs for aëration is impeded, so arterial blood is not duly supplied to the brain and heart and other organs.   Hence where
death results, it happens from syncope rather than from asphyxia;
though if the clot be of such a size that no blood can enter the
pulmonary artery, then death necessarily happens immediately from
suffocation.

The course of the symptoms can perhaps be best shown by
referring to the case to which allusion has already been made.
This patient had a favourable labour of some eight hours' duration; and when left by me at midnight, about an hour and a half
after the birth of her child, was in a favourable condition.   The
pains of parturition had been very severe; but although the use
of chloroform was suggested, the inhalation of it had been declined.
Prior to my departure and afterwards, brandy with arrowroot was
given; and at about two A.M. the lady expressed herself as feeling
comfortable, and quietly fell asleep.   She passed a good night;
but on the following morning, at eight A.M., I was hastily summoned, as a most severe and distressing attack of dyspnœa had
just set in.   On my speedy arrival, the breathing was found to be
hurried and gasping, the surface of the body pale and cold, the
pulse frequent and small and intermittent, and the patient exceedingly faint as well as frightened.   Indeed, the state of collapse
was very alarming; but the administration of some brandy with
ether and ammonia, and the application of a large linseed poultice
with mustard in it, gave sensible relief in about three-quarters of
an hour.   I could only venture to place the stethoscope over the
apex of each lung, but I thus learnt that the respiratory murmur
was natural; and hence this fact combined with the tumultuous
action of the heart, seemed to point out the latter as the seat of
obstruction.   The most perfect quiet was enjoined; the urine was
withdrawn by a catheter; and small quantities of essence of beef,
ammonia, and brandy were given at short intervals.   At the end of
the day, the extract of belladonna was freely applied over the breasts;
so as to check, or possibly to prevent, the secretion of milk.

Now the foregoing symptoms were quite sufficient to teach me,
even if the fact had not previously been learnt from the writings
of others, that cases of this description must generally terminate
quickly in death.   Certainly in this instance it was clear, that very
little more was required for the obstructed heart to become quite
paralysed.   We know that patients prostrated by acute diseases, and
also parturient women, have died suddenly after an attempt to sit
up in bed or to pass a stool, and the fatal event has been referred
simply to fainting; but it seems very probable that the real cause

may have often been the sudden blocking-up of one of the cardiac orifices, or of the pulmonary artery, by a mass of fibrin.*

When the clot obstructs the circulation by its situation in the *left* cavities of the heart, or in the aorta, death, if it occur, either takes place suddenly from syncope because no blood can circulate; or it may be delayed for some hours and happen from coma. The symptoms then are violent action of the heart, great congestion of the lungs with dyspnœa of a suffocative character, expectoration of a bloody and frothy mucus, a leaden hue of the surface, with coldness of the extremities. Supposing the patient to recover from the first urgent stage, the symptoms will gradually merge into those of valvular obstruction of the left side. Such a condition might be diagnosed by the sudden appearance of a murmur where the heart had previously been healthy, and where there had existed no signs of endocarditis. It must be remembered, that concretions have more than once been found to exist on both sides of the heart at the same time; and the symptoms have then chiefly resembled those which arise from deposition in the right cavities.

Suppose fibrinous concretions are discovered in any of the *arteries* or *veins*, it must be granted that possibly they have formed at the parts where they are found. For example, Dr. Humphry records, amongst other cases, that of a pale and anæmic and very weak girl, who was being dressed by her friends in order that she might be taken out of the hospital. Suddenly she fell fainting, and quickly died. During her stay in the ward the right arm had been swollen, and had been kept hanging out of bed, as the patient found this position, with the head inclined towards the right shoulder, the most comfortable. On examining the body there was slight emphysema of the lung, but otherwise the organs were healthy. The right innominate, subclavian, and internal jugular veins were each obstructed by a large clot. That in the innominate vein was firm, of a buff colour, scarcely tinged with red, and adherent to the vessel's coats : in the jugular vein the clot was soft, and looked like a mixture of blood and pus.

But it must also be remembered, as before stated, that the concretions which form in the heart can be carried by the blood, wholly or in part, into some artery which they block up; and thus the supply of blood to an important organ may be suddenly cut off, producing alarming and even fatal results. Where the particles are minute they will perhaps be borne onwards into the capillaries, so as merely to give rise to local congestion and stagnation. Supposing that the masses soften and break up, there is no reason why the disintegrated portions by mingling with the blood should necessarily contaminate it. The injurious effects

* Further on, in the section on hydatid tumours of the liver, (vol. ii. part viii.), the history of a case will be found which distinctly illustrates the correctness of this suggestion.

which result from the solidification of fibrin within the body are
of a mechanical nature. At all events, it is difficult to imagine
why coagulated fibrin should possess any poisonous properties,
as has been taught.

The effects which have been found to ensue from a fibrinous
deposit being carried from the *left* side of the heart, are as
follows :—In several instances, softening of the brain, ending in
hemiplegia, owing to the plugging of the middle cerebral artery ;
paralysis and loss of sensation in the arm, from the obstruction
of the brachial and ulnar arteries ; temporary loss of power in one
of the lower extremities, which has become relieved on the solution of the clot, or on the establishment of the collateral circulation;
disease of the kidney, the issue of obstruction of the renal artery;
and disease of the spleen. The consequences which follow from the
propulsion of masses of fibrin from the *right* side of the heart are
shown in the lungs, by the presence of coagula in the pulmonary
arteries and different kinds of deposit in the pulmonary tissue.
Upon this principle can be explained the occurrence of some forms
of pneumonia, gangrene of the lung, &c. Obstruction in the pulmonary capillaries is indicated by œdema or infiltration of the
lung tissue, and by pulmonary apoplexy. In the same way Mr.
Paget has shown, that particles of cancerous matter may be
brought from remote organs to the right side of the heart and
thence transmitted to the lungs ; where they become arrested in
the pulmonary capillaries, and so induce stagnation and subsequent changes in the blood.

Prognosis.—This must always be very guarded. For the patient not unfrequently dies outright, simply from the formation
of the clot and consequent obstruction. Or, when arising in a
serious disease—such as croup, the occurrence of thrombosis is
like enough just to turn the balance and prevent recovery;
though there may be only retarded, not annihilated, circulation.
Again, this event sometimes hastens death in an incurable disease,
such as cancer ; when, without a complication of the kind, the sufferer might survive for many months. And then, lastly, by cutting
off the main supply of blood to a limb the clot may induce gangrene;
the distressing effects of which will certainly be recovered from with
difficulty, if at all. Thus the sources of danger exist not only in
the interruption of the blood-current, but also in the morbid condition of the system produced by the disturbed nutrition of a
limb or organ.

Post-mortem Appearances.—When a fibrinous deposit is found
in the heart, it often becomes a question whether this was produced during life or after death. Supposing the fibrin to have
separated after death—the blood being stagnant—it forms only a
light-coloured layer on the upper part of a red clot. On the contrary, when the deposition has taken place during life—the blood
being in motion—we find a mass which is modelled to the cavity

containing it, which is adherent to the walls, and which is grooved by the blood that has passed over it. In some instances also, the solidified fibrin has been seen lining one of the cavities of the heart like a false endocardium; or else, forming an additional coat to the aorta or other large vessel, without obstructing it.

According to some writers the fibrinous masses, or thrombi, occasionally soften in their centres; and they are then discovered containing a fluid of a dirty reddish-brown colour, or of a lighter hue resembling pus. Examined microscopically no pus-corpuscles can be found in this fluid, and hence it is a puriform—not a purulent substance. If the process of softening goes on to a great extent, there may be seen only an outer shell or cyst remaining. Occasionally, it is said, the walls of this cyst get ruptured; and the contents becoming mingled with the blood, poison this fluid as effectually, and give rise to the same typhoid symptoms, as if disorganized matter had been injected directly into a vein. Without denying the possibility of this occurrence, I must say that it seems to me to be one which only happens very rarely. It need scarcely be pointed out, that this event is very different to the so-called poisoning of the blood from the presence in it of disintegrated portions of fibrin.*

Treatment.—Sufficient has been already said to prove, that the indications which lead to a rational treatment are very different in different cases. Thus, in some urgent instances, all our efforts have to be directed to keeping the patient alive at the time, without caring for the after-consequences. In other cases, the relief of pain, the compensatory establishment of a collateral circulation, and the prevention of the transference of fresh emboli, are the objects to be held in view. Or, again, the attempt is sometimes made to produce solution of the clot, or its partial organization. While in a fourth class (according to some physicians), the poisoning of the system by the purulent and ichorous destruction of the clot, will have to be combated.

The remedies upon which we have learnt to rely are few, and it must be confessed that their action is uncertain. When there is great prostration, stimulants will of course be needed : either ammonia, or ether, or brandy usually proving very valuable. Then in all instances, the strictest quiet must be imposed ; both as regards the position or movements of the patient, and the absence of every circumstance calculated to prevent repose. The sick room is to be freely supplied with pure air. Such nourishment as essence of beef, raw eggs, and milk ought to be freely administered ;

* The nature and size of this treatise preclude my entering into many arguments which need discussion on this interesting matter ; but I would refer those who wish to investigate it further, to the writings of Virchow, Cohn, Richardson, Gulliver, Humphry, Paget, Kirkes, and John W. Ogle. There are also two excellent articles on this subject in the *British and Foreign Medico-Chirurgical Review*, for July 1861 and January 1863.

these being given in small quantities, frequently repeated. Bleeding, leeching, blistering, or purging must not be thought of.

The admirable series of experiments by Dr. Richardson has taught us that all the alkalies are resolvent—*i.e.*, they lead to solution of nitrogenous tissue. This gentleman's researches prove, that after death from the alkalies and from antimony and from many of the alkaloids (as strychnia, morphia, and atropia) there is the same fluidity or partial fluidity of the blood, the same dissolution of the blood corpuscles, the same softening of the soft parts, the same absence of cadaveric rigidity, and the same extensive but simple vascularity of mucous surfaces and vascular organs. In the carbonate of ammonia we have an admirable agent : since it is not only possessed of the same power as the other alkalies, but it has also the valuable property of exciting the heart and circulation, as well as the muscular system. This agent, freely diluted, may then always be administered unless there is evidence that it is present in excess in the blood and breath ; while very often it may advantageously be combined with bark (F. 371). The conclusion must not be drawn from these remarks that ammonia is the agent which keeps the blood, in the living body, in a fluid state. Before this view was abandoned by Dr. Richardson himself, the theory had been deemed wholly untenable by several authorities. Nevertheless, those who most differed from him still allowed he had proved that ammonia is contained in the blood in larger quantities than was previously supposed, and that added to coagulated blood (out of the body) it is capable of again rendering it fluid.

Another remedy of great value in these cases is opium ; for it not only quiets the circulation, but it relieves pain and calms the depressing fears as well as the nervous restlessness. The dose must be sufficient to accomplish these objects. And lastly, to remove that low state of health which both favours thrombosis and the degeneration of tissues injured by a clot when formed, we must trust to a good nourishing diet, the effects of pure air, and the administration of quinine (F. 379) or of sulphurous acid (F. 48).

Where the result is successful, the practitioner had better be prepared to find that the necessarily tedious convalescence has excited the displeasure of the patient's friends, who are generally unreasonable in proportion to their inability to comprehend the simplest facts in medical science. Annoyance at this circumstance will, however, be lessened by remembering the great danger from which the sufferer has been rescued ; as well as by recollecting that if the physician now and then gets blame where he deserves great credit, he also frequently receives much higher praise than is merited.

11. **HÆMATOZOA.**—In the writings of old authors, from the time of Pliny, cases are to be found recording the presence of animalculæ in the blood [*hæmatozoa*, from Αἷμα = blood + ζῶον =

an animal]. The physicians of the present day have also published examples of this occurrence; but while the statements of some of these gentlemen have been confirmed by independent observers, those of others have been refuted. Thus, Bushnan has reported the case of a boy affected with influenza, in whose blood worms half an inch long were detected an hour after bleeding. According to Rhind, however, these were merely the larvæ of the *Tipula oleracea*, a fly which is so abundantly found in summer in ditch and river water; or, according to Von Siebold, they consisted of the red larvæ of the *Chironomus plumosus*, frequent in water-barrels. Of course they were accidentally introduced into the blood after its withdrawal from the body. Again, Goodfellow met with an instance, in which animalculæ, varying in length from $\frac{1}{8000}$th to $\frac{1}{3000}$th of an inch, were present in the blood of a fever patient; but it is impossible to say what they really were.

The *Distoma hæmatobium* (Bilharzia hæmatobia) was first discovered by Bilharz, in Egypt, during 1851; where it is so common, that nearly half of the adults are supposed to be infected with it. This entozoon inhabits the vena portæ, as well as the mesenteric and hepatic and bladder and intestinal veins. Its habitat is the blood; and hence it may be carried into other parts than those just mentioned. It is not hermaphroditic, the two sexes being very dissimilar. The male is much larger than the female, being about half an inch in length. On the under surface of the cylindrical body, extending from just below the ventral sucker to near the end of the pointed tail, is a kind of groove or deep slit (canalis gynæcophorus); in which the female is lodged during copulation. The latter is more filiform and narrower, though rather longer, than the male. Moquin-Tandon is in error in believing that the female is the superior, and that she lodges the male. These remarkable parasites are very prevalent in those persons who drink the unfiltered waters of the Nile, and who consume fish from this river in a half putrid state. The symptoms produced are those of general constitutional disturbance; together with diarrhœa, chlorosis, pyelitis, bloody-urine, &c. Death ultimately ensues from vital exhaustion; or earlier from some complication like pneumonia, ulceration of the intestines, &c. This hæmatozoon is probably also the cause of a peculiar form of hæmaturia which is somewhat prevalent in Southern Africa and in the Mauritius. The principal remedies which have been used against these trematode helminths are calomel and turpentine; though the efficacy of such drugs must be very problematical. More benefit will probably ensue from attempts to mitigate the symptoms as they arise. Relief can often be given where a cure is hopeless.

A second species of Bilharzia (*Bilharzia magna*) has been discovered by Dr. T. S. Cobbold in the portal system of an African monkey—the Cercopithecus fuliginosus.

The *Hexathyridium venarum* (Polystoma sanguicola) is about three lines in length. This helminth has been detected in venous blood, as well as in the sputa of two young persons suffering from hæmoptysis.

MM. Gruby and Delafond have often detected a species of microscopic thread-worm in the blood of the dog. These filariæ are found in great numbers, they have a diameter less than that of the blood discs, and they circulate in the most minute capillaries. In about four or five per cent. of dogs, the blood is said to be verminous. It has been proposed to give to this hæmatozoon the name of *Filaria papillosa hæmatica canis domestici*.

Andral discovered true *hydatids* in the pulmonary veins of a man aged fifty-five; but it is very doubtful if they were developed there, having been probably introduced through some perforation in the walls of the vessels. And lastly, it is no doubt true that the *Fasciola hepatica* (the liver fluke) has been found in the vena portæ. M. Duval, a physician at Rennes, while dissecting the body of a man forty-nine years of age, came upon a large specimen in the trunk of the portal vein, in the midst of a little fluid blood. In tracing the hepatic divisions of the vein he discovered four or five other helminths of the same kind; all of which were about one inch in length, and half an inch in width. There were none in the mesenteric branches which form the portal vein, and no disease was detected in the liver—or, indeed, in the body—excepting the flukes. The fasciola hepatica and the distoma lanceolatum are often found together in great numbers in the gall-ducts and bladder of the sheep and other graminivorous animals, producing a disease known as the *distemper* or *rot*.

II. SCURVY.

Scorbutus, or scurvy, is a complex morbid state caused by long-continued privation of fresh succulent vegetables or fruits, or their preserved juices. Insufficient animal food, the excessive use of salt meats, sameness of diet, foul drinking-water, inattention to personal cleanliness, exposure to impure air, mental despondency, and the ill-effects of previous attacks of ague or dysentery,—these can all exert a predisposing influence, but nothing more. Such conditions will also intensify the ravages of this disease, though they cannot by themselves produce it.

Of late years scurvy has been seen with comparative rarity in this country; although examples of it are occasionally met with amongst the aged inmates of asylums, workhouses, &c., who have perhaps been long living on tea with bread and butter. After the failure of the potato crop in 1846, numerous instances occurred amongst the working classes in many parts of the United

Kingdom. In our navy this disorder has been gradually becoming extinct since the year 1795, when an Admiralty order was first issued for furnishing the fleet with a regular supply of lemon juice. But bad cases still not unfrequently occur in the mercantile service;* recent Arctic navigators have also suffered from it ; while both the English and French armies in the Crimea were attacked with it to a remarkable extent. The mortality from scorbutus was formerly frightful ; more seamen dying from it than from all other causes put together, not omitting the accidents of war. Thus, Admiral Hosier sailed from England for the West Indies, in 1726, with seven ships of the line, and twice lost his whole crew by scurvy. Again, two years after Lord Anson's memorable expedition sailed from England in 1740, this disorder had proved fatal to four out of every five of the original crews. So likewise, in 1795, the safety of Lord Howe's Channel fleet was seriously endangered by its virulence. Now by taking care to supply the men with fresh succulent vegetables or fruits, or their preserved juices, the circumnavigation of the globe may be accomplished without the loss of a hand from it. When, therefore, a sailor dies from scurvy, some one ought to be as responsible as if the fatal event were due to criminal neglect. At the present time, the ships to and from India and China, which are at sea from ninety to one hundred and fifty days, are said to be those which produce most sufferers from this preventable disease. It rarely begins to manifest itself under fifty or sixty days from the time of leaving port.

Our knowledge of the *pathology* of this disease is not very precise. There can, however, be little doubt that the blood is altered in composition ; but if it be asked what ingredients are deficient, or in excess, or deteriorated in quality, we can only point to statements which appear very contradictory. The red corpuscles are probably much diminished, while those present may be imperfectly organised ; the albumen being also lessened, and having its solubility increased. Perhaps the saline constituents are deficient in amount, the water and fibrin being increased. Dr. Aldridge holds that the real cause of scurvy is a deficiency in the food of certain minerals which are essential to the existence of nearly all the proximate principles by which the animal structure is built up.

* Dr. Robert Barnes, in his Report on Scurvy in the Merchant Service (*Sixth Report of the Medical Officer of the Privy Council, with Appendix*, 1863), shows that during the twelve years, 1852-63, no less than 1058 cases of this disease have been admitted into the Hospital ship "Dreadnought;" the total number of in-patients for this period being 25,486. In the year 1863 alone, this institution received 86 cases of scurvy : 1 patient in every 23 of the whole number admitted being afflicted with this preventable disease.— Since the publication of this Report, the admissions for scurvy into the "Dreadnought" have been as follows :—For 1864, 83 cases with 2 deaths ; 1865, 102 cases with 4 deaths ; for 1866, 101 cases with 7 deaths ; for 1867, 90 cases with 5 deaths. Of the 18 fatal cases, in 15 there were complications. (Letters to the Author from Mr. Harry Leach).

These principles are phosphorus, sulphur, lime, potash, and soda. And he finds that both seeds and flesh are usually deficient in sulphur and the alkalies. Dr. Garrod in some measure confirms this view; for while attaching little importance to the absence of sulphur and soda, he still believes that the blood contains an inadequate amount of potash, and that all antiscorbutics owe their virtues to the quantity of this salt they contain. He says, moreover, that scorbutic patients will recover when some of the salts of potash are added to their food, without the use of succulent vegetables or milk.

The *symptoms* of scurvy show themselves gradually; commencing with a peculiar dirty pallid condition of the skin, and a somewhat leaden hue of the features. Almost simultaneously, or even previously in some instances, there is a sense of lassitude and indolence, mental anxiety, and an offensive state of the breath. Petechiæ appear on the legs; complaint is made of a kind of rheumatic stiffness of the muscles, as well as of wearying pains in the bones; and there is also a pale exsanguine appearance of the gums, with dyspnœa on the least exertion. The appetite, however, often continues good, and digestion is well performed; while in the very aged, the callous and toothless gums remain healthy all through the disease. Hemeralopia and nyctalopia—peculiar forms of partial amaurosis, possibly due to imperfect nutrition of the retina—have now and then been noticed amongst the earliest symptoms. Then, in the second stage, the symptoms are all intensified. The countenance gets sallow and of a dusky hue; the gums swell, are spongy, of a livid colour, and bleed on the slightest touch; the teeth loosen; and the breath becomes still more fetid. As the disease still further advances, the debility greatly increases; the dyspnœa often becomes most urgent; the gums frequently slough; and hæmorrhages occur from the gums and mouth and nose, from the stomach and intestines. Ecchymoses, or effusions of blood beneath the skin, also appear, especially on the lower extremities and trunk; many parts of the body becoming so greatly discoloured with bruise-like marks that the patient appears as if he had been severely beaten. The legs swell, and attempts to move them give pain; indurated tumours occasionally form in the extremities, from the effusion of a fibrinous material into the connective tissue, or between the bone and periosteum; there is stiffness and contraction of one or more joints; and putrid fungoid ulcers arise, which have a tendency to bleed copiously. Moreover, trifling abrasions are apt to take on an unhealthy action, and to become converted into fetid ulcers; while, without care, bed-sores will form. There is also horrible despondency; the skin is dry and rough; the urine is scanty; in some instances there has been spontaneous salivation; while there is at one time diarrhœa, and at another constipation. Unless relieved, the heart's action gets very feeble; and at the end of some weeks the patient either sinks from a sudden sharp attack of diarrhœa or dysentery, or from extensive effusions of bloody serum into the pleuræ or pericardium, or he more slowly dies from exhaustion.　In many instances, too, some slight exertion has been immediately followed by fatal syncope ; at times, probably, from the formation of a thrombus or clot in the heart or in one of the large arteries.

In the *diagnosis* of pure scurvy no difficulty is likely to arise, since there is only one affection with which it can be confounded —purpura.　From this it is to be distinguished by the gradual way in which the symptoms come on, and the cause ; for purpura often appears suddenly, and is in no way due to abstinence from fresh vegetables.　In purpura there is no sponginess or lividity of the gums, the skin of the trunk is seldom of a dusky hue, nor is the disease prevented or cured by antiscorbutic remedies.

But it must be recollected that the symptoms of scurvy are often masked by its being associated with dysentery, typhus, typhoid fever, pneumonia, &c.　Thus, I believe that during the first six months of the British army being in the Crimea, the hospital returns showed but an insignificant number of cases of scurvy; though many of the medical officers remarked, that almost every admission was complicated by the existence of the scorbutic taint.　It was subsequently that pure scurvy broke out so disastrously both amongst the French and English troops.

The *treatment* resolves itself into keeping the patient warm in a pure atmosphere, while we administer some one or more of the well-known antiscorbutics.　The chief agents of this class are lemon or lime juice,* oranges, shaddocks, sauer-krout, salads, watercresses, potatoes, greens, onions, carrots, radishes, dandelion, common sorrel, pickles, &c.　Dr. Lind in his work on scurvy, published in 1757, clearly proved the efficacy of oranges and lemons in preventing this disease ; though his earnest suggestions to the Government were but little heeded for nearly forty years. To check the hæmorrhage, gallic acid (F. 103) may be required, or what will sometimes answer better—iron alum (F. 116) or tincture of perchloride of iron (F. 101) ; for the purging, the liquid extract of bael (F. 97), or a mixture of rhatany or catechu (F. 96,

* For the preservation and mode of using lime or lemon juice the following Notice to Ship Owners was issued by the Board of Trade in September 1865:— (1) Every ship on a long voyage should be supplied with a proper quantity of lime or lemon juice.　(2) The juice having been received in bulk from the vendors, should be examined and analysed by a competent medical officer. All measures adopted for its preservation are worthless, unless it be clearly ascertained that a pure article has been supplied. (3) Ten per cent. of brandy (S.G. 930) or of rum (S.G. 890) should afterwards be added to it.　(4) It should be packed in jars or bottles, each containing one gallon or less, covered with a layer of oil, and closely packed and sealed.　(5) Each man should have at least two ounces (four tablespoonfuls) twice a week, to be increased to an ounce daily if any symptoms of scurvy manifest themselves.　And (6) the giving out of lime or lemon juice should not be delayed longer than a fortnight after the vessel has put to sea.

97); and to strengthen the gums, either an astringent gargle (F. 250, 252) should be recommended, or the tannic acid lozenges (half a grain in each) of the British Pharmacopœia. In addition to these remedies, plenty of milk, raw eggs, nourishing soups, pounded meat with potato or cabbage or onion, together with wine or cider or perry or ale must be allowed. Spruce beer (F. 7) has been found especially useful, and is an agreeable drink. Then, as soon as the state of the gums and the digestive organs will permit of it, good and copious meals of ordinarily prepared fresh meat and vegetables should be given.

If we believe in the soundness of the views of Drs. Aldridge and Garrod, and if we wish to administer physic, or if we have not the power to regulate the diet, we may employ the acid tartrate, chlorate, or phosphate of potash—F. 61, 356, 358, &c. The nitrate of potash must be avoided; since according to Dr. Bryson, it has been found to exert a most injurious influence. Opium is sometimes needed to give sleep, and to relieve irritability. Quinine and steel often produce excellent results in hastening recovery. In all severe cases the recumbent posture should be strictly maintained; as fatal syncope is not unlikely to arise from any cause which in the least degree impedes the force of the heart's action. Moreover, the occurrence of bed-sores will have to be guarded against by putting the patient on a water mattress.

When Dr. Kane was in the Arctic Regions, and had several of his crew struck down with scurvy, he applied his medical knowledge to good purpose. He says,—"Among other remedies which I oppose to the distemper, I have commenced making sundry salts of iron; among them the citrate and a chlorohydrated tincture. We have but one bottle of brandy: my applying half a pint of it to the tincture shows the high value I set upon this noble chalybeate. My nose bled to-day, and I was struck with the fluid brick-dusty poverty of the blood. I use iron much among my people : as a simple remedy it exceeds all others, except only the specific of raw meat : potash for its own action is well enough to meet some conditions of the disease, and we were in the habit of using freely an extemporaneous citrate prepared from our lime juice ; but as our cases became more reduced and complicated with hæmorrhages, iron was our great remedy." And again, mentioning the fortunate capture of a couple of rabbits, he adds, that by keeping them carefully covered up, they reached the ship sufficiently unfrozen to give about a pint of raw blood. It was "a grateful cordial to Brooks, Wilson, and Riley ;" three of the worst cases.*

To prevent an outbreak of scurvy in individuals so circumstanced that its occurrence is to be feared, attention must be paid to the following points. Supposing that fresh animal and vegetable food cannot be obtained, care ought to be taken that everyone is daily supplied with some antiscorbutic principle—such as is found

* *Arctic Explorations*, pp. 286, 288. London, 1861.

in lemon juice and other materials already described. The air which is breathed must be pure. The quarters, huts, tents, cabins, &c., of the troops or sailors are to be dry, warm and wholesome and properly drained. A fair amount of bodily exercise is to be taken every day ; clothing wet from perspiration or rain or snow being afterwards changed, if possible. And lastly, with men in camp, or compelled to winter in the Arctic Regions &c. every encourage ment is to be given by the officers to games in the open air. Foot-ball, racing, hunting, sleighing, and such like do much to keep off disease of all kinds. A great deal may also be done to lessen the monotony of long evenings by supplying interesting books, music and singing, and drafts or chess or backgammon ; while private theatricals form an almost endless source of amusement, what with the rehearsals and different arrangements which such performances of necessity entail.

III. PURPURA.

This disease probably consists of some morbid state of the blood and capillary vessels ; though the precise nature of the alteration, in its early stage, is unknown. The result is, however, that the red blood corpuscles become disintegrated, while the contents of these cells are of course diffused. Hence purpura [so called from Πορφύρα = a purple dye] may be said to be characterized by the occurrence of sanguineous effusions into the cutaneous and mucous tissues of the body ; producing red or claret-coloured maculæ, which die away to be succeeded by fresh eruptions in adjoining patches of skin. When the hæmorrhagic spots are very small, they are termed *petechiæ ;* when larger, perhaps owing to the fusion of several petechiæ, they are known as *vibices ;* while where there are considerable patches of extravasated blood, the blotches are spoken of as *ecchymoses.* All these marks have this character in common, —they do not disappear or fade on the use of pressure.

Purpura was placed by Willan in the class of exanthematous diseases. He enumerated five varieties of it. These are *purpura simplex, p. urticans, p. hæmorrhagica, p. senilis,* and *p. petechialis* or *contagiosa.* Such a subdivision seems, however, to be a very un-necessary refinement. It is sufficient to adopt the two old divisions generally employed in the present day,—viz., that of purpura sim-plex and p. hæmorrhagica. The first is frequently a trifling affec-tion ; which has its origin in mal-assimilation, and can usually be soon corrected. Not so with the second variety. For in addition to the cutaneous hæmorrhage being frequently considerable, the blood is often poured out freely beneath the mucous membranes ; while if there be much degradation of this fluid, copious effusion may take place into the serous cavities, the stomach and intestines, the air tubes, or the bladder, &c.

The *causes* of purpura are obscure. Sometimes it seems due to the excessive use of salt provisions, or of pork preserved in nitrate of potash. The disease known as " black leg," which occurs amongst the lumber men on the Ottawa or grand river of Canada, is merely a form of purpura; being produced by a diet of bread with tea, and pork saved from decomposition by packing in saltpetre. In several instances the origin of purpura can be traced to insufficient food, with the other ills of poverty; to chronic exhausting affections; to ichorhæmia; to degenerations of the liver or spleen; to Bright's disease; to intemperance; and to long-continued mental anxiety. One of the most troublesome cases, as regards duration, which I have seen, was due to a daily loss of blood from large hæmorrhoids. The patient had consulted other physicians without deriving any benefit from the remedies suggested; but he had never mentioned the piles. He thought they were of no consequence; although he never went to stool without losing a tablespoonful of blood, and frequently much more. I am not sure that purpura has not occasionally some connexion with a nearly worn out syphilitic taint : a taint sufficient to produce anomalous symptoms difficult of explanation, and yet not powerful enough to give rise to any of the ordinary secondary or tertiary symptoms. Possibly also this morbid state of the blood will be found to arise in cases of chronic poisoning by arsenic, mercury, &c.

The *symptoms* in simple purpura are often unimportant. They consist almost entirely of successive eruptions of red spots, with more or less evidence of impairment of the functions of digestion and secretion. In a typical example of the more critical form of this disease, the chief points which attract attention are the great languor and debility; the patient's appearance testifying that he is very much out of health. There is a sallow, rather than a dusky, complexion; and sometimes a slightly puffy state of the features. Bleeding from the nose is common. In addition, we find much mental depression; bad appetite, sometimes alternating with an inordinate craving for food; pains about the epigastrium; palpitation of the heart; together with attacks of giddiness on making any exertion, dimness of vision, faintings, constipation, &c.

The petechiæ, or vibices, or ecchymoses generally appear on the legs first, and then on the trunk. They are of variable size, from minute dots like flea-bites, to patches several inches in extent; while they are occasionally of a scarlet colour, and sometimes of a dark livid hue, giving the appearance presented by recent contusions. As they fade away, they assume a dirty yellow tinge. In exceptional cases there are severe pains in the muscles, as well as in the textures around the joints; the suffering being usually attributed to rheumatism. Occasionally I have found that as a fresh crop of petechiæ has come out, the pains have been much relieved; the latter again getting aggravated as the spots have died away.

The mere fact that the prominent feature of purpura is an exudation of blood from the cutaneous capillaries, would lead us to fear that simultaneously hæmorrhage might take place into the substance of the mucous membranes, &c.; and not only is such the case, but it is this occurrence which renders purpura hæmorrhagica a dangerous affection. As a rule, in fatal cases, blood is found copiously effused into the mucous lining of the whole digestive tract from the mouth to the anus; beneath the serous membranes of the heart, lungs, and abdomen; between the arachnoid and pia mater, or even into the cerebral substance; into the urinary passages; as well as into the muscular and glandular tissues. Another characteristic change, moreover, is to be detected in the spleen; which is enlarged and softened, as well as studded with pale yellow spots. By some authorities this condition of the spleen is regarded not as the effect of the disease, but as its cause.

Purpura may be complicated with, or it sometimes occurs during the progress of, other diseases. Thus, it has been met with in rheumatism and gout; in urticaria, eczema, and other skin diseases; in dropsy; in various important affections of the liver, kidneys, &c.; and as a sequela to the different eruptive and continued fevers.

The *treatment* should consist in the exhibition of full doses of sulphate of soda with sulphuric acid (F. 143), or of castor oil, until the bowels are thoroughly cleared. Then, according to circumstances, recourse is to be had to quinine and iron (F. 380); or to the mineral acids (F. 376, 378, 379); or to quinine, steel, and arsenic (F. 381); or to phosphate of iron, &c. (F. 405, 406). A good nourishing diet, fresh fruit or vegetables, a fair allowance of stout or ale or wine, and rest in a pure atmosphere, will be indispensable. The oil of turpentine, in small but frequently repeated doses (F. 50), has been strongly recommended where there is internal hæmorrhage. A tincture prepared from the inner bark of the common larch (Larix Europæa), administered in fifteen minim doses every three or four hours, would at least prove more agreeable. As a rule, however, I feel more confidence in a mixture (F. 103) containing the gallic and aromatic sulphuric acids.

IV. HYDROPHOBIA.

Of the diseases which may arise from inoculation with poisons generated by unhealthy animals, hydrophobia ["Υδωρ = water + φοβέω = to dread], or rabies [*Rabio* = to rave], is the most remarkable as well as the most distressing. It is, indeed, a fearful malady; not only on account of its almost universal fatality, but also because of the horrible suffering it gives rise to. Rabies is generally believed to occur spontaneously in the canine and perhaps in the feline races ; but it is not unlikely that this opinion is opposed to truth. Certainly, the disease is only communicated by inoculation with the saliva to other animals and to man.

Pathology.—The symptoms, together with the absence of any constant structural change, seem to show that this disease depends upon some peculiar alteration in the blood ; this alteration affecting the nervous system, and especially the medulla oblongata with the three divisions of the eighth pair. The poison, when absorbed, may reasonably be supposed to slowly effect some change in the blood, while at the same time the morbid material increases in quantity and virulence. The process by which this occurs has been compared to that which happens in fermentation. According to some authors, a double zymosis or fermentation takes place ; first in the part wounded, and secondly in the system at large. The question is often asked,—Is the disease due to the slow operation of the poison on the system, or to the mental anxiety which the patient undergoes from the consciousness of his danger? Although our knowledge of the nature of this affection is very imperfect, still I know of no reason for believing that anxiety will give rise to hydrophobia any more than it will produce variola or syphilis. But just as we meet with imaginary cases of the latter (syphiliphobia), so we read of mental or hysterical hydrophobia—to be cured by bread pills. Whether in a rabid animal other secretions than the saliva are poisonous is not absolutely certain ; but it is exceedingly probable that they are so.

Stage of Incubation.—Speaking with much latitude, the stage of *incubation*, or of *delitescence* as it is sometimes called, may be said to vary from thirty days to eighteen or twenty months ; the duration perhaps depending upon the virulence and quantity of the poison, as well as upon the constitution and age of the party inoculated. The period appears to be shorter in very young persons than in those more advanced in years. Exceptional cases are recorded where the symptoms have set in as early as the eighth day ; while others are known in which their appearance has been delayed for four, five, and seven years. In one instance, related by Dr. Bardsley, it is said that twelve years intervened between the bite and the first hydrophobic symptoms.* Probably, in the greater number of cases, the latent period has lasted from one to two months.

In 1862, M. Renault published the results of some experiments which had been conducted with the object of learning the time of incubation in the dog. From these it appears, that of 131 dogs bitten by mad dogs, or inoculated with hydrophobic slaver, 63 remained well at the end of four months. The disease was developed in the other 68 after intervals varying from five to one hundred and twenty days. Thus,—

* *Medical Reports of Cases and Experiments, &c.,* p. 237. London, 1807.

In 25 dogs the disease set in between the 5th and 30th day.

31	„		30th „	60th „
7	„		60th „	90th „
5	„		90th „	120th „

Symptoms.—The pathognomonic signs of hydrophobia, in the human subject, are:—Cramps of the muscles of the pharynx and thorax; spasmodic action of the diaphragm; a great dread of fluids; a recurrence of paroxysms of phrensy on attempting to drink, or on exposure to a current of air; a flow of viscid saliva ("hydrophobic slaver"); restlessness and terrible anxiety; delirium, with exhaustion or coma, ending in death.

To consider the symptoms at greater length, we will suppose that a man has been bitten by a rabid animal. After the lapse of the period of incubation, the short stage of *recrudescence* sets in. Complaint is usually made of mental uneasiness, chilliness, languor, and lassitude; there is restlessness also, loss of appetite, and more or less headache. Sometimes a sensation of numbness, or even of great soreness in the bitten part is experienced. But in any case the precursory symptoms are followed at the end of one, two, or three days by the *confirmed* or *hydrophobic* stage of the disease. This commences generally with considerable agitation and garrulity, peculiar rapid movements of the eyes, frequent sighings, nausea, and fever; to which rapidly succeed stiffness of the neck, difficulty of breathing and swallowing, a horror of liquids, and a frightful sense of suffocation. The face has an expression of great alarm. There is an excessive secretion of tenacious saliva, causing frequent hawking and spitting; each expectoration perhaps being accompanied by a shudder. In addition to sleeplessness, spectral illusions are common. Amongst other symptoms of general hyperæsthesia, there is sometimes priapism with seminal emissions; or in women, there may be nymphomania. A frequent desire to pass urine is repeatedly noticed. There now set in violent spasmodic convulsions of the whole body; the paroxysms being occasioned especially by the sight of liquids, or the sound of running water, or any attempt at drinking. The impetuous terror inspired by the sight of water has been well described by Dr. Marcet, who, in relating the history of a case of hydrophobia, says :—" On our proposing to him to drink, he started up and recovered his breath by a deep convulsive inspiration; yet he expressed much regret that he could not drink, as he conceived the water would give him great relief, his mouth being evidently parched and clammy. On being urged to try, however, he took up a cup of water in one hand and a teaspoon in the other. The thought of drinking out of the cup seemed to him intolerable; but he seemed determined to drink with the spoon. With an expression of terror, yet with great resolution, he filled the spoon, and proceeded to carry it to his lips; but before it reached his mouth his courage forsook him, and he was obliged to desist. He repeatedly renewed the attempt, but with no better success.   His arm became rigid and immovable whenever he tried to raise it towards his mouth, and he struggled in vain against this spasmodic resistance.   At last shutting his eyes, and with a kind of convulsive effort, he suddenly threw into his mouth a few drops of the fluid, which he actually swallowed.   But at the same instant he jumped up from his chair, and flew to the end of the room, panting for his breath, and in a state of indescribable terror."[*]

About the *second day* the symptoms become more severe.   The thirst gets distressing, and yet the patient dare not attempt to drink.   " Miserrimum genus morbi ; in quo simul æger et siti et aquæ metu cruciatur : quo oppressis in angusto spes est."[†]   The viscid saliva clings to the fauces.   There is uneasiness or pain at the epigastrium, and flatulence.   The countenance is anxious, and indicative of horror or despair ; the forehead is perhaps covered with a cold clammy sweat ; and there is generally much mental distress, with excessive irritability, though the intellect remains perfect.   Then, as the fatal issue quickly approaches, the sense of suffocation grows more urgent ; while the surface of the body has become so sensitive that a draught of cold air, or the lightest touch, will suffice to bring on convulsive paroxysms.   The senses of hearing and vision get morbidly acute.   The saliva is more difficult to expel, though the attempts at spitting are incessant ; or the secretions of the mouth flow away at the angles of the lips, owing to the dropping of the lower jaw from paralysis.   Occasionally there is frequent micturition, but only small quantities of urine are passed.   And then, at length, the terror becomes succeeded by wild delirium, which ends in exhaustion and death.   Sometimes there is a great mitigation of suffering for a few hours before death. The patient becomes tranquil ; perhaps falls into a quiet sleep, or into a state of deep coma, and then dies without a struggle.

Prognosis.—Very few cases of recovery are known.   The general duration of the disease is from two to four or even six days, counting from the commencement of the confirmed stage. The deaths registered in England from hydrophobia during the eleven years, 1856 to 1866 amount to ninety-three.   More than one-third (36) of these occurred in 1866 alone ; the largest number in any single year since registration was commenced.   In 1851, the fatal cases amounted to twenty-five.   Considering that the population during the middle of the year 1866 was estimated at 21,210,020 we have an approach to two cases of hydrophobia to each million of people.   In 1865, however, the fatal cases did not bear half this proportion.   There is every reason to believe that only a small number of those bitten by rabid animals suffer from hydrophobia.   When the bite is inflicted through the clothes, the

* *Medico-Chirurgical Transactions*, vol. i. p. 138   London, 1809.
† Auli Cornelii Celsi Medicinæ.   Liber v. (*Medicamenta, et Morbi his Curandi*).   Cap. xxvii.   Written when Celsus was between 30 and 35 years of age, probably 18 A.C.

latter will possibly remove the virus from the teeth. As with other poisons too, some individuals may be more susceptible to its influence than others. John Hunter mentions an instance in which of twenty-one persons bitten by a dog, only one suffered. The bite of a rabid wolf appears to be more dangerous. M. Troilliet states that of seventeen persons bitten by a wolf, ten died; and on another occasion out of twenty-three, thirteen perished. Moreover, it is possible that an attack of hydrophobia can entirely go off after the premonitory symptoms have commenced. Dr. Elliotson relates—*Lancet*, May 1829—the following instance:—Two little girls were bitten in the face by the same dog, while they were standing at their father's door. She who was bitten the second became hydrophobic and died. The other, at exactly the same time, experienced precisely the same premonitory symptoms as her sister—heaviness and general indisposition—but they all went off.

Mr. Youatt has proved that hydrophobia has occasionally a favourable termination in the dog. In this animal, the prominent symptoms are an alteration in the bark, which becomes a kind of howl; a rough staring condition of the coat; a peculiar movement of the eyes; together with a continued biting and swallowing of straws, hairs, pieces of paper, &c. Usually there is no fear of water. On the contrary, drink is greedily sought; although the spasms of the pharynx may prevent its being swallowed. If there is a falling of the lower jaw from paralysis, the bark is lost; a form of disease which is consequently spoken of as *dumb rabies*. Death usually occurs between the third and eighth days.

Morbid Anatomy.—The rigor mortis is of short duration. The depending parts of the body are usually very livid. The fauces and pharynx are vascular, and sometimes covered with lymph. The lungs will perhaps be congested, and the bronchi loaded with tenacious frothy mucus. In some cases, the stomach and intestines have presented evidence of partial inflammatory action. But the most constant morbid appearances are detected in the brain and spinal cord; the meninges being congested, fibrinous coagula being present in the sinuses, the ventricles containing a slight excess of fluid, and blood or serum being effused around the cervical portion of the cord. Occasionally there has been a complete absence of any discoverable lesion in the body.

Treatment.—This must be prophylactic, for the cure of the disease seems in the present state of medical knowledge almost hopeless.* The wounded part is to be excised as soon as possible after

* The wonder-working herb with which the Arabian physicians treat this disease has not yet arrived here. Well might Mr. Palgrave be told marvellous stories of this plant, when one hydrophobic patient after taking it discharged "several little dogs! and then recovered. Nay, the narrator professed to have seen these extraordinary puppies, and described their size, colour, form, &c., with great circumstantiality."—*Narrative of a Year's Journey through Central and Eastern Arabia* (1862-63). Second Edition, vol. ii. p. 33. London, 1865.

the bite ; care being taken to remove every portion touched by the animal's teeth, and to obtain a clean raw surface. Even if some days have elapsed from the infliction of the wound, excision had better be resorted to. The operation can do very little, if any, harm; while by the aid of chloroform it is rendered painless. The wound is then to be thoroughly washed by a stream of water long poured over it ; while lunar caustic ought afterwards to be applied. Mr. Youatt prefers the nitrate of silver freely used, to every other caustic ; and he also recommends that after its application the wound be quickly healed, though many authorities advise that it should be kept open by irritating ointments. Subsequently, it might be worth while to prescribe a course of Turkish baths ; so as to aid the elimination of any poison which may have been absorbed prior to the use of the knife.

In treating the disease itself, I would resort to subcutaneous injections of atropine, or of morphia, or of both in combination, to quiet the nervous system ; as well as to the administration, either by the mouth or rectum, of solutions of the sulphite or hyposulphite of soda or magnesia. The reputed power of these agents in neutralizing blood-poisons is worth testing, seeing that nothing better can be suggested. At the same time, sulphur fumigations can be employed. Ice should be given to suck ; and perhaps its application to the upper part of the spine might afford relief. Copious enemata of warm water will possibly mitigate the thirst.

Enormous doses of opium have failed to do any permanent good ; and the same must be said of belladonna, prussic acid, Indian hemp, curara, subcutaneous injections of atropine, and tobacco. Dr. Todd kept a patient under the influence of chloroform for about eight hours ; but it did not seem to retard the fatal termination. So severe are the sufferings, however, that it is a great point to give even temporary relief. Dr. Marcet's patient said imploringly—"Oh, do something for me. I would suffer myself to be cut to pieces ! I cannot raise the phlegm ; it sticks to me like bird-lime." And after trying to collect himself, he again exclaimed—" Gentlemen, don't ask me questions, I cannot say more, my feelings cannot be described !" When the case is seen early, it might perhaps prove beneficial to induce free perspiration by the vapour-bath. If the theory of a double zymosis be true, it may do good to lay open the cicatrix and induce suppuration in it. Tracheotomy has been proposed ; but it would be a useless piece of cruelty to resort to it, unless the patient seemed threatened with early death from spasm of the glottis. In one case where it was had recourse to, and in which the horror of liquids had been most intense, opening the trachea allowed drinks to be partaken of freely.

The practitioner should remember that inoculation through the saliva of a patient with hydrophobia seems by no means impossible. He ought consequently, to carefully guard against this secretion coming in contact, directly or by towels, with any scratch or abraded surface upon his face or hands.

V. GLANDERS AND FARCY.

The disease known as glanders in the human subject, may be defined as a malignant febrile affection, which is very contagious and possibly infectious. It is due to a specific poison received from glandered horses, asses, or mules. Glanders and farcy are essentially identical, both having their origin in the same poison. But where the effects of the morbid agent are manifested in the nasal cavities, the disease is known as *glanders;* while when the lymphatic system suffers, it is called *farcy.*

In the *horse*, glanders is a disease which has long been recognised; for, according to Mr. Youatt, few veterinary writers have published a more accurate account of it than was given by Hippocrates 2300 years ago. It is a loathsome and incurable malady; beginning in this animal with a contagious, constantly-flowing, aqueous discharge from the nostril—commonly the left. In the second stage of the disease, the discharge becomes viscid and glutinous; then it gets purulent, and the neighbouring glands, especially the submaxillary, begin to enlarge; spots of ulceration soon appear on the membrane covering the cartilage of the nose; and the poor beast loses flesh and strength. His hair also comes off, the appetite fails, and there is a more or less urgent cough. As the disease steadily advances, the ulcers increase in size; the discharge is rendered bloody and offensive; the membrane lining the frontal sinuses inflames and ulcerates; the forehead grows tender; more of the absorbents are involved; the conjunctivæ swell and suppurate; little tumours appear about the face and soon ulcerate; and farcy is now superadded, or the glanders degenerates into farcy. The progress is henceforth rapid. The deep-seated absorbents are soon affected; one or both of the hind legs swell to a great size; while the discharge increases in quantity and fetidity. In short, the animal seems to present a mass of putrefaction, until at length he dies completely exhausted.

Farcy in the horse is an inflammation of the lymphatic glands and vessels, giving rise to small tumours called " buttons," or "farcy-buds," that gradually suppurate. The ulcers which form have the same character as the glanderous ones in the nose; while the virus they secrete is just as contagious. By slow degrees this virus poisons the whole system; all the capillary absorbents become inflamed; the legs and head swell enormously; and generally the disease surely runs on to a fatal termination.

In *man* the symptoms which result from the absorption of the poison may show themselves as acute or chronic glanders, or as acute or chronic farcy.—The *acute glanders* is attended by suffering somewhat similar to that which occurs in the horse. The prominent symptoms are fever, great debility, and pains of a rheumatic character in the limbs; there is a profuse offensive discharge from the nostrils; while a number of pustules and tumours form in different parts of the body, which have a great tendency to suppurate and become gangrenous. This peculiar pustular eruption, which looks more like that caused by croton oil inunction than anything else, does not occur until about the twelfth day: it is accompanied by profuse fetid sweats, and sometimes by the formation of black bullæ. Abscesses appear in the neighbourhood of the joints; the nose, eyelids, and face swell and perhaps ulcerate; the urine is often albuminous and loaded with renal casts; while the constitutional disturbance is shown by great weakness and delirium. The disease generally proves fatal before the twentieth day. After death, the mucous membrane lining the nasal fossæ has been found in a state of gangrene, or else it has been covered with numberless small pustules. Acute glanders is considerably more common than the chronic form. It occurs for the most part in grooms, stable-men, &c. Of fifteen cases, the histories of which were collected by Rayer, fourteen died. The length of the period of incubation is rather doubtful, but it is probably from two to eight days.*

Chronic glanders runs its course much more slowly to a disastrous termination; the fatal event being perhaps delayed for several months, or even a year or two. The symptoms consist especially of a discharge from the nostril, of offensive perspirations, and the formation of abscesses in the neighbourhood of the large joints. There is gradually increasing loss of flesh and strength; the prostration which occurs being favoured by attacks of diar-

---

* Dr. Manquet of Tours has related a frightful case of glanders and farcy attacking a pregnant woman. The patient was a rag-picker, living in a filthy atmosphere. The disease was caught from a miserable pony, which had been allowed to feed frequently off the same dishes with the family. The following is Dr. Manquet's summary of the train of events in the woman's illness:—
" Acute pleuro-pneumonia, masked at the outset by accessions of intermittent fever of a double tertian type. On the eighth day, resolution of the pulmonary inflammation, which is replaced by an extremely painful articular rheumatism. Pustular eruptions on the legs: fluctuating subcutaneous tumours in the long axis of the limb, and in the course of the lymphatic vessels (farcy). On the eleventh day a malignant pustule on the nose, which tumifies, reddens, violaceous œdema, phlyctænoid erysipelas. In four days a confluent eruption occupies all the face, and reaches as far as the right shoulder (glanders). Numerous abscesses (farcinous poisoning). Discharge from both nostrils: glandular engorgement. Fever very active towards the end: state of typhoid prostration: petechial spots over the whole body. Spontaneous accouchement on the thirteenth day: infant living (though premature). Death (of the mother), in a condition of putrefaction of the head, on the fifteenth day of the illness, the eighth of the glanderous affection." The infant lived twenty-four hours, and seems to have succumbed to mere feebleness.

rhœa and sickness.   Out of three reported cases only one recovered.

In *acute farcy*, the inflammation begins in the lymphatics leading from the part wounded, and is followed by swelling of the glands and extensive suppuration in the subcutaneous areolar tissue. Great exhaustion soon sets in, from which, however, the patient may recover. But if a pustular or gangrenous eruption appear, together with the glanderous discharge from the nostril, the case may be looked upon as hopeless. In fifteen examples of acute farcy death resulted in ten.

Chronic farcy produces the following effects. Suppose a groom has a slight abrasion on one of his fingers, and that it comes in contact with a little of the discharge from a glandered horse. A few days subsequently, a painful sore appears, which is poulticed. In a day or two an eschar forms; on removing which a deep, unhealthy ulcer is seen. Similar ulcers form about the head, upon the arm, in the course of the absorbents, and in the axilla. The health begins to suffer; while unless the patient can take plenty of nourishment and perhaps remove to the sea-side, symptoms of acute glanders will soon set in and destroy him. This unfavourable result may, however, be often averted; for out of seven cases only one died.

In *Equinia mitis* there is more or less constitutional disturbance, with a pustular eruption. If this be abundant there is high fever, followed by prostration. The disease is due to contagion from the discharge of a horse affected with the grease. The *grease*, in the horse, consists of an inflammation of the sebaceous glands of the heels. It has a tendency to spread to deeper tissues, giving rise to ulceration and large fungoid granulations. The fore-feet may be affected, but much more frequently it arises in the hinder. It is contagious; and as it is the result of gross neglect and mismanagement it is never seen in the stables of respectable people. Consequently, equinia mitis is a disease unknown to grooms, coachmen, and jockeys; though occasionally the drivers of the wretched animals seen with dung-carts, in brickfields, &c., suffer from it. A cure may be effected by cleanliness, warm bathing, disinfecting lotions, mild aperients, quinine, and nourishing food.

For the *treatment* of acute glanders all kinds of remedies have been ineffectually employed. Under these circumstances it is incumbent upon the physician to give a trial to any plan of treatment which affords a hope, however slight, of cure. The investigations of Dr. Polli of Milan, on the action of sulphurous acid, have already been referred to, but the following experiment is especially worthy of recollection. Two dogs were inoculated with the discharge of glanders through the skin. To one ninety grains of sulphite of soda were administered daily; to the other, no remedy was applied. The wound in the former healed up in a few days: in the latter animal, it opened and yielded a sanious discharge, and general infection followed. From this, the conclusion seems justifiable that the sulphite of soda or magnesia (F. 48) should be tried in man. It ought, however, to be commenced at the onset.

In chronic farcy a cure has been effected by large doses (from grs. 10 to 15, thrice daily,) of iodide of potassium and bark. Arsenic with strychnia has been recommended. Quinine might prove useful. Stimulants, good nourishing food, and pure air, will be necessary in all cases. It will also be advisable to open the abscesses; and to syringe the nostrils or wash the ulcers with plenty of water containing a little chloride of zinc, or solution of permanganate of potash, or some other disinfectant solution. The internal administration of carbolic acid, together with the application of lotions containing this medicine to the ulcers, might be anticipated to have a beneficial effect. Then, in a few cases, we could perhaps try to assist in eliminating the poison through the skin, by the repeated use of the vapour bath.

As regards *prophylactic treatment* it is only necessary to recommend free cauterization of the inoculated tissue; together with the administration of the sulphite of soda or magnesia. Fumigation with sulphurous acid gas (SO_2) ought also to be employed.

VI. FURUNCULAR INFLAMMATIONS.

1. BOILS.—A boil or furunculus [as if *Fervunculus*, from *Ferveo* = to burn] is a circumscribed hard tumour, small but very painful, caused by inflammation of the true skin and subjacent areolar tissue. Suppuration takes place slowly and imperfectly; the skin ulcerates, and allows of the escape of a little pus; and then in two or three days a slough of the connective tissue (the core) is discharged from the centre. Boils most frequently form on the back of the hand, the nape of the neck, the armpit, the nates, about the vulva, or on the thighs. In many cases, three or four are met with in different situations, at the same time; successive crops appearing, to the great annoyance of the patient.

Causes.—A boil is always to be regarded as evidence of malnutrition. Hence the most common causes are a residence in an impure atmosphere; insufficient or improper food; sexual excesses; over-work or mental anxiety; and, in short, anything which leads to deterioration of the blood. The young and old seem to suffer equally; and somewhat more than those in the prime of life.

Treatment.—Locally, warm water dressing or poultices should be applied. The most ancient poultice that we read of was made from figs; being used for a boil when Hezekiah was "sick unto death."* Unless the pain be very great, or the tissue over the

---

* "And Isaiah said, take a lump of figs: and they took and laid *it* on the boil, and he recovered."—2 Kings, ch. xx. ver. 7.

swelling coarse and thick, I am convinced that it is better to let the boil break, rather than to open it with the knife. The former plan is never attended with inconvenience; whereas improper interference has more than once led to severe attacks of erysipelas.

Then, in addition to removing the cause of the unhealthy inflammation, the bowels should be cleared out by an active aperient (F. 144, 148, 150). After its operation a good nourishing diet must be allowed, with a moderate quantity of wine or pure beer. As a tonic nothing suits better than quinine (F. 379), or one of the mineral acids with bark (F. 376). When there are successive crops of boils, with or without any obvious cause, no remedy is so efficacious as a trip to the country.

2. STYES.—A stye or hordeolum (*Hordeolus*, dimin. of *Hordeum* = barley) is merely a small boil, of the size and firmness of a barleycorn, situated at the edge of the eyelid. It often forms in strumous and other weakly children. Fomentations and water dressing will bring it to a head; and assist the exit of a drop or two of pus, with a small slough of connective tissue. Quinine or bark or steel, with good diet and cod liver oil, commonly suffice to remove the constitutional cause. If the excretions are offensive and insufficient in amount, one or more doses of a mild aperient (rhubarb and magnesia) will be needed.

3. CARBUNCLES.—A carbuncle or anthrax (from ʺΑνθραξ = a coal) consists of severe inflammation of a circumscribed portion of the skin and subjacent tissue, with infiltration of unhealthy lymph. The swelling which results is hard, flattened and more or less circular in shape, and of a dull-red colour; it is tender and very painful; while it varies in diameter from half an inch to six or seven inches. The surrounding skin gets unduly sensitive, of a purplish tint, and burning hot; while there is a severe throbbing or dull aching pain in the whole of the affected part. As the mischief progresses, the centre of the tumefaction suppurates; at first a doughy feel being communicated to the touch, with subsequently an indistinct sense of fluctuation. Then, the skin ulcerates in several small spots; from which openings a bloody purulent fluid, with shreds of sloughy connective tissue and lymph, can be squeezed. The openings gradually coalesce, until an unhealthy looking ulceration of some size is produced: the discharge increases and gets thinner; while all the greyish sloughs separate from the living tissue and come away. If the case progress favourably, healthy granulations spring up; and the wound daily becomes smaller and smaller until it closes. A well-marked permanent cicatrix remains to show the extent of the mischief.

Carbuncles are most frequently situated about the nape of the neck, or on the back; the next most frequent sites being the shoulders, sides of trunk, abdominal wall, buttocks, back of the

arm and fore-arm, and upper or lower lip.   They are rare in
childhood and youth; generally occurring in individuals who have
passed the middle period of life.   Men suffer at least twice as often
as women.

Causes.—As boils are due to a vitiated state of the blood, so
carbuncles have their origin in a similar though exaggerated condition.   Sometimes they occur as sequelæ to one of the continued
or eruptive fevers; or they arise in individuals weakened by renal
disease.   They are common in diabetes : the first which forms may
prove fatal, if the patient's diet be too restricted in consequence of
over-attention to the state of the urine.   Not unfrequently, carbuncles have appeared to be partly due to an unhealthy condition of
the atmosphere and season.   Lastly, irritating liniments, resinous
plasters, and blisters, will give rise to them in cases where the
predisposing influence of debility is present.

Constitutional Symptoms.—For a day or two prior to the appearance of the carbuncle the patient notices that he is not well:
there is a sense of malaise, with languor and chilliness.   As the
inflammatory action manifests itself, the constitutional disturbance
becomes marked in proportion to the extent of the morbid process;   and there is headache, confusion of intellect, irritability
from the pain, a sallow complexion, a feeble rapid pulse, and a
thickly-furred tongue.   The bowels are usually constipated, but
occasionally there is diarrhœa with offensive and unhealthy stools.
The urine sometimes contains sugar.   Occasionally we find violent
fever and delirium, extreme prostration setting in early.   A fatal
result may ensue from exhaustion, from ichorhæmia, or from an
extension of the disease to important tissues.   If the Registrar-
General's Report for ten years (1857 to 1866) be examined, it will
be found that the annual average mortality in England and Wales
from this disease is 237.   Carbuncles, unlike boils, are generally
solitary.

Treatment.—Linseed poultices, or water dressing, or anodyne
fomentations should be early employed; since they afford more
relief than any other applications, and hasten suppuration.   A
crucial incision down to the base of the swelling, by removing the
tension, often gives ease;   and it may be had recourse to even
before suppuration has become established.   This is not to be regarded as a rule, to be carried out in all cases; but rather as a plan
to be resorted to with judgment and discretion.   In the old and very
nervous, where there is an unconquerable dread of chloroform, I
have not seen reason to regret trusting to fomentations, without
recommending the knife.   Subsequently, when the sloughs have
all come away, a stimulating lotion (F. 264) will promote granulation and cicatrization.

Mr. French has recommended subcutaneous incisions, both for
boils and carbuncles.   The extent of the induration being ascertained, a tenotomy knife is passed horizontally underneath it ; the

blade of which is then turned upwards, and the hardened structure cut through to the utmost extremity of the induration, avoiding the skin. The disease is thus arrested in one direction; and to prevent its spreading in the other, a second puncture at right angles with the first is to be made, thus forming a subcutaneous crucial incision. When any bleeding which may happen has ceased, the whole surface of the tumour is to be covered with collodion. Immediate relief is felt, and the patient is at once able to pursue his ordinary avocations.

Mr. Prichard, of Bristol, has helped to revive the caustic plan of treatment. He not only thinks very highly of it, but is a strenuous opponent of the crucial incision. In whatever stage the carbuncle may be, this surgeon takes a stick of potassa fusa, and rubs it freely into the centre until an eschar is fully formed. The diameter of the skin destroyed is about one-fourth or one-third of the indurated mass. A strong solution of iodine in collodion (F. 205) is then applied to the circumference of the swelling, so as to destroy the erysipelatous element of the disease. Poultices are avoided; a dressing of turpentine ointment (Brit. Phar.) being applied. Great care is afterwards taken to let the slough come away without dragging or cutting it; while attention is paid to ensure cleanliness. To prevent the pain of this proceeding, Dr. Arnott's freezing mixture of pounded ice and salt can be applied to the surface for five minutes before its adoption; or the more recent plan of producing local anæsthesia by the ether spray, as recommended by Dr. Richardson, deserves a trial.

As regards the general remedies our treatment resolves itself into insuring free excretion by the kidneys and liver and intestinal glands, while supporting the strength. Podophyllin (F. 160), nitric acid and taraxacum and senna (F. 147), purified ox bile and jalap or colocynth (F. 170), or the citrate of magnesia (F. 169), or the sulphate of manganese with colchicum (F. 172), are very useful in the first stage; but care must be taken not to induce diarrhœa. Then, chlorate of potash and tincture of perchloride of iron (F. 402), or the mineral acids and bark (F. 376), or ammonia and bark (F. 371), or quinine (F. 379), or steel and arsenic (F. 381), will prove very beneficial. Once or twice I have likewise ordered some preparation of oxygen (F. 370), and it has seemed with advantage. Such remedies, together with easily-digested food (cream, milk, raw eggs, essence of beef, mutton chops, &c.), and stimulants in accordance with the necessity for them, will probably lead the case to a successful issue. It is often necessary to relieve the pain with opium; a full dose (F. 314, 317, 340), once in the twenty-four hours being better than oft-repeated small quantities.

4. MALIGNANT VESICLE. — This contagious and fatal disease (*Malignant Pustule, Charbon*), has long been familiarly known

to practitioners abroad ; but in this country it has attracted less attention. Examples of it, however, have occasionally been described
in the medical journals. Thus, in September 1852, Mr. Harvey
Ludlow gave an account in the *Medical Times and Gazette,* of six
cases which had been under treatment in St. Bartholomew's Hospital. More recently Dr. William Budd has written some excellent
papers on the subject.*

Symptoms.—In most instances there is the following train of
events :—At first, the formation of a small pimple or vesicle on
some exposed part,—often the upper lip, or other portion of the
face. In scratching to relieve the unbearable itching or stinging
sensation, the vesicle gets broken ; and then, at the end of twenty-
four or thirty·six hours, there is found considerable swelling with
some discoloration. The carbuncular inflammation now rapidly
increases in severity ; while the tissues in the neighbourhood of
the original pimple swell enormously, become of a brawny hardness, get cold and lose their vitality, and assume a black colour.
There is a constant drivelling of saliva, the breath gets peculiarly
fetid, the pulse becomes feeble and rapid, the respiration seems
embarrassed, profuse clammy sweats cover the body, and delirium
with great prostration sets in ; death often resulting, with all the
symptoms of general blood-poisoning, within eight days from the
commencement of the attack.

Pathology.—This disease has long been the cause of great
mortality amongst sheep, oxen, horses, and other animals ; being
known under the names of "joint-murrain," "black quarter,"
"quarter evil," "charbon," "sang," "spleen gangrene," &c. It
is conveyed to man either by direct inoculation, or by eating the
flesh of cattle which have suffered from it ; while, in some instances, flies or other insects have carried the poison from the
diseased beast and inoculated him. Many facts also prove that
the virus is retained in the hair, hides, hoofs, fat and tallow of
animals killed by it. Although the vesicle, in man, is usually
situated on a surface habitually exposed, it is not necessarily so.
Mr. Robert Harper has reported a case where it was on the penis ;
the patient, after dressing diseased sheep, having held this organ
during micturition without previously washing the hands. For
inoculation to take place, it is probably necessary that there should
be some abrasion or slight wound ; though it is by no means certain
that it may not occur without this, in parts where the skin is
thin. Women rarely suffer from malignant vesicle ; most of the
victims having been adult men, who had previously appeared
healthy.

Treatment.—It is generally agreed that a cure can often be
effected by decided treatment at an early period of the disease.
One or more incisions should be made through the affected tissue,

* "On the Occurrence of Malignant Pustule in England." Reprinted
from the *British Medical Journal.* London, 1863.

and a strong caustic applied,—such as potassa fusa, or the acid solution of nitrate of mercury, or the actual cautery.   Afterwards the part had better be dressed carefully with a lotion of carbolic acid.   As regards the constitutional remedies I would recommend the most reliance to be placed on full doses of quinine and steel with some mineral acid (F. 380), or on steel and chlorate of potash (F. 402), or on the sulphite of soda or magnesia (F. 48). At the same time it will be necessary to allow alcoholic stimulants, milk or cream, raw eggs, and essence of beef (F. 2, 3), &c.   The patient's bed must be placed where there is a free current of fresh air, regardless of the nurse's fear that he will catch cold.

VII.   HÆMORRHAGE.

1. INTRODUCTION.—The escape of blood from the vessels in which it is naturally contained constitutes hæmorrhage [Hæmorrhagia, from Αἷμα = blood + ῥήγνυμι = to break out].   There is extravasation of all the component parts of the blood, not merely an exudation of one or more of its constituents impregnated by the colouring matter—hæmatin.   For several years it has been maintained that blood may exude (as sweat does from the skin) through the unbroken surfaces of organs, without any rupture in the coats of arteries, capillaries, or veins; and in this way most of the cases of hæmorrhage which come under the notice of the physician have been accounted for.   Dr. Todd first taught me to doubt the occurrence of hæmorrhage by *exhalation*; for he argued, that if the blood corpuscles (which measure about $\frac{1}{3000}$ of an inch in diameter) could pass through pores in the capillaries, such openings must be large enough to be detected by the microscope.   More recently, Virchow has insisted upon the fact of the vascular system being everywhere closed by membranes, in which it is not possible to discern any porosity; and hence he asserts, that although we cannot, in every individual case, point out the exact site of the rupture, yet it is quite inconceivable that the blood with its corpuscles should be able to pass through the vessel's walls in any other way than through a hole in them.   And yet, in spite of all this, it seems highly probable from the microscopical observations of Dr. Cöhnheim that we are wrong.   By placing frogs under the influence of woorali poison, and then tying the femoral vein, this gentleman has been able to trace the phenomena of capillary congestion and ecchymosis in the transparent web of the frog's foot. In this way he has seen, as others have done by adopting his proceedings, the red blood corpuscles making their way through the apparently unbroken walls of the capillaries into the adjoining tissues.   Dr. Charlton Bastian, who gave an account of Cöhnheim's observations to the members of the Pathological Society in April 1868, describes the process as one of adherence of the corpuscles

to the capillary wall; this being succeeded by the protrusion of a minute tag of the corpuscle through the wall, and this again by a larger and larger portion until the whole has escaped. In the year 1846, Dr. Augustus Waller in describing the appearances presented on a microscopic examination of the tongue of the living frog, notices the passage of the corpuscles through the coats of the vessels. He, however, seems to have taken it for granted that there was a rupture. His words are,—" I consider therefore as established,—1st, the passage of these corpuscles de toute pièce through the capillaries; 2ndly, the restorative power in the blood, which immediately closes the aperture thus formed."*

Many *classifications* of hæmorrhage have been attempted. The chief subdivisions made by authors in the present day are these:— (1) *Traumatic* when a vessel has been directly divided, and *spontaneous* when the bleeding has resulted from some constitutional cause. (2) *Symptomatic* when clearly a result of some disease, as tubercle, cancer, &c., *idiopathic* or *essential,* when no such connexion has been perceptible. Or, (3) *active* hæmorrhage when congestion or inflammation has preceded the flow, and *passive* where there have previously existed signs of debility, with poverty of blood. Moreover, hæmorrhages have been termed *constitutional* where they occur at intervals, and seem to be of service to the general health, as in the bleeding from piles in plethoric people: they are often called *vicarious* when supplemental of some other hæmorrhage, as where a woman has a periodical bleeding from the nose in place of the usual catamenial discharge: and they are sometimes spoken of as *critical* when the flow of blood occurs during the progress of some disease, producing marked good or bad effects.

The *causes* of hæmorrhage are heat, violent mental emotions, muscular exertion, the use of stimulants, and exposure to various irritants. A predisposition to it appears sometimes as if it were hereditary, and then there is said to be the hæmorrhagic diathesis. Mechanical obstacles to the circulation are powerful causes of blood extravasation. This is a fact which is exemplified in the case of valvular disease of the heart; in hypertrophy of the left ventricle of the heart, with some impediment to the passage of blood through distant capillaries; as well as in those affections of the liver which —by obstructing the flow of blood through the inferior vena cava and the vena portæ—produce congestion of the whole portal system, and as a consequence hæmorrhage into the stomach or bowels. Morbid states of the blood—as, on the one hand plethora, on the other anæmia—are also favourable to hæmorrhage. Degeneration of the tissues forming the coats of vessels is a frequent cause. And lastly, diseases of certain organs—as of the kidneys and liver and spleen—also tend to produce the hæmorrhagic tem-

* *The London, Edinburgh, and Dublin Philosophical Magazine and Journal of Science.* Vol. xxix. p. 287. London, July to December 1846.

perament, by exercising some deleterious influence upon the composition of the blood.

The *seat* of the hæmorrhage, speaking with a permissible degree of latitude, may be said to vary with the patient's age. Thus, bleeding from the nose is most common in youth; from the lungs and bronchial tubes, the stomach, the urinary passages, and the uterus in adults; and from the cerebral vessels and rectum in advanced life—between the age of sixty and seventy.

The *symptoms* necessarily depend upon the cause and seat and extent of the loss, as well as upon the condition of the patient. Where signs of plethora have previously existed, with headache, heat of skin, and a full bounding pulse, a moderate hæmorrhage may prove at the time beneficial; whereas, in cases of asthenia, every ounce of blood that comes away serves but to increase the vital depression. The effects which should raise the practitioner's fears are,—depression with rapidity of the pulse, pallor of the face, deep sighing, and loss of vision; coldness of the extremities; syncope on attempting to sit up; great restlessness; and wandering or delirium. Sometimes there is no loss of consciousness, even though the powers of life are almost exhausted; and then amongst the many unmistakeable symptoms of approaching death, I know of none more alarming than the patient's feeble expression of perfect ease and contentment, and his desire to be let alone.

Concerning the *hæmorrhagic diathesis* (in which there is probably a watery condition of the blood, a deficiency of fibrin, and a delicate condition of the coats of the vessels but particularly of the capillaries) it will be sufficient to say that it is equally manifested in male and female children; though during adult life men seem to suffer from it more frequently than women. This habitude may be hereditary; or it can be induced by insufficient food, with residence in a close and damp situation. From time to time I meet with or read of cases where this state appears to me to be connected with an unnatural condition of the spleen,—seen either in the form of disease, or of some congenital malformation or malposition. The diathesis is indicated by the existence of a tendency to ecchymoses from slight pressure, to dropsy, to painful swellings around the joints, &c.; as well as by the occurrence of spontaneous hæmorrhage from the umbilicus a few days after birth, from the nose or gums in youth, and from the urinary passages or rectum in after years. At all ages too, there is a fear lest death should happen from the failure to check bleeding after the infliction of the most trifling wound; as from a leechbite, biting the tongue, the extraction of a tooth, a laceration from a fall, or even rupture of the hymen.

The *prognosis* is unfavourable in cases of hæmorrhage where the blood escapes into a serous cavity, or into the substance of an organ, or when there is the hæmorrhagic diathesis. In other instances it is generally favourable, death very rarely resulting. The obstetric physician especially, cannot but frequently feel surprised at the large quantity of blood which is lost without the patient succumbing.

With regard to the general principles of *treatment* it must be first noticed, that as a rule it is desirable to suppress the hæmorrhage. Some authorities affirm that there is danger in stopping a discharge which may almost be called habitual; but I have seen nothing to lead me to acquiesce in this opinion. On the contrary, I regard it as a fallacy. In the course of years, many elderly people have come under my notice who have been injured, and greatly inconvenienced, by the frequent bleeding arising from piles. Of course, however, when such cases are interfered with, it is necessary to guard against congestions of internal organs; which may be best done by attention to the diet, and by taking care that the bowels act regularly. The few exceptional instances where attempts to arrest a bleeding would be hazardous, are found in plethoric people, who seem occasionally to be relieved from a threatened fit of apoplexy by a timely attack of epistaxis. With so-called vicarious hæmorrhages the attempt is to be made to procure the flow from the natural seat.

In endeavouring to control any form of hæmorrhage we ought to keep the patient as quiet, mentally and bodily, as possible. His apartment should be cool; he must rest on a mattress without much covering; his diet ought to be simple but nutritious, cold or even iced drinks being freely allowed; while the position of his body is to be such, that the afflux of blood to the bleeding organ will be impeded.

Our chief resources are then to be found in the use of astringents. One of the best of these agents is *cold;* and therefore ice is to be applied locally, while it can also be freely swallowed. A valuable and most efficient drug, is *gallic acid;* given in doses of ten to twenty grains every two or four or six hours. The efficacy of this astringent is often increased by combining it with fifteen or twenty minims of the *aromatic sulphuric acid.* The *ammonio-sulphate of iron* (ammonia iron-alum) is an excellent styptic, from which I have seen the best effects in hæmoptysis; while in all cases I think it is more to be relied on than the tincture of perchloride of iron to prevent any return of the bleeding. The *mineral acids* quicken coagulation, and hence either of them (especially the sulphuric) may often be used with advantage. *Alum* and *sulphuric acid* have answered well in several instances. *Ipecacuanha* appears sometimes to exercise a favourable influence on internal hæmorrhages, but it must generally be given in doses of one grain every thirty or sixty minutes until a feeling of nausea is produced. In cases of hæmorrhage from the lungs or stomach, the act of vomiting would probably do harm; though I have often seen it work marked good in flooding after labour. The *acetate of lead* was long recommended as an efficacious styptic, but I now never use it until after gallic acid has had a fair trial. This latter failing, acetate of lead in five grain doses, administered at short intervals with a draught of vinegar and water, has appeared useful (F. 117). I have no faith whatever in this salt when given in the ordinary small doses. *Ergot of rye* is particularly indicated in many forms of uterine hæmorrhage; whether this occur in the form of flooding after labour, or in consequence of the presence of some foreign body within the cavity of the womb. The officinal liquid extract of ergot, in doses of twenty or thirty minims, frequently repeated, can usually be trusted to. Although a decided opponent to the use of secret remedies, yet it must be allowed that *Ruspini's styptic* now and then succeeds where other remedies fail. The *oil of turpentine* has also been esteemed a good astringent, especially in bleeding from the lungs, stomach, or kidneys. Ten or twenty minims may be given in mucilage every two or three hours; while sometimes it can be beneficially used in the form of inhalation, or as a stupe (a hot and moist flannel sprinkled with the oil) to the walls of the chest or abdomen.

For obstinate cases *mercury* (Hg) is a very valuable remedy. At one time I thought the beneficial effects were not induced until salivation was effected; but further experience has led me to believe this to be an error. The officinal *liquor hydrargyri perchloridi* may be given in doses of one to two fluid drachms (gr. $\frac{1}{16}$ to gr. $\frac{1}{8}$) every three or four hours, until a good effect ensues. This metal (Hg Cl$_2$) is contra-indicated where there is any predisposition to pulmonary or renal disease.

When the hæmorrhage has been excessive and has produced dangerous exhaustion, *opium* proves invaluable. It not only acts as a stimulant to the heart's action; but—as suggested by Dr. W. Griffin—it probably sustains, in those who seem to be dying from loss of nervous power in the brain consequent upon the insufficient supply of blood, that natural tension of the cerebral vessels which is required. As a general rule, I prefer the extract of this drug in doses varying from one to three grains; while it is better usually to combine it with cordials.

Formerly *bleeding* was resorted to, in order that while the force of the heart's action became lessened, the current of blood might be diverted from the affected structure. When there is organic disease, venesection is usually most objectionable; while in no case does it possess such advantage over other remedies as to lead to its recommendation.—If there be constipation, purgatives of *sulphate of soda*, or of *sulphate of magnesia and sulphuric acid*, or of castor oil, should be administered.

Lastly, it must be remembered that in very severe cases—particularly such as occur in obstetric practice—when other means fail, and there is loss of consciousness with inability to swallow stimulants, we can still resort to *transfusion*. This operation is probably of considerable antiquity. According to Sismondi, phy-

sicians in 1482 were persuaded that the blood was the seat of life;
so that they believed that if the vital fluid of a child could be put
into the veins of an old man, the latter would be rendered young
again. On this principle, the charlatan Cottier made Louis the
Eleventh bathe in children's blood, while it is related that he even
caused the king to drink of it.   Sismondi at the same time remarks,
that several children were the victims of an attempt to pass their
blood into the veins of Innocent the Eighth.*   Villari, also,
speaking of the state of profound exhaustion and somnolency into
which Innocent the Eighth had fallen, notices that a Jew doctor
proposed to restore the exhausted vitality by the transfusion of the
blood of a young person; " an experiment that hitherto had only
been made on animals.   Accordingly, the blood of the decrepid old
pontiff was passed into the veins of a youth, whose blood was
transferred into those of the old man.   The experiment was tried
three times, and at the cost of the lives of three boys, probably
from air getting into their veins, but without any effect to save
that of the Pope.   He expired on the 25th April 1492."†   As to
the precise truth of these statements nothing is known.   But if
they are correct, it certainly seems clear that the practice of the
Jew doctor did not spread.   Hence, when the operation was revived
about the middle of the seventeenth century, it was regarded with
enthusiasm as the grand discovery of the time.   The Germans have
asserted that one of their countrymen, Libavius, suggested the
idea in 1606.   The French have claimed it for the anatomist Denis,
who is said to have tried it upon man in 1666 or 1667.   While in
this country it is popularly believed that the credit of proposing it
is due to Dr. Richard Lower; who performed transfusion on animals at Oxford, in 1665. One point is irrefutable, that on the 23rd
November 1667, several ounces of the blood of a young sheep
were transfused into the veins of Arthur Coga, by Dr. Richard
Lower and Edmund King; the operation being performed at
Arundel House, in the presence of the Fellows of the Royal Society, and with such advantage that the man wished it repeated
three or four days afterwards.‡ The benefit, unhappily, was not of
long duration.   Extravagant expectations soon led to the operation
being abused.   In France such disastrous results ensued that in a
short time its practice was forbidden by law, save with the approba-
tion of the physicians of the Paris faculty. And then, as it was found
that disease could not be cured nor youth renewed by injecting the
blood of the young into the bodies of the aged, the operation was
set aside. Thus it remained in abeyance for more than a century,

    * *Histoire des Francais.* Par J. C. L. Simonde de Sismondi.   Tome
neuvième, p. 221.   La Haye, 1837.
    † *The History of Girolamo Savonarola and of his Times.* By Pasquale
Villari. Translated from the Italian by Leonard Horner, F.R.S.   Vol. i.
p. 144.   London, 1863.
    ‡ *The Philosophical Transactions of the Royal Society of London, from
their commencement in 1665 to the year 1800.* Abridged, with notes, &c.,
vol. i. p. 203.   London, 1809.

until again brought forward by Blundell in 1818. As to the best mode of performing transfusion but little need be said. Fresh human blood is always employed now; though authorities vary in opinion as to whether it should be defibrinated or not. The advantages of removing the fibrin are chiefly that the danger of injecting clots is avoided, while blood so treated is said to be more highly charged with oxygen than that taken pure from the veins. In either case, the syringe employed is to be completely filled, so as to exclude even a bubble of air. Then, its nozzle being introduced into either of the patient's veins at the bend of the arm, the operator must take care to proceed very slowly; for one of the great dangers of transfusion consists in forcing in the blood too rapidly. With regard to the quantity of blood to be employed, it may be remembered that the operation should be stopped when the patient has rallied; which will generally occur when from three to twelve ounces have been injected.

2. **CEREBRAL HÆMORRHAGE.**—Until recently the terms cerebral hæmorrhage and apoplexy have been generally employed synonymously. It is, however, highly necessary to draw a distinction between the two. For, inasmuch as apoplexy in the proper signification of the word, may occur quite independently of any extravasation of blood within the cranium, so the latter frequently takes place without giving rise to apoplectiform phenomena. When the hæmorrhage proves to be considerable, the victim is indeed struck down suddenly,—he has a fit of apoplexy. It sometimes happens for example, that the effusion is very abundant; the blood first poured out into one of the corpora striata or one of the optic thalami, passing into the lateral ventricle of the same side, filling it, and then breaking down the septum lucidum so as to flow into the opposite lateral ventricle. In such a case, the profound coma that sets in can only terminate in death at the end of an uncertain number of hours. But where clots of a more moderate size are formed in the nervous tissue, there may be no impairment whatever of the senses. The symptoms are then limited to paralysis of the side of the body opposite to that hemisphere which is the seat of mischief.

In cerebral hæmorrhage the blood will be effused externally on the surface of the brain, or internally within the nervous tissue itself. With the first variety—sometimes spoken of as meningeal hæmorrhage—the blood is found either between the bones of the skull and the dura mater, or in the sac of the arachnoid, or in the meshes of the pia mater. The most common cause of external hæmorrhage is mechanical injury—such as blows, falls &c. Spontaneous rupture of the coats of a vessel in one of the membranes, especially where there has been any aneurismal dilatation, may happen, however. In the cerebral hæmorrhage which sometimes occurs during childhood, the blood is generally poured into the cavity of the arachnoid. The symptoms produced by meningeal hæmorrhage vary according to the extent of the loss. Speaking generally, it rarely gives rise to paralysis; owing perhaps to the pressure acting uniformly upon the contents of the cranium. When only a small quantity of blood is effused, absorption may speedily take place and recovery ensue.

Hæmorrhage into the substance of the brain is uncommon in the young. Yet it occurs now and then in youth, and even during childhood, where there is chronic renal disease; more especially if there be likewise some hypertrophy of the left ventricle of the heart. Aneurisms of the cerebral vessels are also met with at all periods between youth and advanced life—between the ages of 14 and 65, these being the extremes in some sixty reported cases of which I have taken note. The amount of blood extravasated in cases of cerebral hæmorrhage varies from a drop or two, producing clots scarcely larger than one or more pin's heads, to several ounces. Although all portions of the brain may be the seat of the effusion, still the more vascular the part the greater must be the liability to hæmorrhage. Consequently, the corpora striata and optic thalami—the superior ganglia of the cerebrum—show the greatest proclivity to this accident, while the corpus callosum and fornix are the least liable to it. The effects produced vary greatly according to the site of the extravasation; the extent to which the nerve-fibres are separated, or bruised, or torn; and the quantity of blood lost. Thus, there may be only temporary mental confusion; or insensibility, passing off after eighteen, twenty-four, or more hours; or hemiplegia, temporary or permanent; or profound coma—preceded or not by convulsions—ending fatally in a few hours.

Récamier, Trousseau, Todd and others have taught, that when complete and absolute hemiplegia occurs suddenly, without loss of consciousness, softening of the brain ought to be diagnosed. Whenever, on the contrary, the complete loss of motor power is attended by deprivation of consciousness—whenever, especially, coma has set in suddenly, then the occurrence of hæmorrhage to a considerable amount should be suspected. Furthermore, where there is perfect loss of motor power, with merely dulness of intellect without actual insensibility, hæmorrhage in connexion with softening will probably be found to be the cause. As already mentioned, the paralysis in hemiplegia is on the opposite side of the body to the hemisphere of the brain which is affected. Blood is rarely poured out into both sides of the brain at the same time; though a large clot sometimes extends into one lateral ventricle, and gradually increases until it breaks into the opposite one. Then again, it is not uncommon after death to find a clot cavity, or cyst, or cicatrix, in each division of the brain; but in such there is almost always evidence to show that the appearances of mischief on one side are more recent than those on the other. Supposing only a small clot to be formed, it can ultimately become absorbed, merely leaving a cicatrix. The extent of motor tract which has been injured being also small, the paralysed limbs will recover. Where this favourable result ensues, it almost always happens that the leg regains its power sooner than the arm; while what is equally inexplicable and even more remarkable, when the arm recovers first, such an event is said to be an unfavourable omen. Certainly, in a few reported cases where the patient has been able to use the arm before regaining the capability of walking, the arm has again lost all motor power at the end of a few months, severe pains have attacked the leg, and death has been preceded by complete imbecility. The pons Varolii being a part absolutely essential to life, since in it the most important nerve fibres converge—transverse fibres between the two hemispheres of the cerebellum and connecting this with the cerebrum, as well as longitudinal fibres linking the medulla oblongata with the cerebrum—so when blood is effused into this structure there rapidly ensues deep apoplectic stupor, paralysis of both sides of the body, and death at the end of a few hours. And then, lastly, hæmorrhage into the cerebellum may take place alone, or combined with effusion into the cerebrum. Either form of extravasation in this organ is far from being common; but when it occurs it very quickly causes death.

On searching for the immediate *cause* of cerebral hæmorrhage, attention must be paid to the composition of the blood, the state of the heart and kidneys and coats of the bloodvessels, and the condition of the tissues of the body generally. With regard to the first, our knowledge is imperfect; but, according to Andral and Gavarret, there is an essential connexion between cerebral hæmorrhages and a diminution of the fibrin of the blood with an increase of the red globules. Rupture of a vessel not unfrequently occurs as a sequel of renal or cardiac disease; when it is probably due in part to an altered condition of the blood, though we know that in Bright's disease the coats of the arteries are also often the seat of some degeneration. Thin or poor blood may be the only cause; in confirmation of which view it may be remarked that a fatal fit occurred in a patient under my care, who for many months had suffered from almost uncontrollable uterine hæmorrhage, due to a fibrous tumour. Mr. Travers met with a case where the attack of hæmorrhage happened while the patient was being bled for pneumonia; and numerous examples are on record of the occurrence of apoplectic stupor at the very time that bleeding was being practised for the relief of hemiplegia. There are many circumstances which render it probable that, in the majority of cases, disease of the coats of the vessels is the cause of the effusion; more especially if, combined with such disease, there be hypertrophy of the left ventricle of the heart, forcing the blood with greater power than the coats of the vessels can stand. Of course the chances of rupture are much increased if the morbid action in the coats of the vessels has gone so far as to give rise to aneurism.   Chronic arteritis by producing pulpy softening, or calcareous or atheromatous deposits (calcification and fatty degeneration), may render the vessels unable to bear the force of the blood-current.   When the nutrition of the nerve tissue becomes diminished, softening ensues ; and the same result sometimes follows from acute inflammation.   The way in which the cerebral arteries get occasionally plugged by a portion of fibrin (an embolus) has been already described.

As regards the *treatment* of cerebral hæmorrhage I have but little to say.   The patient is to be kept quiet : the sitting posture is more favourable than the horizontal.   Nourishing food is to be allowed in such quantities as can be digested.   Attention should be paid to the intestinal and renal excretions to this extent, —that if the bowels are confined, an aperient had better be given ; while where there is retention of urine, a catheter must be employed.   No benefit whatever, but on the contrary great mischief, is likely to arise from bleeding, strong purgatives, emetics, and deprivation of nourishment.

At about the end of twenty-four or thirty-six hours from the commencement of cerebral hæmorrhage there frequently·sets in a certain amount of febrile action.   The face becomes flushed, the skin hot, the respiration somewhat hurried, and the pulse frequent —perhaps hard or wiry.   In such cases, simple remedies are still the best.   A few doses of the solution of citrate of ammonia can be given, if medicine be thought desirable ; but a free allowance of soda or potash water, iced water, tea with milk, &c., will prove quite as serviceable.

3. OTORRHAGIA.—Hæmorrhage from the ears [*otorrhagia,* from Οὖς = the ear + ῥήγνυμι = to burst out] arises from several different causes.   The chief are the following :—1. *Fracture of the base of the skull,* by which a communication is established between the sinuses of the dura mater and the middle ear.   The membrana tympani being ruptured, the blood escapes externally.   If both petrous bones be injured, there will be hæmorrhage from both ears. The occurrence of bleeding, on one or both sides, is generally regarded as a symptom of very unfavourable import.   2. *Wounds and ulcerations of the auditory canal ;* whether produced by earpicks or other instruments, insects, foreign bodies voluntarily introduced, or old hardened ceruminous concretions.   3. *Granulations, polypi, and abscesses of the auditory canal.*   The proper use of the ear speculum will show which of these conditions is actually present. 4. *Caries and necrosis of the petrous portion of the temporal bone, with destruction of the membrana tympani.*   If the walls of the carotid canal be involved a spiculum of bone may wound the internal carotid artery, and cause fatal loss of blood.   5. *Rupture of the membrana tympani ;* which can occur during the ascent of high mountains, or in the descent of low valleys, or in going to any

great depth in a diving-bell, &c.; during violent sneezing or vomiting; or during a paroxysm of hooping cough or asthma. In these
cases the air is violently forced through the Eustachian tube into
the tympanum, the delicate membrane of which gives way
where it is least capable of offering resistance—near the insertion
of the handle of the malleus. And 6, otorrhagia will perhaps be *a
vicarious hæmorrhage*;—i.e., it is said that this form of hæmorrhage
may replace the catamenia, or a long continued bleeding from
piles or old ulcers, though as far as my own experience goes I have
never known of such an occurrence.

4. **EPISTAXIS.**—Probably every one remembers the frequency
with which, in his school-days, he suffered from a " bloody nose,"
and the famous plans by which old ladies were wont to cure it.
Unless this bleeding comes on during the progress of some disease
—as hooping cough, continued fever, anæmia, &c. it is seldom at
all troublesome in youth.

But epistaxis ['Επιστάζω = to drop upon] should generally give
rise to much anxiety when it occurs in advanced life. If there be
a tendency to apoplexy, or if the patient be afflicted with heart-
disease, the bleeding is not unlikely to prove beneficial for a time.
Even then it is an occurrence of serious import; for it may indicate disease in the coats of the bloodvessels at different parts of
the body, and possibly prove to be the first threatening of a more
serious attack of hæmorrhage into some internal organ. Moreover,
no advantage whatever is gained by a bleeding from the nose when
this sets in during the progress of disorders which injure the
quality of the blood; as in renal and hepatic and splenic diseases,
in fever, in scurvy and purpura, &c. Exhausting epistaxis will
sometimes prove the immediate cause of death in cases of leucocythemia, when this affection is approaching a fatal termination.

The bleeding seldom takes place simultaneously from both nostrils. It is either a transitory occurrence, or it is continuous, or it
ceases and returns after an uncertain interval, or it happens periodically. The blood flows in drops, or in a complete stream; while it
not only comes from the nostrils in front, but may pass posteriorly
into the mouth and fauces. As regards adults, males suffer from it
more often than females. It can be caused by direct violence, by
whatever obstructs or greatly quickens the circulation, by morbid
states of the blood, by congestion of neighbouring parts, by the suppression of some habitual discharge, by an ulcer on or through the
septum of the nose, by exfoliation of the bones assisting to form
the walls of the nostrils, as well as by polypus and disease of the
pituitary membrane.

As to the *treatment*, care must be taken to discriminate between
those cases where interference is requisite, and the contrary. Supposing the aid of the practitioner is needed, it will be better to have
the patient sitting upright in a cool apartment, and with the neck

unconfined by collars, &c.   Dr. Négrier says he has always found
the bleeding arrested by making the patient raise one or both of the
arms above his head, and letting him hold them in that position
for some time.   This simple plan failing (for, like all infallible
remedies, it seldom answers), cold applied to the neck and back
may, by reflex action, check the discharge ; or cold water, or ice,
can be applied directly over the nose and forehead.   External
compression of the nostril with the fingers sometimes succeeds,—
usually by favouring the formation·of a clot.   In urgent cases I
have successfully swabbed the nostril with a saturated solution of
perchloride of iron ; and have likewise seen injections of infusion of
matico, or of alum and water, or of the tincture of perchloride of
iron and water, or of the iron-alum in solution, do good.   Plugging the nostril with charpie, or with cotton wool soaked in
some astringent lotion, often stops the flow ; and so does the
passage of a styptic rod made with equal parts of tannin and cacao
butter (F. 424), or the employment of tannin mixed with a little
alum as snuff.   But these expedients proving useless, the posterior orifice of the nostril must be plugged ; a proceeding, however, which is very annoying to the patient.   It is easily accomplished by introducing a gum-elastic catheter, with a piece
of waxed twine passed through its canal so as to project at the
eyelet-hole, along the nostril into the pharynx ; the end of the
ligature being then brought through the mouth by means of a pair
of forceps, and made tight to a piece of sponge.   By removing the
catheter and pulling the nasal end of the twine, the |sponge plug
will be firmly drawn into the posterior nares ; from which position
it should not be removed for forty-eight hours.

With regard to internal remedies, the condition of the patient
must be our guide in selecting either the perchloride of mercury
(F. 27), or gallic acid (F. 103), or ammonia iron-alum (F. 116),
or one of the mineral acids with bark (F. 376), or the tincture
of perchloride of iron (F. 101), or oil of turpentine (F. 102).
Sometimes mild laxatives (F. 142, 143) may be required ; or if
there be any liver derangement, nitric acid and taraxacum (F. 147)
will do good.   The diet is to be nourishing ; consisting of animal
food, with a fair amount of potatoes, watercresses, and ripe succulent fruits.

5. STOMATORRHAGIA.—Discharges of blood from the
mouth and throat [stomatorrhagia, from Στόμα = a mouth + ρήγνυμι
= to break out], seldom give rise to any trouble, except when they
occur during the last stages of scurvy or purpura, or after the
excessive abuse of mercury. In some few instances, the small veins
about the inside of the cheek and pharynx have become varicose ;
and when their walls have ruptured, severe or fatal bleeding has resulted. Ulcers about the tongue and fauces rarely bleed much ; but
once or twice glossitis terminating in gangrene has produced
hæmorrhage which has only ceased with death.

Dr. Condie of Philadelphia has recorded a case where the blood flowed from the mouth in a stream, and on the gums being wiped with a sponge, it "was seen to start up at every pore from the whole surface." Now this would by many be regarded as an example of *hæmorrhage by exhalation ;* just as the occurrence of cutaneous bleeding, where the blood is said to appear like a dew upon the skin, has been explained. Remembering the observations of Cöhnheim, it is necessary to criticise these views very cautiously. Still I cannot but think, that in such instances as have just been mentioned there is probably no hæmorrhage, strictly speaking. The discharge is simply an exudation of serum, which is coloured by the red matters of the dissolved or ruptured blood corpuscles.

It is worthy of note that prisoners, malingerers, hysterical females, and others, often feign hæmoptysis by pricking their gums, sucking out the blood, and mingling it with saliva and phlegm. This imposition will be readily detected on examining the mouth, as well as by noting the absence of all signs of either thoracic or abdominal disease.

The *treatment* of stomatorrhagia has to be conducted on the general principles already laid down. Medicines need not be administered unless the use of a cold astringent wash, or of tannic acid lozenges, or of ice, fails to stop the bleeding.

6. **HÆMOPTYSIS.**—The term hæmoptysis [Aῖμα = blood + πτύω = to spit] is only to be applied to those cases where the blood escapes through the mouth from the larynx, trachea, bronchial tubes, or air-cells of the lungs. Sometimes the blood is poured into the air-sacs of the lungs without any external discharge, and then the disease is generally spoken of as *pulmonary apoplexy.*

In by far the greater number of cases, hæmoptysis is merely symptomatic of tubercular phthisis ; though it may also, and not unfrequently, be due to disease of the heart—especially of the left cavities, impeding the free return of blood from the lungs. Very rarely it arises from some ulceration about the air-passages ; from inflammation, abscess, gangrene, or cancer of the lung ; from the detachment of fibrinous casts of one or more of the small bronchial tubes; and from aneurism of the great vessels, particularly the aorta. Moreover, it is generally believed that this form of hæmorrhage, in women, may be connected with some irregularity or suppression of the catamenia ; though I have seen no cases of the kind, save where there was reason to suspect tuberculosis. When there exists a predisposition to hæmoptysis, it can often be immediately brought about by anything which hurries the circulation, by congestions of various important organs, by violent coughing, playing on wind instruments, ascending high mountains, tight lacing, &c.

The discharge, when proceeding from the lungs, is often preceded by pain or oppression about the chest, a sense of heat and soreness beneath the sternum or between the shoulders, lassitude and mental depression, flushings of the face, a salt taste in the mouth, dry cough, and more or less dyspnœa with palpitations. On other occasions I have noticed that there has been a complete absence of premonitory symptoms, with the exception of an infrequent and perhaps labouring pulse. The quantity of blood which will be expelled varies from a streak on a pellet of mucus, or a minute clot or two, to one or many pints. As it comes up, if in any appreciable quantity, it is generally frothy and of a bright florid hue. It is usually expectorated with a variable amount of coughing; though when the bleeding is excessive, the blood is often gulped up or vomited. Occasionally, the diagnosis can be aided by shaking out the clots in water; when they will perhaps be found distinctly branched, and forming casts of the bronchial tubes. Hæmoptysis occurs in about two-thirds of all the cases of phthisis, and it does so under two circumstances. Thus, it may happen from the active congestion of the first stage of tubercular deposit causing rupture of one or more small vessels, when it is to be regarded more as a warning of coming mischief, rather than as a proof of the lung being irremediably injured : or it can take place when the tubercles have begun to soften, and the coats of some vessel have been destroyed by the spreading of the ulceration. The hæmorrhage very rarely destroys the patient at once; though in the cases which I have watched, it has frequently seemed to hasten the fatal termination of phthisis.

Half a dozen exceptional cases of tubercular phthisis are known, where the hæmorrhage has had its origin in a rupture of an aneurism of one of the branches of the pulmonary artery. Sometimes, the aneurismal tumour has been developed, as it were, in a tubercular cavity; the sac of the aneurism probably filling the vomica completely prior to rupture. In other instances, a varicose dilatation of the vessel has been found, perhaps extending for a couple of inches. On rupture of these aneurisms death may of course happen immediately; but in the cases which have been reported there have usually been occasional attacks of severe hæmorrhage for a few weeks before the patient has succumbed from exhaustion.

In dilatation of the bronchi, without any coexisting tubercular disease, small quantities of blood are often expectorated with the sputa. But every now and then it happens, in these cases, that the hæmorrhage is abundant; and I believe a few instances have happened where such hæmoptysis has proved fatal.

Many examples of aortic aneurism have been reported where there has been rust-coloured expectoration; or where the sputa have been tinged with bright blood; or where there have been one or more gushes of blood, for weeks or even months before the disease has proved fatal by complete rupture, or by inducing laryngeal suffocation from pressure of the sac on one or both recurrent nerves. In the well-known case of Mr. Liston, hæmoptysis to the extent of several ounces occurred in July 1847; after which

there was a freedom from almost all symptoms until October,
when cough set in with rusty sputa. Death took place in
the December of the same year. At the autopsy, there were found
three or four perforations of the trachea, communicating with
the sac of the aneurism ; the openings having become blocked up
with portions of the clot.

In *pulmonary apoplexy* (an absurd name, for there is no sudden
stroke, no loss of sensation or power of motion) the blood is
effused into the air-cells, and occasionally into the smaller bronchial tubes, where it coagulates. There are two forms of this
affection,—one where the effusion is *circumscribed,* and we find
small and hard masses in the substance of the lungs, varying in
size from a pea to a small orange; the other, in which the blood
is *diffused* through the broken-down pulmonary tissues. Extravasation of blood into the air-cells of the lungs most frequently arises
from disease of the heart, particularly of the mitral orifice ; but it
may possibly be due to some affection of the pulmonary tissue or
vessels, or to such an impoverished state of the blood as occurs in
scurvy, fever, &c. Whether the blood come from ruptured bronchial arteries, or from the plexuses formed by the pulmonary capillaries on the septa of the air-cells, is undecided : most probably it
is sometimes from one source, sometimes from the other. Occasionally the internal bleeding is attended with spitting of blood.
If only a small quantity be extravasated, the patient recovers ; but
if the loss be excessive, symptoms of internal hæmorrhage with
great dyspnœa will manifest themselves, and most probably end
fatally. Auscultation often tells us nothing in these cases.
Nevertheless, if we can fortunately listen before the blood coagulates, we perhaps shall find large crepitation from the air-bubbles
passing through the fluid and bursting ; while subsequently there
will be dulness on percussion, with absence of all respiratory
murmur in the affected portion.

A few special remarks are called for on the *treatment* of hæmoptysis. The hæmorrhage should always be checked as quickly
as possible ; and for this purpose, after enjoining strict quiet and
rest in bed with the head and shoulders elevated, I have found no
remedy so efficacious as gallic acid. This agent should be given
in the proportion of ten or fifteen grains, every two or three or four
hours, according to the urgency of the symptoms ; sometimes
commencing with thirty grains for a dose in five or six ounces of
water, with half a drachm of the aromatic sulphuric acid. When
there are indications of great anæmia, from five to ten grains of the
ammonio-sulphate of iron (F. 116) may be preferable to the gallic
acid. Sucking small pieces of ice does great good ; and occasionally the application of cold over the chest is useful, though
the effect of this practice must be watched. In one instance,
where frightful quantities of blood were being brought up, the violence of the discharge could only be checked by pouring cans of

cold water over the chest. Certain authorities state that a tea-spoonful of common salt dissolved in a little water, or taken dry and swallowed as best the patient can, seldom fails to stop the bleeding for a time; others advise bleeding, leeching, antimony, or digitalis; some prefer the ergot of rye, or turpentine, or emetics of ipecacuanha; many, again, recommend dry cupping over the chest, or the application of turpentine stupes; while a few speak highly of the use of a ligature round the limbs, so as to impede the return of blood through the veins.

The patient is not to be reduced by low diet. Strong essence of beef, milk or cream, cold tea, and raw eggs are to be allowed; while there is not the least objection to solid animal food &c. if there be any desire or appetite for it. And although many cases will do well without stimulants, yet there are others where alcohol in some form or other is really needed. Good claret, or carlowitz, or ofner, or tokay, or port wine, in proper quantities, at proper intervals, will often prove useful. For it must be recollected that not only is it necessary to stop the hæmorrhage, but our remedies have to be so ordered as not to encourage the extension of the disease which has set it going.

To prevent the recurrence of the bleeding in diseases of the air-passages or lungs, I have some confidence in the inhalation of atomised astringent fluids. Tannic acid (F. 262) has especially seemed serviceable when thus employed. It will also be necessary to relieve any cough which may be present by anodynes—especially by morphia (F. 346, 347). Meanwhile, every endeavour ought to be made to improve the general health. If change of air be thought advisable, care should be taken to select a fitting locality. To send an individual just recovering from hæmoptysis, perhaps due to a slight deposit of tubercle, to a mild relaxing watering place, is simply to invite the hæmorrhage to return. A dry and bracing climate, or a long sea voyage in a large and well appointed ship, may prove very serviceable; whereas a residence in a warm and humid atmosphere can only be productive of most mischievous results.

7. **HÆMATEMESIS.**—This term, signifying strictly vomiting of blood [Αἷμα = blood + ἐρέω = to vomit], is generally employed to denote hæmorrhage from the stomach. The blood is usually vomited in large quantities, is not frothy, is sometimes mixed with food, and is often of a dark colour from admixture with the hydrochloric acid of the gastric juice (all acids blacken the blood). Hence it presents marked differences from the blood in hæmoptysis; which is brought up by coughing in mouthfuls at a time, is of a florid red colour, is frothy, and is frequently mixed with sputa. Moreover, in hæmoptysis the hæmorrhage is generally preceded by cough, dyspnœa with palpitation, tickling in the throat, and a peculiar sensation in the thorax.

To make the distinction more clear, the chief signs of each variety may be thus tabulated :—

In *hæmoptysis* :—
  Dyspnœa; pain or heat in chest.
  Blood coughed up in mouthfuls.
  Blood frothy.
  Blood of a florid red colour.
  Blood mingled with sputa.
  Absence of melæna.
  Bronchial or pulmonary symptoms.

In *hæmatemesis* :—
  Nausea; epigastric tension.
  Blood vomited profusely.
  Blood not frothy.
  Blood dark coloured.
  Blood mixed with food.
  Melæna very common.
  Gastric or duodenal symptoms.

Hæmatemesis occurs every now and then without any appreciable cause ; or perhaps it happens to be vicarious of some other hæmorrhage, especially of the catamenia ; or it results from changes in the blood itself, as in scurvy ; or it arises from aneurism of one of the abdominal vessels, the sac communicating with the bowels ;* or it may be owing to congestion of the stomach from some impediment to the free passage of the blood, such impediment being due to disease of the heart, liver, &c. Thrombosis of the portal vein (arising either from disease of the coats of the vessel, or from obstruction of its canal by the compression of cancer or cirrhosis or abscess) has on more than one occasion proved to be the cause of fatal hæmatemesis. But the most direct provocative of this form of hæmorrhage is either passive congestion of the walls of the stomach, or simple or malignant ulceration. In simple ulceration, the blood most frequently comes away slowly, in small quantities, and often after a meal; though sometimes a large vessel is laid open, and a gush of blood takes place which possibly proves fatal. So also in the ulceration of a cancerous mass the bleeding is usually slight. When from any causes the extravasation is moderate, the vomited matters are said to resemble " coffee-grounds."

Hæmatemesis is more common in women than in men. It is generally preceded by a feeling of oppression and weight, by dull pain or tenderness, in the epigastric and hypochondriac regions ; as well as by a sense of anxiety and faintness. Often there is only nausea, dizziness, and lowering of the pulse in frequency and

* Dr. Gairdner has recorded (*Clinical Medicine*, p. 495. Edinburgh, 1862) an instructive example of aneurism of the superior mesenteric artery ; which opened in the duodenum twenty-two months before death, causing repeated and very copious hæmatemesis. The symptoms and history closely resembled those of gastric ulcer. And there was this remarkable circumstance, that between the patient's admission (she was a servant girl, sixteen years old) into the Edinburgh Royal Infirmary on the 4 January 1848 and her death on 28 November 1849, complete convalescence took place. This was somewhat interrupted by an ulcer on the leg, amenorrhœa, and dyspepsia; but the hæmatemesis did not recur after the 7 February 1848. On the day of her death she fell down suddenly in the street with an attack of syncope. At the autopsy it was found that the aneurism had burst into the peritoneum, in the cavity of which more than 3 lbs. of blood had been extravasated. The duodenal opening was closed.

force. The hæmorrhage commonly produces great depression; owing partly to that alarm which is always engendered by "spitting of blood," and partly to the quantity of blood lost.

In gastric hæmorrhage, the blood frequently passes into the intestines, and is voided per anum; or part will be vomited and part expelled with the fæces. When the intestinal evacuations contain blood, whether this comes from the vessels of the stomach or only from those of the intestines, the patient is said to be suffering from *melæna* [Μέλας = black]. As this name implies, the evacuations are often black, and sometimes resemble tar; but the dark appearance is by no means constant, and does not occur if the blood comes away too quickly to be acted upon by the intestinal juices. Cirrhosis of the liver, or any disease which produces obstruction of the portal system, necessarily gives rise to congestion of the gastric and intestinal veins; a condition which often terminates in the extravasation of large quantities of blood that are expelled with the stools. Amongst the other less common causes of melæna may be mentioned enteritis, dysentery, intussusception, simple and carcinomatous ulcerations, aneurismal and other tumours, &c. It must not be confounded with bleeding from the rectum, owing to the presence of a polypus or of hæmorrhoids.

The *treatment* of acute hæmatemesis should consist in enjoining abstinence from solid food, with perfect rest in the horizontal posture; while cold acidulous drinks, ice, strong essence of beef, and perhaps some astringent Hungarian or Greek or Bordeaux wine may also be prescribed. If the patient be prostrated, enemata of beef tea with port wine or brandy and a little opium will do much good. With respect to drugs, a mixture of gallic acid with the aromatic sulphuric acid (F. 103) will often answer well. The oil of turpentine is thought by some to be a specific (F. 102). In one case, a single dose of a concentrated solution of the perchloride of iron (one teaspoonful in glycerine) effected a cure. Prolonged application of cold to the epigastrium is occasionally useful.

Where the bleeding is chronic, or when it is continuous but slight in amount, the mineral acids with bark (F. 376) will often do more real service than any other remedies. Quinine and iron, however, prove very valuable in some instances (F. 380). Cream, raw eggs, essence of beef, various broths, and perhaps cod liver oil, ought also to be allowed. As regards cases of melæna, where there is no gastric disease, active purging will be necessary; and hence a full dose of calomel and jalap or of podophyllin (F. 140, 160) should be given, followed by the common black draught or castor oil. Subsequently the mineral acids with bitters (F. 378) may be tried.

8. **HÆMATURIA.**—Hæmaturia [from Αἷμα = blood + οὖρον = urine], or hæmorrhage from the mucous membrane of the urinary passages, may proceed from the kidneys or bladder or urethra. It is common in the early stages of those forms of renal disease

which have their origin in a morbid state of the blood : hence, as we shall see by and by, it is a frequent result of acute desquamative nephritis.   It may also arise from malignant disease of the kidney or bladder ; from the presence of a calculus either in the kidney, ureter, bladder, or urethra ; from cystitis ; or from renal inflammation, as well as from granular degeneration. A blow over the loins has caused it ; while irritating medicines, such as oil of turpentine and cantharides, can also produce it.   Occasionally it sets in during the course of rheumatic fever, pneumonia, continued fever, malignant small-pox, scurvy, &c., just as epistaxis does. Having more than once seen urine contaminated with the menstrual discharge mistaken for real hæmaturia, it will hardly be deemed superfluous to give a word of caution.   As a rule, therefore, in any case of suspected renal disease occurring in woman, the practitioner should not venture on stating a positive opinion while the patient has her courses on.

Urine containing blood in comparatively small quantity will be found of a peculiar smoky hue, or even of a black colour (owing to the action of the acid of the urine on the hæmatin), and loaded with albumen.   If the escape of blood be free, the colour may vary from a port-wine hue to a bright arterial tint. The *distinction between renal and vesical hæmorrhage* is important.   Dr. Prout states that when the " blood is derived from the *kidney*, it is in general equally diffused throughout the whole urine ; on the contrary, when derived from the *bladder*, the blood for the most part comes away in greater or less quantity at the termination of the discharge, the urine having previously flowed off nearly pure."   Sir Thomas Watson has also remarked that the expulsion of slender, cylindrical pieces of fibrin, which have evidently been moulded in the ureter, is characteristic of hæmorrhage from the kidney or commencement of the ureter.   Moreover, in hæmorrhage from the secreting portion of the kidney (not the pelvis), the urine on being examined microscopically is usually found to contain casts of the renal tubes formed of coagulated blood (often spoken of as *blood-casts*) ; while there is also seen the delicate round renal epithelium, with casts composed of epithelial cells and blood corpuscles.   When the bleeding is from the bladder, the blood corpuscles are observed mixed with the flat scaly vesical epithelium ; and the urine contains also more or less muco-purulent matter.   Supposing malignant disease to be the cause, cancer cells will not unfrequently be found in the urine, and so determine the diagnosis.   If there be one or more calculi, the hæmorrhage will be lessened or entirely checked by rest, and increased or reproduced by any jolting exercise.   While where the blood comes away in drops or in a stream, unmixed with urine, the urethra is in all probability its source.

During the last year or two, the histories of a few cases of *intermittent* or *paroxysmal* hæmaturia have been recorded in the medical journals.   Though of rare occurrence, this disorder did not escape the observation of Rayer, of Elliotson, &c. The pathology of it is involved in doubt. The precise cause of it is unknown. Sometimes this affection is apparently connected with marsh miasma, the blood appearing at regular intervals, and perhaps being accompanied by imperfect rigors. This form can often be cured by full doses of quinine or arsenic. In other instances, it seems to have had its origin in simple exposure to cold; and in these the usual remedies for malarial poisoning are valueless. The urine is quite healthy, except at the time of the attack. Then it is found of a deep brownish-red colour; it contains an excess of urates and mucus; a variable (as regards quantity) precipitate of albumen is thrown down by heat or nitric acid; while no blood corpuscles can be seen on a microscopic examination, but only disorganized blood constituents and possibly tube-casts of disintegrated blood. The blood elements seem to come from the kidneys; and possibly as an exudation from the Malpighian bodies. The absence of blood corpuscles looks like an indication that there has not been a rupture of any vessel.*

A peculiar form of hæmaturia is sometimes met with in Egypt, Southern Africa, and the Mauritius, which is probably due to the Distoma hæmatobium. The eggs of this parasite are to be found in the urine, and sometimes the perfect entozoon may be discovered. The parasite is probably introduced into the system by drinking the waters of the district without filtering them.

The *treatment* will vary with the circumstances under which the hæmorrhage occurs. Where there is malignant disease, or a calculus at any part of the urinary tract, astringents should be resorted to; the best being the tincture of the perchloride of iron, gallic acid, Ruspini's styptic, the diluted sulphuric acid, &c. The fear of causing strangury must prevent the use of turpentine. Where there is some morbid poison in the blood, or actual renal disease, we ought to rest the kidneys, and promote elimination by the skin and bowels; for which purpose hot air or vapour baths, warm water

---

* Among a few other examples of paroxysmal hæmaturia which have fallen under my notice is the following. It may be mentioned here, as I have not met with anything of the kind in previous cases of abdominal section. Briefly, the facts are these :—On the 25 February 1868, I removed two ovarian tumours from a young lady, 19 years of age. The urine had been previously examined, and found to be quite natural. After the operation, the catheter was employed for several days. On the 26th the urine withdrawn appeared clear and healthy. There was sickness during the day and night; but no shivering—not even chilliness. On the 27th, at 10 A.M., Dr. Peplow drew off more than half-a-pint of very bloody urine. At 3 P.M. I emptied her bladder myself, taking away a pint of urine which was loaded with blood. On boiling, it became almost solid from coagulation of albumen. Examined microscopically, a quantity of dark granular matter was found with some nucleated epithelium; but no blood corpuscles could be seen, nor any tube-casts. At 11·30 P.M. I again introduced the catheter. The urine was then clear and pale and acid, the specific gravity being 1012 : no deposit was produced by boiling, or by adding nitric acid. There was no return of the hæmaturia subsequently.

baths, and purgatives, will prove the most effectual. Simple drinks, especially plain water, should be taken very copiously. Hæmorrhage from the urethra will often be checked by the application of ice; or by passing a large bougie, and leaving it in the passage for some hours. Lastly, in vesical hæmorrhage, a solution of alum or of tannic acid, of such a strength as to have a styptic taste, may be injected into the bladder; while the iron-alum can often be advantageously administered at the same time.

9. **UTERINE HÆMORRHAGE**. — Hæmorrhage from the uterus is a symptom of so many different diseases, that, to consider it properly, one ought to write a treatise on the various functional and organic derangements of this organ. Two forms of uterine hæmorrhage have to be distinguished, viz., menorrhagia and metrorrhagia. The term *menorrhagia* [Μῆνες = the menses + ῥήγνυμι = to burst out,] should only be applied to cases of increased menstrual flow; although it is very often employed to signify any sanguineous discharge from the uterus other than the normal monthly escape. *Metrorrhagia* [Μήτρα = the womb + ῥήγνυμι,] is the technical expression for hæmorrhage occurring from the uterus, independently of menstruation.

The *catamenia may be abnormally increased* from conditions which produce attenuated blood; as tuberculosis, granular degeneration of the kidneys, affections of the spleen, anæmia owing to prolonged lactation, &c. Another common cause is excessive congestion of the ovary and uterus during the maturation and escape of the ovule. The same result also ensues from any great excitement at the monthly period, or excessive sexual indulgence at other times; from metritis and ovaritis; from the approach of "the change of life;" from the hæmorrhagic diathesis; as well as from such relaxation of the uterine tissue as is often associated with abrasion of the lips of the cervix. Moreover, where there is structural disease of the uterus—*e.g.* fibroid tumour, polypus, or cancer— the menstrual flow frequently merges into uterine hæmorrhage, and thus proves most troublesome. It is frequently very disheartening in the treatment of fibroid tumour to find, that just as the strength is being regained the monthly period comes round; the flow, by its excess, prostrating the patient, and undoing all that has been accomplished in the preceding two or three weeks.

The diseases which give rise to *uterine hæmorrhage,* properly so-called, are principally cancer; polypi, whether cellular or glandular or fibrous; as well as fibroid tumours, especially such as produce enlargement of the uterine cavity, or which impede contraction of the muscular fibre cells and other structures composing the wall of the uterus. Then this condition may be occasioned by congestion of the uterus or ovaries; by inflammatory engorgement or hypertrophy of the whole uterus, or of the cervix and labia only; and by fungoid degeneration of the mucous membrane lining the

uterine cavity.   Among the more exceptional causes of hæmorrhage
we must not omit to mention pelvic hæmatocele; subinvolution,
as well as chronic inversion of the uterus; and the retention in the
womb of any portion of a product of conception,—such as a vesicular
mole &c.   Either of the foregoing affections may produce frequent
attacks of bleeding, or a constant loss.   The blood comes away
steadily, drop by drop, with occasional small coagula, so as to
saturate three or four napkins in the twenty-four hours; or there
are gushes at intervals, with large clots; or the loss at times becomes
so severe as to amount to flooding.   The practitioner must also
remember the frequency with which còpious hæmorrhage proves to
be the precursor of abortion; no less than the constancy with which
it indicates more or less separation of the placenta—perhaps owing
to placenta prævia—in the latter months of pregnancy.
    On making a few remarks upon the *treatment* of these cases, it
will be necessary to confine them to the steps to be adopted for
controlling the hæmorrhage; since the proceedings required for
removing its cause will hereafter be treated of.   At once, therefore, it may be said that astringents are the remedies chiefly to be
trusted to; and the best of these are gallic acid and cinnamon,
either alone or in combination, or with the aromatic sulphuric
acid (F. 103, 104).   Some authorities advise the acetate of lead :
if used, it should be given in larger doses than are ordinarily employed (F. 117).   Where any inflammatory action exists, mercury
will be a good agent to employ; and, as before mentioned, I prefer
the solution of corrosive sublimate (F. 27).   The ergot of rye has
no styptic property; though when the bleeding is due to a flabby
state of the uterus, this drug does considerable good by inducing contraction.   There is no objection to administering it in combination
with astringents (F. 103).   Supposing there is anœmia as a cause
of the loss, the ammonio-sulphate of iron proves very efficacious
(F. 116); more so, in my opinion, than the perchloride of iron.
The latter, however, is sometimes serviceable (F. 101).   Every
now and then we meet with cases where the discharge of blood is
excessive, though we can detect no cause for it, and where no kind
of astringent or tonic has the least effect.   In such I have found
most benefit from corrosive sublimate, or some other preparation of
mercury; the infusion of digitalis, in half-ounce or ounce doses, as
strongly recommended by Drs. Dickinson and Robert Lee, having
given me nought but disappointment.
    The local remedies to be resorted to are of considerable impor-
tance.   The principal are as follows :—A favourite remedy is the
application of cold water over the pubes.   To be of any service, ice
in a bladder should be employed.   Napkins dipped in vinegar and
water, soon get converted into offensive fomentations.   The frequent
introduction of small lumps of ice up the vagina, or the use of
enemata of very cold water, will often prove efficacious.   The same
remark applies to vaginal injections of tannic acid or infusion of

matico; especially if the patient's hips be so raised that a portion of the fluid can be retained at the top of the vagina. I have also seen great good follow the employment of astringent vaginal pessaries (F. 423); or the use of galvanism where there is a want of muscular contraction; or the introduction of sponge tents up the canal of the cervix, and through the internal os (F. 426). Thes plans failing, or it seeming probable that they will fail if tried, recourse should be had to plugging the vagina firmly with some soft material like cotton wool; or with a sponge soaked in vinegar; or with an elastic air-ball enclosed in a case of spongio-piline, which is capable of exerting considerable pressure on being distended. Plugging the os uteri only, with lint or cotton wool, does not succeed as well as might be anticipated; for the foreign body seems to cause contraction, so that it is soon expelled into the vagina. In several instances where there has been troublesome hæmorrhage from the upper part of the interior of the uterus, I have succeeded in stopping it with the styptic rod of tannin and cacao butter (F. 424). The passage of this rod into the uterine cavity is easily accomplished; while in no case has its retention and dissolution in the uterus produced any unpleasant symptoms. The patient is of course to be kept quiet in bed in all cases; the diet &c. being such as has been advised in managing the other important varieties of hæmorrhage.

VIII. INFLAMMATION.

Every part of the body is liable to inflammation [*Inflammo* = to burn], and much of the premature extinction of human life is due to it. Hence a knowledge of the various phenomena of this morbid process—their causes and relations and effects, may be said to constitute the master-key to the comprehension of the nature of a large amount of disease.

Now although inflammation is here spoken of as "a morbid process," it is not to be inferred that its effects are not frequently most salutary. By it many morbid poisons are gradually expelled from the system, wounds which do not unite by the first intention are healed, fractured bones become firmly knitted together again, and so on. A portion of skin and connective tissue, as in the case of a boil, inflames and degenerates and dies: yet the inflammatory process, by its continuance, not only leads to the casting-off of the slough, but also to the reproduction of healthy tissue.

No useful or indeed correct definition of inflammation can be given at present. It may only be said that it is sometimes a destructive, sometimes a formative process; and that it consists essentially of an excessive proliferation of cells, accompanied by marked symptoms of local and constitutional disturbance. In vascular structures, when inflamed, it can be seen that there is congestion and stagnation of blood, with morbid adhesiveness of the corpuscles, in the capillaries of the affected tissues; these vessels being at first contracted, but subsequently becoming dilated. There is also an exudation of liquor sanguinis through the walls of the vessels, with or without extravasation of blood cells; the exuded matter undergoing certain important changes according to the texture in which it occurs, the coexisting local or general disease, and the severity or extent of the inflammatory process itself.

Causes.—Inflammation occasionally arises unexpectedly, and from causes unknown. In other instances it will be found to have been produced by some mechanical or chemical irritant; or by the action of cold; or by some morbid poison received into, or generated within, the system. It is now admitted by many as probable, that inflammation is not an affection of the capillaries, nor an altered state of the nerves, nor a change in the blood; but that it is a form of abnormal nutrition—that where it has its seat, the series of changes by which the tissues should be renovated becomes deranged. It is said to be *acute* when it runs its course rapidly, and is attended with severe constitutional and local disturbance; *chronic,* when its phenomena are less strongly marked. *Subacute* inflammation is marked by symptoms which are intermediate between acute and chronic, and which do not attain any great severity. By some authors the term *latent* has been applied to those cases in which internal inflammation proceeds silently and treacherously, and without manifesting signs by which its existence might be suspected. And then there are certain *specific* inflammations, examples of which may be seen in scrofula, gout, rheumatism, syphilis, the exanthemata, &c.

Pathology.—The study of the pathology of this complex morbid process shows that it consists in a derangement of the normal nutritive changes, leading to loss of function in the elements of the tissue involved.—"The conditions of the healthy maintenance of any part by nutrition, are," observes Mr. Paget, " 1st, a regular and not far-distant supply of blood; 2nd, a right state and composition of that blood; 3rd (at least in most cases), a certain influence of the nervous force; and 4th, a natural state of the part in which nutrition is to be effected. All these are usually altered in inflammation."* The *supply of blood* to the affected texture is increased; the vessels are dilated and elongated, so that such as were previously invisible come into view, owing to their distension with red corpuscles; there is a tendency to stagnation—an agglomeration of the red corpuscles into masses so that the vessels get choked, all blood movement through them being stopped—in many of the turgid vessels; while when lymph is effused, and begins to be organized, new vessels are formed in it. Every student, in the pursuit of microscopic investigations, has watched with delight the circulation in the healthy web of the frog's foot;

* *Lectures on Surgical Pathology.* Second Edition, p. 219, London, 1863.

and doubtless must have noticed that as the blood flows through the vessels the red corpuscles are most abundant in the middle of each stream, being surrounded by liquor sanguinis. On applying a drop of any irritant to the web, however, the stream gets more loaded with the blood cells, the clear margin of liquor sanguinis gradually disappearing; while coeval with this, the rate of movement lessens. As the work of the irritant becomes more appreciable to the tissue, these two conditions (increase of cells and diminution of circulation) become more and more manifest, and the vessels enlarge; the blood corpuscles, exhibiting a tendency to adhere to each other and to the walls of the vessels, until the latter are blocked up and there is *stagnation* or "*stasis.*" Around such an area of capillary stasis there may be seen *congestion*,—a condition differing from stagnation to this extent, that the accumulated blood corpuscles impede but do not stop the flow of blood through the vessels; while outside the congested district there is *determination* or fulness and rapid movement of blood. Then, as the result of this, we know that the liquor sanguinis exudes through the walls of the vessels; or sometimes even the coats rupture, and extravasation of blood corpuscles ensues.

Again, in inflammation, the *purity of the blood* is frequently more or less disturbed. According to Mr. Wharton Jones, the most constant change is an increase of the fibrin in the plasma; less constant but yet frequent, a diminution of the red corpuscles; and still less constant an increase in the colourless corpuscles. But then, these alterations can happen independently of inflammation, increase of fibrin and diminution of red corpuscles being a normal result of pregnancy; while on the other hand, "the essential phenomena of inflammation may occur when the blood of the body generally is in a perfectly healthy state."[*] It is probable, however, that this latter event is only observed when the inflammatory action falls short of a certain extent and intensity. With regard to the *nervous force*, it is generally said not to be normal; but how it is changed we no more know than we can explain how it operates in ordinary nutrition. And, lastly, the *healthy condition of the part itself* is altered in the inflammatory state; this change being due to more or less degeneration from hindered nutrition, as well as to the penetration of such inflammatory products as lymph and pus into the elemental structures and the interstices between them.

Symptoms.—For some eighteen centuries the distinctive external marks of the inflammatory process have been said to be the combination of pain, swelling, heat, and redness:—"Notæ inflammationis," says Celsus, "sunt quatuor, rubor et tumor, cum calore et dolore." The antiquity of this formula, however, must not lead to its too rigid adoption. In several of the cases which

---

[*] "On the State of the Blood and the Bloodvessels in Inflammation," by T. Wharton Jones, F.R.S. *Guy's Hospital Reports.* Second Series, vol. vii. p. 76. London, 1851.

come under the physician's notice such a combination of pheno-mena is absent; while not only is this so, but occasionally we may be unable to discover any one of them. Pericarditis in an aged person, for example, has often run its course without giving rise to pain or any appreciable increase of heat. Yet after death, though no one of the symptoms will perhaps have been detected during life, unmistakable evidence of inflammatory action has been found in the presence of an excessive exudation of liquor sanguinis.

Then in speaking of the constitutional symptoms, great stress is always laid on the occurrence of a remarkable buffiness of the blood, and fever. As regards the *blood* it will be found when drawn from the body to exhibit, after standing and coagulating, the *buffy coat*; *i.e.*, the upper portion of the clot consists of fibrin unmixed with red corpuscles. It must be remembered, however, that this appearance is not characteristic of inflammation; for it generally arises when, from any circumstance, the fibrin coagulates more slowly, or the corpuscles subside more rapidly, than in healthy blood. It is also frequently found in the blood of plethoric persons, and in that of pregnant women. Sometimes the surface of the buffy coat is contracted and concave : the blood is then said to be both buffed and cupped. As soon as the inflammatory action reaches a certain degree, the nervous and vascular systems become affected; the general derangement which ensues being described as *inflammatory* or *symptomatic fever*, or as *constitutional disturbance*. This fever manifests itself by depression, chilliness followed by heat, frequency of pulse, headache, a furred tongue, thirst, and loss of appetite. Repeatedly, the chilliness amounts to shivering; while it is generally allowed that the onset of sponta-neous inflammations is more frequently attended with rigors, than that of inflammation due to external injury. The intensity of the inflammatory fever will depend upon the nature of the tissue affected, the extent of the mischief, and the constitution of the patient. It is sometimes so slight as to escape notice; though always well marked when the nervous and circulating systems have not previously been enfeebled by disease or age.

The chemical examination of the *urine* shows a certain varia-tion from the normal composition. Thus, the *chlorine* being chiefly derived from the chloride of sodium taken with the food, its amount will of course depend on the quantity of salt thus con-sumed. Hence, in acute inflammatory diseases where there is always complete anorexia, we should expect to find the chlorine con-stantly diminishing, until the morbid action has reached its highest point; an increase occurring as restoration to health gradually takes place, and as the power of assimilating food returns. Ac-cordingly this is what really happens in all acute diseases, except in the case of intermittent fevers. The investigations of Neu-bauer and Vogel have shown, that the secretion of chlorine is usually increased during the paroxysms of these fevers, and some-times for a short time after them ; though the mean daily quantity is somewhat less than normal.   This point will be found further noticed in the sections on *Intermittent Fever* and *Pneumonia*.   In chronic disorders, the quantity of chlorine will likewise depend on the amount and nature of food taken, the strength of the digestive organs, and the non-separation of it from the body by watery stools, &c.   Extra mental or bodily labour will also temporarily increase the secretion of chlorine.   The proportion of *urea* secreted with the urine depends upon the extent of the tissue metamorphoses.   It usually happens at the commencement of most acute febrile diseases that the quantity is increased, although the patient has no animal food.   After the disorder has reached its culminating point, the amount becomes less than normal; but it increases as convalescence gets established.

When the inflammation goes on to suppuration, the commence-ment of this event is commonly marked by the occurrence of shivering, and the constitutional disturbance is then called *hectic fever* ; the leading symptoms of which are frequency and weakness of pulse, alternations of chilliness with heat and flushing followed by sweating, an excessive wasting of the body, and daily increasing debility.   Hectic fever also accompanies other diseases, as all forms of phthisis, dysentery, &c.

Termination or Effects.—The most favourable termination is *resolution*,—the complete restoration of the part to its normal state.   The term *delitescence* is now and then employed when the phenomena disappear suddenly and rapidly.   If the inflammation only change its seat from one part to another there is said to be *metastasis.*

Then the effects of this process will perhaps be *formative ;* that is to say, new particles or granules or cell-growths result, which are susceptible of further development.   In this way we have serous effusions, varying in quantity from a few drachms to many pints ; blood effusions, chiefly arising from the rupture of new vessels in freshly formed material ; and the exudation of coagulable lymph or fibrin, which may become a nidus-substance for the growth of new elements.   On the contrary, the effects may be *destructive :* this is seen in suppuration, when pus cells are developed from the elements of the degenerating tissue ; in ulceration, a progressive softening and disintegration of successive layers of tissue ; and in sloughing, gangrene, sphacelus, or mortification.

Where inflammation attacks the connective tissue, all the results of inflammatory action are likely to occur.   So also when the larger glands and the solid viscera of the body suffer.   In in-flammation of the serous membranes, we expect there will be exudation of serous fluid and coagulable lymph or fibrin—in other words, that it will prove adhesive inflammation.   The synovial membranes are less liable to this disease than the serous, and coagulable lymph is seldom poured out. The mucous membranes are rarely affected by the adhesive form of inflammation; but when attacked the inflamed membrane pours out serous fluid, or viscid mucus, or pus, or blood—as is well seen in pneumonia, in which the extravasated red corpuscles give a pathognomonic rusty tinge to the sputa.

Treatment.—The general principles only admit of being laid down, so extensive is the subject; but their importance is such that they deserve attentive consideration. In the commencement the cause of the inflammation should, if possible, be removed. Attempts may then be made to obtain resolution: or, if this seem impossible, the next best termination, which, in cases of external inflammation, will generally be suppuration; in internal, sometimes suppuration, sometimes adhesion. The important point, then, for consideration is this :—How are these desired results to be best attained? For very many years but one answer has been given to this question. The reply has been—by the adoption of the *antiphlogistic regimen;* which consists essentially in the use of low diet, bloodletting, active purging, counter-irritation, mercury, and antimony. It is to be feared that such remedies still find favour with some practitioners. I cannot but hope, however, that the more closely disease is studied, the smaller will become the number of those who recommend the use of these devitalizing agents. As my own experience has grown, so have I become more and more imbued with the persuasion that inflammatory action is not a fire to be put out by subtracting or withholding fuel. In the shape of general propositions it may be affirmed,—that when an inflammation is established it is not possible to cut it short by antiphlogistic remedies : that general bleeding, unless carried to a very dangerous extent, will not sensibly diminish the amount of blood in an inflamed part : that bleeding will not render an impure blood pure : that depressing agents favour the extension of the morbid action, and deprive the system of the power of rallying from the effects of the disease : that in critical instances of inflammation there is depressed nervous power, together with impaired action of the heart : finally, in all cases a determined lowering plan of treatment is found to be very badly borne in the present day, whatever may be said to have been the case in former times.

The theory has found favour with some pathologists that inflammation, as we now see it, is of a different type to that which formerly existed; perhaps being more readily excited by mal-nutrition, being more prostrating, and possibly being more dangerous to life through its incapacitating the system for the same degree of reaction as that which formerly followed an attack. In other words, the febrile symptoms accompanying inflammation are said to have altered from an inflammatory to a typhoid character. This view was originally ably suggested by Dr. Alison, who certainly said all that was possible in favour of such an argument.* On the contrary, its soundness has been well disputed by Professor J. Hughes Bennett;† who has consistently maintained and taught that inflammation is the same now as it has ever been, that the analogy sought to be established between it and the varying types of fever is fallacious, and that bloodletting and antiphlogistic remedies have been all along opposed to a sound pathology. As these opinions cannot be discussed with sufficient fulness in these pages, I would especially recommend the perusal of Dr. Alison's and Professor Bennett's very admirable essays to my readers. At the same time it is right to say I agree with the conclusions of Dr. Hughes Bennett. Many circumstances have led me to do so. Thus, amongst other points, I am thoroughly sceptical as to the soundness of the assertion which has been made that the human race is degenerating. Tubercular affections, the special result of deteriorated constitutional powers, are not more rife than they were. On the contrary, taking into consideration the increase of the population, the Reports of the Registrar-General for the last ten years show a decline in their mortality to some extent in England. Yet if it were true that the physical powers of mankind are on the wane, such a result would hardly be possible.‡ Count Cavour died at the age of fifty from over-work,

---

* *Edinburgh Medical Journal*, May 1857.   † *Idem*, March 1857.

‡ The discussion very much resembles that which has often taken place as to the stature and strength of men at different epochs. Dr. Graves (*Studies in Physiology and Medicine*, p. 180. London, 1863) remarks upon this curious fact,—"That from the most remote ages there has existed a singular propensity among mankind, to disparage the size of their contemporaries, and to represent it as diminutive, when compared with that of preceding generations. We find traces of this opinion in the works of various writers from the time of Homer and Hesiod down to the present period; indeed this is carried so far in the ancient authors, that whenever an old man speaks of the stature and physical powers of men it is only for the purpose of descanting on the degeneracy of the human race, and of referring with much complacency to the feats of superior strength and activity which he witnessed among the tall and athletic companions of his youth. That this opinion is not borne out by facts, is proved by the measurement of human bones found in the most ancient burial-places, by considering the stature of the Egyptian mummies, by the examination of ancient armour, and lastly, by inspection of the buildings designed for the abode and accommodation of mankind in former ages." And again the same author observes,—"With respect to the strength of men, the same opinions have prevailed as with regard to size and stature. It has been asserted, that the men of the present time have degenerated from the vigour of their ancestors; and it is also maintained, that civilized man is inferior in strength to the savage who roams the wilds of Africa or America, Neither of these opinions appears to be well founded; bodily strength is the result of health, exercise, and a proper supply of wholesome food."

The reader who feels any interest in this strange controversy may also refer to the writings of Geoffroy Saint-Hilaire. He tells us (*Traité de Tératologie*, tome i. p. 170. Paris, 1832) that, in 1718, Henrion, a zealous supporter of the view that the men of ancient times were of larger stature than their present descendants, formed a table or chronological scale of the variations of the human stature from the Creation to the Chris-

though it is much to be feared bleeding had much to do with his premature death. "Like most Italians, he firmly believed in the efficacy of bleeding, and was accustomed to be bled in every case of illness."* Just one week before his death, after walking about his estate at Leri, he got chilled; and not feeling better the next morning, had himself bled. On the following day he was also bled, apparently without advice; and then on the next day but one, he again lost blood by the wish of his physician. The death of this statesman seems to have directed the general attention of his countrymen to the subject of bleeding. And this attention was not given too soon; for in 1861 the lancet appears to have been as freely used in Italy as it was formerly in England, when some of our hospital out-patient rooms were compared to slaughter-houses. Dr. Borelli, in particular, has attempted to show his confrères that the depletory treatment of disease is injurious : and, in some articles contributed during 1863 to the Sardinian *Gazetta Medica*, he accounts for the necessity of substituting tonics and restoratives for antimony and purgatives and bleeding, by adopting this convenient change of type theory. Hence it becomes necessary for the supporters of this hypothesis to allow, that while disease in Great Britain has undergone this change some twenty or five-and-twenty years since, it is only since 1860 that it has done so on the Continent. Then again, there is no connexion between the type of epidemic disorders, and that of organic diseases. The type of the former has always varied. Indeed there is but little uniformity in the progress of a single epidemic. Take that of cholera, for example. At the commencement of the pestilence the great majority of those attacked, die : towards the close of it, by far the greater number of cases recover. But pneumonia, pericarditis, peritonitis, are in all respects the same diseases now that they were (to speak only of facts within my own knowledge) twenty years ago. And moreover, if Dr. Alison be correct in all his assumptions, we must grant that not only the type but the cause of disease has changed : since, if we are to place implicit reliance upon the experience of Cullen, Gregory, Mason Good, and others, upon some points on which they are likely to have erred from the imperfection of the means of diagnosis, we surely must credit their statements where simple observation alone was necessary.

tian era. According to this Adam was 123 feet 9 inches high, and Eve 118 feet 9 inches and 9 lines; Noah was 20 feet lower than Adam; Abraham, was between 27 and 28 feet in height; Moses 13 feet; while Hercules measured 10, Alexander 6, and Julius Cæsar 5 feet. The human race thus progressively diminishing, were it not for the interposition of Providence, would have dwindled to the size of microscopic beings by this time. These reveries of the learned Henrion were founded on the tradition of the Rabbins, according to which Adam was at first 900 cubits high; but after he had sinned, God caused a considerable diminution of his size.

* *Cavour. A Memoir.* By Edward Dicey. Second Edition, p. 234. London, 1861.

Nevertheless, only some sixty years ago—to take one example from many—inflammation of the brain was supposed to be the constant cause of insanity; and the greatest men of the day believed that it invariably required lowering measures. At Bethlem Hospital the system of treatment consisted of bleeding, purging, and vomiting in the spring months:—" A certain day was appointed on which the patients were bled, another when they were purged, another when they were vomited. They were bled in May and again in June; *the precise time depended on the weather*. All this had been the practice for many years, and no better practice, it was stated, was then known."*

Again, for how many years were the sympathetic disorders of pregnancy attributed to plethora and bleeding resorted to, when in fact they were due to anæmia. Yet no one will argue that the blood of a woman with child is different now to what it was fifty years ago. The experiments of Andral and Gavarret showed that the mean normal proportion of blood globules is about 127; that the essential character of plethora is that this proportion is greatly increased; while in pregnancy it may be said to be always diminished. Practitioners then began to remember that they had found but little advantage from bleeding in the disorders arising from the progress of gestation; though many, perhaps, like Dr. Sangrado, attributed their want of success to not having practised depletion to a sufficient extent.

But something more may be said upon the practical bearings of the question—*i.e.*, upon the treatment of inflammation. On this point I think it may be remarked that those practitioners who have ventured to study the phenomena of acute inflammation for themselves, regardless of theories belonging to the past, and caring little whether disease has changed its type or not, are now mostly agreed that our treatment must be confined to simply attempting to guide the morbid process to a favourable termination; just in the same way as we at present try to conduct cases of typhus, small-pox, scarlatina, &c., through their natural progress, without making heroic and unprofitable efforts to cut short the disease. This object is to be obtained by supporting the vital powers, instead of lowering them : by avoiding undue interference, as well as by assisting the excretion of effete products. If this be true, it necessarily follows that during the early stages of the attack all sources of irritation ought to be removed, so that the patient may enjoy perfect quiet of body and mind ; the sick-room should be well ventilated, and kept at a temperature of about 60° Fahr.; the diet had better be light, and ice or cold water freely allowed ; sedatives are generally to be administered if there be pain or much irritability ; while if the febrile excitement be great, salines and refrigerants may be ordered. Aperients will be needed where

* *Further Report of the Commissioners in Lunacy to the Lord Chancellor*, p. 78. London, 1847.

fæcal matters have accumulated in the intestines ; but they are not
to be employed as derivants,—*i.e.*, to draw blood from the inflamed
tissue to the alimentary canal, since it is merely a mischievous
delusion to suppose that they can have this effect.   When the
pulse becomes soft, or at all irregular, or small, good broths and
essence of beef and other nutrients are to be administered ; milk
and cream and raw eggs will often prove invaluable ; while directly
there are indications of general weakness we may be sure that
wine is required, in quantity varying from two or three to twelve
ounces in the twenty-four hours.   Where great exhaustion sets in,
more especially if there be wandering or delirium, brandy must be
substituted for wine.   In all acute disorders the various organs are
much weakened, so that their functions are either partially or
entirely arrested.   To give food when there is a perfect loathing
of it, is worse than useless.   But we may advantageously administer alcoholic stimuli, either to retard the destructive metamorphosis of tissue, to afford to the system the elements for the
generation of heat, to repair the circulating energies, to supply
a stimulus to the nervous system, or simply empirically—because experience has proved the great value of such remedies
when judiciously prescribed, without teaching us how they act.
And then, lastly, as the period of crisis approaches, Dr. Hughes
Bennett's example can be followed of giving a diuretic—half a
drachm of spirit of nitrous ether, with or without ten minims of
colchicum wine—thrice daily, to favour the excretion of urates ;
whilst, when a crisis occurs by sweating or diarrhœa, care is to
be taken not rudely or unnecessarily to check it.

When disease is treated in accordance with the plan just
sketched out the physician soon learns, that if his prescriptions
are somewhat tame they certainly do not aggravate the intensity
of the morbid action ; that the mortality of inflammatory affections
as compared with that of former years, is greatly lessened ; while
where recovery follows, it does so with the intervention of a much
shorter period of convalescence than when the opposite system is
practised.   As a matter of fact, the success of the method is apparent from the following :—During the fifteen years ending in
May 1863, Dr. Bennett had thus managed all the cases of pneumonia which had been under his care in the clinical wards of the
Royal Edinburgh Infirmary, amounting to one hundred and fifteen ;
of which number one hundred and twelve were dismissed cured,
and three died.   Rather more than half of these were cases of
simple uncomplicated pneumonia, the average duration of which
was some 13½ days.   About one-sixth were double uncomplicated
cases, their average duration being 20 days.   If we examine seven
of the complicated examples it will be found, that one supervened
on bronchitis and emphysema, two on typhus fever, one on bronchitis and pleurisy, one on pleurisy with effusion of eight weeks'
standing, one on rheumatism with heart disease, and one on severe

rheumatism with endocarditis and pericarditis; the average duration of the pneumonia in these seven being 21½ days. The three fatal cases were all complicated: the first, with uncontrollable diarrhœa and follicular disease of the mucous membrane of the small intestines; the second, with persistent albuminuria and anasarca; and the third, with delirium tremens and universal cerebral meningitis.

Contrasting this result with that obtained from an opposite course of proceeding, it seems to me that all doubt on the subject must be removed. Thus, during ten years—from 1 July 1839, to 1 July 1849—648 cases of pneumonia were treated, by different physicians, according to the rules then enforced by all writers, in the Royal Infirmary of Edinburgh; of which number 388 were cured, 38 relieved, and 222 died. Again, of 107 cases, recorded by M. Louis in 1835, and treated by bleeding and tartar emetic, 32 died. So, of 648 cases treated by Rasori, in the hospital at Milan, by large doses of antimony, 143 died. Andral, in his *Clinique Médicale*, tells us that pneumonia is one of those diseases the treatment of which is at once most simple and most efficacious. The principal remedy is copious bloodletting; neither children, adults, nor aged persons being spared. Yet of the 65 examples narrated to prove the soundness of his principles, no less than 36 ended fatally. Moreover, Laennec, who bled moderately at the commencement of the disease, regarded the mortality as one in six or eight. And lastly, Dr. Dietl treated 380 cases of primary pneumonia, in the Charity Hospital of Vienna, thus:—85 by venesection, one death in every 5 resulting; 106 by large doses of tartar emetic, with one death in 5·22; and 189 by diet only, with one death in 13½, all the fatal cases moreover being complicated. The account given by Dr. George W. Balfour, in 1847, of Skoda's axiomatic defence of his views,—viz. that pneumonia was a disease which tended not to dissolution but to resolution, seems to have been the starting point of the greatest change in medical practice which is likely to be seen in the present age. It was after this that the foregoing statistics were collected, and that a new era commenced.

At the same time that bleeding as an antiphlogistic remedy should be rarely if ever practised, it may be remembered that a small loss of blood will often be beneficial, particularly in relieving excessive pain, and in moderating attacks of dyspnœa due to some obstruction to the circulation in the heart or lungs. As Dr. Bennett remarks:—"I have often been struck, especially in cases where large thoracic aneurisms cause these symptoms, with the small loss of blood which will occasion marked relief. The same result may be hoped for in other cases where the congestion is passive, even when that is associated with active repletion of blood, followed by exudation. But I need scarcely remark that this mere palliative object of bloodletting is not the ground on which the practice has hitherto been based, and that in this point of view it requires to be very differently explained." The same observations apply to the use of tartar emetic; which is perhaps valuable in small doses, and combined with other neutral salts, to favour excretion by the skin, kidneys, or intestines; but most injurious when employed in the heroic way often recommended.

With regard to the use of mercury, there appears to be every reason to believe that its utility in controlling inflammation or in promoting absorption of the effused products, has been very much overrated; and indeed it seems highly probable that inflammatory diseases will progress more favourably without the use of this medicine than with it. Some practitioners even now, however, would be afraid to treat pericarditis or iritis without blue pill or calomel; although more than twenty years have elapsed since Dr. John Taylor's valuable contributions to clinical medicine were published,* in which it was clearly shown that the opinions then current on this subject required revision. For example, of the cases of pericardial inflammation on which this excellent physician founded his observations, four got well without any treatment; while in twelve, ptyalism was not succeeded by any abatement of the mischief. Moreover, in six others, ptyalism was followed by pericarditis; in three, by endocarditis; in two, by extensive pleurisy; in four, by pneumonia; and in one, by erysipelas and laryngitis. Again, in one instance, the pericarditis and pneumonia both increased in extent after ptyalism; while in only one was salivation followed speedily by relief, and in two or three by a gradual diminution. More recently, Dr. Henry W. Williams† has cured sixty-four cases of iritis, of every degree of severity, including its idiopathic, traumatic, rheumatic, and syphilitic varieties, without a dose of mercury; the treatment having chiefly consisted in sustaining the general system, in relieving pain by narcotics, and in keeping the pupil dilated by belladonna.

From all this the conclusion appears quite evident, that in the treatment of acute inflammatory diseases practitioners must be content to trust more to that natural tendency to recovery which is present, and less to heroic remedies, than they have been in the habit of doing; for it is highly probable, that though we may be able to guide inflammations to a successful termination, yet we cannot cut them short, while any rude attempts to do so will merely increase the patient's danger. The risk of all inflammations being in proportion to the weakness of the patient, the amount of blood-poisoning, and the complications which arise, it surely cannot be wise to go out of our way to produce debility and thus favour the occurrence of toxæmia. But the fact is, and it ought never to be lost sight of, that "the body possesses a perfectly marvellous power whereby it protects itself against diseases, wards off some, cures in the best and speediest way many of those that have set in,

* *The Lancet.* London, 17 May 1845, to 31 October 1846.
† *The Boston Medical and Surgical Journal,* vol. lv. pp. 49, 69, 92. 1856.

and by a process of its own brings others more slowly to a favourable issue.   This innate power is called the *vis Naturæ medicatrix*,
being justly appreciated by physicians and philosophers, and highly
praised by them.   Of itself, it is sufficient to cure numerous diseases ;
in almost all, its influence is beneficial ; and, moreover, the remedies
that are in their own nature the best, are only of use in so far as
they stimulate and direct and control this inherent virtue."*

IX. DROPSY.

Dropsy [formerly more correctly called *hydropsy*, from ᾽Υδωρ –
water + ὄψις = the appearance] may be defined as an accumulation
of watery or serous liquid in some one or more of the natural
serous cavities of the body, or a diffusion of this fluid through the
interstices of the connective or areolar tissue, or a combination of
both.   The accumulation is sometimes an indirect consequence of
inflammation, though more frequently it occurs quite independently
of this process.

Dropsy is an important symptom of disease.   Being a result of
over-distension of the bloodvessels and particularly of the veins
and their capillaries, it will be found to arise from many different
conditions.   In general terms it may be said, that there is either
some mechanical impediment to the circulation ; or an altered
condition of the blood,—either an excess of water, or an accumulation of excrementitious matters.   Very commonly all these conditions coexist : in other words, there is impeded circulation, with
blood rendered poor by a relative excess of water, while it is also
contaminated with the elements of the bile or urine owing to
hepatic or renal inefficiency.   Consequently, each case of dropsy
will present two classes of dangerous symptoms, viz. those due to
the original disease, and those produced by the effusion.

Supposing the cerebral ventricles are distended with water, we
say the patient has *hydrocephalus*.   When serous fluid occupies the
pleura or the pericardium, we technically speak of the diseased
condition by the term *hydrothorax* in the one case and *hydropericardium* in the other.   If the cavity of the peritoneum be the seat
of the collected water, the complaint is called *ascites*.   Dropsy
of the tunica vaginalis testis is termed *hydrocele*.   Should the connective tissue of one region only become infiltered with serous
liquid, the part is said to be *œdematous* ; while *anasarca* is the term
applied to the more or less general accumulation of serum in this
tissue throughout the body.   Lastly the combination of anasarca
with dropsy of one or more of the large serous cavities is known
as *general dropsy*.

* *Conspectus Medicinæ Theoreticæ*. Auctore Jacobo Gregory, M.D.
Editio Quinta.   Sect. 65, 66.   Edinburgi, 1815.

Now, to understand the manner in which dropsy originates, it must be remembered that from all the internal surfaces of the healthy body a kind of excretion or oozing forth of fluid is constantly taking place, accompanied at the same time by absorption. Consequently, when the two processes of exhalation and absorption are properly balanced, the surfaces will merely be kept moist. But suppose that the balance, from some cause or other, is disturbed. Imagine exhalation to take place more rapidly from the surfaces of one of the shut sacs, or absorption more slowly, than in health ; or while exhalation is going on, let the power of absorption cease : under either of such circumstances it is clear that dropsy must result. It is probable that absorption takes place by the lymphatics, by the lacteals, and by the veins ; the first removing the worn-out particles of the body, the second taking up the chyle from the alimentary canal, while the third imbibe the fluid exhaled from serous membranes. In dropsies, the veins and their capillaries are chiefly in fault. . Assume, for example, that owing to the pressure of a tumour there is obstruction to the circulation through the principal vein of a district. The backward pressure which results must affect the veins, capillaries, and arteries; though in the natural order of events the veins and their capillaries may be supposed to suffer first. The resulting congestion prevents these distended vessels from taking up more fluid ; while to relieve the turgidity, effusion of serum takes place through their coats. This effusion occurs most freely through the capillaries and small veins, because their walls are the most easily permeated.

When dropsies arise from defective absorption, they are called *chronic* or *passive* dropsies : when from excessive exhalation of serous fluid, *active* or *acute*. Those due to cardiac or renal disease slowly producing some alteration in the blood, with obstruction to the circulation, are usually of the first kind ; those caused by cold, by sudden checking of the urine or perspiration, by the poison of scarlatina, &c., of the second.

The *causes* producing those conditions on which dropsy depends, are firstly, any circumstances which can induce irritation or congestion of secreting tissues—as cold ; the sudden retrocession of exanthematous eruptions ; and the poison of gout, rheumatism, &c. Secondly, whatever weakens the tissues or impoverishes the blood—as insufficient food, loss of blood, exhausting diseases, malaria, and scurvy. And thirdly, anything which obstructs the circulation and produces venous congestion—as obliteration of the veins; the pressure of inflammatory products and of tumours ; as well as organic diseases of the heart, lungs, liver, spleen, and kidneys.

The *symptoms* of dropsy will vary somewhat according to the morbid state which has originated the effusion. It is now generally admitted that blood deteriorated by an undue proportion of water, or blood charged with excrementitious materials, or blood containing a large excess of colourless corpuscles, has its circulation through the capillary vessels much impeded. As this impediment is most felt at the parts furthest removed from the influence of the heart's action, and where the force of gravity in the common position of the body is greatest, so it is in these districts that the transudation of serum through the coats of the choked-up vessels first occurs, while the process of absorption is also arrested. Hence, the dropsy in these cases often begins in the form of œdema about the feet and ankles. If the disease be not arrested in this stage, the œdematous state extends up the legs and thighs; the scrotum and penis, or the tissues about the vulva, get infiltrated; and ascites soon follows. Considerable suffering is produced by the dyspnœa; which is urgent in proportion to the amount of anæmia, and the extent to which the action of the diaphragm is interfered with by the abdominal effusion. The urine is scanty, and often contains an excess of urates; but it is only albuminous where the kidneys have become secondarily implicated. And then there are such other symptoms as palpitation, deficient perspiration, mental distress, thirst, constipation, daily-increasing weakness, &c., which need not be further dilated on here, as they are not peculiar to dropsy from anæmia.

Disorganization of the mitral or of the aortic valve, or of both, is the most frequent cause of cardiac dropsy. The spoilt valve sooner or later interferes with the circulation to an extent which cannot be overlooked. At first, perhaps, there is only shortness of breath on any exertion being made, together with palpitation and debility. Then, the feet and ankles begin to swell; the skin putting on a peculiar white and glistening appearance. As the effusion extends upwards, rest in the recumbent posture becomes impossible; while only unrefreshing dozes or snatches of sleep can be obtained. The heart's action gets daily more and more embarrassed; and a confused or indistinct systolic murmur is detected. The lungs become greatly congested; and moist crepitating râles are especially heard over their lower and posterior portions. Frothy sputa, sometimes streaked with blood, are coughed up. The eyeballs protrude: the alæ of the nose distend widely with each expiration. The urine is scanty: unless the circulation through the kidneys be much interfered with, there will not be found any albumen. In the same way, if the hepatic circulation be unimpeded, there will be little or no peritoneal effusion. But in either case, the general symptoms increase in severity. The dyspnœa becomes most urgent. And death generally occurs from apnœa, the dropsical pulmonary tissue gradually becoming useless for its natural functions.

In hepatic dropsy, ascites is the most significant symptom. Whether the original disease be of the form of congestion and hypertrophy of the liver, or chronic hepatitis, or cirrhosis, or cancer, the dropsy will generally commence in the form of effusion into the peritoneum.   The œdema of the extremities sets in sub-sequently.   As the ascitic fluid increases, so those symptoms of hepatic disease which have shown themselves for some time pre-viously become more marked and severe.   The attacks of sickness, the constipation and unhealthy stools, the sallow or jaundiced skin and conjunctivæ, the urine loaded with bile or urates, the restless-ness and weakness, as well as the wearying pain and fulness and tenderness in the right hypochondrium,—all these results of a greatly impeded flow of blood through the portal system of vessels point to the liver as the origin of the suffering, and tax the skill of the practitioner to the utmost for their relief.

Acute renal dropsy, or acute inflammatory dropsy, arises when the functions of the skin are suddenly suppressed, thus allowing cer-tain morbid materials to accumulate in the blood and so to set up inflammation in the secreting tubes of the kidneys.   Typical examples of this form of dropsy are seen when, from exposure to cold, the action of the skin is checked during the stage of desqua-mation in scarlet fever ; compelling the kidneys, as it were, to remove a poison from the system which is particularly obnoxious to their tissues.   In such cases, the urine either gradually or all at once, becomes scanty and of a dark brown colour ; while on being tested, it is found loaded with albumen.   About the same time general dropsy sets in.   There is effusion of serum, more or less copious, into the connective tissue all over the body, as well as into the serous cavities—especially the peritoneum.   This is followed, in cases about to prove fatal, by complete suppression of urine, with all the symptoms of uræmic poisoning—convulsions, coma, &c.   Death, however, is an exceptional occurrence in these instances ; unless the renal inflammation has been so severe and extensive, that the tubes have become universally choked with epithelium and fibrinous exudation.

Cases of chronic renal disease are frequently accompanied with dropsy.   This usually only happens, however, at a late stage, when the composition of the blood has got altered, and when the circu-lation through the kidney has become obstructed.   There is œdema of the connective tissue, followed by effusion into the pleuræ or peritoneum.   In these instances, the tendency to dropsy is in-creased by the coexistence of valvular disease of the heart.

The *prognosis* in dropsy generally will depend upon the cause. Where there is no organic disease of important viscera, a cure can be frequently effected.   In cases of spontaneous recovery, the disappearance of the effusion is accompanied by abundant sweating, profuse diuresis, or diarrhœa with copious watery stools.   Where the kidneys or heart or liver are permanently affected, the dropsy can sometimes be, at least temporarily, removed.   Death may ensue from the dropsy ; or from some inflammatory intercurrent disorder,—as pleurisy, or peritonitis, or enteritis ; or from the primary organic disease.

The *treatment* of dropsy will be discussed in speaking of the different disorders of which it is the consequence. But it may here be remarked, that in all cases two indications necessarily require to be followed—viz., the cure of the effusion which is only the symptom of other disease, and the relief of the disease itself. For the former we trust chiefly to diuretics, purgatives, diaphoretics, emetics, and the mechanical removal of the fluid by tapping and acupuncture. At the same time it is necessary to maintain, as far as is practicable, the general nutrition of the system.

One of the most celebrated of the ancient Greek physicians, Aretæus, was of opinion that success in the treatment of dropsy was due more to accident and the favour of the gods than to re-medial measures. And if by "success" a permanent cure of the organic affection be meant, no doubt the observation will still apply. Nevertheless, it must be remembered that in dropsy due to a fatal disorder, the patient may succumb to the former, long before the latter would in its uncomplicated course destroy him; and hence if this distressing symptom can be relieved or removed, life will probably be very materially prolonged.

Many authors on tropical diseases describe certain complicated cases of general dropsy under the name of BERIBERI, OR THE BAD SICKNESS OF CEYLON.* This obscure disease is almost unknown to pathologists in this country; though it is a frequent cause of death among European and native troops at Ceylon, and convicts in Indian jails. It would appear that a residence of some eight or twelve months in a district where it is endemic is necessary for its development. From the writings of Drs. Morehead, Aitken, and Waring, &c., I gather that the *symptoms* of this affection are chiefly great and progressive weakness, marked anæmia, lassitude and faintness, anxiety, numbness of the surface generally, with stiffness and œdema of the lower extremities. The trunk and face then become swollen, there is difficulty of breathing, the limbs get almost paralytic, and there is vomiting—sometimes of blood. The urine is almost suppressed, the thirst is great, the pulse is intermittent and frequent; and then flutterings or palpitations are experienced with a sense of suffocation, probably in consequence of the effusion of serum into the pleuræ and pericardium. Great exhaustion naturally follows; and within two or three weeks from the commencement, there is in most instances death. Occasionally the fatal event occurs suddenly and unexpectedly,—probably from embolism. The *morbid appearances* afterwards found are anasarca, œdema of the lungs, hydrothorax, hydropericardium, ascites, and cranial effusion. Cold and wet are the exciting *causes*, and hence beriberi occurs not unfrequently towards the close of the rainy season; while a watery condition of the blood, ill-health

* The name *Beriberi* is that given by the Malabars to this disease. *Beri* is the Singalese for weakness, and by iteration implies great weakness.

generally, and the consequences which follow a neglect of sanitary laws, are the predisposing conditions. Sometimes the effusion is encouraged by coexisting heart, liver, or renal disease; and often the persons affected are favourably circumstanced for the development of scurvy—that is to say, they have a scorbutic diathesis.

By way of *treatment*, attention to the means which prevent anæmia will be advisable, with chalybeate drinks, warm clothing, &c. Then, if the vascular action be not much depressed, purgatives may be cautiously used, as elaterium; or diuretics can be trusted to. I would suggest that a combination of digitalis and steel (F. 393) might prove serviceable. The vapour or hot-air bath often seems to be very useful. Probably the wet-sheet packing (F. 136) would produce greater action of the skin with less languor. Stimulants (especially gin) will generally be required, together with milk, soups, animal food, &c.

There are two remedies, much esteemed in parts of India, which ought not to be forgotten. Of these, *Treeak Farook*, the ingredients of which are unknown, but which acts as an aperient and diuretic when combined with rhubarb, is the best. *Oleum Nigrum*, prepared from the seeds of Celastrus Nutans, Benzoin, Cloves, and Nutmegs is less employed. The dose of the former is from 5 to 15 grains; while of the latter 10 minims will be needed to produce a stimulant and diaphoretic effect.

X. CANCER, OR CARCINOMA.

1. **GENERAL PATHOLOGY.**—There is scarcely an organ or tissue in the body which may not be attacked by cancer [*Cancer* = a kind of ulcer] or carcinoma [Καρκίνος = an eating ulcer]. This disease is not half as fatal to men as it is to women. The liability of the breast and uterus to be affected by it is considerable; otherwise cancer would seem to be more common in men, since the skin and bones and digestive organs are more prone to it in the male than in the female sex.* It is very uncommon in children; but when it occurs in them it is generally located in the bones or in the eye, or more rarely in the testicle or ovary.

A cancer may be described as a local manifestation of a specific disease of the blood; the morbid growth having incorporated in it peculiar materials which accumulate in the blood, and which the development or extension of the growth will tend to increase.† As

* In England, during the eleven years 1856—1866, the deaths registered from cancer amounted to 78,479. Thus, beginning with the year 1856, the numbers run 5859, 6201, 6433, 6676, 6827, 7276, 7396, 7479, 8117, 7922, and 8293. Of the 8293 in 1866, the *males* counted 2532; a considerable proportion (1345) dying between 55 and 75 years of age. The *females* amounted to 5761; the period of greatest mortality being between the 45th and 65th years, in which time 3008 perished.

† *Lectures on Surgical Pathology*, by James Paget, F.R.S., &c. Second Edition, pp. 384 and 766. London, 1863.

it is of constitutional origin, so the removal of the local manifestation does not effect a cure; but the cancer returns either in the seat of the original disease, or in some other structure. Moreover, when the primary affection has existed for a variable period, secondary deposits are very apt to be formed in the lymphatic glands, lungs, liver, spleen, &c. It is in these two respects especially (the reappearance of the disease after operation, and the contamination of the neighbouring lymphatic glands, &c.), that cancerous growths differ from benign tumours; although amongst the latter there are certain bodies which do recur and which are consequently known as recurrent tumours, while simple growths can also give rise to glandular enlargements by the irritation they set up. For these and other reasons which will presently be mentioned the foregoing definition of cancer does not meet with universal acceptance; since some authorities now assert that the disease is at first local, though at an early period it becomes general.* Any way, the practical point is that the surgeon does not seem to be consulted while the affection is only local; for otherwise the assertion made in France that cancer is completely incurable could not have been successfully maintained, as it has been.

Although the tendency of cancer, however, is to increase constantly and rapidly until life is destroyed, yet in a very few instances, it becomes latent; that is to say, after the disease has reached a certain line of development it remains in a state of repose or suspension, neither advancing nor receding. Sir B. Brodie refers to a case where the cancer was quiescent for twenty-five years; Dr. Babington knew an instance in which scirrhus of the mamma became stationary for twenty-four years; Dr. Maurice H. Collis has seen two examples of scirrhus of the breast, each of which lasted for twenty-nine years; and Sir Astley Cooper attended two women in whom the period of latency was respectively seventeen and twenty-two years. Equally rare is the spontaneous cure of cancer by inflammation, ulceration, and sloughing; or by fatty or calcareous degeneration. Yet it is certain, that through these means at least temporary, if not permanent, recoveries have been effected. And when we consider the matter fairly, the wonder is that a cancerous growth does not undergo spontaneous cure more frequently, rather than so very seldom. All cancer cells have a period of development, growth, and decay; but unfortunately, though they perish, they leave behind germs which perpetuate the structure. In a monograph *On the Healing Process of Cancer in the Liver*, published by Bochdalek of Prague, in 1845, is described a

---

* Several other theories have also been proposed to explain the nature of cancer. Thus, some have believed that the disease is of hydatid growth, —that independent organized parasites of the entozoa class are produced. Broussais with his followers regarded the malignant growth as the result of inflammatory mischief. A third theory assumes that the diseased part has the functions of a gland; secreting from the blood, and thus removing from the system, the cancer poison.

mode of cure as it sometimes occurs in this organ, the disease breaking down into a purulent-looking matter; so that the fluid portion becoming absorbed, the whole shrinks together merely leaving a small inert fibrous or fatty mass.

On submitting any cancerous growth to a minute examination, it will be found to consist of peculiar nucleated cells called "cancer cells," and of their free nuclei; together with a milky fluid or semi-fluid mixture, termed "cancer juice." The more dry and juiceless the growth, the less is its malignancy. The cancer cells and juice are either infiltrated into previously healthy tissues, or they are contained in a stroma or bed of new fibrous tissue. The cancer cells are of various shapes, being round, oval, fusiform, triangular, or elongated into one or more sharp processes; they vary in size from the $\frac{1}{700}$ to the $\frac{1}{3000}$ of an inch, the medium being $\frac{1}{1000}$; and they chiefly resemble in structure and aspect the secreting gland-cells. On magnifying a specimen of scirrhus about two hundred diameters, the cells will be seen containing a comparatively large, regular, oval or round, and well-defined nucleus. Sometimes two nuclei exist in the same cell; and each nucleus has one or two nucleoli. Moreover, mingled with these cells, we find free nuclei, and numerous degenerated cancer cells; some of these cells appearing withered and full of oil globules, others being transformed into granular matter—in the débris of which the nuclei lie loose. Whether cancer originates in the multiplication and abnormal development of the connective tissue cells, as taught by Virchow, Weber, Klebs, and others; or whether it essentially results from the proliferation of the epithelial cells lining the acini or follicles or tubules of the affected organ, combined with an hypertrophy of the connective tissue corpuscles, is uncertain. This latter view, originated by Cornil and supported by Waldeyer, seems probable. According to the last-named authority, when the epithelial cell-growth is much in excess, soft medullary cancer is the product; where the hypertrophy of the connective tissue greatly exceeds the epithelial proliferation, we have scirrhus; while if both conditions occur in nearly equal proportions, firm medullary cancer is the consequence.

Lebert has insisted that the cancer cell is pathognomonic—that it can be distinguished from every other kind of cell growth, and that it positively indicates the nature of the formation. Dr. Hughes Bennett and Müller consider, on the other hand, that no single element is diagnostic. Hence, their opinion seems to confirm that generally entertained—viz., that the microscope is merely an aid to diagnosis; but that, conjoined with a consideration of the progress and form and general appearance of the morbid growth, the use of this instrument may frequently enable us to arrive at a correct conclusion as to the nature of any particular tumour.

Dr. Wilks, writing in 1858, states his conviction that cancer has no peculiarities which can always distinguish it from other morbid growths, or even from many healthy structures.   He suggests, that if we make a list of different abnormal structures arranging them according to their rapidity of growth, disposition to spread, propagation, &c., those at the top of the scale may be called cancerous; but no boundary line can be drawn between the last which is styled cancer, and the next on the list which has acquired some other name.   Or again, if the term malignant be applied to the highest on the list, semi-malignant to those below, and innocent to the lowest, that still no clearly defined lines can be made between these divisions.   Allowing the truth of these observations, I would still venture to point out that broad distinctions have been sought for where none could be expected.   For just as there is a border-line so faint between the animal and vegetable kingdom that it is often difficult to say decidedly to which world a particular zoophyte belongs, so we may arrange the different phases of health and disease with such method that it cannot be said where one terminates and the other commences.   And yet practically there is but little difficulty.   As was well remarked by Burke, though no one can say where twilight begins or ends, there is ample distinction between day and night.

The question is still sometimes raised whether simple or benign tumours ever undergo degeneration into cancerous growths. Many surgeons believe this to be impossible, but more evidence is needed before this conclusion ought to be finally accepted.   At all events, there appears little or no reason why cancer cells should not be infiltrated into the tissues of non-malignant growths, as readily as into the textures of a healthy gland; unless indeed it be that the former are generally very much firmer and less vascular than the latter.

2. **VARIETIES OF CANCER.**— There are two principal varieties, and six sub-varieties of malignant disease,* most of the latter being probably mere modifications of the former.   They consist of,—

Scirrhus, or Hard Cancer.
Medullary, or Soft Cancer.
　Epithelial Cancer.
　Colloid, Gelatiniform, Alveolar, Cystic, or Gum Cancer.
　Melanoid, or Black Cancer.
　Osteoid Cancer.
　Hæmatoid Cancer, or Fungus Hæmatodes.
　Villous Cancer.

A scirrhous cancer never becomes medullary or epithelial, nor

* To avoid any error, it should be mentioned that the terms "cancer" and "malignant," employed in the text, are regarded as synonymous. The expression "malignant" is so generally used, that provided a definite meaning be attached to the word, I cannot see how any good would arise from abandoning it.   Moreover, it is convenient, since it allows us to speak of the *degree* of malignancy of any particular variety of cancer.

does the converse happen.   But a medullary or an epithelial cancer may become melanoid or hæmatoid; a scirrhus or a firm medullary will sometimes become osteoid; or either of the two chief forms can assume the colloid character.

In all forms of cancer there is one general sign which is looked upon as pathognomonic.   This is known as the cancerous cachexia. It is recognised by the peculiar dirty-yellowness of the skin, the sharp contracted features, and the general loss of flesh, which constitute it; the detection being made more clear by noting the prostration of strength, the absence of all energy, and the despondency which accompany it.   The general aspect of the patient is indescribable; but when once observed attentively, it will generally be afterwards appreciated without difficulty.   According to some authorities, this cachexia precedes the local manifestation; but my own experience leads me to agree with those who regard it as a secondary effect, and as being a measure of the general systemic mischief.

A rough comparison of tubercular with cancerous disease, showing how they resemble each other and how they differ, is not without interest.   The following are the chief features of such a sketch :—It is doubtful if tubercle and cancer are to be structurally distinguished from each other in their early stages.   There is no end to the number of tubercles which may be scattered through the body, as there is no limit to the masses of cancer which can invade the different organs.   Tubercle has an early tendency to die; fatty degeneration gradually progressing from the centre to the circumference of the tubercle, until the whole softens down and gives rise to a cavity or "vomica."   In cancerous tumours there is a like tendency to fatty degeneration; the morbid tissue undergoing disintegration leading to the formation of increasing ulcerations.   Cancerous parents transmit a tendency to cancer to their offspring; whereas phthisical men and women seem more frequently to communicate a tendency to cancer to their children, rather than a disposition to tubercle.   In tubercle despondency is the exception, the patient frequently seeming to be unaware of the gravity of the disease until it is far advanced; but with cancer there is great mental depression from the very commencement, and often before there is any local manifestation of disease.   In tubercle night sweats and diarrhœa are prevalent; while in cancer they are rare.   With tubercle there is at any early date an increased temperature of the body, besides an abnormal frequency of pulse; neither of these conditions being present in cancer.   Tubercle is principally a disease of early life and youth; cancer, of adults and the aged of both sexes.   There is a tubercular facies as well as a cancerous facies, but they bear no resemblance to each other.   And lastly, a progressive loss of flesh and strength takes place in both diseases.

A. SCIRRHUS, OR HARD CANCER.—This is the most frequent form of cancer.   It is seen occasionally in the stomach, in the upper

part of the rectum, and elsewhere; but most frequently, by far, in
the female breast. Three varieties are recognised,—the simple, the
atrophic, and the lardaceous. The first, or simple scirrhus, is
characterised by tardy growth, great hardness, and a tendency to
produce excessive induration of the tissues implicated in the infiltration. In the second, or atrophic variety, the tissues of the
affected gland get gradually much contracted; so that the hard
diseased portion appears to draw into its substance the healthy
surrounding tissue by numerous radiating bands or lines. The
affected gland finally becomes puckered up, until nothing seems to
remain but the stony tumour. This tumour seldom acquires a large
size. The third, or lardaceous kind, is easily distinguished by the
development of fat which takes place with the disease; so that the
affected gland is rendered larger than it was, and communicates a
brawny feel to the touch. Regarded from a clinical point of view
the distinction of these three varieties of this form of cancer is not
of much importance. They all present the same constitutional
symptoms, run the same destructive course, and require the same
general treatment.

In the breast, scirrhus [$\Sigma\kappa\iota\rho\rho\grave{o}\varsigma$ = indurated] is found as an
infiltration affecting part or the whole of the mammary gland. The
diseased mass is extremely hard, correspondingly heavy, and in-
elastic; while the increase in size is no tgreat, for the part of the
gland affected is frequently not much larger than it was in health.
The nipple gets gradually drawn in, while the surrounding areola
is also somewhat retracted; though these events are not peculiar to
mammary cancer, for I have seen them produced by simple inflammation of the gland tissue. After a variable period, the tumour
with the proper tissues of the breast in contact with its surface,
and the skin which is often adherent to it, ulcerate; a foul and
excavated and spreading sore, with everted edges, being formed,
from which there is a constant sanious discharge, and very often
sharp attacks of hæmorrhage. The ulceration sometimes extends from the skin inwards; sometimes from the substance of
the cancer outwards. The amount of suffering varies; occasionally the pain being comparatively slight, though generally it is
severe and lancinating, and consequently most exhausting.

As the local mischief advances, so the health fails; while the cancerous cachexia becomes fully established. The disease spreads to
the lymphatic vessels and glands in the axilla. Secondary cancerous deposits, which are more frequently of the nature of encephaloid than scirrhus, may occur in almost every tissue of the body.
They are most common in the pleuræ, lungs, liver, glands of the
mesentery, bronchial glands, and long bones. The state of the
patient is pitiable. Together with great bodily suffering, the mind
is harassed at the knowledge of the distressing nature of the
malady. At night there is hectic fever, with dry skin and parched
mouth. Without narcotics sleep is impossible. Attacks of nausea

and vomiting are common and urgent. There is often a tickling cough. The emaciation increases daily. The countenance is not only pale and anxious, but it presents a slight leaden hue; while the features have become pinched, and the lips and nostrils slightly livid. Pains, constant and worrying like those of rheumatism, extend over the body, especially to the back and lower part of the spine; the hips and shoulders being also the seat of wearying aches. As the pressure of the enlarged axillary glands obstructs the circulation through the arm, so the whole extremity swells to a surprising degree. Lying by the patient's side, supported on a pillow, this limb is as useless as a log of wood—indeed it is only a painful incumbrance. Care has to be taken to prevent bed-sores. All appetite has long ceased; though there is often much thirst. The force of the circulation diminishes almost hourly. There is forsooth life, but then it is life encumbered with everything that is undesirable. At length, the looked for release draws nigh. Not unfrequently, death happens a few days earlier than is expected; either owing to a sudden increase of the exhaustion, or from thrombosis, or from suppression of urine and uræmia. With other instances, the sufferings are increased by the setting in of pleurisy and accompanying effusion, or of pneumonia. But most commonly the system seems to be thoroughly worn out; a short period of freedom from pain and misery ensues—without loss of consciousness; and then a calm sleep follows, from which there is no waking on this earth.

Scirrhus of the breast is very rare in men. The only example which has been under my charge, so far as can be recollected, was in a gentleman sixty-eight years of age; whose mother and two sisters had died of mammary cancer. The disease occurs in women most frequently between the ages of forty-five and fifty.

Records, made by Mr. Paget,* of 139 cases of scirrhus of the breast, watched to their conclusions, or to their survivals beyond the average duration, give the following results:—In 75 not submitted to operation, the average duration of life, after the patient's first observation of the disease, has been 48 months. In 64 submitted to operation, and surviving its immediate consequences, the corresponding average has been a little more than 52 months. The longest duration of life, in the former class, has been 216 months; in the latter class, 146: the shortest in the former was 7 months; in the latter 7½.

B. MEDULLARY, OR SOFT CANCER.—Medullary [*Medulla* = pith or marrow], or encephaloid ['Εγκέφαλος = the brain], or cerebriform [*Cerebrum* = the brain + *forma* = a model] cancers are of two kinds —soft and firm; the former being the most frequent. In either condition they are found in about equal proportion as separable tumours, or as infiltrations. As *separable* tumours, when occurring in the testicle, the breast, the eye, the intermuscular and other spaces in the limbs; as *infiltrations*, when occupying the

* *The Lancet.* London, 19 January 1856.

substance of the uterus, the alimentary canal, the serous membranes, and the bones. The course of both varieties in their fatal career is rapid; the average duration of life, from the patient's first observation of the disease, being little more than two years. Moreover, they occur at an earlier age than other kinds of cancer, being sometimes met with before puberty. The *soft medullary tumours* are commonly round or oval; and present to the touch a sense as of the fluctuation of some thick fluid, so that the most experienced practitioners are often deceived. Such growths are very vascular; the material composing them resembles brain substance, partially decomposed and broken up; they yield abundance of cancer juice on being pressed or scraped; and they frequently contain extravasated blood. The *firm medullary cancers*, on the other hand, are elastic and tense, but not presenting the stony hardness of scirrhus. In their shape and size they resemble the soft variety. They are also found to possess distinct investing capsules, or they may extend into the substance of organs.

Medullary cancer of the breast is so rare in this country that, even in our museums, specimens are but seldom seen: on the Continent, however, this form appears to be more common. The lymphatic glands are much more frequently primarily affected with medullary cancer than with scirrhus.

a. *Epithelial Cancer, or Cancroid Epithelioma.*—Some difference of opinion exists as to whether this disease is really a form of cancer; or whether it is not an affection *sui generis*, consisting of an infiltration of cells of scaly epithelium, with a serous liquid different from cancer juice. Hence some authors (Hannover) speak of it as "epithelioma;" others (Alibert) as "cancroid;" while others again (Paget) describe it as epithelial* cancer. In its clinical history, it certainly resembles cancer; inasmuch as it returns after being removed by operation, it is prone to incurable ulceration, it affects the lymphatics seated near it, and it ultimately destroys the patient. On the other hand, it is peculiar in two respects—it is very little liable to multiplication in internal organs, and it appears often to be produced by local causes only. As pathologists seem divided upon this question, it will be better to treat of it in this place, as if it were undoubtedly a true form of cancer; a plan which has the unfortunate recommendation of being probably correct, while it is certainly convenient.

The disease is generally located in or beneath some portion of skin, or of mucous membrane; especially upon those parts of the latter which most closely approach the skin in structure, as the lips, eyelids, prepuce, vulva, &c. The most common seats consequently are the lower lip, the tongue, the larynx, the nymphæ, the labia majora, the glans penis and prepuce, and the cervix and lips of the uterus.

* From 'Επὶ = upon + θηλὴ = the nipple. Properly, therefore, the epidermis of the nipple; but now used generally for the layers of cells forming the cuticle.

Formerly, it often attacked the scrotum of chimney-sweeps; but since the Act of Parliament made the use of machinery imperative, the soot-wart has been less frequently seen. Epithelial cancer, wherever and however produced, may commence as a warty growth, or as a slight induration which speedily ulcerates. In the former case, its growth is comparatively slow; in the latter, it makes rapid progress, the ulceration extending in all directions, and destroying every tissue (even bone) which it meets with. The lymphatics become involved; and then gradually the chief symptoms of the cancerous cachexia manifest themselves. Its origin appears sometimes traceable to the irritation of soot, to that set up by the use of a clay pipe without a varnished mouth-piece, to that caused by retained secretions under the prepuce—as in phimosis, &c. Moreover, cases have been recorded which seem to show that a simple wart or pimple, when constantly picked or fretted, may undergo development into epithelial cancer. But it would be premature to assert, at present, that these causes are alone sufficient to excite the disease. That they can set it up when there exists a constitutional tendency to cancer is granted. And very possibly they may do more: only, this point has yet to be proved.

True "cauliflower-excrescence of the uterus" is, in all probability, always a variety of epithelial cancer. Commencing on the surface of the labia uteri in the form of small papillary or villous eminences, these elevations by their gradual growth and expansion and branching take on the peculiar cauliflower appearance. It is a rare disease; so much so, that during the six years I was physician to the Hospital for Women, there came under my care—according to the observations which I have recorded—59 cases of carcinoma of the uterus amongst the out-patients, only one of which was an example of cauliflower excrescence; the remaining 58 being instances of medullary cancer, or of scirrhus, or more frequently of epithelial cancer not assuming the appearance of an excrescence.

Care must be taken to distinguish epithelial cancer from rodent ulcer and from lupus. *Rodent ulcer* has generally a somewhat circular shape, with indurated margins; and it gradually spreads in all directions. It most frequently attacks the eyelids, next to these parts the nose or cheeks, and very rarely the auricle of the ear; while in some cases it has occurred on the vulva, and in other regions. Then it does not affect the lymphatic glands; it does not destroy life, or only does so very slowly; and the general health is not injured for a long time unless there be pain or hæmorrhage. This ulcer occurs about the middle period of life, equally in both sexes; and it can be permanently cured. If a portion of the edge of the sore be minutely examined, it will be found to consist of fibrous tissue, and not of cell-structures. As regards *lupus* it is to be recollected that it commences frequently by the formation of a dull red tubercle, which has its seat most often on the ala or tip of the nose; the resulting ulceration is slow, it is superficial, only involving the skin, and its edges are not indurated; it seldom commences after the middle period of life; and it has a great tendency to heal spontaneously.

Epithelial cancer occurs much oftener in the male than in the female sex, and is most common after the age of 50. When once established it gradually progresses to the destruction of life, but more slowly than medullary cancer; rather less than four years being the average duration of life from the commencement. The degree of malignancy seems greater when the disease is seated on the tongue or on the penis, than when on the scrotum or the lower extremities. Moreover, the removal of the affected part by operation probably gives a better chance of recovery than the excision of any other variety of carcinoma. The essential character of this disease may be said to be, that it is composed of cells of epithelium and their nuclei. The cells vary in size and shape; and are infiltrated, together with a juice or serous fluid, into the interstices of the affected tissues.

b. Colloid Cancer.—This variety of disease—to which the names of colloid [Κόλλα = glue], alveolar [*Alveolus* = a little trench], cystic [Κύστις = a bladder], and gelatiniform [*Gelatina + forma*] cancer have been applied—consists of a clear viscid substance somewhat resembling soft gelatine or gum. Its most frequent primary seats are the stomach, intestinal canal, omentum, and peritoneum; though it sometimes invades the breast, the glands of the neck, or the periosteum of the long bones. Secondarily, it affects the lymphatic glands, lungs, &c. A section of a colloid cancer presents to the naked eye a clear, soft, gelatinous mass, intersected and surrounded by tough fibrous-looking tissue; the intersections, when numerous, forming small cysts or cavities filled with colloid matter. Such a cancer often attains considerable size. Thus, in the Museum of King's College there is a preparation showing a tumour of this nature, connected with the omentum, as large as a cocoa-nut. The disease probably always occurs as an infiltration, superseding the natural tissues of the affected part as it grows. It occurs equally in both sexes; it is very rare in children; and in its progress and symptoms it corresponds with other cancers, save that it less frequently ulcerates.

Colloid matter may form independently of cancer, as happens sometimes in the thyroid gland in bronchocele, and in some multilocular ovarian tumours. The latter often attain an immense size; but they may be removed by operation without any fear of the return of the disease.

c. Melanoid Cancer.—Melanotic [Μελανόω = to grow black], melanic, or black cancer, is generally medullary cancer modified by the superaddition of a black pigment. Scirrhus sometimes becomes associated with melanosis, and still more rarely epithelioma does so.

d. Osteoid Cancer.—The nature of osteoid ['Οστέον = a bone] cancers may be best expressed, according to Mr. Paget, by calling them ossified fibrous or medullary cancers; and by regarding them as illustrating a calcareous or osseous degeneration. Their growth is usually from some bone, and especially from the lower part of the femur. Their general history corresponds to that of the scirrhus and medullary varieties of cancer. They are as malignant and as quickly fatal as the medullary; and they give rise to secondary deposits in the connective tissue, lymphatics, lungs, &c.

e. *Hæmatoid Cancer.*—Hæmatoid [Αἷμα = blood + εἶδος = form] cancer—fungus hæmatodes—is probably a soft medullary or other cancer, the substance of which has become more or less infiltrated with blood. When it protrudes through the skin it forms a large vascular mass, somewhat resembling a clot of blood. As can be imagined, while ulceration goes on the attacks of hæmorrhage are frequent and frightful.

There are certain *sanguineous cancerous tumours*, which on account of their rarity have hardly received the attention they merit. These growths are rich in bloodvessels, and in splenoid tissue analogous to the placenta. Most of them are situated in or near the bones, they are very vascular and often pulsatile, and they look like a piece of spleen or of raw soddened meat. They recur after extirpation, while generally their growth is rapid. I have seen only one instance of this form of malignant disease; and in this case the tumour grew into the cavity of the mouth from the side of the lower jaw. It was removed by Sir William Fergusson, but soon returned. Again it was excised, but how far this last operation proved successful I do not know.

f. *Villous Cancer.*—Villous [*Villus* = shaggy hair] cancer is a variety of medullary and perhaps of epithelial cancer, occurring most frequently on the mucous membrane of the urinary bladder. The histories of cases of this disease coincide with those of medullary cancers.

3. CAUSES OF CANCER.—With regard to the causes of this disease but little is known. All classes of society are equally subject to it; the rich and poor, the idle and industrious, the gay and the melancholy, all suffering from it in equal proportions. The only probable predisposing causes may be thus stated: (1) Descent from a phthisical parent, as will again be referred to. (2) Descent from a cancerous parent. Lebert traced an hereditary tendency in about one-seventh of a certain number of cases: Sibley found it in 8¾ per cent. (3) Age. The greater proportion of cases by far, in men, occur between the 55th and 65th years. in women, between the 45th and 55th. Under maturity, cancer is rare in both sexes. (4) Sex; for the disease is twice as common in women as in men. (5) Child-bearing; for out of 92 cases of uterine cancer, the histories of which I published in 1863, no less than 80 had borne children. Of these, one was the mother of "several" children; while the others had had 497 pregnancies amongst them, or an average of about 6¼ to each. This is at least 2¼ above the proportion in England. And (6) although cancer is not contagious in the ordinary sense of the term, yet there are some grounds for entertaining an opinion that if fresh cancer cells be introduced into the blood, they may be deposited and propagate themselves. Dr. Druitt says,—"The experiment has been tried on dogs by Langenbeck and by Lebert; and cancerous tumours were found in various parts, when the animals were killed some time afterwards; yet it must be remembered that some of the tumours found in these cases may have existed before the inoculation."[*] The experiment of Langenbeck, however, was carefully repeated by Vogel, but without producing the same result; while Gluge also failed in his attempts at inoculation.

A fair consideration of the foregoing shows, that our knowledge of the causes of cancer is very slender. In the great majority of cases the patient is unable in any way to account for its origin. Very frequently, in scirrhus of the breast especially, the tumour is only discovered by accident. And it is almost certain, that mental anxiety, peculiar temperaments, particular occupations, injuries, &c., have nothing to do with producing the cancerous diathesis. Tubercle is deposited in the most active organs; cancer, on the contrary, attacks an injured or weak part. Hence it not unfrequently seems to follow a blow, or an attack of inflammation. For many years past, in listening to the histories of patients afflicted with cancer of the uterus, I have been struck with the frequency with which they have told me of the loss of one or more of their relatives from phthisis. My attention having been thus excited, careful enquiries have been made in all the cases of carcinoma which have come under my observation. And the result has been, that I have much less frequently been able to trace a hereditary tendency to this disease, than to phthisis. Sometimes where the father or mother has died of phthisis, one or more of the children have suffered similarly, and one or more from cancer. I have had under my care, at the same time, a young man of the age of 24 with tubercular disease of the lungs, while his sister has been my patient with cancer of the breast: these two being the only offspring of a mother who had died of inherited phthisis at the age of thirty, but whose father was alive and healthy. This proneness to cancer in the offspring of tubercular parents has also been noticed by Mr. Zachariah Laurence, who seems rather inclined to entertain the opinion that there may be some connexion between the two diseases. At all events he says that of 40 patients, the subjects of scirrhus or encephaloid, 15 knew of one or more blood-relations having died from phthisis.[†] Mr. Weeden Cooke has pushed the enquiry much further. From his experience he believes that phthisical parents

---

[*] *The Surgeon's Vade Mecum.* Seventh Edition, p. 112. London, 1856.
[†] *The Diagnosis of Surgical Cancer.* Second Edition, p. 62. London, 1858.

beget cancerous offspring, while cancerous parents have phthisical children.* An examination of the histories of 79 examples of cancer of the breast which have been under this gentleman's observation shows, that three-eighths of these cases occurred in persons having phthisical relatives.

4. **TREATMENT OF CANCER.**—The treatment of cancer is at present, as far as I positively know, in just the same unsatisfactory condition as was that of phthisis only a few years ago. But inasmuch as we have sure grounds for believing that well-defined cases of pulmonary consumption, which would have been regarded as utterly incurable a few years since, are now sometimes restored to health by the aid of medicine ; so we have every reason to trust that at no distant day cancer may be made to yield to some remedy, or combination of remedies, yet to be discovered. In the meantime very much may be done to relieve the patient's sufferings, and to prolong life.

PALLIATIVE TREATMENT.—The great point is to keep up the constitutional powers to as near the standard of health as the disease will allow ; which can best be done by tonics, nourishing food, pure air, warm clothing, great cleanliness, removal of offensive discharges, mental occupation, and by preventing or relieving pain. In carrying out this important indication the physician will not only be deservedly earning the gratitude of his patient, but he may likewise, by kindness and judicious advice, be preventing him from consulting those callous charlatans who will make the most solemn assertions of their ability to cure him, until he either sinks into the grave, or has expended every guinea that he possesses. Moreover, it is the positive duty of the practitioner to make every effort to give even temporary relief. The remark of Bacon, though of universal application, should have especial weight here. He says,—" I esteem it the office of a physician not only to restore health, but to mitigate pain and dolors, and not only when such mitigation may conduce to recovery, but when it may serve to make a fair and easy passage."

The best course to pursue, in addition to adopting all those generally known hygienic measures for the maintenance of health, is to do all that is possible to relieve pain ; to improve the blood by tonics and nutritious food ; and to check the growth of the cancer and the contamination of the system by suitable remedies.

First, *as to the Relief of Pain.*—This is a most important object ; inasmuch as the great bane of cancer, next to its tendency to destroy life, is the acute physical suffering to which it gives rise. And not only is this so, but it is certain that the more intense the pain, the more rapidly will the patient succumb. Many practitioners appear insufficiently impressed with these facts ; and they hesitate to effect a certain good by the proper administration

* *On Cancer : its Allies and Counterfeits,* p. 85. London, 1865.

of sedatives, lest they should check the secretions, destroy the appetite, or produce other doubtful evils. So much benefit, however, has resulted from the free use of anodynes in my hands, that a reconsideration of this subject cannot be too strongly urged. Drugs of this class have a most favourable influence upon the mind as well as on the body ; while they enable us to prolong life, by rendering that life bearable. Moreover, the more carefully the phenomena of this disease have been studied at the bed-side, the more probable it has appeared to me that if a cure for cancer be ultimately discovered, it will be found amongst agents possessing narcotic properties. On one point I feel certain, that the irritation of malignant ulcerations by caustics and astringents is most injurious in every way, while the application of soothing remedies is just as beneficial. In making this remark it is necessary to explain that I am not referring so much to the total destruction of cancerous growths by potential escharotics, as to their irritation by the superficial application of these agents. And, if we think of the matter, it cannot but seem probable that nothing is so likely to increase cell-growth as stimulation and heat. If we take cancer of the uterus, for example, in whatever stage the disease may be, the local use of nitrate of silver, of acid solution of nitrate of mercury, of lotions containing bromine or iodine, or of caustic potash can only prove irritating and set up bleeding or other mischief. On the contrary, sedatives employed to the seat of disease are of great service. A compound of opium, conium, and belladonna is invaluable. These agents, mixed together with sufficient oil of theobroma, can be readily applied by the patient herself, in the form of a pessary (F. 423).

The mode in which the narcotic is administered is a matter of no little moment. As a general rule, I believe the least efficient plan is to give it by the mouth ; but if *opium* be prescribed in this way, I would recommend the extract to be used in the form of pills, in preference to any other preparation (F. 343). Frequently it will be better, in order to avoid producing constipation, to give this drug in combination with belladonna (F. 344). The dose at first should be small ; but week by week it must be increased, as the system gets gradually accustomed to it. In this way, large quantities at length become needed ; but I have never seen anything but good from even such an amount as twenty-five or thirty grains in the course of the twenty-four hours. *Morphia* can also be given by the mouth ; either in the form of pills (F. 343), or in combination with chloroform and Indian hemp and ether and hydrocyanic acid, &c. (F. 315, 317). But of all the methods for exhibiting the agents under consideration no one plan is so valuable as the *subcutaneous injection of morphia*. By this process the most complete and speedy relief is afforded ; generally with the great advantage of not deranging the stomach. Considerable caution, however, is necessary with the first injections, even when the

patient has been taking morphia by the mouth for some time;
and certainly it will be advisable for the practitioner to feel his
way by commencing with only a small dose—one-third or a quarter
of a grain.   The reason for such care being needed is the fact, that
while none of the morphia can be lost it is at once absorbed :
whereas, when introduced into the stomach this drug gets diluted
with the gastric fluids, and probably is not completely taken into
the system for an hour or more.   In some instances one injection
in the twenty-four hours will suffice to ensure a good night's rest,
with a comfortable calm day; but in others it has to be repeated
every twelve hours (F. 314).   *Aconite* and *atropine* may be employed
in the same way, though if possible with greater precautions.   The
exhibition of one or two minims of the officinal liquor atropiæ
sulphatis (min. 1 = gr. ₁₀₀ of the salt), mixed with the solution of
morphia, not only increases the efficacy of the latter as a destroyer
of pain, but causes a more refreshing sleep than the morphia alone.
Next in value to hypodermic injections I would place *enemata*, or
suppositories; for making which the extract or liquid extract of
opium, or the solution of morphia, had best be employed (F. 339,
340).   There may be cases where *conium* or *henbane* can be advantageously administered; but usually these anodynes, unless combined with opium, have seemed to me very uncertain and inefficient.
    Secondly, *the improvement of the blood by tonics and nutritious
food* has to be considered.   With reference to tonics none are generally so beneficial as the various preparations of *bark*.   The compound tincture of cinchona, or the tincture of yellow cinchona, or
the liquid extract of yellow cinchona, in full doses, may be recommended; either of these restoratives being combined with ammonia
or ether (F. 371), or with the mineral acids (F. 376) where there
is any tendency to hæmorrhage or to night sweats.   *Ferruginous
tonics* seem seldom to agree so well as the bark, but there is often
no objection to employing both.   Thus, a draught with acetic acid
and cinchona or quinine can be given night and morning ; while
the reduced iron, or the ammonio-citrate of iron, or steel wine, or
some similar preparation, can be administered during dinner in the
middle of the day (F. 380, 394, &c.).   *Cod liver oil* is frequently
very useful (F. 389); proving a valuable adjunct as a kind of food.
Where its use is indicated but the stomach rejects it, attempts
must be made to procure proper digestion by the simultaneous
administration of *Pepsine* (F. 420).
    As regards *diet*, only the most nutritious food should be allowed.
Wine, beer, milk, whey, cream, raw eggs, broths and soups, fish
and other animal food, are all necessary (F. 1, 2, 3, 5, 15, 17, &c.).
And where there is so poor an appetite that but small quantities
of these matters can be taken, it will often be advantageous to use
some of them as enemata (F. 21, 22, 23).   Under these circumstances, the opium already recommended had better be mixed with
the nourishment ; so as to avoid teazing the patient with more injec-

tions than are absolutely needed. At the same time it is to be recollected, that though the appetite be bad, there is generally a desire for fluids. Taking advantage of this, I am in the habit of ordering large quantities of good milk. When it seems apt to turn acid on the stomach, it will be as well to give it with soda or Vichy or lime water (F. 14). The addition of a lump of ice to each tumblerful makes this mixture agreeable, as well as grateful to the irritable stomach.

Thirdly, *we have to try and check the growth of the cancer and the contamination of the system.* And here it must be confessed that our ignorance is great, for we know of no mineral or vegetable product which possesses the required power. Iodide of potassium, iodine, mercury, iodide of lead, bromide of potassium, bromine, iodide of iron, iodide of arsenic, arsenious acid, puccoon, and a host of similar remedies have been tried only with the result of proving their worthlessness. It seems indeed like the labour of Sisyphus to continue the employment of such agents. They do no real good, to say the least ; and it is to be regretted that their use cannot be emphatically and finally condemned. Unfortunately nothing much more promising can be suggested ; but the medicines which have appeared to me more nearly to fulfil our purpose than any others are *belladonna* and *acetic acid* in combination. A more extended experience is required before it can be right to speak of these agents with greater confidence. I commenced the use of belladonna unwillingly, because it was long since recommended, and was not thought to exert much influence for good. But in moderate doses, continued for several months, it has certainly been very serviceable in my hands ; its utility having been augmented by giving it with full doses of acetic acid. And I would especially recommend that when a cancerous growth has been removed by excision or caustic, the patient should perseveringly take the belladonna and acid for a very long time afterwards. Made into a mixture with bark or quinine or cascarilla (F. 376, 383), we have an excellent tonic ; while the combination appears to have the power of moderating abnormal cell-growth.

By many, the preceding remarks will be deemed somewhat disheartening. But in the present state of medical science, the practitioner must be content to give relief to bodily suffering, and to afford mental tranquillity ; without expecting to effect a cure of this fearful disease. It is in no slight degree gratifying to be able to accomplish only as much as this. And therefore while striving to increase our knowledge, let us remember that if the foregoing remedies be carefully and perseveringly used, peace of mind with bodily ease will be given ; and thus life may be prolonged even for a few years.*

* As illustrative of the correctness of these observations, the following case may be related :—Mary Stanning, thirty-two years of age, married but never pregnant, came under my care at the Farringdon Dispensary, on the 20 March 1851, suffering from scirrhus of the rectum. Finding that I could not cure her, she applied and was admitted into one of our metropolitan hos-

CURATIVE TREATMENT.—In attempts to effect a cure, one of three plans has usually been followed: viz., either complete and thorough excision; removal by the use of potential caustics; or the promotion of absorption by methodical compression, sometimes combined with the application of intense cold.

First, *as to Excision.*—A general opinion can only be formed with great difficulty, since the views of surgeons on this head are much divided. Still I think there are few who will deny, that as a rule, extirpation by the knife is quite insufficient to effect a cure. The operation may relieve the local distress, and will probably prolong life for a few months; while as the use of an anæsthetic renders the proceeding painless, it may perhaps occasionally be worth while resorting to it to gain these objects. Nevertheless, on the other hand, it must not be forgotten that the operation itself will possibly prove fatal; while in some cases it certainly appears to increase the malignity of the disease. Thus, Dr. Walshe points out that " excision of a cancerous tumour seems to awaken a dormant force. Cancers spring up in all directions, and enlarge with a power of vegetation almost incredible." Again, of the cases of cancer of the tongue which have been described by authors, the most frightful are those where the disease has returned after operation. Thus Mr. Weeden Cooke says that " the disease reappears with intense malignity, not only in the tongue itself, but in all the neighbouring glands. The tongue sloughs more rapidly and bleeds profusely, the glands enlarge to an enormous size, interfering with the powers of deglutition; they then ulcerate, and discharge serum, or pus, or blood, rapidly destroying the patient by a hideous death. This is the rule in patients operated on: it is the exception in cases treated only constitutionally." With regard to the *time* at which, if an operation be determined upon, it should be performed, authorities differ. Some surgeons recommend excision when the disease is first discovered; others, as I think erroneously, advise delay. Mr. Spencer Wells, in laying down some precepts as to the use of the knife, observes—" It is not to use it in the early stages of cancer, not to use it unless the cancer is actually ulcerated, or growing so fast that the skin is about to give way. In such cases, especially where an open cancer gives

pitals, which she left in an apparently dying state in April 1852. On the 28 of the same month I was sent for; and found her very low, and as if she could not live many hours. The eminent surgeon under whose treatment she had been in the hospital wrote to say that he had heard M. S. was under my care, that she was dying, and that he would like to be present at the postmortem examination. By attendance to the hygienic rules laid down in the text; by the occasional exhibition of bark, of steel, and other tonics; by the employment of wine and nourishing food; and by the daily use of large quantities of opium, this patient slowly improved. She was able to get about, to keep her rooms clean, &c.; and although her sufferings at times were acute, yet she generally was tolerably free from pain until the last few weeks of her life. She died on the 18 June 1856.

great pain, and is wearing away the patient by bleeding or profuse fœtid discharge, the knife is used in the hope of relieving suffering, and prolonging not saving life. In some other cases, where a cancer causes great mental anxiety to a patient, you may remove it at her earnest entreaty, after explaining fairly the danger of relapse."* Now knowing with what difficulties this subject is surrounded, it is necessary to speak with considerable diffidence of the views of others. But it does not strike me that these rules are those which ought to be generally followed by the profession, and I am not even sure that Mr. Wells adopts them. However this may be, my own opinion is that excision can only be resorted to with any prospect of success if the tumour be small and comparatively circumscribed, if the lymphatics be unaffected, if the skin and muscles be non-adherent, and if the cancerous cachexia be not developed. And even in these cases, it is necessary that a free dissection be made; at the same time removing, if possible, a portion of the adjacent texture, which though it look sound to the naked eye may yet contain a few cancer cells or their nuclei. It must also be doubted whether it is advantageous to procure union of the wound by the first intention ; for many of those cases which have remained healthy during a more than ordinary length of time after operation, have had profuse suppuration set up by it. Moreover, the patient ought not to be lost sight of for many months afterwards ; for whether removal be effected by the knife or by caustics, it will be advisable, as before recommended, to administer belladonna, and to attend to the diet, &c.

While speaking of the knife it had better be mentioned, that several attempts have been made to destroy malignant tumours by lowering their nutrition ; with which object practitioners have tied the chief nutrient artery of the affected part. No real success has attended these efforts. Nor could it well be expected, remembering how readily the collateral circulation would be established after the operation. Section of the principal nerve going to the diseased structure has also been had recourse to, chiefly in the hope of relieving pain.

Secondly, *as to Removal by Caustics.*—This method has found both advocates and opponents in the present day; the latter class probably being the most numerous. Be that as it may, however, the process certainly possesses many important advantages. Thus, if properly employed, there is not the least danger to life ; I have never known it to be followed either by erysipelas or pyæmia ; while it may be found beneficial in deeply ulcerated, and some other cancers, where the knife is objectionable. My own experience with this plan of extirpating scirrhus and medullary tumours of the breast has been gradually increasing during the past few years, and the more I see of the practice the greater is my opinion of its merits. It frequently

* On Cancer Cures and Cancer Curers. *The Medical Times and Gazette.* London, 11 July 1857.

does not prevent the disease returning, but then it allows each recurring growth to be destroyed before attaining any size.* The

* As examples, I quote the following from my case books :—Mrs. S. æt. 47. 13 *June* 1864. Clin. Med. v. 57. Has a scirrhus of left breast, the size of a fowl's egg. Catamenia only been on twice in last 20 years. Palliative treatment failing to retard growth, I removed the tumour on the 25 March 1865, after about seventeen daily applications of the saturated solution of acid sulphate of zinc (F. 198). From the 24 *Feb.* 1865 until the 8 *Feb.* 1866, a pill of quinine and belladonna and conium was taken twice daily. On the latter date, I reapplied the caustic to a swelling the size of a bean which had formed in the cicatrix. In a few days it came away : the pill was still to be continued. On the 9 *May* another small growth had appeared which was again attacked with caustic. The pill was replaced by a mixture of citric acid with bark. On 6 *July*, I found the disease returning in the nipple. As it increased it was removed with caustic, the wound being nearly healed by October. In *December* she was ordered a mixture of belladonna, acetic acid, and bark. On the 1 *Feb.* 1867, there was another growth in the old cicatrix, and caustic was applied ; while at the end of *October* two small tumours were found, which were removed as before. From this time, all has gone on well. There has been no return of the complaint. The cicatrix is soft and supple. She says (6 *November* 1868) that she is quite well, and her appearance confirms her statement. The mixture has been taken continuously for twenty-three months, and she is not to give it up yet.

Mrs. G. æt. 59. 25 *November* 1864. Clin. Med. v. 239. Has a soft medullary cancer of right breast, as large as an orange. As she could get no relief, she submitted to its removal by the caustic, as in previous instance, on 11 *March* 1865. So deep was the growth, that the cartilages of two of the ribs where they join the sternum became exposed. All did well, however. Belladonna was taken in a pill until 8 *March* 1867, when it was discontinued as she felt quite well and the cicatrix was healthy and soft. On 2 *July* 1868 this patient continued well.

Mrs. P. æt. 52. 28 *July* 1865. Clin. Med. 3276. Scirrhus of left breast, which has been growing rapidly since first discovered six months ago. The zinc caustic was first applied on 20 August. Tumour came away on 4 September. On 14 *July* 1867 she remained perfectly well, and had just married for the second time. The cicatrix was barely to be distinguished.

Mrs. G. æt. 47. 20 *October* 1865. Clin. Med. v. 478. Has a movable scirrhus of right breast. Caustic was applied daily for about twelve times : on 14 *November* the tumour was loose in the poultice. 12 *June* 1868, I found two or three little tubercles in the old cicatrix. Has been taking acetic acid, belladonna, and bark since 7 December 1866 ; and is to continue doing so, together with cod liver oil. On 31 *October* 1868, it was remarked that the tubercles are no larger : no pain. General health better than it was three months back. Is continuing the mixture and oil.

Miss W. æt. 21. 10 *June* 1864. Clin. Med. v. 501. Has a very solid tumour, size of a walnut, in right breast. Is very nervous, as her mother's sister died of cancer of uterus. 30 *November* 1865, I found the tumour as hard as a stone, larger, tender to the touch, and the seat of occasional shooting pains. On 16 *December* 1865, the tumour came away, after seven daily applications of zinc caustic. Belladonna (gr. ¼) was ordered daily, and taken for some months. 10 *September* 1868, she told me that she was and long had been perfectly well. Cicatrix supple and healthy.

Mrs. H. æt. 49. 7 *December* 1866. Clin. Med. 3882. Ulcerated medullary cancer of right breast. An eminent hospital surgeon has told her that she "has a very bad cancer, for which nothing can be done." 29 *December*, tumour came away, after five very free applications of the zinc caustic. On 1 *April* 1867 my report says that the caustic has had to be applied to some small cancerous nodules : the slough came away to-day. General health has greatly improved. *March* 1868, my notes say that last month, two or three

chief agents which have been tried are the arsenical pastes, chloride of zinc, chloride of bromium, sulphate of zinc, manganese cum potassâ, the strong mineral acids, and the concentrated alkalies. The *arsenical pastes* cannot be employed without great caution, inasmuch as their action is not merely local but pervades the whole system. M. Manec, of the Salpétrière Hospital in Paris, has largely used them; for he believes that arsenic has a peculiar destructive affinity for cancerous growths, and that its action does not extend to healthy tissues. His formula—perhaps the best one which can be tried, consists of one part of arsenious acid to seven or eight of cinnabar, with four of burnt sponge, made into a paste with a few drops of water. He does not employ it to a surface of greater extent than the size of an English florin at each application; and he states that the quantity of arsenic absorbed from such a surface never produces unpleasant symptoms. Should severe pain arise, it will be mitigated by applying bladders of ice and salt. Dr. Marsden was in the habit of using an arsenical mucilage (F. 199); and I believe that he placed considerable reliance on its efficacy.

The *chloride of zinc* is a valuable agent, especially as there can be little to fear from its absorption. The epidermis must first be destroyed by a blister or by strong nitric acid; and the caustic is then to be applied (mixed according to F. 197), in quantity varying with the amount of destruction required. Dr. Fell's plan of treatment consists in the use of the chloride of zinc, combined with a perennial plant known among the North American Indians by the name of puccoon, but described by botanists—owing to the bloodlike juice which exudes from it when cut—as the Sanguinaria Canadensis (F. 197). The chloride of zinc is the essential agent, however, and this creates a superficial slough; which slough is daily scored to a certain depth by several incisions with the knife, strips of linen covered with the caustic being afterwards laid in the furrows. At each dressing, the tumour is destroyed deeper and deeper; until at length it becomes converted into a large eschar, which separates by a line of demarcation according to the general principles of surgery. Together with this local application, the general health is attended to; a nourishing and sustaining diet is allowed; and the puccoon is administered thrice daily in half-grain doses. Frequently also, Dr. Fell combines with this

suspicious tubercles were found about the old cicatrix. They were easily destroyed: wound healed, and looks quite healthy. 4 *September* 1868, remains well. Has been taking a mixture of acetic acid, belladonna, and bark since beginning of treatment; and is still to persevere with it. Has become quite stout.

The foregoing are a few of what may be called successful cases. In addition, I have more recent instances which seem to be going on well. Contrariwise, I could quote others, where the same line of treatment has failed completely to save life. It is distinctly to be understood, however, that I am not recommending any infallible practice; but only one which frequently prolongs existence, which occasionally leads to a restoration to health lasting for some years, and which has no serious disadvantage beyond producing pain that can be considerably mitigated by subcutaneous injections of morphia and atropine.

drug the sixteenth of a grain of iodide of arsenic, and one grain of conium.

The *chloride of bromium* has been highly praised by Landolfi, who uses it made into a paste with flour, or combined with other caustics (F. 197). The proper method of applying the paste is on a piece of linen cut to the size of the part to be destroyed. At the end of twenty-four hours the rag is removed; the slough separates after a few days; and the sore is then dressed with charpie soaked in a solution of chloride of bromium—grs. 10 to 20 in water fl. oz. 12. The patient takes a pill morning and evening, containing one-tenth of a grain of the chloride. I have tried this plan in one instance of cancer uteri; but while the local disease seemed to be much diminished by it, the patient died with all the constitutional symptoms unrelieved.

The anhydrous *sulphate of zinc* has been strongly recommended by Sir James Y. Simpson; who says, that when it is applied to an open and diseased surface it acts as a safe, most powerful, and manageable caustic. In these remarks I can entirely coincide. It may be employed in the form of a dry fine powder; or as a paste made with an ounce of the salt to fl. dr. j. of glycerine; or as an ointment—one ounce to 120 grs. of lard. When used in either way to an open or ulcerated surface, the part to which it is applied is rapidly destroyed to a depth corresponding to the thickness of the superimposed layer; the slough usually separates on the fifth or sixth day; and there is left behind, if the whole morbid tissue be removed, a red and granulating and healthy wound which rapidly cicatrizes. Until all the disease is destroyed, the applications must be repeated. The sulphate of zinc will only act as a caustic to a broken or open surface. Hence, when the epithelium is entire, this must be removed by a small blister, or by a strong acid, or by the supersulphate of zinc (F. 198). The application of the caustic gives rise to local pain and burning in most instances, but never to any marked constitutional disturbance.

The *manganese cum potassâ* is much used by Mr. Weeden Cooke in ulcerated cancer. It is said to be efficacious, causes but little pain, removes all unpleasant odour from the sore, and does not injure the general health. This agent may be employed as a powder, or made into a paste with water; while it must be applied in a layer as thick as the tissue to be destroyed. By means of carrot poultices the eschar is encouraged to drop off in three or four days; when, if necessary, the manganese is reapplied until the diseased mass is all destroyed. Then the subjacent healthy tissues are made to granulate and cicatrize by the aid of a slightly stimulating lotion of chlorate of potash. With regard to the *strong mineral acids* and the *concentrated alkalies* but little need be said. If the former be used, sulphuric acid, made into a paste with saffron, will prove the most efficacious: if the latter, the Vienna paste (F. 204).

Thirdly, there remains for consideration the plan which chiefly has for its object *the promotion of absorption by methodical com-*

pression, with or without the application of intense cold. Now pressure is supposed to act beneficially in cancer by diminishing the supply of blood, and hence of nourishment to the tumour; by depriving the cells of the space necessary for their growth; by injuring them from direct violence; and by promoting their absorption. Since compression was first proposed by Mr. Samuel Young, in 1809, numerous cases have been treated by it by different surgeons; and certainly the results seem to have been more favourable than those produced with many other modes. The pressure, however, must be methodically and perseveringly applied; the most unobjectionable method being by Dr. Neil Arnott's apparatus, which consists of a spring, an air-cushion, supported by a flat resisting frame or shield, with a pad and two belts. "The effects produced by pressure are," says Dr. Walshe, "removal of existing adhesions, total cessation of pain, disappearance of swelling in the communicating lymphatic glands, gradual reduction of bulky masses to small, hard, flat patches, or rounded nodules (which appear to be, both locally and generally, perfectly innocuous), and in the most favourable cases total removal of the morbid production. The relief of pain afforded by the instrument is, without exaggeration, almost marvellous; this effect being insured by the peculiar softness and other properties of the air-cushion, the medium through which the pressure of the spring is transmitted to the surface."*

The efficacy of intense cold depends on its arresting the circulation, producing some change in the microscopic cells, and in its altering the vitality of the part. Congelation not only gives relief from pain, but is said to suspend the progress of the disease; though its influence in the latter respect is generally allowed to be very slight. In cancer of the uterus, the frigorific mixture—equal parts of ice and salt, may be applied by means of a gutta percha speculum for fifteen or thirty minutes, once a day or even oftener. I have used it in a few instances only; for, although it was found to allay pain, yet it did not seem to possess the least potency as a means of cure.

XI. RODENT ULCER.

Rodent ulcer [*Rodo* = to gnaw] was first described by Dr. Jacob, of Dublin, as a "Peculiar ulcer of the Eyelids." It is sometimes spoken of as Lupoid ulcer; a term, however, which had better not be adopted, since it is liable to mislead. Equally unadvisable is it, in my opinion, to speak of the disease as rodent *cancer;* for the affection has none of the general or local characteristics of the true cancerous ulcer. Rodent ulcers are most frequently met with on the face; especially about the eyelids, or over the malar bone, or on the upper lip. They are also sometimes formed on the scalp, and at the vulva; while in more than one instance I have seen this disease on the lips of the uterus.

* *The Nature and Treatment of Cancer*, p. 211. London, 1846.

This peculiar ulcer generally has its origin in some small and irritable pimple; or less frequently in a wart, or an old cicatrix. The tendency to ulceration is manifested very slowly; or it should rather be said, that several months elapse between the commencement of the disease and the time when it starts actively upon its destructive course. The affection commonly begins by the ugly wart, or the cicatrix, cracking; or the surface of the pimple gets abraded. At all events, a little sanious discharge escapes and forms a thin scab. The irritation set up by this scab, slight though it be, leads to its being picked off. A patch of excoriation is thus disclosed; which again scabs, is again scratched off, and so on until a small ulcer is revealed. As this enlarges, it presents some singular features. Thus it is found to have hard and rounded and elevated margins, with an indurated and irregularly excavated floor; it slowly but steadily spreads in circumference, and to a less degree in depth; while from its uneven and somewhat glazed surface a scanty ichorous matter escapes, which is free from smell. There is very rarely any discharge of pus or blood: if pain be experienced it is seldom acute. The surrounding skin is natural. As the ulceration with its hardened wavy border extends, so it destroys every structure in its course. Skin, connective tissue, muscles, nerves, vessels, bones,—all seem to melt away before it. Hence the most frightful disfigurement results. No description is needed of the appearance which must follow from the destruction of the lip and gum and alveolar processes of the maxilla; or from the laying open of the nasal cavities; or from the erosion and exfoliation of the walls of the orbit, with the consequent collapse of the eye; or from the penetration of the disease through the skull to the membranes of the brain. All the time this serious mischief is gaining ground, the lymphatics and their glands remain healthy; or if the latter enlarge, they only do so to a slight extent owing to irritation or some accidental inflammation. Moreover, no similar disease springs up at other parts of the body. The general health is maintained too, in a surprising manner; so that until the last few months of life the patient's strength seems undiminished, he is able to eat and sleep well, and he could occupy himself in his accustomed duties were it not for the repulsiveness of his appearance. When death occurs, it is due to exhaustion; this being sometimes rapidly increased, towards the end, by attacks of hæmorrhage. The disease is rare before the fiftieth year: it occurs equally in both sexes.

When a rodent ulcer comes under treatment at such a stage that an operation is feasible, a permanent cure may be effected by complete excision. The same result can also be obtained by the use of potential caustics,—chloride of zinc, the supersaturated sulphate of zinc, potassa fusa, &c.; although great care must be taken to destroy every particle of affected tissue. Frequently, the caustic will have to be applied more than once; but there is no objection to this being done while the patient is under the influence of an anæsthetic, the subsequent pain being mitigated by the subcutaneous injection of morphia. The combination of excision with the transplantation of a healthy portion of skin from the forehead or other district, so as to prevent deformity, has produced excellent results in the hands of some surgeons.

XII. LUPUS.

By the word Lupus [*Lupus* = a wolf] is understood a spreading, tuberculated, inflammatory disease of the skin. It commences in the form of indolent little swellings or tubercles, which have a tendency to progress slowly to ulceration ; but whether these tubercles become absorbed, or whether they ulcerate, there is always left a permanent seamed scar. This unsightly affection occurs in those who have not reached the middle period of life,— mostly in young women with florid complexions. There can be little doubt that it is dependent upon, or connected with, the scrofulous diathesis. According to Virchow the tuberculated substance of lupus is composed of young and soft and vascular granulation tissue ; while it arises in the connective tissue of the derma, and spreads inwards to the deeper structures. After a time, the centre of the tubercle softens and breaks down, an open sore or ulcer resulting.

There are two *varieties* of this disease, viz. the chronic form or lupus non-exedens, and lupus exedens. This division is perhaps convenient ; but I agree with Mr. Hutchinson that the difference between the two forms is chiefly due to the part affected. In a lecture on this subject he says,—" If lupus attacks the nose, it will affect both skin and mucous surface; and as there is in the alæ of the nose little else, except the opposed layers of these tissues, if they both ulcerate, destruction of the part must result, and the disease will earn for itself the name of exedens. If lupus attack any level surface of the skin, it will cause the formation of indolent tubercles, with but little ulceration, but still resulting in a scar, and here it will be called non-exedens. The difference depends solely upon the anatomical peculiarities of the part attacked."* It is not, however, denied that the degree of ulceration varies in different cases ; but then it does not do so to a greater extent than happens in separate lupus patches on the same subject.

The form known as *chronic lupus* generally commences on the cheek, or upper lip, or lobe of one ear, or on some part of the trunk or extremities, as a small and reddish-coloured tuberculated substance ; around which other little tumours are gradually pro-

* *Clinical Lectures and Reports, by the Medical and Surgical Staff of the London Hospital.* Vol. ii. p. 128. London, 1865.

duced. Very slowly these effusions blend into a patch, which has the appearance of a yellowish brown gelatinous structure beneath the cuticle. As this disorganized tissue becomes absorbed in the course of years, the deep fibrous structure of the cutis or true skin is rendered apparent; and thus is produced an irremediable seamed cicatrix. Very often the absorption proceeds irregularly; a scar being seen at one part of the patch, while there are tubercles at another—especially at the edges whence the disease slowly spreads. In these cases there is no ulcer or even any excoriation; the cuticle remaining entire. Associated with lupus non-exedens, small erythematous patches are sometimes observed on different parts of the skin of the face or of the extremities. Mr. Erasmus Wilson has seen them on the fingers; having the appearance of chilblains, for which they have been mistaken. These blotches may occur without any other lupoid disease. They vary in size, but seldom exceed an inch in diameter. Each patch is usually slightly raised, is circular, and of a purplish hue. The patches give rise to depressed white cicatrices. Owing to these characters, this condition has been described as *lupus erythematosus*. According to some authors, the erythematous form of lupus is believed to be the consequence of inherited syphilis; but no satisfactory evidence in support of this view can be adduced.

In *lupus exedens*—or *noli me tangere*, as it used to be called—the morbid action almost always commences on the nose. There are the same dull brown or red-coloured tubercles, merged into patches; the surfaces of which crack and become excoriated. The fluid that exudes forms a thin scab; while underneath this, suppuration and ulceration slowly go on, spreading from the middle of the softened tubercle. As successive crusts form and fall off, so the destruction of the tubercle and skin and sometimes of the deeper tissues progresses. Leisurely but surely the devastation increases. As the ulceration extends, so there are often soft tubercles developed on the surrounding skin. The general appearance becomes frightful. The alæ nasi disappear, the bones perish, and the cavities of the nose are laid open. One or both of the lower eyelids will perhaps be drawn down on the cheeks, while the lips are perhaps drawn upwards. Indeed there is no end to the cruel deformity which may be produced; cases being on record where the face is said to have consisted of little more than one large and repulsive-looking cicatrix.

In the *treatment* of both forms of lupus recourse must be had to constitutional and local remedies. With regard to the former, it is necessary to bear in mind that agents which impart tone to the system are needed. The diet ought to be nutritious; animal food twice a day, with plenty of milk night and morning, being most valuable. On the same principle, cod liver oil proves serviceable. Country air has a favourable effect. Arsenic acts well as a tonic, though it is doubtful if it possess any special efficacy. Still, I have usually prescribed it in this disease; almost always giving it, however, in combination with quinine and iron (F. 381, 399), or with a mixture of the phosphates of iron and lime and soda, &c. (F. 405), or with the hypophosphite of soda and bark. In exceptional cases, a prolonged course of the liquor hydriodatis arsenici et hydrargyri (F. 51); or of the green iodide of mercury (F. 53); or of the red iodide of mercury (F. 54); or of iodide of potassium in decoction of sarsaparilla, or in bark, (F. 31); or of iodide of iron (F. 32): for such, one or other of these medicines has seemed to be required.

The local remedies are of the greatest importance. In lupus exedens, the only hope of checking the destructive ulceration lies in the free use of powerful caustics. The best of these are the chloride of zinc, nitric acid, the acid solution of nitrate of mercury, and pure carbolic acid. Suppose we decide on the employment of the first of these, it should be thus applied:—Every scab is to be peeled off, and the exposed sore cleaned and dried. If there be bleeding, pressure with the finger and lint will stop it. Then the caustic is to be thoroughly rubbed into every part of the ulcer, but especially to the edges; inasmuch as it is from the margins that the morbid action extends. Unless a healthy granulating surface results, the caustic is to be again had recourse to at the end of ten or fourteen days; the sore being dressed with simple stimulating lotions, or with a lotion of the glycerine of carbolic acid and water, in the meantime. For the destruction of the tubercles and patches of diseased tissue in chronic lupus, caustics are also required. None are better than the chloride of zinc, or the acid solution of nitrate of mercury, or caustic potash, or carbolic acid. Some practitioners prefer a strong solution of iodine in glycerine. As in the management of rodent ulcer anæsthetics and sedatives have been recommended, so in the present case the patient is not to be deprived of the relief which the exhibition of these drugs is capable of yielding.

XIII. SCROFULA.

The term Scrofula [from *Scrofa* = a sow; because swine were supposed to be especially subject to swellings in the neck] is employed to designate an idiopathic constitutional or blood disease; which may result either in the formation of tubercle, or in some specific form of inflammation or ulceration. The condition of system that lies at the root of these varieties of one widely prevalent disease is commonly spoken of as the scrofulous, strumous, or tuberculous diathesis. Hitherto, in the Reports of the Registrar-General the tubercular order of diseases has included scrofula,

tabes mesenterica, phthisis, and hydrocephalus.* A more clear
and scientific arrangement is made in the "Provisional Nomenclature of Diseases" adopted by the Royal College of Physicians of
London. According to this there are two varieties of scrofula to
be considered:—(1) Scrofula with tubercle. (2) Scrofula without
tubercle.

1. SCROFULA WITH TUBERCLE.—Scrofulous diseases with
tubercle comprehend more especially tubercular meningitis, tubercular pericarditis, phthisis pulmonalis, acute miliary tuberculosis
tabes mesenterica, and tubercular peritonitis. The word *tuberculosis*,
[from *Tuberculum*, dim. of *Tuber* = a knob or excrescence] had better
be used to designate the production of tubercle; while by *scrofulosis*
should be meant that deteriorated constitutional condition which
is the fountain-head of local tuberculous manifestations. These
manifestations consist in the growth of the peculiar substance,
named *tubercle*, in the tissue of the arachnoid, or pleura, or pericardium, or peritoneum; in the lymphatic glands, particularly the
mesenteric; and in the textures of the lung, spleen, liver, or kidney.
In 1317 cases of tuberculous disease examined by Willigk, the
following was the order of frequency in which various organs were
found affected:—Lungs, intestines, mesenteric glands, larynx, lymphatic glands, peritoneum, spleen, kidneys, pleura, liver, air-passages, bones, genital organs, brain, cerebral membranes, urinary
passages, pericardium, stomach, bowels, skin, muscles, tongue,
pharynx, œsophagus, pancreas, and heart.

Owing to the frequency of tubercular disease in the lungs, and
the marked degree of wasting with which it is attended, the expressions pulmonary tuberculosis, tubercular disease of the lungs,
phthisis, and consumption have usually been regarded as synonymous. Greater precision, however, has now become necessary.
By and by I shall define phthisis, or pulmonary consumption, as a
disease of the lungs which is characterised at first by condensation,
and subsequently by degeneration and softening and excavation,
of more or less extensive portions of pulmonary tissue; these local
changes being accompanied by such general results of imperfect
nutrition as loss of flesh and strength, with a gradually increasing
tendency to death. The disease is not necessarily connected with

* The deaths from all causes in England and Wales for the year 1866,
with an estimated population of 21,210,020 were 500,689: of which number
considerably more than one-seventh happened from scrofulous affections in
one form or other. Thus there died of,—

Scrofula	2,901		The Tubercular *Order*
Tabes Mesenterica	6,377	72,425	of the Constitutional
Phthisis	55,714		*Class* of Diseases.
Hydrocephalus	7,433		

This number, it must be noticed, is quite independent of 77,249 deaths from
other disorders of the lungs, pleuræ, bronchi, or larynx; some of which are
not unlikely to have been more or less closely connected with the strumous
cachexia.

the formation of tubercle. The consolidation and softening are often tubercular, without doubt; but they may also be the consequence of some form of inflammation and condensation (chronic pneumonia, ulceration, simple abscess &c.) of the pulmonary structure. In short, the word phthisis can be conveniently employed as the general designation for a condition of the lungs and system which arises from three or four different diseases; just as it is expedient to use the expression dyspepsia to indicate the prominent symptom of several dissimilar conditions of the stomach attended with one like result.

The peculiar substance whose presence constitutes tubercular disease is found in two forms,—as grey, or miliary, or true tubercle; and as yellow or crude tubercle. The *grey* tubercles are tough, soft, compressible, and semi-transparent; and by the microscope are seen to be composed of minute irregular-shaped bodies, with hyaline basis or connecting substance. The resemblance they bear to millet-seeds leads to their being spoken of as miliary tubercles. The *yellow* tubercle is found in larger masses, presenting an opaque cheesy appearance. It is now generally believed that these two varieties merely represent different stages of the same substance, the grey being sooner or later converted into the yellow deposit. The change is supposed to be due to fatty degeneration; the oil or fat communicating the yellow colour. With more favourable cases the grey instead of retrograding into yellow tubercle, becomes dry and dense and shrivelled into a contracted fibrous-like mass. Occasionally this latter change is associated with calcareous degeneration. Although most of the cheesy matter found in disease is of a tubercular nature, yet all does not possess this character. It may be a product of pneumonia, or a syphilitic deposit, or a result of embolism, or of suppuration.

Of course there has been a vast amount of speculation as to the mode of formation and nature of tubercle. One class of pathologists maintains that this substance is only a retrograde metamorphosis of pre-existing structures, tissue elements, or morbid products. According to Virchow tubercle is a degenerative cell proliferation—the proliferation of badly nourished connective tissue cells. There is a complete correspondence between the corpuscles of tubercle and those of the lymphatic glands. Hence, tubercle is defined as a growth resembling lymphatic structure; that is to say, it must be classed among the lymph tumours or those which are constructed after the pattern of lymph glands, and which stand in close relation to connective tissue formations. Another explanation, and that to which several authorities (Rokitansky, Lebert, Ancell, and Hughes Bennett) subscribe, is that tubercle consists of an exudation of the liquor sanguinis, presenting marked differences from the simple or inflammatory exudation on the one hand, and the cancerous exudation on the other. As the blood is dependent for its constitution on the results of the primary digestion in the alimentary canal, on the secondary digestion in the tissues, and on the healthy performance of the function of respiration, so it is argued by Dr. Bennett that the causes of the tubercular exudation are to be sought in the circumstances which operate on, or influence, those results :—" The successive changes which occur for the purposes of assimilation in the healthy economy may be shortly enumerated as follows :—1st. Introduction into the stomach and alimentary canal of organic matter.   2nd. Its transformation by the process of digestion into albuminous and oily compounds : this process is chemical.   3rd. The imbibition of these through the mucous membrane in a fluid state, and their union in the termini of the villi and lacteals to form elementary molecules : this process is physical.   4th. The transformation of these, first, into chyle corpuscles, and, secondly, into those of the blood, through the agency of the lymphatic glandular system : which is a vital process.   It is from this fluid, still further elaborated in numerous ways, that the nutritive materials of the tissues are derived, so that it must be evident if the first steps of the process are imperfectly performed, the subsequent ones must also be interfered with.   Hence we can readily comprehend how an improper quantity or quality of food, by diminishing the number of the elementary nutritive molecules, must impede nutrition."*

From the chemical analysis of tubercle, it appears to consist of animal matter and earthy salts; the former being principally albumen and cholesterine, while the latter consist chiefly of insoluble phosphate and carbonate of lime, with the soluble salts of soda.   The precise nature of the change in the blood which occurs in tubercular disease is unknown ; but it would seem that the aqueous part is increased in proportion to the solids, while the red corpuscles are especially diminished.   Tubercle has a low and feeble vitality, having a tendency to pass into early decay (molecular death) ; this being apparently caused by the density of the tubercular growth and the mutual pressure of its particles, but especially by its occluding the capillary vessels within its sphere of action, so that it is essentially bloodless.   As it goes on to break up or soften, so it manifests a tendency to cause its expulsion by inducing disorganization and ulceration of the tissues involved in its growth.   Where each group of tubercles softens, an excavation or cavity is formed.   The destructive or ulcerative tendency may, however, be sometimes checked ;* as is proved by the occasional detection in the deadhouse of lungs marked with cicatrices.   The testimony of Laennec, Carswell, Bennett, and Sir James Clark also goes to confirm the truth of this observation ; and although I have heard physicians of repute state that they have never cured a case of consumption, yet I am sure that a considerable number of cases now recover after well-directed treatment.   There are three ways

* *On the Pathology and Treatment of Pulmonary Consumption.*   By John Hughes Bennett, M.D., &c.   Second Edition, p. 33.   Edinburgh, 1859.

in which it is probable that a cure may result,—either by the conversion of the tubercular matter into a cretaceous or calcareous substance; or by the expectoration of the exudation, the collapse of the ulcerated walls, and the cicatrization of the cavity; or by the ulcerated walls becoming covered with a false membrane, and forming a chronic cavity. In any case it is of course inferred that the blood is rendered healthy, and consequently that the production of tubercle is stopped.

A necropsy of a tubercular patient is seldom made without finding fatty degeneration of the liver, kidneys, or arteries; but whether these degenerations stand in the relation of secondary dependence upon the tubercle-forming diathesis is uncertain.

Since the year 1865, when M. Villemin's experiments on the *inoculation of tubercle* were laid before the French Academy of Sciences, much attention has been paid to the artificial production of tubercular disease in animals. This pathologist experimented on rabbits; taking them in pairs, inoculating one by placing portions of fresh tubercle under the skin, and leaving the other alone. Both being then kept under exactly the same conditions, the inoculated rabbit was found after a certain time to be tuberculous, while the other animal continued healthy. However often repeated, the results were the same. Other experimenters came forward, including Lebert, and confirmed them. M. Villemin also experimented on rabbits with the materials of carbuncle, phlegmonous abscess, cancer, cholera stools, and typhoid lymph; but in no case did the same effects follow as with the matter of tubercle. Then, during 1867, Mr. Simon laid before the Pathological Society several specimens of tubercular disease in rabbits, the product of inoculation with tuberculous matter. About the same time, a paper was read on this subject at the Royal Medical and Chirurgical Society by Dr. William Marcet. This gentleman's experiments appear to have been conducted partly to show, that in inoculation we possess another means of diagnosis. His conclusions are as follows :—(1) The inoculation of guinea-pigs with the expectorations of patients suffering from phthisis, will in a certain stage of the disease, and possibly throughout, give rise to the formation of tubercles in the operated animals. (2) If two or more guinea-pigs inoculated with human expectorations brought up by coughing should die from tubercular disease, or on being killed at least thirty days after inoculation should exhibit tubercles, this may be considered as a direct and positive evidence that the person whose expectorations were inoculated was suffering at the time from tubercular phthisis. (3) If two or more guinea-pigs be inoculated with the expectorations of a person in the third stage of phthisis, and if these animals do not die of tubercular disease or exhibit any tubercles when killed fifty days after inoculation, it may be considered that the softening of tubercles and the secretion from the pulmonary cavities are arrested; and consequently that the patient is in a fair way of recovery. (4) Other materials besides the pulmonary expectorations taken from the human body in certain stages of phthisis, as blood and pus, appear to be also possessed of the power of causing the formation of tubercles in guinea-pigs, when inoculated to these animals. (5) The spleen appears to be the first, and the lungs one of the last organs, in guinea-pigs, to be attacked with tubercular disease.

The discussions which followed the publication of the foregoing principles have led to the subject being investigated by Dr. Andrew Clark, Dr. Sanderson, and Dr. Wilson Fox. And briefly stated the result comes to this,—that the inoculation of the rodentia with other materials than tubercle will render the animals tuberculous. In the experiments of Dr. Wilson Fox, 117 guinea-pigs and twelve rabbits were inoculated with various materials. Of the 117 guinea-pigs 58 proved tubercular; 6 were doubtful; and 53 failed. Those cases were only reckoned as successful in which three of the following organs were shown to be affected, viz. the lungs, bronchial glands, liver, spleen, peritoneum, intestines, or lymphatic glands. The animals had all been kept under conditions as natural as possible, and had been well fed and attended to. The most common effect was the production of cheesy matter, usually encapsuled under the skin; the next change was an enlargement of the lymphatic glands in the neighbourhood of the inoculation, the glands showing on section scattered lines and streaks of cheesy degeneration; the lungs were the organs next most frequently affected; and then the bronchial glands. In all the cases, the growth was one resembling lymphatic structure, consisting of masses of round cells or nuclei embedded in a homogeneous tissue. Supposing these experiments are satisfactory, the opinion of Villemin and his followers that tubercle is a specific growth, producible by itself alone, will have to be abandoned. During Dr. Fox's experiments it was found, that pieces of thread charged with vaccine lymph, simple setons, portions of putrid muscle, pus from various sources, sputa, &c. gave rise to the usual constitutional symptoms of tubercular affections, as well as to growths not distinguishable from tubercle.*

* These results are curious when compared with the views of some authors of note on the effects of inoculation with variolous matter and vaccine lymph. As all evidence, at the threshold of this important enquiry, is deserving of attention, I note the following references. In doing this, I am merely helping to collect materials which are to be sifted. The data are much too scanty for any conclusions to be drawn.

Dr. John Fordyce when giving an account of the virtues of Peruvian bark in scrofulous cases (*Medical Observations and Inquiries*, by a Society of Physicians in London, fourth ed. vol. i. p. 184, London, 1776) cites the history of a young lady, 16 years old, who was inoculated for the small-pox. This proved of a favourable kind, and she soon recovered; but "for some weeks after had a few troublesome sores near the places where she had been inoculated, during which time, although she often took physic, a great part of the right parotid swelled considerably, as well as the glands on each side of the neck." In a few weeks the sores healed, and the swellings disappeared, under treatment.—Again, Dr. W. Rowley (*Seventy-four Select Cases &c.*, second

Some of the substances proved more powerful in producing this material than others; none being more potent than the material of indisputable tubercle and the so-called tubercular pneumonias.

The *causes* which have been most frequently assigned for tuberculosis are hereditary influence, syphilis, debauchery, bad air, improper food, and a cold damp atmosphere. As regards hereditary influence, it may be noticed that if by this is meant that there is a certain poison or strumous virus transmitted from parents to children, the position is hardly tenable; but, on the other hand, if it be only understood that the children of tuberculous parents are more liable to have the disease developed in them on the application of the exciting causes than the children of healthy parents, as was the opinion of John Hunter, the position is most probably true. That it is not contagious seems to me certain; notwithstanding that even now some few practitioners in all countries, and many of the common people in the southern parts of Europe, entertain a contrary opinion. This question as to contagion has always been brought forward at intervals, since the time when Aretæus taught that there was a risk in conversing, face to face, with a scrofulous subject. And now it is again exciting attention; chiefly in consequence of the bare hypothesis submitted to the profession by Dr. William Budd in October 1867, that tubercular consumption is a true zymotic disease, due to "a specific morbific matter," which is propagated from one person to another, and so disseminated through society. But with all deference I must say, that nothing which I have observed leads me to agree with Dr. Budd. Indeed, that tubercle is a disease of a specific nature, in the same sense as typhoid fever, scarlet fever, typhus, syphilis, &c., appears to be one of the most untenable propositions which could have been started. Whether this opinion will have to be modified by Dr. W. Budd's explanations (none having as yet been given) remains to be seen. Many authors have imagined that a syphilitic taint in either

edition, p. 47, London, 1779) says—"I have seen several instances where inoculation has produced the King's evil; therefore we should be very cautious what subject we take the matter from." He mentions one case apparently in support of this view.—Antonio De Haen, a great opponent of inoculation, believed that inoculated small-pox was a frequent cause of scrofula. (*Opuscula omnia medico-physica.* Tom. iii. De methodo inoculandi variolas &c. Neapoli, 1778).—And lastly, Barthez and Rilliet (*Traité des Maladies des Enfants*, deuxième édition, tome troisième, p. 399, Paris, 1854) have expressed their opinion, that vaccinated children are more disposed to tuberculosis than the non-vaccinated. Thus of 208 vaccinated children, 138 died tuberculous, and 70 non-tubercular. Of 95 non-vaccinated children, 30 were tubercular and 65 not so. As the conclusions of Messrs. Barthez and Rilliet with regard to the significance of these figures do not seem very clear, it will be better to give their own words:—"Nous ne regardons nullement la vaccine comme une cause de tubercules; car jamais nous n'avons vu l'affection chronique lui succéder immédiatement; nous constatons seulement que les enfants vaccinés meurent plus souvent tuberculeux que non tuberculeux, et que le contraire a lieu pour les enfants non vaccinés. Nous en concluons que la vaccine favorise très probablement la prédisposition aux tubercules." (p. 400).

parent will induce tuberculosis in their offspring; while some have even maintained that this disease is only a degenerated species of syphilis. There may be said, however, to be but little truth in either of these suppositions; tubercular affections and syphilis being very different diseases, quite independent the one of the other. Neither does the development of tubercle appear to be influenced by climate or temperature: the inhabitants of the tropics and of the arctic regions are sufferers from it. But it is to diseased nutrition, however brought about, that we may refer the production of scrofulosis and tuberculosis. And it is to insufficient, innutritious, or improper food, that the vast majority of cases of diseased nutrition are due; though it will also arise from almost constantly breathing a vitiated atmosphere, from long continued sorrow and mental depression, or from want of cleanliness and healthy exercise.*

The *symptoms* which precede the occurrence of tuberculosis are generally indicative of disorder of the digestive organs. Dr. Wilson Philip first noticed that there were some forms of indigestion which ended in phthisis; and it has more recently been proved

---

* A most singular narrative confirmatory of these views has been given by Laennec. It runs thus:—" I had under my own eyes, during a period of ten years, a striking example of the effect of the depressing passions in producing phthisis; in the case of a religious association of women, of recent foundation, and which never obtained from the ecclesiastical authorities any other than a provisional toleration, on account of the extreme severity of its rules. The diet of these persons was certainly very austere, yet it was by no means beyond what nature could bear. But the ascetic spirit which regulated their minds, was such as to give rise to consequences no less serious than surprising. Not only was the attention of these women habitually fixed on the most terrible truths of religion, but it was the constant practice to try them by every kind of contrariety and opposition, in order to bring them, as soon as possible, to an entire renouncement of their own proper will. The consequences of this discipline were the same in all: after being one or two months in the establishment, the catamenia became suppressed; and in the course of one or two months thereafter, phthisis declared itself! As no vow was taken in this society, I endeavoured to prevail upon the patients to leave the house as soon as the consumptive symptoms began to appear; and almost all those who followed my advice were cured, although several of them exhibited well-marked indications of the disease. During the ten years that I was physician of this association, I witnessed its entire renovation two or three different times, owing to the successive loss of all its members, with the exception of a small number consisting chiefly of the superior, the gate-keeper, and the sisters who had charge of the garden, kitchen, and infirmary. It will be observed, that these individuals were those who had the most constant distractions from their religious tasks, and that they also went out pretty often to the city, on business connected with the establishment. In like manner, in other situations, it has appeared to me that almost all those who became phthisical, without being constitutionally predisposed to the disease, might attribute the origin of their complaint to grief, either very deep or of long continuance."—*A Treatise on Diseases of the Chest and on Mediate Auscultation*, by R. T. H. Laennec, M.D. Translated from the French by John Forbes, M.D. &c. Fourth Edition, p. 303. London, 1834.

The following evidence on this head is also deserving of attention, more especially as it may be feared that there is a tendency in the present day

by Mr. Jonathan Hutchinson and others, that the peculiar feature
of this dyspepsia consists in the difficult assimilation of fatty
matters.   Sugar and fat and even alcohol "turn acid," giving rise
to sour eructations and heartburn and flatulence.   Besides this
important warning it is stated by many authorities that persons
possessing the strumous diathesis manifest certain peculiarities.
The chief of these are,—a coldness of the body and extremities; a
dull white, but very delicate skin; and a rounded graceful outline
of the face, with a delicacy of feature and rosy hue of the cheeks,
strongly contrasting with the surrounding pallor and giving to the
countenance, especially in women, a characteristic beauty. The hair
is also said to be usually blonde or auburn; while the eyes are
large and blue, projecting and humid, with the pupils habitually
dilated, and the sclerotics of a pearly whiteness. The eyelashes are
long; unless they have been destroyed by that inflammatory action
which causes swelling and eversion of the edges of the eyelid, and
which is known as ophthalmia tarsi.   Moreover, scrofulous subjects are thought to be remarkable for the development of the head,
of the alæ nasi, and of the upper lip; as also for the large size of
the lower jaw, and the milk-white teeth which early become carious.
It is asserted too that the breath is habitually sour and fetid; the
neck being long and rounded, the chest narrow and flat, the shoulders
high, the abdomen large and prominent, the limbs thin, and the
flesh soft and flabby. The opinion is very commonly entertained, that
in youth all such persons manifest great cerebral activity; that they
are impatient and passionate; that their intellectual system is
largely developed; and that although many have more imagination
than judgment, yet a few are profound and capable of sustained
mental exertion.   There are not many cases, however, where the
actual appearances will correspond with this description. The most
constant peculiarities are the paleness and coldness of the body,
and the tumidity of the abdomen.

Tubercular diseases may set in at any period of life, though they
are peculiarly the affections of childhood and youth. Perhaps the liability to them is greatest from three to fifteen, and from eighteen to
thirty-five or forty.   Their development is favoured by all conditions which tend to render the blood unhealthy; such as malformations of the chest, defective structure of the lungs, a small heart,

---

unduly to increase the severity of prison discipline.—" In all parts of Europe,"
says Dr. Baly, formerly physician to the Millbank Penitentiary, " the proportion of deaths has been much greater among criminals in prisons, than amongst
persons of a corresponding class out of prison; and the increased mortality
is due to various forms of scrofula, and especially tubercular phthisis.   The
causes which contribute to this result are cold, poorness of diet, deficient ventilation, want of sufficient bodily exercise, and dejection of mind.   In a great
number of cases of phthisis in this prison, apparently hopeless, the disease
was immediately checked on the release of the prisoners, many of whom entirely recovered."   Quoted from Dr. William Addison,—*On Healthy and
Diseased Structure*, p. 48.   London, 1849.

diseased nutrition, continued anxiety and grief, sexual excesses, &c. When these causes act upon a frame hereditarily predisposed, the disease is almost sure to be developed ; but it is not certain, though it is very probable, that they can give rise to it where there is no such predisposition.

Tubercular diseases are not only preceded but are frequently accompanied by a disordered state of the primæ viæ,—such as "biliousness," acid eructations, flatulence, irregular action of the bowels with pale and clay-like evacuations, a distaste for fatty food, and a generally bad appetite ; conditions which are so constant, that some authors speak of them as *strumous dyspepsia*. Then we find paleness and puffiness of the face, with swelling of the lips and nostrils, and purulent discharges from the ears ; vesicular eruptions about the head ; enlargement of the glands of the neck and of the tonsils ; disagreeable exhalations from the skin, especially of the feet and axillæ ; feebleness and rapidity of the pulse ; together with weakness and progressive loss of weight. The muscles are soft and flabby ; the mucous membranes are irritable, and apt to become spotted at parts with aphthæ ; the nervous suscepti- bility increases ; the sleep is seldom sound ; the physical powers decline ; and the force of the circulation diminishes, so that there is coldness of the extremities. Moreover, together with a dimi- nished power of maintaining the animal heat, there is general un- easiness or irritability with a susceptibility to attacks of simple fever. As the disorder progresses, so all those symptoms which arise from depraved or impoverished blood, and from enfeebled vital energies, are strongly manifested. In women, the catamenia become irregular or entirely cease.

The *temperature of the body*, as taken by the thermometer kept in the axilla for five minutes, is found to be continuously raised above the normal standard in all cases while the production of tubercle is going on, quite independently of the organ affected. This elevation often reaches 103° or 105° Fabr. ; while it some- times does so before any evidence can be obtained of local disease. As a rule, the higher the temperature is raised, the greater is the severity of the constitutional disease, and the greater is the amount of tubercle produced. On the other hand, as the formation of tubercle ceases, so the temperature falls towards the normal standard. This standard may be said to be 98°, a variation of two or three tenths of a degree above or below this being of little or no moment.

It is a matter of common observation that many tuberculous patients, while daily losing flesh and strength, are yet very san- guine in expecting recovery ; though unfortunately they generally imagine a cure is to be effected without any great exertion on their own parts. Perhaps there is no other critical disease where it is more important to impress upon the sufferer the absolute necessity for steady perseverance in the use of remedies ; and the hopelessness of giving way to that want of energy and determination, which many try to excuse by the expression of their devout desire to "trust in Providence."

Remembering what has been said upon the hereditary nature of tuberculosis it should be noticed, that there are three points to be particularly attended to in order to prevent its transmission. These are,—(1) To obtain well-assorted marriages—the marriages of parties in sound health and vigour, and not related by blood to each other. (2) Where this disease exists in the parents, or in either of them, great care must be taken to maintain the health of the mother during the period of utero-gestation. She should wear warm clothing, take regular exercise in the open air, avoid heated rooms and late hours, sleep in a large room, and have a plain nourishing diet. (3) On the birth of the child, every means ought to be taken to strengthen its general health, and to counter-act the hereditary influence, by attention to the food, air, cloth-ing, &c. If the mother be free from the strumous habit, she may suckle her offspring, but otherwise a young and healthy nurse should do so. At the age of nine or ten months the infant ought to be weaned and fed on cow's or goat's milk, a small quantity of light nutritious vegetables, and a little good broth. Dr. Paris strongly recommended milk impregnated with the fat of mutton suet, which he ordered to be prepared by enclosing the suet in a muslin bag, and then simmering it with the milk. The child must be clothed in flannel; should live in apartments which are well-ven-tilated and well-lighted; ought to have plenty of exercise in the open air; and once daily should have a cold sea-water bath, or a tepid bath with bay salt dissolved in it. Ill-arranged, badly drained, close-smelling, damp houses must be avoided; as well as all those localities which are generally regarded as unhealthy.

The regulation of the food and occupation and residence of those adults who have any tendency, hereditary or acquired, to tubercular disease, ought never to be neglected. The necessary rules which the physician should lay down for the guidance of such persons will be obvious from a consideration of the concluding re-marks of this section. The normal vigour of life not only depends on the healthy condition of the nervous centres, the heart, the lungs, and the digestive system; but it can only be maintained by all these organs acting harmoniously in a properly developed frame. Consequently where one system is weak, judicious attempts must be made to strengthen it. The remarkable change which can be wrought by a course of physical training will often prove very beneficial, provided the amount of exertion gone through is suited to the age and strength of the individual. This amount ought to vary not only in proportion to the soundness of the lungs and heart &c., but also in relation to the development of the whole body. A perfectly healthy man should have, as a rule, a certain weight in proportion to his height and age; although it is difficult to say exactly what this weight should be. Some rough conclusions at least, can be drawn from the table by Dr. Hutchinson in the chapter on tubercular phthisis, as well as from the following. This exhibits the relative growth of the human body (males) in height and weight, from eighteen to thirty years of age. It has been constructed by Mr. J. T. Dawson from observations upon 4800 prisoners at the Borough Gaol of Liverpool.

Age.	HEIGHT.			WEIGHT.		
	Average.	Maximum.	Minimum.	Average.	Maximum.	Minimum.
	ft. in.	ft. in.	ft. in.	st. lbs.	st. lbs.	st. lbs.
18	5 4·34	5 11	4 10½	8 10·79	10 10	6 6
19	5 4·94	5 11½	4 11	9 4·11	12 8	7 4
20	5 5·11	5 11	5 1	9 5·58	12 8	7 13
21	5 5·57	5 11¾	5 0¼	9 5·02	13 0	7 3
22	5 6·17	6 1	5 0¼	9 12·41	13 2	7 0
23	5 6·17	6 1	4 11	10 2·95	12 12	7 12
24	5 5·94	6 1	4 9	10 2·	12 12	7 12
25	5 6·30	6 0	4 11	10 5·65	13 8	8 2
26	5 6·28	6 1¾	4 9¼	10 1·06	13 8	6 12
27	5 6·38	5 11¾	5 1	10 4·75	13 10	7 12
28	5 6·65	6 1	5 1	10 2·62	13 2	7 7
29	5 7·02	6 0½	5 1¼	10 5·53	13 12	8 4
30	5 6·36	6 1	5 0½	10 1·55	14 1	8 1

An examination of this table shows that the results do not indicate a progressive increase in height or weight. For instance with regard to height, Mr. Dawson remarks,—" The average height of 185 men at 24, is less than that of 200 men at 23, and 100 at 26 give a lower average than 200 at 25; while 100 at 30 give a lower average then 95 at 29.''* Still these are the best results at present available. And my object in quoting them will be attained, if I succeed in leading the practitioner to pay that attention to the subject which is necessary; so that when he finds a decided disproportion between the age and height and weight of a patient, he may not rest satisfied until he has discovered the cause of such misrelation. With regard to the disease under consideration, the question is very important; since one of the most constant, as well as one of the earliest, results of the deposit of tubercle is a steady and progressive loss of weight.

For remarks on the *treatment* of scrofula with tubercle, the reader must refer to the directions which are given in the sections on phthisis, hydrocephalus, tabes mesenterica, &c. But it may be summarily stated that the object always to be kept in view is to improve the faulty nutrition, so as to promote the formation of healthy blood, and thus prevent the fresh production of tubercle; while we also endeavour to favour the absorption of that which

* *Journal of the Statistical Society of London,* vol. xxv. p. 24. London, 1862.

has been formed. These indications will be best carried out by the use of a diet containing as much properly cooked animal food, milk or cream, and raw eggs as can be assimilated; by the long continued employment of cod liver oil; as well as by the exhibition of drugs which check undue acidity when it prevails, and which will aid digestion where this function is imperfectly performed. The utility of such special remedies as bark, preparations of steel, the alkaline hypophosphites, iodine, topical counterirritants, change of climate, &c. will all be dwelt upon by and by. Suffice it to add here that the tuberculous patient ought never to be allowed to breathe air which is in the slightest degree impure; that out-door exercise, on foot and on horseback and in an open carriage is of the greatest importance to him; that his clothing is to be such as will protect the body from changes in temperature, flannel being worn next the skin throughout the year, with the addition of a chamois leather jacket over the flannel vest during cold weather; that the functions of his skin are to be maintained by bathing in water of a suitable temperature, followed by friction; and that he should devote eight or ten hours out of every twenty-four to sleep, on a horse-hair mattress, in a warm and dry and properly ventilated room.

2. SCROFULA WITHOUT TUBERCLE.—Scrofula, or external scrofula, or struma, or tabes glandularis, or king's evil, manifests itself chiefly by glandular swellings, more or less extensive ulcerations, and indolent abscesses. Cases of scrofulous ophthalmia are very far from uncommon; while the same must be said of strumous diseases of the bones and joints.

Inflammation of the lymphatic glands—strumous adenitis—is one of the most frequent consequences of the scrofulous habit. The glands of the neck, and those about the base and angle of the lower jaw, are more frequently affected than any others. The subjects of this form of morbid action are especially young children, although it is not a rare affection of strumous adults. There are rarely any premonitory symptoms to attract notice; the first indication of the disease being an indolent swelling of one or more glands without marked constitutional disturbance. The enlargement often remains stationary for months or even years; but if from any cause the mischief suddenly increase, and especially if a tendency to suppuration become manifested, then the system suffers considerably. The already unhealthy patient becomes irritable and restless; a low kind of fever is set up; the tongue gets furred, the bowels are costive, and the appetite fails; while the urine is found scanty, and loaded with urates. Unhealthy discharges also often take place from the ears, nose, and eyes; while in female children there is frequently a troublesome form of vaginal leucorrhœa. Where the general health is already very bad, or when it gradually becomes so, the inflamed glands rapidly undergo disorganization; the surrounding skin and connective tissue becoming involved, and extensive indolent ulcerations resulting. The site of these ulcers, when they have healed, is ever afterwards indicated by unsightly cicatrices.

The constitutional treatment of these cases is much the same as that required in the early stages of scrofula with tubercle. Nutritious food, cleanliness, and residence in pure air are the requisite measures. Hence we prescribe mutton and beef, potatoes and watercresses, raw eggs, milk and cream, cod liver oil, warm or tepid or cold baths, and sea air. Iodine in different forms is often given,—iodide of potassium, iodide of ammonium, iodide of iron; but as a rule I have more confidence in quinine and iron, chlorate of potash with bark, arsenic and steel (F. 399), and chemical food (F. 405). Locally, benefit now and then arises from the use of the officinal iodine liniment; or from the ointment of iodide of lead, or that of iodide of cadmium, or that of red iodide of mercury diluted with an equal proportion of lard. It has been suggested, that these enlarged glands can often be dissected out with advantage; but I have had no experience of this practice. When suppuration takes place, the treatment will have to be the same as for an abscess.

Scrofulous ulcers are a common indication of the cachexia under consideration. They are more often seated about the neck, shoulders, arms, or hips, than elsewhere. By their gradual extension, extensive tracts of skin may be destroyed. The efforts at repair are always slow and imperfect; for if any granulations appear they are sure to be exuberant and flabby, while the subjacent tissue is boggy and readily broken down by pressure with a probe. The general health, bad from the beginning, daily deteriorates. The only hope of cure is from the constitutional treatment just recommended. Cicatrization is sometimes procured after destruction of the unhealthy tissue by strong caustics,—such as nitric acid, or potassa fusa. A lotion of carbolic acid (ten grains of crystals to each ounce of water) can be recommended.

Strumous abscesses often commence insidiously in the connective tissue, or they have their origin in the suppuration which repeatedly follows glandular inflammation. They are apt to become indolent; or they suppurate imperfectly; or they burrow deeply in all directions. Hence, long sinuses are formed; from which there exudes a thin sanious pus. Although hasty interference is to be deprecated, yet frequently these abscesses have to be opened with the knife. This is advisable, partly because their cure will be thus expedited; but chiefly for the reason that the linear cicatrix which results is less disfiguring than the rough and irregular scar that follows from allowing the skin to ulcerate. Moreover, by a neglect of this advice, when the abscess has occurred over one of the long bones, such as the shaft of the tibia, periostitis and necrosis have occurred.

Strumous ophthalmia occurs in children between the time of weaning and the end of the ninth or tenth year. Its chief symptoms consist of slight conjunctival and sclerotic redness; with the formation of little phlyctenulæ or pustules, and often of ulcers, on the cornea. There is a copious lachrymal secretion; with irritability of the nasal and buccal mucous membranes. The great intolerance of light (photophobia) is almost a pathognomonic feature. It causes spasmodic contraction of the eyelids; and makes the child hide its head, or sit in a dark corner, or shade the eyes with a handkerchief. Both eyes are usually affected. In addition, there are swellings of the lips, eruptions behind and within the ears, as well as disordered intestinal secretions. The hot tears while they flow over the cheek, set up irritation; a troublesome eczematous rash often resulting.

The management of these cases will tax the skill and vigilance of the nurse as well as of the doctor. The absolute necessity for constitutional treatment need not be again insisted on. Great attention must be paid to cleanliness. Warm bathing of the eyes, and fomentations, are very serviceable. A drop or two of wine of opium may be placed in each eye night and morning; or sulphate of zinc or alum collyria (F. 291) can sometimes be advantageously prescribed. Frequently, however, sedative applications (F. 290) are more serviceable. The application of spermaceti ointment to the edges of the eyelids at night is necessary, to prevent their becoming agglutinated. In obstinate cases small flying blisters to the temples, or behind the ears, should be ordered. It is remarkable sometimes to witness the rapidity with which the eyes improve as discharges are established from the skin at the back of the ears. In the house, also, a green shade ought to be worn; while out of doors a gray or blue veil is absolutely necessary.

Caries, or ulceration of bone, due to scrofula has no particular features distinguishing it from that produced by other causes. The liability to it, however, should not be forgotten; while care ought to be taken not to mistake its early symptoms for those of rheumatism.

XIV. RICKETS.

Rickets, or rachitis, or rhachitis, or osteomalacia infantum, is a constitutional disease; being characterised by a softening of the bones, superadded to many of those conditions that result from impaired assimilation. There is general debility, flaccidity of the muscles, and a sluggish state of the nervous system. Owing to the diminution of the earthy matter in the bones, the form of different parts of the skeleton gets much altered. This alteration is possibly caused by the action of the muscles, but more probably it arises in consequence of the limbs bending under their own weight or under that of the body.   The long bones are usually most affected; their shafts being curved, and their cancellous extremities thickened.   There is frequently also that peculiar condition of the spleen and lymphatic glands, known as amyloid or albuminoid degeneration; the liver being likewise many times found similarly affected.

The disease is essentially one of early childhood : it is very rarely congenital : it has no direct relationship with scrofula, or cancer, or syphilis.   The cachexia usually becomes first apparent between the sixth and the twelfth month after birth.   Whether there is any essential identity between the rickets of childhood and the mollities ossium of adults is uncertain.   My own belief is that these osseous degenerations are, to say the least, very closely allied.   The important peculiarity which is relied upon as showing a distinction between rickets and mollities ossium, viz., that the former is remediable, while no treatment checks the latter from running into a state of fatal fatty degeneration, seems to admit of explanation.   During childhood the development and growth of the bones are amongst the most important of the processes which are carried on in the system.   While this development is going on, it surely can easily be influenced; that is to say, it may be checked, or retarded, or urged on in an abnormal course.   But when ossification is complete, then alterations either in a right or wrong direction are made with much more difficulty.   Structural disease if thoroughly established is perpetuated; while it much more easily runs on to fatty degeneration than does similar disease in childhood.

Causes.—Anything which induces imperfect assimilation of food and impaired nutrition of the body may act as a cause of rickets.   Hence, this affection is sometimes met with in such weakly children of wealthy parents, as suffer from defective action of the vital forces.   Like scrofula, however, it is essentially a disease of the poorer classes.   Insufficient, and especially, improper food; the constant respiration of foul, impure air; residence in damp, dark, cold, or filthy dwellings : these and all similar circumstances, readily serve, in all probability, to generate rickets. Again, the children of parents who have weakened themselves by sexual excesses, or who have married too early or much too late in life; or of those whose constitutions have been impaired by syphilis, or by a strumous taint, or by unhealthy occupations; as well as the offspring of delicate anæmic mothers : all such children are, doubtless, predisposed to this disease.   I do not mean by this that rickets is hereditary; but merely that the health of the parents has an effect on the health of the child, so that if the former be bad the latter will be disposed to quickly fail when the exciting causes of disease are brought into action.

M. Guérin, from numerous experiments on animals, has proved the possibility of inducing artificial "rickets" at will, by merely separating the young too early from their mothers, and supplying them with food suitable only for the adult. There is no question that in these cases of improper feeding partial starvation is induced, both by the imperfect assimilation of the food, and by the diminution of digestive power which is brought about. That the same result can be produced in the human subject by the same means no one who attends the hospital out-patient room will doubt. The infant mortality in Lancashire has long been excessively high, the occupations of the poorer women causing them to neglect their children. During the cotton famine (1862-63), this mortality was greatly diminished; for the mothers being unemployed had plenty of time to attend to the feeding of their offspring, while as the resources of the parents became diminished the children were not stuffed with unsuitable artificial food. And it must be remembered that excessive mortality is only a portion of the evil which care will remove. The effects of partial starvation are not simply most fatal to large numbers during infancy, but prove highly injurious by laying the foundation for future suffering in those who escape immediate death. With an ill-developed body we commonly find a weak nervous system, and consequently a low form of intelligence; so that individuals thus constituted are unable to make any stand against the first inroads of physical no less than of moral disease.

Symptoms.—The earliest indication that some morbid process is going on in the system is generally shown by languor with an occasional feverish condition of the body, sadness and irritability of the temper, copious perspirations about the head, and general tenderness of the trunk and extremities. Soon there is some swelling of the abdomen, gastro-intestinal irritation and diarrhœa, general debility and wasting, with slightly painful tumefaction of the wrists and knees and ankles. The transition from apparent health to disease is gradual, and occasionally only marked by the presence of slight ailment; so that the practitioner must be on his guard. Some time always elapses between the commencement of the morbid process and its certain detection. And even when the cachexia may be early recognised there is commonly an interval of several months before any deformity can be noticed.

The long bones are amongst the first to exhibit a change from the natural form; the femur bending forwards and outwards, and the tibia generally outwards—*bow-legs.* In some instances the knees bend inwards, while the feet are thrown outwards—*knock-knees.* The clavicle, humerus, radius, and ulna are always much curved, and sometimes twisted. The thoracic deformity is usually well-marked; the back being flattened, the sternum thrust forward, and the natural curve of the ribs lessened. The child is said to be *pigeon-breasted.* The flat bones also get thickened, and there is a real (not simply an apparent) enlargement of all the extremities of the bones. Pelvic deformity is common, while the spine gets contorted in various ways; but both of these results occur at a much later period than the curving of the long bones. The head appears disproportionately large; the face becomes pale, and the features attenuated; while the eyes look unnaturally bright, and have a staring expression. The respirations are quickened; and the pulse gets frequent and feeble. The appetite is bad or capricious, and the powers of digestion much impaired. The stools are pale or slate-coloured, and very offensive : perhaps the food passes through the intestines only half digested. The urinary secretion is more abundant than in health, and loaded with earthy phosphates—especially phosphate of lime; the excess being probably due to this salt being gradually drained from the osseous system. There is no doubt that all the tissues lose their tone, and become weak and flabby, as the disease progresses; though the chief signs are shown by the osseous system. Thus the bones are always found more or less soft, spongy, and pliable; owing to the diminution of their earthy constituents, particularly of the phosphate of lime. This softening of the bones may be so great that they can easily be cut or bent; but there is never that extreme softening sometimes observed in cases of mollities ossium in adults, in which there seems to remain but little of certain bones beyond a lot of greasy adipocere in a case of periosteum. On an average, in rickets, the affected osseous tissue contains two-thirds less of earthy matter than should be present. The lime salts are not only less freely taken up by the bones or periosteum, than in health, but part of those already deposited in the osseous texture are reabsorbed and excreted in the urine.

In addition to the foregoing symptoms, it has been noticed that rickety children manifest a tendency to chronic hydrocephalus; to catarrh, or bronchitis, with pulmonary collapse; to laryngismus stridulus; to urinary calculi; as well as to albuminoid infiltration of the spleen, lymphatic glands, liver &c. Where the emaciation and anæmia are great, it will generally be found that the tissues of one or more important organs have become infiltrated with albuminoid or amyloid material. Occasionally, where death has occurred from anæmic convulsions, I believe that an albuminoid degeneration of the kidneys has been the source of the mischief. In many instances there is obstinate diarrhœa, which is probably due in part to the large amount of free acid constantly generated in the alimentary canal. This acid also often interferes with the assimilation of milk, causing this important food to be vomited or passed in the stools in the form of indigestible masses of curd.

During the last stage of the disorder the child may either slowly sink from exhaustion, or from some cerebral or thoracic or abdominal disease. More frequently, however, a happier result is obtained. The functions of the body are at first slowly, but afterwards rapidly, restored to a normal state. The earliest signs of improvement are generally, a more healthy condition of the secretions and excretions, and an increase in the tone and powers of the system. As the appetite improves, the flesh becomes firmer; the languor, dulness, and febrile symptoms all subside; growth proceeds rapidly; and the tumidity of the abdomen disappears. The disease of the bones too is now arrested, and healthy osseous matter actively deposited at those parts where the weakness has been the greatest, i.e., at the part where the curvature is the most marked. As the general health daily improves, so the bones become firmer and harder; until at length only the deformities produced by the curvatures remain, to show during life how the individual has been once affected.

M. Guérin divides the term of rickets into three periods, viz., a, the stage of incubation; b, the stage of deformation; and c, the stage of transition of the organs and functions to a healthy condition. Of 346 cases of rickets observed by this author,—3 had arisen before birth, 98 in the first year, 176 in the second, 35 in the third, 19 in the fourth, 10 in the fifth, and 5 in the sixth. Of these, 148 were males, and 198 females. The average period of incubation was six months, during which a marked train of deranged actions manifested themselves. The total duration of the disease is from one to two or three years, or longer.

Diagnosis.—This is sometimes difficult in the early or precursory stage, as the symptoms closely resemble those presented by scrofula in one or other of its various forms. The enlargement of the ends of the long bones, producing tumefaction of the knees, ankles, wrists, &c., serves to aid the diagnosis; while the subsequent curvature confirms it, since softening of the bones during childhood only occurs in rickets.

In almost all rickety children it will be noticed that the fontanelles close late, being found widely open instead of ossified at the end of the second year of age. The commencement of teething is also deferred; the two central temporary incisors of the lower jaw not making their appearance until between the tenth and twelfth months, instead of the beginning of the seventh. The children are also backward in walking and talking; their growth looks stunted; and their intellectual powers are below the average.

Prognosis.—When uncomplicated, a favourable result may be expected from judicious treatment; but where there is considerable deformity, together with great loss of vital power, recovery will be doubtful. The earlier during infancy that the disorder occurs, the more unfavourable is the result likely to be; inasmuch as the general cachexia is then usually very severe. About 2 per cent of all the deaths occurring in England under 5 years of age are returned as due to rickets. This small proportion, however, must not be regarded as a proof that the danger of the disease is inconsiderable. Death directly from rickets is not common: death from its complications is frequent. Without doubt, the fatality of bronchitis, pleurisy, laryngismus stridulus, chronic hydrocephalus, infantile convulsions, diarrhœa, &c., is greatly increased by the rickety cachexia.

Treatment.—To prevent the occurrence of rickets in delicate children, or in the offspring of weakly parents, the treatment must be commenced at birth. It is usually very simple, and consists in attention to the following points :—The infant is to be fed only at the breast for the first eight months of life; by the mother if she be strong and sound, by a vigorous wet-nurse if the maternal health prove indifferent. As the result of a large experience I may say positively, that I have never known a rickety child to have been properly fed during the first year of its existence. If farinaceous food be given as the infant reaches the eighth or ninth month, "Liebig's Food" (F. 4) is to be selected. About the same time good beef tea, as well as the gravy out of a joint of beef or mutton may be allowed; followed after some weeks by the yolk of a lightly cooked egg, custard pudding, and subsequently by a little underdone mutton minced very fine or pounded in a mortar. During this period, attention is to be paid to cleanliness, and to suitable clothing; it being important that every young child should be warmly clad, and almost always with flannel next the skin. And then, the residence ought to be healthy; care at least being taken that the nursery is properly heated and ventilated, so that pure air may be breathed night and day.

When the cachexia is established, much can be accomplished by a well-directed course of remedies. In all instances, attempts must be made to check any complications—as catarrh, laryngismus stridulus, dyspepsia, diarrhœa, &c. that may be exhausting the system; at the same time that everything is done to strengthen the constitutional powers. Tepid chalybeate, or oak bark (F. 126), or sea water baths, or daily sponging with salt water; pure air— especially sea or country air; good nourishing diet, with an abundance of milk; ferruginous tonics, sometimes in combination with quinine; and cod liver oil, taken continuously for many weeks or even months: such are the remedies on which I chiefly rely. Where milk (whether of the cow, goat, or ass) cannot be digested, it should be given with lime water, or cream can be tried; or, these disagreeing, whey may be used as an inferior though still useful substitute. In bad cases I have seen benefit from the administration of restorative soup, or of raw meat simply minced (F. 2). With regard to the preparation of steel to be employed I know of none equal to Parrish's syrup of the phosphates of iron, lime, soda, and potash (F. 405). Supposing the bowels to become so constipated as to require physic, the most gentle aperients are to be ordered,—rhubarb, syrup of senna, or half a teaspoonful of castor oil in beef tea. That bane of the nursery, grey powder, is very seldom needed; while antimonial wine and all such lowering medicines are to be positively interdicted.

If, during convalescence, the child shows a marked liking for any particular kind of food, the desire should be gratified if possible. Sometimes there is a great desire for sweets, sometimes for salt, sometimes for fat and butter,—tastes which may rather be encouraged than otherwise.

Several years ago M. Piorry stated that he had long been in the habit of administering phosphate of lime with advantage to rickety children suffering from curvature of the spinal column. He recommended it in the form of very fine filings of fresh bones ; giving about one ounce daily, in milk, or in rice-milk. M. Piorry did not attribute all the improvement observed to this salt, as a highly nutritious diet was simultaneously employed. But it seemed certain, that in several patients in whom the spinal column had continued to deviate more and more every year, and who were subjected during several months to good regimen, free exposure to light, a dry and warm temperature, and especially to the use of the phosphate, the progress of the affection had become completely arrested. Now it likewise appears probable that this remedy may prove useful in all forms of rickets, as well as in the osteomalacia of adults, and in women threatened with the softening of the bones during pregnancy. The insolubility of the phosphate of lime has hitherto prevented its direct administration ; but it has been suggested that this objection can be removed by uniting the phosphate with carbonate of lime, when a soluble combination and valuable remedy results.

With regard to the use of irons and splints and other mechanical contrivances for supporting the legs of rickety children, several surgeons object to them, because they believe that the limbs subsequently become straight spontaneously. There seems, however, reason to doubt the correctness of this opinion ; and hence I am disposed to recommend the employment of some well-fitting apparatus in many cases. I have never seen any harm arise from the patient wearing light irons for a few hours every day during attempts at walking, provided they are made with joints corresponding to the hip and knee and ankle; so that while affording efficient support (for the legs bend because they cannot carry the weight of the body) they need not unnecessarily interfere with the natural movements. When there is any tendency to curvature of the spine, a reclining or recumbent position must be adopted for many hours of each day ; while if necessary, properly made stays or some other kind of spinal support, should be resorted to.

XV. TRUE LEPROSY.

This disease, of peculiar interest from its great severity and wide prevalence in remote ages, has lately excited considerable attention inasmuch as it is believed to be on the increase in the West Indies and in some other of our colonies. Of rare occur-

rence in the British Islands, still a few instances have been reported which serve to show that leprosy may become developed in
our own climate in the present day.   Most of the examples,
however, that have been seen in this country have occurred in
individuals who have long resided in some part of Africa or Asia,
even if they happen to be natives of Great Britain.   In Norway,
the disease—known under the name of Spedalskhed—is endemic:
at the last census in 1864 the number of lepers in that kingdom
was 2182.   This affection is likewise endemic in Greece.   At
every part of the south of Europe, cases are frequently met
with; but Spain and Portugal seem to have a larger proportion of leprous poor than most other European countries.
Wherever it has been witnessed, the features of true leprosy
(*Tsaraäth of the Jews, Elephantiasis Græcorum, Lepra Elephantia,
Eastern Leprosy, Black and White Leprosy*, &c.) have been found to
be the same.   There appears to be a stage of incubation, certainly
lasting for months and perhaps for years, attended with general
malaise and depression and occasional attacks of feverishness; a
period of persistent cutaneous eruption and discoloration; and a
stage of disordered innervation, with degeneration and death of
the affected tissues.   All observers agree in describing two forms
or modifications of this disease,—the tuberculated and the
anæsthetic (*Elephantiasis Græca Tuberculata*, and *Elephantiasis
Græca Anaisthetos*).   In the former, the morbid action appears
chiefly to attack the cutaneous and mucous surfaces; in the latter,
the nerves and nervous centres.   Either variety may exist alone,
or both may be present at the same time, or one form may succeed
the other.   On these grounds, the Committee appointed by the
Royal College of Physicians to draw up a Report on Leprosy has
recommended the arrangement of the two forms of this disorder
into the "tuberculated" and the "non-tuberculated."   Under the
latter head are included those modified cases sometimes designated
leucopathic, where there are white spots or blotches on the skin
which are more or less anæsthetic; as well as such as have an
eruption in the form of annular spots not unlike those of common
lepra, but with their centres anæsthetic, while the distinctive
characters of leprosy are present.

    Causes, Terminations, &c.—The commencement of leprosy is not
limited to any particular age.   According to Drs. Danielssen and
Boeck, the tuberculated form begins to manifest itself most
frequently between ten and forty years of age, and the anæsthetic
variety between the tenth and thirtieth year; but both kinds have
been seen at every period of life between early childhood and old
age.   The same authorities state, that the average duration of the
tuberculated form among the patients in the hospital at Bergen
from 1840 to 1847 was between nine and ten years: of the anæsthetic form, between eighteen and nineteen years. With both varieties, but especially the non-tuberculated, the morbid action some-

times remains stationary for several years.   In leprosy, as in other constitutional diseases which run their course slowly and which are indicative of a depraved habit of body, death happens quite as frequently from some intercurrent mischief as from the original malady.   Many lepers die of chronic diarrhœa or dysentery, of bronchitis or pneumonia, of nephritis, as well as of intermittent and remittent fevers and erysipelas.   Occasionally, death has taken place quite suddenly, without any sufficient cause being discoverable at the autopsy.   When the disease itself destroys life, it may do so by the thickening of the tissues of the glottis producing apnœa ; or by hæmorrhage from one or other of the ulcerations ; or by convulsions and coma due to the influence of the morbid state of the blood on the nervous centres.

There is a very general belief amongst the best observers in all parts of the world that leprosy is hereditary, though it also occurs where no such influence can be traced ; and that it frequently skips over one generation to reappear in the next.   At the Bergen Hospital it was noticed that the hereditariness seemed to be more frequent on the maternal than on the paternal side ; while it was also more diffused in the collateral than the direct line.   The evidence may be said to be conclusive that it is not contagious, nor transmissible by sexual intercourse.   The male sex appears to be more liable to the disease than the female ; but the testimony on this head is contradictory.   Very probably false deductions have been made, owing to all the facts not being known.   All writers agree, however, that the lowest classes of society are the most liable to leprosy ; while if it is not directly caused, it is certainly greatly aggravated and its progress hastened, by improper and insufficient food, personal uncleanliness, intemperance and sexual excesses, as well as by residence in malarial districts or in damp and ill-ventilated dwellings.   Taken generally, lepers are as filthy and degraded in their mode of life as they are miserable and destitute.

Symptoms.—The chief features of the Mosaic leprosy are described in the thirteenth chapter of Leviticus, in which will be found " the laws and tokens" whereby the priest is to be guided in discerning this dreaded affection.   Here we notice (verses 24 and 25) what may be regarded as an indication of the commencement of the disease in an erythematous rash.   In this respect, the same feature marks the onset of *tuberculated* leprosy in the present day.   The general feverishness which occurs in all acute cases towards the end of the latent period, ushers in an erythematous eruption ; on the appearance of which, the fever subsides. Where the disease makes its approach very gradually, there may be an absence of all fever.   There will be one pinkish or purplish-red spot, or several ; if several, they either remain isolated, or they run into patches.   After a time, this rash perhaps subsides. There is an interval of freedom ; followed, however, by another attack of fever and a fresh eruption, more severe and extensive than the first.   This suspension of morbid action and aggravated re-development may possibly occur several times.   At length, the serous portion of the blood escapes into the intervascular tissues at the site of the exanthematous spots; giving rise to hard and semi-transparent elevations or tubercles.   Exudation also occurs into the superficial spongy stratum of the true skin, causing thickening and an appearance of great coarseness; as well as into the neighbouring connective tissue, producing œdema.   About the same time, an excess of brown pigment is deposited in patches.   Then the brawny-looking skin slowly undergoes a gelatiniform degeneration; while as portions of this degenerated material get atrophied, so white spots and cicatrices are left, though there has been no wound or ulcer.   The alæ of the nose, the integuments of the cheek, the tissues of the lips and ears, become swollen and bloated. There is a copious mucous discharge from the nostrils.   The eyes present a livid watery appearance, the conjunctivæ being in parts congested; while the lids get tumid and flabby, little nodules are formed on them, and their edges are sometimes everted.   The hairs of the head and face assume a yellowish-brown or reddish tinge at first, and subsequently become white : often they fall off in considerable quantity.   The mucous lining of the nose, mouth, palate, glottis, and throat is all engorged and pulpy-looking, while here and there it is spotted with little tubercles which may ulcerate; so that there is an abundant secretion of viscid saliva or of mucopurulent matter, with hoarseness or loss of voice.   The nails become discoloured and squamous.   Glandular tumours form ; the inguinal glands swelling first and most extensively, and then those of the axilla.   An unpleasant kind of greasy sweat often exudes from the surface of the whole body, but especially from the swollen hands and feet.   The skin is not insensible to the touch : perhaps a sense of heat and itching is complained of.   Muscular cramps are common.   Until now the venereal passion may have been excessive.   As the tuberculated masses increase in size and spread over the neck and chest, the trunk and extremities, so a lethargic condition of the mind and body gets developed.   The general aspect is repulsive.   Headaches are complained of; the extremities are contorted and swollen and useless; the testicles waste ; and absorption takes place of the bones of the palate and of the nose, so that the latter organ becomes flattened.   Complications now arise : there is frequently albuminuria, dysentery or chronic diarrhœa, or some bronchial or pulmonary mischief.

During the progress of the foregoing series of changes, complaint is often made of pain.   This may at first be slight, so that it will possibly be looked upon as of a rheumatic or neuralgic character.   But while the tuberculated masses have been forming in the skin, a congestion of the capillary vessels of the sheaths of the nerves has been taking place; producing an exudation of a viscid gelatinous material into the sheaths and connective tissue, and thus distending the nervous trunks to double their size. In this way we can account for the occurrence of hyperæsthesia followed by anæsthesia; the pressure of the congested skin and distended capillaries at first causing great pain, while the subsequently increased compression from exudation benumbs the sensibility. According to Mr. Erasmus Wilson the neurotic affection begins at the periphery, and proceeds towards the centre; the cutaneous nerves being first destroyed, then the nervous trunks that supply those nerves, and slowly and by degrees the nervous centres— the spinal cord and brain. At first and for years these morbid changes are attended with fugitive and shooting pains; but ulti- mately they terminate in perfect insensibility, so that the knife can be used without pain, or a taper may be held to the affected skin without being discovered by the patient.

The *non-tuberculated* form of leprosy commences by the forma- tion of one or two circumscribed patches on the hands, or face, or feet. These patches are shining and wrinkled and rather paler than the surrounding skin; while they are so devoid of sensibility that the application of a hot iron is not felt. Frequently, large bullæ form on these patches. These bullæ break and leave ulcers, which usually scab and heal. Slowly, the affected parts spread; and as they do so certain constitutional symptoms arise. The pulse be- comes infrequent, and slow or labouring; the mental faculties get sluggish or benumbed; there is a sensation of coldness of the surface; there is constipation, though the appetite is voracious; and the ends of the fingers and toes seem glazed, as well as rather swollen and stiff. As months, or perhaps years pass on, the cuticle cracks in different places and desquamates; while frightful ulceration, un- attended with any pain, occurs on portions of the extremities. The integuments about the small joints seem to slough off in large flakes; the interior of joint after joint gets exposed; and there is a constant sanious discharge from the numerous wounds. The bones of the toes or fingers get exposed, loosening as they do so; until after a time, one phalanx after another comes away, leaving behind granulating sores which ultimately heal. The hands and feet, thus deprived of portions of osseous support, get contorted into all kinds of shapes. Ultimately the limbs may become entirely use- less, the patient being obliged to crawl about from one part of the room to another. The axillary and inguinal glands swell. The temperature of the body gets much reduced; the thermometer sometimes showing a diminution to the extent of 20° Fahr. There is ozæna, and the surface exhales a loathsome fetor. The sensibility of both mind and body gets greatly blunted; so that until the sufferer is relieved by death, there is a mere animal life, his loathsome state being usually more distressing to those who witness it than it is to himself.

Morbid Anatomy.—The reports of Drs. Danielssen and Boeck on the changes found after death in the leprous patients at the

Bergen hospital are so important, that no apology is necessary for directing attention to the following summary of them. In the developed stage of the *tuberculated* variety, the corion or cutis vera of the affected parts is tumid and thickened ; while on squeezing it between the fingers a viscid or gruelly fluid exudes. The subcutaneous connective tissue is infiltrated with a gelatinous or lardaceous effusion, firmly adherent to the corion. The subcutaneous veins and nerves are thickened and enlarged from the deposit of this effused matter on their outer surface. In the advanced stage, the nerves, especially when lying near to ulcerations, are much thickened and enlarged ; in consequence of congestion and inflammation of their sheaths. The mucous lining of the nares and fauces and larynx is swollen ; while it is occupied with tubercles, and often ulcerated. The opening of the larynx is frequently the seat of morbid deposit, so that the rima glottidis is sometimes nearly closed up. Tubercles are occasionally found on the mucous lining of the trachea and large bronchi. The cervical glands are occasionally much enlarged. The substance of the lungs is seldom altered ; but the pleuræ are often much thickened from tuberculous deposits, as is the peritoneum. The mesenteric glands are very generally more or less enlarged. Isolated rounded ulcers are occasionally found on the inner surface of the intestines. The liver is now and then the seat of tubercles. The kidneys are almost always affected in the advanced stage of the disease ; the morbid changes being usually those characteristic of albuminous nephritis. Within the cranial and vertebral cavities no distinct or uniform morbid changes have been detected,—neither in the substance of the brain or spinal marrow, nor in their investing membranes.

When the *anæsthetic* form has been completely developed, and the paralysis of the muscles as well as of the skin has become decided, the skin is often found much attenuated, all the fatty matter has disappeared, and the substance of the muscles is atrophied. The connective tissue in the parts surrounding the seat of ulceration or necrosis is infiltrated with a serous or lardaceous deposit. The nerves which traverse this infiltrated tissue, as well as the deep-seated ones, are excessively swollen ; their sheaths being filled with a firm albuminous matter in which the ultimate nervous filaments are imbedded. These alterations are considered to be the result of inflammation of the nerves, and are identical with those found in the tuberculated form of the disease. The axillary and inguinal glands are often much enlarged. The nervous centres are commonly the seat of notable alterations. Especially, there is congestion of the posterior or dorsal veins of the spinal marrow ; effusion of an albuminous serum within the arachnoid membrane, and between it and the dura mater ; adhesion of the arachnoid to the pia mater ; and consolidation or hardening of the substance of the spinal cord at the parts affected, which most frequently happen to be the cervical and lumbar regions. Generally, the cord is also somewhat contracted in size ; but sometimes it is so atrophied as not to be much larger than a quill. The cineritious substance is altered, having acquired a dirty yellow colour so as nearly to resemble the medullary substance. The roots of the nerves within the vertebral canal are coated with albuminous exudation. Sometimes the axillary and ischiatic plexuses, and the principal nerves issuing from them, are visibly atrophied. The morbid appearances discovered within the cranial cavity appear to be similar to those which exist within the spinal cavity, though they are observed in a less decided or advanced degree. Whenever there had been well-marked anæsthesia of the face, the Casserian ganglion was always seen to be the seat of some change. There was usually a sero-albuminous effusion around it, many times so considerable that the distended dura mater bulged out at the part ; while the nervous filaments of the ganglion seemed to be glued together by the exuded matter.

With respect to the condition of the blood in both the tuberculated and the anæsthetic forms of leprosy, the most marked change from the normal standard appears to consist in the excessive quantity it contains of albumen and fibrin. These, it will be remembered, are exactly the elements, more particularly the albumen, in the morbid effusion with which all the pathological alterations, characteristic of the disease, are connected.

Treatment.—Although cases of recovery are not unknown, yet as a rule this disease is incurable. The patient's hope of a cure may, however, be increased by removal from a malarious to a high and dry salubrious district ; by allowing a nutritious, wholesome, palatable, and digestible diet ; and by insisting upon strict attention to personal cleanliness. The use of baths is very advisable ; but it is uncertain whether any special good can be derived from arsenical, sulphur, or iodine baths. I should certainly be inclined to give the arsenical baths a fair trial ; administering them on alternate days with the wet-sheet packing (F. 136).

With regard to ordinary drugs those on which most reliance may be placed are cod liver oil, quinine, and steel. The efficacy of arsenic and iodine must be allowed to be doubtful. A long continued course of purgatives has sometimes appeared beneficial. In two instances of tuberculated leprosy which I saw at St. John's Hospital for Skin Diseases, and notes of which I am enabled to give here through the courtesy of Mr. J. L. Milton, more relief seemed to be derived from the use of aperients with nourishing food, than from various other plans of treatment.* In the selection

---

* *Case* 1. Thomas C——, æt. 18, was admitted into St. John's Hospital, under the care of Mr. Milton, on 16 April 1867, suffering under well-marked symptoms of leprosy. He is of Irish parentage, but was born in the Madras Presidency. When a lad he was sent over to Ireland to be educated. Four years after leaving India, in May 1863, the disease first commenced as a pricking sensation in the extremity of the right little finger; this pricking being gradually followed by complete insensibility. During the next two years

of aperients it will be better to trust to the most simple. Few perhaps will answer better than the sulphate of soda; none can

the anæsthesia steadily spread till, on the inside of the arm, it reached the armpit. In the winter of 1865 tubercles began to appear on the forehead and then under the eyes: the nose, chin, and cheeks were next invaded. Anæsthesia now attacked the left leg, all the lower part of which became insensible. Subsequent to this the right leg was affected in the same way. Bronzed spots, accompanied by tubercles, now made their appearance on different parts of both legs and thighs; while the left arm likewise became slightly affected.

At the time of his admission, the face was entirely covered with dirty reddish-brown tubercles which were of all sizes from that of a split pea to the bigness of half a small walnut. They were smooth and painless; on some few of them thin small scales were seen. There were several of these tubercles on the under part of the chin and on the sides of the neck, but none on the back of the latter. Nearly the whole of the right arm was covered with brown stains of every depth of hue; there were some on the left, but much fewer and smaller. These stains varied in size from that of a pea to that of a crown piece. In every part that showed a stain sensation was lost. He used when at school to amuse himself by cutting these places with a knife and never felt any pain from doing so, though they bled. The legs were even more extensively affected by spots and anæsthesia than the arms; the patches too extended over the thighs, whereas the upper arms were pretty free.

With one short interval the patient remained in St. John's Hospital up to the middle of June 1868. During this period there was but very little change, and that little was always for the worse. Now and then the disease appeared to be stationary, but there has never been any lasting improvement. The hue of the skin has become darker, the tubercles have spread a little, a firm scale has formed over one elbow, while a large firm crust occasionally appears on the outer side of the left nostril; but with these exceptions the symptoms have not materially changed. He says he has always noticed that the complaint gains ground in winter, and is better or at least stationary during summer. Except occasional attacks of pain in the right arm and liver and diaphragm, at times very severe, he has not suffered much.

The medicines tried were iodide of potassium, strong decoction of sarsaparilla, the Zittman treatment, calomel and black draught, steel, nitric acid, and a preparation of quinine and carbolic acid. Of all these, the iodide and the purgatives were alone beneficial. The others were either useless or injurious; except the calomel and black draughts which repeatedly checked the progress of the disease and relieved the pains. Had brisk purgatives been given persistently and from the first, it is thought that some benefit might have resulted; but as Mr. Milton had had no previous experience of their effects in this disease, he was afraid of the action of such powerful medicines on a weakened constitution.

The urine was several times analysed and examined microscopically, but except very extraordinary variations in the amount of the nitrate of urea nothing unusual was seen: it contained no albumen and no blood. Mr. Milton could detect no change in the blood; and Mr. Robert Taylor who examined a specimen, found it quite normal.

Case 2. George H——, aged 38, entered St. John's Hospital, under Mr. Milton's care, on 17 May 1867. He was suffering under anæsthetic and tubercular leprosy in a very aggravated form. The disease began more than eight years previously, and according to his account followed a severe attack of ringworm which almost entirely covered him with patches from an inch to a foot in diameter. Nearly a year after this his face became remarkably flushed and puffy. Finding that he got no better, he came home on leave and placed himself under the care of an eminent physician in Dublin. He rebe worse than such as contain one or other of the different preparations of mercury. With regard to this metal its use may indeed be positively forbidden ; since the universal experience shows that it acts most injuriously in whatever form it is tried.

Perhaps no article in the materia medica has been more freely employed in this disease than arsenic. The Hindu doctors have long used it very extensively. Mr. Palgrave tells us that the Arabs suffer much from leprosy, which sometimes assumes the blotchy form called " Baras" and sometimes the hideous " Djedām." Under this latter, " the joints first swell, then break out into sluggish yet corroding ulcers, and at last drop piecemeal, while frightful sores open in various parts of the body, especially about the back and loins, till death comes, though after too long delay. The ' Baras' also, though never fatal, may lead to superficial ulceration." The natives have hit on a vigorous " though too often an unsuccessful specific in the sulphate of arsenic, or yellow arsenic, for so they call it ; and now and then they cure with it, occasionally killing by an overdose or smearage."* Even these " now and then" cures must, however, be looked upon with suspicion ; for although a leper will possibly have recovered while taking arsenic, yet it requires a much larger amount of evidence than can be adduced to lead to the belief that there was any connexion between the medicine and the cure.

Lastly, Drs. Danielssen and Boeck say they have found, in the anæsthetic form of the disease more especially, that the repeated application of cupping glasses and moxas along the course of the spinal column has proved of marked advantage in relieving the lesions of innervation ; whether these agents have been adopted during the stage of increased or of diminished sensibility.†

covered and went back to Trinidad, but the disease reappeared and gained ground rapidly. His case was treated in Trinidad with arsenic in large doses and purgatives ; under which the improvement was so considerable that at one time he thought he was getting rapidly well. Unfortunately the treatment was neglected, and a relapse ensued. He came home again, but becoming worse and worse, quitted Ireland and entered St. John's Hospital.

At this time he was in a dreadful state. The tongue was tubercular and fissured, the voice thick and hoarse, the nose sunk in, the mucous membrane of the lips ulcerated away, the muscles of the arms and legs shrunk to the last degree, the hands incurved, and nearly all the skin stained with the characteristic hue of leprosy. The tips of the fingers were ulcerated ; while the skin of the face was tuberculated and dirt coloured, and there were large tenacious crusts upon it. He was put upon purgatives, and at first seemed to derive great benefit from them : in particular the ulceration of the lips entirely healed up. Here too Mr. Milton was afraid to continue the remedies ; but when they were left off the symptoms relapsed, and when they were tried again the progress under them was slow. At length he grew dissatisfied ; and was accordingly transferred on the 22 January 1868 to the Middlesex Hospital, where he died quite suddenly on the 14 April.

* *Narrative of a Year's Journey through Central and Eastern Arabia* (1862–63). Second Edition, vol. ii. p. 34. London, 1865.

† The foregoing remarks have necessarily been made as concise and practical as possible. But if it be desired to follow up the study of this

XVI. MELANOSIS.

Melanosis is a very rare disease; and consequently our knowledge concerning it is not very extensive. It is characterized by the deposition in various tissues of the body, of a black or dark-brown substance; whence its name,—from $\mu\ell\lambda\alpha\varsigma$ = black + $\nu\acute{o}\sigma o\varsigma$ = disease.

Melanotic formations may take place in various parts of the body, may present much variety of form, and may owe their production to different agents. They are divided by Dr. Carswell into two great groups:*—(1) True Melanosis, of which there is only one class. And (2) Spurious Melanosis, of which there are three kinds—a, that arising from the introduction of carbonaceous matter; b, from the action of chemical agents on the blood; and c, from the stagnation of the blood.

1. TRUE MELANOSIS.—This disease has its seat most commonly in the connective and adipose tissues; but it is also found, though rarely, in the mucous and serous membranes, in tendons and cartilages, as well as in the osseous system—particularly the bones of the cranium, the ribs, and the sternum. The organs it most commonly affects are the liver, lungs, spleen, pancreas, lymphatic glands, brain, eye, kidneys, testes, uterus, ovaries, rectum, and mammæ. Moreover, melanotic matter has been detected in the blood—particularly in that taken from the minute veins of the liver. Andral states that he has met with it in the false membranes formed on serous surfaces. The black pigment granules of melanotic matter may be infiltrated through a cancerous tumour (melanotic cancer), or through a benign growth. In short, melanotic disease

disease at greater length, the reader will find much valuable matter in the following works:—An essay by Mr. Robinson in the *Medico-Chirurgical Transactions*, vol. x. p. 27. London, 1819.—Antiquarian notices of Leprosy and Leper Hospitals in Scotland and England, by Professor Simpson, *Edinburgh Medical and Surgical Journal*, October 1841, January and April 1842. The number of this Journal for January 1842 also contains a paper on tubercular elephantiasis by Dr. T. B. Peacock; while that for July 1842 has one by Mr. J. Kinnis.—*Traité de la Spedalskhed ou Elephantiasis des Grecs*, par D. C. Danielssen et Wilhelm Boeck, Paris, 1848.—Cazenave's *Manual of Diseases of the Skin*, translated from the French by Dr. T. H. Burgess. Second Edition, p. 314. London, 1854.—*Report on Leprosy by the Royal College of Physicians.* Prepared for Her Majesty's Secretary of State for the Colonies. London, 1867.—*On Diseases of the Skin, A System of Cutaneous Medicine*, by Erasmus Wilson, F.R.S. &c. Sixth Edition, p. 587. London, 1867.—An account of two cases in the *Guy's Hospital Reports.* Third Series, vol. xiii. p. 189. London, 1868.—In the *Bible,* the chief description occurs in chapters 13 and 14 of Leviticus. But there are also notices of lepers and leprosy in several of the other books, especially in the 5th chapter of Numbers; in the second book of Kings, chapter 5; the second book of Chronicles, chapter 26; as well as frequently in the New Testament, —the gospels of St. Matthew, Mark, and Luke.

* *Pathological Anatomy.* Section on Melanoma. London, 1838.

has a great tendency to extend to different parts of the body through the lymphatic system.

Varieties.—Dr. Carswell describes four minor forms of true melanosis:—(1) The *punctiform*, in which the black colouring matter appears in minute points or dots, grouped together in a small space, or irregularly scattered over a large surface; this variety being more frequently seen in the liver than in any other organ. The gland looks as if it had been freely dusted with charcoal. (2) *Tuberiform melanosis* (the most common and conspicuous of all the forms) may occur in the majority of the different organs, if not in all; as well as on serous surfaces, such as the pleura and peritoneum. The tumours vary in size from a pin's head to an orange; they are either single or aggregated together, in the latter case producing irregularly-shaped masses of great bulk; they are seen enclosed in a membranous covering, or they will be non-encysted; and co-existent with them the punctiform variety is found in the liver, lungs, and kidneys. (3) *Stratiform melanosis* occurs only on serous membranes. The black matter is frequently so small in quantity, that the tissue on which it is deposited may merely appear as if stained with it; or it will be more abundant, so as to give rise to a distinct layer of the consistence of firm jelly. This form is much more frequently met with in the horse than in man. (4) *Liquiform melanosis* is chiefly produced in natural or morbid cavities. Dr. Carswell says that he never saw it in man as a product of secretion; but that he has met with it in consequence of the destruction of melanotic tumours, and the effusion of their contents into serous cavities. The accidental cavities in which it has been found have been chiefly ovarian cysts.

It is probable that the melanotic matter is deposited in a fluid state, and that it acquires consistence by the absorption of its more liquid parts. It has never been found solid in serous cavities, where its diffusion is not impeded by unyielding tissues; but in the liver and lungs the tumours may have about the same consistence as a lymphatic gland. The black matter is almost tasteless and odourless; and chemical analysis shows that it is essentially composed of the constituent elements of the blood. According to M. Foy, it is the colouring matter of the blood highly carbonized.

Symptoms.—In subcutaneous melanosis the peculiar appearance of the tumours or nodules removes all difficulty as to diagnosis. But the symptoms accompanying melanotic deposits in internal organs are rarely well marked; so that their presence is often only ascertained after death. Dr. Copland states,* that as far as the symptoms have been recorded, and as far as he could observe them in a single case, melanosis is characterized by a gradual sinking of the vital energies, a cachectic habit of body, and a dusky ash-coloured countenance. There is also a marked change in the nutritive functions; this deterioration slowly giving rise to emaciation,

* *A Dictionary of Practical Medicine*, vol. ii. p. 830. London, 1858.

dropsy, weakness of the pulse, and night-sweats towards the termination of the disease. Occasionally, when the lungs have been affected, there has been a blackened mucous expectoration.*

* A very interesting example of extensive subcutaneous melanosis was under the care of Sir William Lawrence, at St. Bartholomew's Hospital, a few years back. From the account which has been published (*Medical Times and Gazette*, p. 225, 27 February 1864), and from a letter with which Mr. Eccles has favoured me, I am enabled to give the following particulars of the patient's history :—J. F., aged thirty-three, was in an emaciated low condition, when admitted on *28th January* 1864. He had been a railway porter for eleven years, was married and the father of two healthy children, and his parents were living. Eighteen months previously he first noticed a lump in each groin the size of a hazel-nut. Six months subsequently another growth, resembling a wart, appeared just below the umbilicus : which increased rapidly in size, was removed by ligature, and left only a black mark. Until two months ago he was strong and well, no fresh nodules having appeared ; but at this time, the hundreds which were found scattered all over him at the date of his entrance into hospital made their appearance, and his health gradually deteriorated. When admitted, the original lumps in the groin were about the size of small eggs ; being hard, nodular, very movable, and apparently consisting of enlarged glands. Scattered over the trunk and the lower and left upper extremities, were innumerable nodules ; which varied from the size of a millet-seed to that of a full-sized pea, and seemed to be situated in the subcutaneous tissue. They were thickest over the abdomen and back ; but, in the thighs, laid chiefly in the course of the vein. Similar nodules were felt in the situation of the lymphatic glands in the neck. He complained of some pain in the right lumbar region, but otherwise did not suffer much, save from a continued sensation of sinking. No blood was detected in the urine, although he said that of late he had passed blood in his water. There was no evidence of the disease being of a cancerous nature. A microscopic examination of the melanotic matter showed only the small pigment granules and the larger pigment cells.—On the 9th February, the day after death through exhaustion, Mr. Eccles made an examination of the body. On reflecting the abdominal integument, the nodules were proved to be, with few exceptions, entirely subcutaneous. They were easily separable from their connexions, were of the consistence of soft putty, and were quite black. One rib, just at its junction with the costal cartilage, was infiltrated, and the bone softened, so as to be easily cut through with a scalpel. Somewhat larger nodules were scattered over the interior of the thorax, beneath the pleura ; and a like condition existed in the pericardium, the cavity of which was filled with a dark serous fluid. Similar deposits were found beneath the visceral layer of the pleura, especially between the lobes, and some of smaller size in the substance of the lower lobes of each lung. The bronchial glands were apparently wholly infiltrated. The heart was studded on its exterior with numerous nodules (very like ordinary dry black currants), which here and there seemed to involve the muscular tissue of the heart. Similar deposits were situated beneath the endocardium, but the valves were unaffected. The liver was only slightly affected, the disease seemingly extending from the surface into the substance of the viscus. The fibrous capsules of the kidneys were greatly affected, especially the right, only a very little of the structure of these organs being apparently implicated. The supra-renal capsules were not examined. The spleen was very firm and small ; but no deposit could be detected. Attached to the omentum were several masses of disease, of which the largest were two lying in the cavity of the pelvis, each somewhat larger than a man's fist. On cutting through these, they were apparently uniform in structure throughout. The intestines were seemingly natural, save that the rectum contained some pinkish-coloured fæces. The brain, orbits, &c., could not be examined ; an unfortunate circumstance, as the

Pathology.—It is still a matter of uncertainty whether true melanosis is not simply medullary cancer modified by the formation of black pigment in its elemental structures. Mr. Paget (writing prior to seeing Sir W. Lawrence's patient) says :—" On this long-disputed point there can, I think, be no reasonable doubt. I have referred to a case of melanotic epithelial cancer : but, with this exception, I have not seen or read of any example of melanosis or melanotic tumour in the human subject which might not be regarded as a medullary cancer with black pigment. In the horse and dog, I believe, black tumours occur which have no cancerous character; but none such are recorded in human pathology."* On the other hand, Dr. Walshe entertains a directly opposite opinion, and for the following reasons :—" 1. That the melanic pigment should in itself constitute cancer is an absurdity : it never even forms a stroma, as the cells continue permanently free. 2. The stroma of many melanic tumours is perfectly distinct in its physical, chemical, and microscopical characters from all cancerous stromata. 3. Many melanic tumours do not contain cancerous juice. 4. The microscopical characters of the pigment-cells and granules are the same in all kinds of growth in which they occur. 5. Melanic tumours, when no ordinary cancerous elements exist in them, cause no local or general symptoms except those dependent on the size and seat of the growth. 6. When melanic tumours produce the local or general symptoms of cancer, they are found either to be composed of encephaloid or scirrhus, wholly or in part impregnated with black pigment. 7. Neither the local nor general symptoms produced by carcinoma are modified in cases in which melanic matter is found to pervade it. 8. The circumstance that melanosis is rarely solitary, is strongly insisted upon by Cruveilhier, as a ground for ranking it with cancer. But tubercle multiplies similarly, yet assuredly tubercle is not cancer."† Unfortunately, I can myself say but little upon this matter; though it seems to me, from a careful study of those recorded cases which are scattered through our literature, that there is great reason to doubt whether melanosis is so closely allied to cancer as many pathologists assert. It is not a very uncommon disease in horses, especially in those of a grey colour; and it is said that in these animals life is scarcely shortened by its presence, though it exhibits the same tendency as in man to multiply itself in different parts of the system.

Melanosis is most often met with in the middle-aged, or even in those advanced in life. Mr. Wardrop, however, has seen it in

man had gradually become blind a few days before his death. The mesenteric glands were affected in the same way as the bronchial; and there were numerous nodules beneath the peritoneum in the sub-peritoneal tissue.

* *Lectures on Surgical Pathology.* Edited by William Turner, M.D. Second Edition, p. 731. London, 1863.
† *The Nature and Treatment of Cancer*, p. 184. London, 1846.

a little girl only two years old, in whom "the humours of the eye were converted into a black gelatinous substance." Where the disease attacks the skin, it will often be found to have commenced in or near a congenital mole or a wart.

Treatment.—On this head there is little to be said that is satisfactory. Indeed, all that can be done is to attempt to relieve and combat the distressing symptoms as they present themselves. The two classes of medicines which will be found most useful are tonics (especially the mineral acids with bark), and cholagogue purgatives. The necessity for good diet, sea air, and a moderate amount of exercise, should also be borne in mind.

2. SPURIOUS MELANOSIS.—There are three kinds of this counterfeit disease. They arise thus :—

a. From the Introduction of Carbonaceous Matter.—This variety of false melanosis—sometimes spoken of as black phthisis—occurs only in the lungs. These organs present a black carbonaceous colour; the bronchial glands are also blackened; while the pulmonary tissue is indurated and friable, infiltrated with black serum, and often broken down into irregular cavities. The discoloration has its origin in the inhalation of the carbonaceous product of ordinary combustion; as well as in the inspiration of air loaded with minute particles of coal. Hence, it is chiefly found in the lungs of those who have worked in coal mines.

b. From the Action of Chemical Agents on the Blood.—In digestion of the coats of the stomach by the gastric juice after death, and in poisoning by acids, the blood contained in the gastric capillaries, as well as that which is extravasated, will generally present a blackish tint. Sometimes the blood is almost as black and thick as tar; while it adheres to the fingers on being handled, and imparts a peculiar impression something like that produced by glycerine. The inhalation of sulphuretted hydrogen gas will also darken the blood in the intestinal capillaries.

c. From the Stagnation of Blood.—Retarded or impeded circulation may produce black discoloration of the blood. When this fluid ceases to circulate in the capillaries of an organ it coagulates, the serum and salts become absorbed, and a black substance remains. The latter probably consists of fibrin and hæmatin. The organs in which the foregoing changes occur are the digestive and the respiratory.

XVII. FATTY DEGENERATION.

The designation of *fatty degeneration*, or *fatty metamorphosis*, is given to a certain class of cases which during life are marked by the occurrence of progressive anæmia with great prostration; and which, after death, are found to be distinguished by the more or less perfect transformation into fat of various important textures, but especially of the muscular fibres of the heart.

Fat is an important element of the human body. There is the adipose tissue, in the cells of which oily materials are naturally stored up for the welfare of the individual. And there are other textures—as the villi of the mucous coat of the duodenum and jejunum, where this element transitorily abounds after the digestion of particular kinds of food. But in the cases about to be treated of, fatty matter is present in abnormal situations; the tissues being more or less converted into this substance. As a consequence of this deterioration there may result the most disastrous lesions. There is, therefore, no connexion between the tendency to form fat around organs, or to the production of obesity, and the change of textures into fat. In the former case we have a condition which may prove preservative, if confined within due limits. In the latter, we recognise only a process of decay and death; the result of some defect in the nutritive functions. A tissue once completely converted into fat (and there is no tissue in the body which may not undergo such conversion) cannot be reconstructed by human aid. The extension of this degeneration, however, can now and then be hindered; while the work of the affected organ may be lightened by well-timed assistance.

A fatty degeneration of one or more of the viscera (most frequently perhaps of portions of the muscular fibres of the *heart*) is very commonly found after death from chronic disease, or even from old age. Inactivity, impaired nervous power, the persistent yielding to some master-passion, over-study, and cessation of function, lead to this change; as does phthisis, excessive or small continuous losses of blood, continued fever, and indeed all wasting diseases. Intemperance is a fruitful source of it; so is long-continued privation of good food and pure air; and so also appears to be a residence in tropical climates.

The fact that the tissues of even more than one organ are in a state of degeneration, must simply be taken as an indication that life is somewhat in peril. Not that death is necessarily imminent; but that the individual, if he would live, will be obliged to exercise great and constant caution. The bloodvessels of the brain may long have their coats affected, and yet offer no impediment to the flow of blood or to cerebral nutrition; but let any sudden strain be put upon them, and sanguineous apoplexy at once results from their rupture.

All varieties of cell-formation may undergo fatty degeneration; the process commencing at first with the production of a few fatty molecules, and continuing until the amount is so great that the cell wall gives way. The *liver* is particularly liable to be thus affected, the hepatic cells becoming enlarged and loaded with oil granules. There are certain forms of *Bright's disease* in which the epithelium of the convoluted uriniferous tubules is found in a state of fatty degeneration; the degenerated epithelium so filling the tubules that they present a yellowish opaque appearance. In fatty degeneration of the *muscular fibres of the heart*, the metamorphosis may go on until all normal structure has disappeared in the portions affected. The same not unfrequently occurs in the internal coat of the walls of *arteries*, the change being often visible to the naked eye in the shape of round or angular white spots; such parts on being minutely examined presenting the usual characteristic appearances. The atheromatous change which happens in the arterial walls of old people—particularly in the aorta, is a form of fatty degeneration; beginning with a low kind of inflammation of the arterial coat, and often ending in softening and ulceration. If an atheromatous patch be submitted to microscopic examination, it will be seen to consist of fat globules, plates of cholesterine, granule cells, and amorphous fragments of tissue. Again, in certain diseases like paralysis, deformities of the limbs, spinal curvature, &c. the *muscular structures of the affected part* may undergo transformation into fat; so that they are observed on dissection to be pale and thin and yellowish, or marked longitudinally with alternate red and yellow streaks. This latter appearance is due to the deposit of fat between the primitive muscular fasciculi, combined with real fatty degeneration. It is a condition which can be well examined in any of the voluntary muscles of over-fed prize cattle. And lastly, about the age of fifty, when old age begins to steal on by slow degrees, the corneæ may be the first to tell the unwelcome truth. The *arcus senilis*, commencing at the upper and outer margin of the clear cornea, and occurring symmetrically in both eyes, is the result of the retrograde metamorphosis under consideration. And this change is of special importance, inasmuch as it is sometimes indicative of a like alteration going on in organs beyond our ken. I say "sometimes," because it is certain that it may exist alone, the tissues of the heart or liver or kidneys being healthy; or the latter may be undergoing fatty degeneration without the arcus being present.*

The designation of *idiopathic fatty degeneration* has been given by Dr. Wilks to a class of cases in which excessive anæmia and debility are the peculiar phenomena during life; and a fatty degeneration of many parts of the body, but more especially of the heart, the characteristic changes detected after death. The term idiopathic is used to disconnect these cases from those instances of fatty change of organs which are found as accompaniments of other diseases.

Perhaps the symptoms and progress of a case of idiopathic fatty degeneration may be made more clear by the sketch of a typical example:—A woman, thirty-five years of age, married but

* The reader who wishes to study this part of the subject more closely should refer to Mr. Edwin Canton's excellent treatise *On the Arcus Senilis, or Fatty Degeneration of the Cornea.* London, 1863.

never pregnant, complains of great and increasing debility. For the last eighteen months she has had much mental anxiety; but her diet has been good, her home healthy, and she has not suffered from any exhausting disease, such as bæmorrhage, diarrhœa, &c. As far as is known she has never had ague, nor lived in a malarious district. She has taken drugs of various kinds without any benefit for almost a year: to her surprise, the favourite antibilious pills have disagreed unmistakeably. The catamenia are regular though scanty, and there is no leucorrhœa; she is thin but not wasted, is weak, and presents a marked pallid aspect; there is no arcus senilis; the pulse beats are only forty, and there is an anæmic cardiac murmur; while the lungs, lymphatic glands, liver, spleen, &c., appear not to be diseased. Moreover, the urine contains neither albumen nor sugar; and on examining the blood microscopically no excess of white corpuscles can be detected. We hope that by the careful administration of a nourishing diet, together with bark or quinine and iron, the symptoms may become ameliorated. But this expectation does not get realized. The strength rapidly gives way: there is neither pain nor anxiety. In a short time, perhaps at the end of a month or two, we find that there have been frequent attacks of sickness and purging; the legs have become slightly œdematous; while she is reduced to such a condition of weakness that she can scarcely raise herself in bed. A few days later she is found in a half-conscious state; and then at the end of some hours death happens. At the autopsy it is noticed that the body is spare, but not wasted as in phthisis: all the tissues are very pale, and the viscera appear bloodless. The brain, lungs, intestines, spleen, and supra-renal capsules, are healthy; as are also the generative organs. The liver, however, is pale and fatty; while the muscular tissue of the heart has undergone an extreme degree of fatty degeneration, presenting a pale mottled appearance to the naked eye. This change is chiefly seen in the left ventricle, which exhibits the appearance of white striæ of fat, every part being occupied by this fatty change: the right ventricle is less affected, and the auricles look healthy. On examining with a quarter inch object-glass some of the fibres from the left ventricle no traces of transverse striæ can be seen, but only a large number of small oil globules, with free fat globules which have escaped from the ruptured fibres. The kidneys are pale, and healthy to the naked eye; but on a microscopic examination the tubules and secreting cells are found to contain a considerable amount of fatty molecules.

Sufficient has now been said to show the importance of a careful examination of this subject, which will be again referred to in treating of the diseases of various organs. Its extensive bearing on the practice of medicine cannot be better summed up than by quoting the words of the late Mr. Barlow, of the Westminster Hospital:—" Who, a short time ago," says this gentleman, " would have dared to assert, unless from some morbid desire to be ridiculed, hæmorrhage of the brain, the heart, the lung, and the placenta was often the result of fatty degeneration similarly affecting these parts and leading to their rupture?   Who could have asserted that ' mollities ossium,' atheroma of arteries, and the arcus senilis, heretofore grand and unmeaning appellations, were only specimens of the same devastation?   Who have affirmed that ramollissement of the brain and softening of the heart were (I say not, invariably) examples of it too?   Who could have spoken of degeneration of the liver and kidneys as conditions associated with, and dependent on general atrophy?   Who could have traced gradual to the same cause as sudden death, as now we can?   Surely, there has been, to speak most modestly, a great and evident advancement in pathology."*—These remarks need no confirmation at the present time, for universal observation has proved their truth.   The entire subject of the various forms of degeneration of tissue, can hardly have too much attention paid to it. When a man is attacked with acute disease—with pneumonia, pericarditis, rheumatic fever, &c. the practitioner naturally thinks of the special treatment which these disorders require.   But a more important matter still is to consider seriously the state of the patient's blood and tissues,—of what is commonly called his constitution.   Thus it is obvious, that the widest possible distinction must be drawn between the management of acute bronchitis occurring in a previously healthy subject, and the same disease affecting an individual with granular kidney or with fatty degeneration of the muscular fibres of the heart.   So also, the ophthalmic surgeon consulted as to the cure of a case of cataract could, I imagine, scarcely advise an operation where the opacity of the lens appeared to be connected with diabetes ; though under many other circumstances extraction would be the means of restoring sight. It is upon the recognition of these and similar points that the future prospects of the art of healing look so promising.   Even as it is, much has been accomplished in this direction.   We are able to see more certainly than our forefathers could what medical treatment will accomplish and what it will not.   And it seems to me that it is owing to this enlightenment—forasmuch as we know that degenerated tissue cannot be repaired by bleeding or mercury or antimony, that recourse is had much less frequently to such active remedies than formerly ; and not because there has been any change in the type of organic disease.

XVIII. AMYLOID DEGENERATION.

The discovery in the animal kingdom of starch, or, at least, of a substance which possesses properties allied to those of the

* *On Fatty Degeneration,* p. 90.   London, 1853.

amylaceous group in the vegetable world, is full of interest to the pathologist and physician. For some few years it has been known that the liver, spleen, and kidneys occasionally undergo a peculiar degeneration, which has been described under the names of the *Lardaceous, Waxy, Cholesterine,* or *Albuminous Infiltration;* though until the publication of the researches of Virchow (1854— 1859), we were not only ignorant of the nature of this substance, but of its exact seat. Even now our knowledge of this morbid process is very imperfect.

What we do know of the matter, as far as I can gather from a careful study of the writings of Virchow, Wilks, Francis Harris, Gairdner, and the author of a very excellent article in the *British and Foreign Medico-Chirurgical Review* for October 1860, together with the observation of the few cases which have been under my charge, seems to be as follows:—In the human body there are to be found, according to Virchow, two allied, but not identical, substances. In the first place we find bodies which, in their chemical properties, are analogous to real vegetable starch, and in their form bear an extraordinary resemblance to vegetable starch-granules, inasmuch as they constitute more or less round or oval structures, formed by a succession of concentric layers. They are in fact *starch corpuscles* or *amylaceous concretions.* To this class belong the little corpora amylacea of the nervous system; the laminated bodies that are discovered in the prostate of every adult man, and which, under certain circumstances, accumulate in large quantities, so as to form the so-called prostatic concretions; and rare substances of a similar kind which occur in certain conditions of the lungs. These formations assume a blue colour by the action of iodine, as vegetable starch does; the blue becoming green if they are mixed up with much albuminous matter, for inasmuch as the nitrogenous material is rendered yellow by iodine, while the amyloid becomes blue, the result must be green. The greater the quantity of nitrogenous matter the browner does the colour become.

In the foregoing instances the starch-like matter lies *between* the elements of the tissues. Very different are the cases of disease, where there is a degeneration of the tissues themselves; in which all their component parts become filled with a *starch-like* or *lardaceous substance* and get gradually infiltrated with it, just as lime is diffused through the tissues in calcification. The change commences in the muscular fibre-cells of the middle coat of the small arteries; the walls of which vessels gradually get thickened, while their calibre becomes diminished. Then the morbid process involves the surrounding anæmic parenchyma; extending until the whole tissue in the neighbourhood of the arteries is altered. This amyloid substance, thus infiltrated, has the peculiarity of not becoming blue under the influence of iodine alone, but of assuming a peculiar yellowish-red colour; though it takes on either a blue or a violet tinge, if the application of iodine be followed by the very cautious addition of sulphuric acid. Hence this material seems less allied to starch properly so called, than to that substance which forms the external membrane of vegetable cells—cellulose; though it differs from this in becoming coloured upon the application of a pure solution of iodine, whilst real cellulose is not at all coloured by iodine alone. Owing to 'this multiplicity of reactions, it is difficult to say to what class the material really belongs; though it has been somewhat generally assumed, from its reaction with iodine and sulphuric acid, that it is analogous to the substances of the amylaceous group. Meckel, in an essay on *Lardaceous Disease*, cites the chemico-physical appearances as favouring the presumption that the material is cholesterine, or some closely allied fat. Virchow and others show, on the other hand, that the substance does not in any way behave like a fatty matter; while the reactions of cholesterine and the apparent amylaceous compound are so different that the two cannot be confounded. Finally, some careful analyses by Kekulé and others have tended to show that there is a very close chemical identity between this morbid material and albumen; and hence it has been urged, that instead of our having to deal with amyloid degeneration of tissue, the substance is almost proved to be *albuminoid* in its nature.

Whatever the particular substance may be, however, the important fact remains, that in the so-called *amyloid*, or *albuminoid*, or *cellulose degeneration*, we have a remarkable constitutional disease; which generally invades several organs at the same time, and renders them incapable of performing their functions. The patients gradually assume a cachectic, broken-down appearance; they lose flesh and strength; dropsy often supervenes; the urine gets albuminous if the kidneys become affected; diarrhœa sets in when the digestive tract is involved; and in spite of remedies death soon takes place.

Where the liver, spleen, or kidneys have been the organs affected, an unpractised eye might fail to detect the alteration in structure unless there is an extreme amount of disease. But when, for example, we incise a liver where the process of amyloid degeneration is far advanced, a feeling is communicated like that experienced on passing the knife through a piece of wax; while the cut surface presents a semi-transparent appearance. The gland is also found increased in size; it has some resemblance to a fatty liver, though its increased weight distinguishes it; a sense on handling is given like that received from a lump of wax; and if the disease be very extensive no trace of normal structure can be distinguished, though in an earlier stage the lobules are seen distinctly mapped out owing to the matter being deposited within the lobule and in and among the secreting cells. Dr. Harris first employed chemical reagents to detect the presence of amyloid in the walls of the intestines; and he noticed that on brushing a solution of iodine over the mucous membrane of the affected portions, innumerable dark-red points corresponding with the villi appeared, which points became changed to a bluish-steel colour on the super-addition of a drop of dilute sulphuric acid.

Virchow speaks of the occurrence of amyloid degeneration of the lymphatic glands as an undoubted fact; and in all probability he is correct. Dr. Wilks, however, with more caution, says, that the change in these organs is not strictly lardaceous, but is either a variety of it, or has a close relationship with it. It produces a lingering form of fatal cachexia. " The enlargement of the glands is in most cases gradual, extending sometimes over a period of two, three, or more years, and often from commencing in the neck in weakly children, is called scrofulous. When the mischief is thus gradual in its commencement, and affecting only part of the glandular system, no marked symptoms ensue, but as time tends to its development in the thoracic and abdominal glands, a slow prostration ensues, terminating in death."* The glands often get an enormous size; they have a peculiar elastic feel; they will form large tumours in the neck and groin; while the posterior mediastinal and lumbar glands may all be affected, or only these latter glands along the course of the aorta may be involved without any affection of the external glands. When these diseased bodies are removed, they are found as distinct tumours, very tough and solid. On making a section of one of them, the cut surface looks to the naked eye as if dotted over with points of wax; and though Dr. Wilks says no effect is produced by the application of iodine, yet Virchow maintains that this agent colours the diseased parts of the gland red, whilst the normal portions are rendered yellow. If when the iodine-red hue is obtained we use sulphuric acid, a blue colour may be procured if the exact proportion of acid necessary to effect this change be hit upon.

Sometimes the disease in the glands is associated with the presence of the peculiar wax-like substance in the spleen, or with lardaceous liver, and with tuberculosis. The symptoms in any case are those of anæmia, prostration, and final exhaustion. The lymphatic glands and spleen being connected with the blood making process, the most injurious results must ensue if a gradual destruction of their texture goes on.

There is only one more important point to be briefly noticed— viz., that amyloid degeneration may either exist alone, or it will be present in connexion with tuberculosis, suppuration, diseases of the bones, or syphilis. Thus, in phthisis, this form of hepatic disease is said to be much more common than fatty liver; while sometimes the amyloid and the fatty degeneration occur together. So frequently has amyloid degeneration been found connected with caries or necrosis, that at one time it was thought the osseous disease exercised some determining influence on the production of the amyloid material. Multiplied researches have proved, however,

* *Guy's Hospital Reports.* Third Series, vol. ii. p. 103. London, 1856.

that amyloid degeneration is as frequently associated with phthisis and syphilis, as with bone disease. So, also, it was considered that Bright's disease often became associated with amyloid degeneration, until it was found that the former was sometimes merely a symptom of the latter affecting the kidneys. While lastly, evidence is accumulating rather rapidly which serves to show that there is some important link between lardaceous disease and long-continued suppuration. The two conditions have now been found connected together too often for such an alliance to be simply accidental.

XIX. MINERAL DEGENERATION.

The process by which mineral matter is infiltrated or deposited in a tissue must be briefly noticed. Every texture in the body is probably liable to mineral degeneration; but it is most frequently observed in the coats of arteries, and in the cartilages. Tubercular and cancerous growths may also undergo this change, while it not uncommonly occurs in fibroid tumours of the uterus.

The importance of discriminating between *calcification* and *ossification* has been well pointed out by Virchow. Formerly both these conditions were spoken of as " ossification." But a structure does not become true bone because it takes up lime into its intercellular substance, and has stellate cells present in it. On the contrary, it is merely " calcified " or " petrified." At the same time it is not to be forgotten that " ossification " does sometimes take place, with the formation of dense or compact and spongy or cancellated tissue, and occasionally even of periosteum.

The coats of large arteries are often found brittle from petrifaction. And this earthy degeneration may not only occur alone, but in combination with fatty degeneration or atheroma. Sometimes plates of mineral matter are discovered embedded in the middle coat of the vessels, rendering them hard and rigid tubes.

All varieties of exudation have a liability to undergo the calcareous transformation; the animal matter becoming absorbed, while the mineral constituents get aggregated and so form laminæ. In this way Dr. Hughes Bennett states that he has seen the gallbladder converted into a calcareous shell, and the pericardium into an unyielding mineral box enclosing the heart. The cardiac valves have thus likewise become petrified.

With regard to fibro-calcareous tumours, Mr. Paget describes two methods by which calcification may advance,—a peripheral and an interstitial. In the former, the most rare, a common fibrous tumour becomes coated with a thin and rough and nodulated layer of chalky or bone-like substance. By the latter method, a similar substance is more abundantly deposited throughout the growth; being often so arranged, that by maceration a heavy and hard mass can be obtained, knotted and branched like a lump of coral. With both forms the change is an earthy degeneration, consisting of a deposit of the salts of lime and other bases, in combination with, or in place of, the fibrous tissue. True bone is not formed in uterine fibroids.

XX. GOITRE AND CRETINISM.

The arrangement of goitre and cretinism in one section is not to be justified simply on the score of expedience. It is almost impossible to doubt the existence of some relation between these two diseases; although what the connecting bond may be, is as yet a matter of conjecture. But that they are often combined together in the same individuals is, of course, indisputable.

1. GOITRE AND EXOPHTHALMIC BRONCHOCELE.— The disease called *Goitre* [perhaps from *Guttur* = the throat] by the Swiss; popularly, in this country, *Derbyshire Neck*, from its prevalence in some parts of Derbyshire; and technically *bronchocele* [from Βρόγχος = the windpipe + κήλη = a swelling], consists of a morbid enlargement of the thyroid gland. This produces an unsightly disease; which, though usually painless, is much dreaded by the inhabitants of those districts where it is prevalent.

The characters presented by the swelling vary according to its duration. It will either be soft, or firm, or very hard. The whole gland may be swollen, or the centre only, or either side. According to Alibert, the right lobe is more frequently affected than the left. The largest goitre that I have measured caused the neck to have a circumference of two feet. The swelling is unaccompanied by pain, and usually gives rise to little inconvenience beyond the deformity which it produces. Sometimes, however, throbbing of the vessels, inordinate pulsation of the heart, great depression of spirits, dyspepsia and sickness are complained of; together with other symptoms indicative of an attenuated state of the blood. Dental caries and deafness are not uncommon. Moreover, distressing sensations may be induced by the pressure of the enlarged gland on the surrounding parts; while respiration and deglutition are rendered painful and difficult by the compression of the trachea and œsophagus. Goitre is much more common in women than in men : almost in the proportion indeed of twelve to one. Sometimes there appears to be a connexion between bronchocele and irregularity of the uterine functions. Thus I have remarked in many cases that the enlargement of the gland is greatest at the catamenial periods, and especially when the flow is scanty. Other authors have also noticed that the disease makes the most progress during the puerperal state; and a few remarkable cases confirmatory of this opinion have fallen under my own observation. Profuse leucorrhœa is a frequent accompaniment of the throat-swelling, whether pregnancy exist or not. The palpable swelling of the thyroid which is sometimes met with in hysteria led Dr. Graves to suggest, that the globus hystericus, or sensation as of a ball rising in the throat, is due to a sudden congestion of this gland. It may be doubted, however, whether this peculiar sense of choking is not more plausibly explained on the supposition of an irregular action of the constrictor muscles of the pharynx, one of the many consequences of deranged innervation.

Wherever goitre prevails, popular opinion regards the water used for drinking as its cause.   Dr. Edmund A. Parkes thinks it is certain, that the water of goitrous districts contains large quantities of lime and magnesia ; being derived from limestone and dolomitic regions, or from serpentine in the granitic and metamorphic districts.   During the ten years, 1843-53, the water used in the food and drink of the prisoners at the Durham County Jail contained large quantities of sulphate of lime, carbonate of lime, and chloride of magnesium.   The men in all classes, whether on low diet or otherwise, suffered extensively from goitre.   The pumping machinery of the well then got out of order, and the water (filtered) of the river Wear was temporarily introduced for the use of the jail.   The effect soon became apparent on the health of the prisoners, and the affections in the neck immediately subsided.   So marked was this result, that the water of the well was analysed by Professor Johnston ; who condemned it as unwholesome and unfit for use.*   Still more conclusive evidence has been brought forward by Mr. M'Clelland ; who affirms, as the result of his personal inquiries, that goitre never prevails to any extent except in villages situated upon, or close to, limestone rocks.†   The facts adduced by this gentleman in confirmation of his opinion are deserving of attention.   At the mountain province of Kemaon, in Bengal, the inhabitants all belong to the same tribes of Hindoos, and are subject to fewer irregularities in their mode of life than any other people in the world.   Yet, while the residents of some of the districts are almost free from goitre, those of other villages suffer extensively.   The tract in which the disease most prevails is the richest and most fertile portion of the province.   The natives themselves ascribe the prevalence of goitre to the quality of the waters.   The following abstract of the proportion of inhabitants of each rock affected with goitre and cretinism, compared with the healthy, proves the probable correctness of this view :—

Granite and gneiss rocks . . . . *Goitre,* $\frac{1}{100}$; *cretins,* none.
Mica slate and hornblende slate rocks . . *Goitre,* none; *cretins,* none.
Clay slate rock . . . . *Goitre,* $\frac{1}{125}$; *cretins,* none.
Green sandstone rock . . . . *Goitre,* none; *cretins,* none.
Calcareous rocks (chiefly Alpine limestone) *Goitre,* $\frac{1}{4}$; *cretins,* $\frac{1}{33}$.

When it is remembered that a district of more than a thousand square miles has been made the subject of the foregoing inquiry, that in every portion of this space the same circumstances attended

* *The Monthly Journal of Medicine,* vol. xx. p. 377.   Edinburgh, 1855.
† *Sketch of the Medical Topography, or Climate and Soils, of Bengal and the N.W. Provinces.* By John M'Clelland, Surgeon, &c. p. 83. London, 1859.

the presence or absence of the disease, surely there must be something more than an accidental coincidence.   And yet the inferences
drawn by Mr. M'Clelland have not been allowed to pass unchallenged.   They have been particularly objected to by M. Chatin,
who mentions that in Savoy there are two villages divided from
each other by only a narrow ravine.   Both villages stand on rock
and soil of the same nature, their elevation is the same, and they
seem subjected to the same influences.   But in one goitre prevails,
while in the other it is unknown: in the first, the water supplying
it contains a trace of iodine; in the second there is no iodine in
the water.   In consequence of such contradictions as these, there
has been a growing conviction in the professional mind that this
disease is due to a combination of circumstances, rather than to a
single cause; and it has been said to be probable that neither a
marshy soil, nor the absence of the sun's rays, nor the configura-
tion of the locality, nor the habits of the people, nor any peculiarity
of the waters, will separately induce goitre.   But in thus attempting
to multiply the causes of this disease we are departing from that
sterling canon of criticism—that the simplest explanation is always
the best.   In the present instance, moreover, there is less room
for doubt than happens to be the case with many medical questions; and hence there is the less excuse for resorting to conjecture.

There is a *cystic variety of bronchocele,* in which cysts are developed in the thyroid body, instead of this gland becoming
uniformly enlarged with solid matter.   The lining membrane of
these cavities is very vascular; so that if they be opened and their
brown-coloured serous contents evacuated, they require to be well
stuffed with lint to prevent hæmorrhage.   As granulations are
thrown out from the walls, the cyst contracts; while ultimately it
entirely closes.   Iodine injections in such cases are not simply
inefficient, but they may prove dangerous.

The first point in the *treatment* of goitre is, if possible, the
removal of the patient from the infected locality.   Then, in
women, care is to be taken that the menstrual functions are regularly established.   As regards therapeutic agents, the introduction
of iodine, by Dr. Coindet of Geneva, has in a great measure superseded all other remedies.   The iodide of ammonium (F. 38) is often
very beneficial; especially if its internal administration be accompanied by its employment locally.   Bromide of potassium, in
thirty grain doses, has been recommended.   Iodide of potassium
is also useful (F. 31); and sometimes cod liver oil, given with it,
aids recovery.   At the same time the tumour should be rubbed
every night with the officinal iodine ointment, or painted with
iodine liniment diluted with an equal quantity of spirit or glycerine.
The iodide of iron (F. 32), quinine and iron (F. 380), steel and
aloes (F. 404), are all valuable medicines.   A nourishing diet
must be allowed, and the hygienic surroundings of the patient
attended to.

A plan of treatment adopted in India by the late Major Holmes seems to have had great success.* This gentleman (who was barbarously murdered during the Indian mutiny) is said to have treated a large number of sufferers. The method, as practised at Fyzabad, Oudh, is as follows :—Three drachms of the red iodide of mercury are carefully mixed in a mortar with nine pounds of suet. Sixty, one hundred-and-twenty, or one hundred-and-eighty grains of this ointment, according to the size of the tumour, are to be rubbed in with an ivory or wooden spatula for about ten minutes soon after sunrise, and the patient desired to sit with the goitre exposed to the rays of the sun. After six or seven hours' exposure, the pain is often considerable, and the surface generally becomes slightly blistered. Some more ointment is then to be gently spread over the tumour, and the person may be allowed to go home ; but he has particular directions not to interfere with the blistered surface, and to attend for a fresh application if necessary, as soon as the skin has healed. Major Holmes usually advised that the ointment should be used but once a year to the same patient. Mr. Whishaw, also of Fyzabad, says that small goitres, such as are seen in England, are cured by one application ; but those of larger size require three or four. He mentions the case of a woman whose goitre measured nearly five feet in circumference, and hung down some inches below her navel. The ointment was used once a month for a year, when she left the hospital ; the swelling having been reduced to the size of a small cocoa-nut. By some of the surgeons of the Indian army it is thought better to employ a stronger ointment than that used by Major Holmes. Mr. Greenhow uses one of the strength of an ounce and a half of the salt to three pounds of lard. A modification of this plan appears well-deserving of trial,—viz. the simple inunction, every other night for some weeks, of the officinal ointment of red iodide of mercury (grs. 16 to the ounce). Care had better be taken not to blister the neck by the too free application of the remedy.

In this country when medical treatment fails, surgeons have attempted to give relief by one of three operations. Thus some cases are recorded as having been cured by the introduction of setons into the diseased gland ; and in three obstinate cases which were unrelieved by the iodide of ammonium, iodide of iron, quinine, &c., I effected cures by passing thin double iron wires, through the glands and leaving them there for a week. With other instances this treatment has failed to effect any good; and unfortunately there are no means by which we can tell beforehand whether the seton will prove beneficial or useless. A little care is necessary in introducing the wires, to prevent enlarged vessels from being pierced. Occasionally the operation of tying the thyroid arteries has been practised ; and these means having failed, attempts have been made to extirpate the gland. To most practitioners, however, the last operation will probably seem unjustifiable.

* *The Lancet*, p. 438. London, 10 October 1863.

The peculiar form of this affection which has been named EXOPHTHALMIC BRONCHOCELE, owing to the prominent condition which the eyes assume in it, is a remarkable disease. Not only is there protrusion of the eye-ball (proptosis oculi), but generally more or less short-sightedness so that objects a few yards off cannot be correctly defined, with sometimes a constant and involuntary motion of the eyeball (nystagmus); the thyroid body, as well as being enlarged, is the seat of strong pulsations; whilst the patient suffers from frequent attacks of palpitation of the heart, with occasionally a loud systolic bruit (anæmic?). For our knowledge concerning it, the profession is indebted to the observations of Dr. Stokes, Sir Henry Marsh, Dr. Graves, Dr. Begbie, Von Basedow, &c. Hence, it has been proposed at different times and at different places to name it " Stokes' disease," " Begbie's disease," " Maladie de Graves," and " Morbus Basedowii." There is nothing to be said in favour of this style of nomenclature; and it is to be hoped that its adoption will be checked, since it can only lead to the starting of questions of priority which are sure not to end in any satisfactory solution.

The triple set of characteristic symptoms must especially be remembered,—the exophthalmia, the hypertrophy of the thyroid, and the cardiac palpitation. Both eyes are as a rule, symmetrically affected; while in exaggerated cases, the globe of the eye is only incompletely covered by the lids during sleep. The smooth tumour of the thyroid seems often to rest on the top of the sternum; bulging on each side of the trachea, and usually being more largely developed on the right, than on the left side. Frequently, however, the swelling is less than in ordinary goitre. The hand applied over the gland detects a pulsation or pulsatory thrill, everywhere: the ear, a continued bruit which is loudest with the systole. The pulsation of the deep-seated vessels of the neck is usually visible. In many instances the heart is enlarged; although, at first, the disturbed action of this organ is merely functional. The tilting of the apex against the walls of the chest seems to be sharper and more apparent than ordinarily. A systolic bruit is often heard at the base of the heart, and in the cervical vessels. The pulse, under the influence of slight excitement, can be at once raised from 90 or 100 to 120 or 130. The general health is always deranged. There is a liability to attacks of giddiness or faintness; the extremities are often chilly; the digestion is disturbed, as shown by a tendency to nausea and diarrhœa; the temper is bad—discontented; the appetite is sometimes voracious, though it frequently fails; and sleeplessness is not uncommon. The termination in recovery may generally be looked for; though it is important to recollect that death has sometimes occurred suddenly as if from serous apoplexy, and sometimes gradually from diarrhœa or exhaustion.

The cause of this disease is unknown. Females, particularly

about the time of puberty, are much more liable to it than males. It is not necessarily connected with uterine derangement. Occasionally it has commenced suddenly after a fright. In one instance I could only trace its production to the violent action of an emetic, which was unwisely taken at the commencement of the catamenial flow to relieve pain. The mode of production of the exophthalmia has not been positively determined. It has been attributed to distension of the intraorbital vessels, pressing the eyeball forwards; to serous infiltration of the areolar tissue behind the globe of the eye; or to an increased growth of adipose tissue in the orbit. Whichever may be the correct explanation (the first, or congestive theory, is the most plausible) it usually happens that the ocular prominence and the thyroid tumour increase or diminish simultaneously; although in cases of recovery, the former usually gets more completely cured than the latter. M. Trousseau believes that this complicated affection (which he describes as " La Maladie de Graves," since he says it was first recognised by this distinguished physician in 1835) is a neurosis; being accompanied by local determinations of blood, and having as its proximate cause a modification of the vaso-motory apparatus. This theory explains the occurrence of disturbance in regions supplied by branches from the sympathetic.

In the management of cases of exophthalmic goitre it is above all things necessary to remove the patient out of the way of every insalubrious influence, and if possible to place her residence in some elevated district such as Malvern; to allow an invigorating diet, with plenty of milk, animal food, and cod liver oil; and at the same time to lessen congestion of the thyroid by such topical applications as ice, cold water douches, and evaporating lotions. The treatment pursued at the principal hydropathic establishments is sometimes especially serviceable. With regard to drugs, more confidence may be placed in digitalis than in any other. Given in full doses, at proper intervals, it calms the cardiac and arterial pulsations, while it seems to impart tone to the heart's walls : its administration is to be stopped when the pulse has fallen to 70. If the practitioner hesitate about this use of the remedy, he may try the effects of the American Wild Cherry (F. 333), the action of which is more gentle. The different preparations of steel have long been recommended, but they do not always agree. With a pulse at 120, a salt of iron will often augment the distress and give rise to urgent dyspnœa. All the iodine and bromine salts prove injurious. They aggravate the exophthalmos, the palpitations and pulsations, as well as the general anæmia; and though they may possibly cause a temporary diminution in the size of the thyroid, yet this is no sufficient set-off for the mischief they effect.

2. CRETINISM.—This is a strange disease,—a sort of idiocy, accompanied by imperfect development and deformity of the bodily

organs, particularly of the head. The disease may be either complete and incurable, or incomplete and curable. Intermediate between these forms there is a degree known as demi-cretinism. Many authorities assert that cretinism has a close but ill-understood connexion with goitre. M. Kœberle, of Strasburg, who has written a work on this subject which is highy spoken of, disputes this connexion. He attributes the disease to a miasmatic poisoning. Just as some marshy lands produce cholera, some yellow fever, and some ague,—so also he believes that cretinism will arise in certain malarious districts under suitable conditions of temperature and moisture. Dr. Macculloch, some years since, hinted that cretinage had its origin in malaria.* But in my opinion the views of M. Bouchardat approach much nearer to the truth. According to this gentleman, endemic cretinism is chiefly due to two causes acting simultaneously,—the connexion of this disease with endemic bronchocele, and consanguineous marriages. In all localities where endemic cretinism prevails, endemic goitre is met with. The goitrous parents have cretinous children, and the offspring of the latter are complete cretins. For bronchocele to be induced a few months' use of impure drinking water will suffice ; but for the production of cretinism it is necessary that insalubrious conditions should extend over several generations. It is certain that most, if not all, cretins are goitrous ; though bronchocele is seen to prevail where there are no cretins.

The cretin is found principally in the valleys of the Alps, the Pyrenees, the Andes, and the Himalaya mountains. In the complete form, the stature is diminutive ; the head of great size, flattened at the top, and spread out laterally ; the countenance is vacant and void of intelligence ; with the nose flat, lips thick, lower jaw elongated, and mouth gaping and slavering. Then the tongue is large, and frequently protruding from the mouth ; the eyes are red and watery ; often there is squinting ; the abdomen is sunken and pendulous ; the legs short and curved ; while the skin is cadaverous or dark-coloured, coarse, and rough. In the females, menstruation comes on at a late period,—on an average about the eighteenth year ; while in extreme examples of this disease, the reproductive powers may remain undeveloped through the whole life. Idiotism of the lowest grade is this cretin's lot. He is deaf and dumb, or blind ; often he is voracious ; while frequently he is addicted to the most disgusting practices.

Demi-cretins and curable cretins have badly formed heads, and very limited mental powers. They are neither dumb nor blind ; though the faculty of speech may be imperfect. By great care they can be taught a certain amount of self-control. But if neglected, they acquire very filthy habits, like the complete cretins ; so as, indeed, more to resemble animals than human beings. I say, if neglected ; for, thanks to Dr. Guggenbühl,—the founder of

* *An Essay on Malaria*, p. 435. London, 1827.

the establishment at Abendberg, near Interlachen, for the treatment of cretins—it has been proved that even for these wretched
beings much may be done. The chief remedies are pure mountain
air ; plenty of exercise ; a simple nourishing diet into which milk
largely enters; wholesome water; the occasional use of such
medicines as cod liver oil, carbonate of iron, phosphate of lime,
valerianate of zinc, &c. ; with moral control, and judicious mental
training.* Dr. Guggenbühl has also directed attention to the highly
arched palate of the idiot, as indicative of atrophy of the base of
the brain ; just as depression of the vault of the cranium shows
imperfect development of the cerebral convolutions. He very properly insists upon the necessity, in training the idiot, of ascertaining the prominent instincts, and the amount of intelligence which
exists ; so as to encourage those faculties which are not altogether
wanting.

XXI. GOUT.

Few disorders have attracted greater attention from ancient
and modern physicians than gout.† Sydenham, who was well able
to describe its symptoms from a personal experience inasmuch
as he suffered from it for thirty-four years, says that "it kills more
rich men than poor, more wise than simple. Great kings, em-
perors, generals, admirals, and philosophers, have all died of
gout. Hereby Nature shows her impartiality : since those whom
she favours in one way she afflicts in another—a mixture of good
and evil pre-eminently adapted to our frail mortality." It has
long been, and is still, a vulgar error, that an attack of gout is
salutary ; helping to prolong life and drive away other maladies.
The truth is, however, that it produces local and general mischief,
which increases with every paroxysm ; and though the evil effects
may at first be inappreciable, yet the physical powers become

* An interesting account of this establishment is given by Sir John
Forbes, in *The Physician's Holiday*. Third Edition, p. 180. London, 1852.
It is necessary to mention, however, that since Sir John's visit in 1848,
the Institution on the Abendberg has been widely condemned ; and it has
been asserted, from actual observation, that not only does it fail to fulfil the
objects it was established to promote, but that Dr. Guggenbühl's conduct as
superintendent is not deserving of professional confidence. At the same time
it is allowed that this physician's efforts were at first most disinterested and
praiseworthy ; and hence it is to be hoped that these efforts will be remembered, while his failings may be forgotten.

† The old Greek physicians named this disorder according to the part
affected. Thus they speak of podagra [ποδάγρα, from πούς = the foot + ἄγρα = a
seizure]; chiragra [χειράγρα, from χείρ = the hand]; gonagra [γονάγρα, from
γόνυ = the knee]; and arthritis [ἄρθρον = a joint] when several articulations
were simultaneously attacked. The term gout seems to have been first used
about the year 1270 ; having been derived from the Fr. *goutte* = a drop,
because it was thought to be produced by a humour which fell *goutte à goutte*
into the joints.

gradually undermined. Of course when the gouty fit is over, the blood is purer and the patient is in better health than before ; but the cause of the attack has produced a permanent and injurious effect,—probably on the kidneys, possibly on the heart.

Gout may be defined as a specific inflammation, having a constitutional origin, and being much favoured by an hereditary taint. It is accompanied by great pain and swelling of the affected joint, fever with general disturbance, and especially by some disorder of the digestive organs. The disease is either acute or chronic. It has a tendency to recur again and again, after variable intervals.

The inflammatory action most frequently invades the ball of the great toe, or the metatarso-phalangeal joint. Thus, out of 516 cases of gout, Sir C. Scudamore found that only the great toe of one foot was affected in 314 ; the great toe of each foot in 27 ; the ankle and great toe of the same foot in 11 ; the outer side of one foot in 10 ; the instep, one or both, in 31 ; the ankle, one or both, in 47 ; while in the remainder, the part was either the heel, tendo Achillis, the ham, knee, wrist, thumb, or fingers.

Symptoms.—The *acute* attack may be preceded by premonitory symptoms, or it will come on suddenly. In the former case, the patient complains for two or three days prior to the seizure of more or less dyspepsia, and especially of heartburn with flatulence ; of dull pain in the left side of the chest, with inability to lie comfortably on that side ; while, in many instances, there is also fluttering irregularity, or intermission, in the heart's action. There are at the same time symptoms of impeded cutaneous action, the skin being dry and hot, and sometimes affected with scaly eruptions or with urticaria ; while the urine is loaded with urates.

Very often, however, there is no warning. The victim goes to bed apparently well ; but about two or three o'clock in the morning awakes with severe burning and throbbing pain in the ball of the great toe, or in the heel, or the fascia covering the instep of the foot, or the thumb. There is frequently a slight rigor succeeded by heat. The pain is most excruciating, but it abates towards the dawn, and the patient falls asleep. On again awaking, the affected part is seen to be red and swollen, while it is exquisitely tender to the slightest touch ; the sufferer is feverish, restless, very irritable, and mentally depressed ; his tongue is white and thickly furred ; his bowels are constipated ; and his urine will be found high-coloured, rather scanty, acid, and loaded with urates or with uric acid, sometimes with phosphates or oxalate of lime, while occasionally it contains a little albumen. When the urine presents much uric acid (which is seldom the case) this circumstance is favourable, since it indicates that the kidneys retain their eliminating power ; and hence it may be hoped, that the blood becoming quickly freed from the excess of this principle, the patient will soon recover. Often the bladder is irritable, so that it has to be emptied frequently ; while the urine in its passage gives

rise to a sense of heat in the urethra.   On the second night the pain
again becomes aggravated; and, perhaps, also on the third.   But
in a few days the attack passes off, the œdema disappears, the
cuticle over the inflamed part desquamates, and the patient regains
his usual health.   Very frequently he is conscious of feeling better
and brighter and more buoyant than he has been for a long time
previously; for though the attack may prove permanently somewhat injurious, it is undoubtedly temporarily curative.

With improved strength and spirits, very little attention is
paid to hygienic rules.   The victim forgets that the disease will return.   At first, a happy time of two or three years may elapse.   With
each paroxysm, however, the interval will shorten; until at length,
perhaps, the patient is hardly ever free from an attack, except it
may be for a few weeks in summer.   At the commencement also,
the disease confines itself to a single joint : by degrees, several
joints in both feet or in the hands suffer.   Deposits (called tophi or
tophaceous deposits or chalk-stones) are formed around and outside the joints, of a material resembling moist chalk, and consisting
chiefly of urate of soda; small spots of which substance can often
also be seen just beneath the skin of the auricle of the ear, and
less frequently on the eyelids or in the integuments of the face.

The disease is generally spoken of as *chronic* gout when the
attacks are almost constant, and the constitution has become impaired by them.   The actual pain, perhaps, is not quite so intense as
in the acute form ; but the distortion and partial or complete anchylosis of the joints, the impairment of the various digestive organs,
and the effects upon the kidneys, render these cases very serious.
The urine is pale, abundant, and of low specific gravity; the quantity
of uric acid is below the healthy average ; and there is often some
albumen.   As in acute, so in chronic gout, the urea is eliminated
in due proportion.   Every now and then the concretions round
the joints give rise to suppuration and ulceration of the skin, and
then masses of urate of soda mingled with pus globules are discharged ; such discharges, however, often proving beneficial to the
general health, unless the ulceration is extensive.

Complications.—In one variety, called by Cullen *retrocedent*
gout, some internal organ becomes affected as the disease disappears from the joints.   The term "metastasis," signifying the
shifting of the disease from one part of the body to another, is
hardly applicable here.   The application of cold to a gouty limb
is one of the most frequent causes of this mishap.*   In cases
where the stomach is attacked we find sickness and vomiting,

* A filthy practice has oftentimes been adopted, even by individuals who
ought to know better, of soaking the gouty limb in urine every night.   The
patient collects his urine for the twenty-four hours, sometimes adds a little
salt or soda to it, and then employs it as a cold foot-bath before going to bed.
The most troublesome case of severe pain in the stomach (probably of a
gouty character) which has ever fallen under my notice occurred in a man
seventy-five years of age, who had adopted this custom for eight months.

hæmatemesis, violent spasmodic pain, with great distress and anxiety. When the retrocession is to the brain, it produces intense headache, lethargy, and sometimes apoplexy or paralysis. In such instances, the membranes of the brain are probably affected by the gouty inflammation. Dr. Alexander has related a marked example of retrocession to the heart. In this instance, a gentleman, suffering severely from gout, applied some snow to the painful joint. At first relief was experienced, but soon a sense of intense burning and constriction around the lower part of the chest was produced. He then suddenly lost sensibility; and was found sitting in his chair, with an almost imperceptible and slow (40) pulse, tardy catching respiration, and with a death-like pallid complexion. His recovery was brought about by the free employment of stimulants and counter-irritants.

Diagnosis.—The diagnosis of acute gout is in general simple enough. It is only likely to be confounded with rheumatic fever, but the following distinctions may serve to prevent any error. In gout the blood is impregnated with uric acid, in rheumatism this principle is absent; gouty inflammation is attended with the deposition of urate of soda in the affected tissues, but nothing of the kind occurs in rheumatism; gout occurs mostly in men, rheumatism in men and women equally; and gout at first only attacks one or two joints—usually the ball of the great toe, while rheumatism affects many and large joints. Then lastly, to obviate all chance of error we ought to take into consideration the general history, with the assigned causes of the disease.

We sometimes meet with puzzling cases where the gouty diathesis seems to be developed in individuals who never suffer from its local manifestations. Thus many obscure pains, which are often regarded as simple local neuralgiæ, are really mere results of the poison of gout in the system; and this is true with regard to several dyspeptic symptoms, pains in the left side of the chest, palpitations of the heart, difficulties of respiration, attacks of syncope, pulsations in the head with giddiness, imperfect action of the liver, and morbid deposits in the urine. So also, scaly eruptions on the skin, urticaria and eczema, hæmorrhagic complaints, pains about the forehead and eyes, occipital headaches, painful congestion of the tip of the nose or of the lobe of one ear, tonsillitis, bronchitis, toothache, and lumbago may all be either due to the gouty diathesis or very materially modified by its existence. The importance of rightly interpreting these symptoms has been particularly insisted upon by Dr. William Gairdner, who believes that the strumous is not more frequent than the gouty habit.

When the health and strength have been much diminished by frequent attacks of regular gout, decided paroxysms are rarely experienced; but the patient suffers severely and frequently from the disease in its irregular forms. The symptoms of anomalous, or misplaced, or atonic gout are then chiefly as follows:—Painful dyspepsia, with heartburn, flatulency, acid eructations, piles, and constipation; frequent attacks of faintness and palpitation of the heart; nervous weakness and great irritability of temper, so that the patient is feared by his relatives, who too seldom make allowance for his weakness and sufferings; frontal headache, with pain in the occiput and nape of the neck; as well as frequent flushings of the cheeks, and sometimes transient attacks of heat and redness about the nose. Moreover, there is often irritability of the bladder, with scanty high-coloured urine; diminished strength, so that a little exercise fatigues, and noise or bustle alarms; a desire for quiet and seclusion; susceptibility to every atmospheric change; and frequent annoying neuralgic pains, with cramps, and an irresistible desire to grind the teeth. Sometimes the teeth are thus actually worn down to the sockets, the uneasy sensations being only alleviated by forcibly grinding them together. As these symptoms continue, the debility becomes greater; until the entire system is ruined. And then, ultimately, the patient either dies from apoplexy; or from hydrothorax; or from pulmonary congestion, caused by the disturbance of the heart's action; or from ascites, due to disease of the liver and kidneys; or even, perhaps, suddenly, from profound syncope; or he gradually sinks exhausted and imbecile.

Causes.—Women are much less liable to this disease than men. It generally begins between thirty and forty years of age; few first attacks being witnessed before twenty, or after sixty. It is very often hereditary. But undoubtedly gout is frequently acquired by a luxurious mode of living, sedentary habits, and overmental toil and anxiety—especially when stimulants are resorted to for the purpose of making such toil more supportable. Where a predisposition to the disease can be traced from the parents or grand-parents, it usually first appears at an earlier time of life than when it has been acquired.

Gout is especially induced by the use of port wine, sherry, strong ale, and porter. In many instances, Madeira, champagne, Burgundy, cider, and perry have a similar influence. An undue quantity of animal food and over-rich diet are frequent causes, especially when combined with the employment of port, sherry, &c. Alcohol in the form of distilled spirits (particularly gin and whisky) has but little effect in producing it: rum is possibly an exception to this rule. In Scotland, where whisky is the chief drink, gout is very seldom seen; those who take this beverage to excess being punished by other, and even more painfully fatal diseases. Everything which, by inducing mal-assimilation of the food, leads to the formation of an excess of uric acid in the blood is an important cause. Thus, all depressing influences—great fatigue, the shock of an accident, a simple blow or fall, cold and damp, venereal excesses, dyspepsia, hæmorrhage, mental anxiety, poverty, &c. may produce an attack, in one predisposed. The spring is the season in which the disease is most apt to occur, while the autumn ranks second.

Plumbers, painters, and others who become the subjects of lead poisoning, seem to be particularly predisposed to gout.

Morbid Anatomy.—On examining the bodies of those who have died after repeated attacks of gouty inflammation, we shall often find important changes in the joints which have been affected, as well as in some of the internal organs.

Now as to the joints, it must be recollected that they are frequently more or less completely anchylosed. Around and within them is the chalky matter (urate of soda) the deposition of which forms the characteristic feature of gouty inflammation; the amount of this salt varying in quantity, but often being so abundant as to produce considerable swelling and distortion. The articulations may even appear as if set in plaster. The synovial fluid is thick and creamy-looking. The ligaments are rigid and contracted. Repeatedly too, the cartilages are quite destroyed, and the bones denuded.

With regard to the internal structures it may be said that we often find morbid appearances in the heart, lungs, coats of blood-vessels, and membranes of the brain. But in these changes there is nothing characteristic of the disease under consideration, and it is probable that they are accidental complications. The kidneys appear to be the organs which are specially affected. Several years ago Dr. R. B. Todd drew attention to the condition of these glands in chronic gout. The gouty kidney is found contracted to one-half or one-third its usual size ; and it has a shrivelled appearance. The capsule is thickened and opaque, and the surface is granular. The decrease in size takes place at the expense of the cortical portion. On making a section of a gouty kidney several white streaks can sometimes be seen, chiefly running in the direction of the tubes of the pyramidal portion ; which streaks, when microscopically examined, are found to consist of crystals of urate of soda. The urine in these cases is generally natural in quantity, pale in colour, of low specific gravity, and contains a variable quantity of albumen. There may be also more or less dropsy with this condition ; while the cases frequently end in uræmic convulsions, delirium, and coma.

A contracted kidney, with albuminous urine and granular and waxy casts, is found in other disorders besides gout; but it is only in this affection that there exists the deposit of urate of soda.

Pathology.—If we analyse the blood in gout we shall find the red globules in their normal proportion, unless the attack has been long and has much depressed the patient, or unless the disease has occurred in a previously debilitated subject. Under either of these circumstances the coloured corpuscles may be considerably diminished. The fibrin is increased in quantity if the local inflammatory action has been severe ; so that it may be augmented to five or six parts in 1000, as happens also in non-specific inflammations. The specific gravity of the serum is lowered in the cases where the disease has been of long standing, as well as in those accompanied with albuminuria; but the important point with regard to the serum is this,—that it invariably contains uric acid in the form of urate of soda in an abnormal quantity. Dr. Garrod points out that in health the merest traces of both uric acid and urea can be detected by very great care in manipulation; but this trace is by no means sufficient to be discovered by the thread experiment. This gentleman says that in several experiments on the blood in gout and albuminuria, where quantitative determinations were made, the amount of uric acid in the 1000 grains of serum was found to vary from 0·025 to 0·175 grain. Hence it seems probable, to say the least, that in uric acid we have found the actual materies morbi.*

The amount of uric acid daily eliminated by the kidneys in health is about eight grains; and it can easily be understood that the same effect ensues from these organs performing their office inefficiently, as from the formation of an increased quantity of this salt in the system. Not that the mere accumulation of urate of soda in the blood will produce the phenomena of gout. For, as Dr. Garrod says,†—" the poison may lie dormant for a considerable time; but when crystallization of the salt takes place in any tissue, inflammation is suddenly lit up by its presence, and a paroxysm of gout ensues."

Treatment.—The treatment of gout naturally divides itself into that proper during an attack, and that to be adopted in the interval. That this malady is curable there can be no doubt; though it has been (and as Dr. William Gairdner insists, ever will be) the *opprobrium medicorum*, where extirpation by means of the medicines of the Pharmacopœia is only aimed at. The fit may be postponed, mitigated, and often shortened by drugs; but only temporary relief from this source must be looked for. At the same time it should not be thought that Cullen's remedies—patience and flannel, are to be trusted to.

It is generally considered that *bleeding* during an *acute* attack is unnecessary. Dr. Gairdner well observes—" I am convinced that bleedings to such an amount as is necessary to subdue inflammation, are much to be avoided in gout. Those who prescribe

---

* *Dr. Garrod's Plan of ascertaining the Presence of an abnormal Quantity of Uric Acid in the Serum of the Blood:*—Take about two drachms of the serum and place it in a flat glass dish or watch-glass. To this add twelve drops of ordinary strong acetic acid, which will cause the evolution of a few bubbles of gas. When the fluids are mixed, introduce two or three threads of cotton, or one or two ultimate fibres from a piece of unwashed huckaback. Allow the glass to stand on the mantel-piece, or on a shelf in a warm room, for from thirty-six to sixty hours, until its contents set, from evaporation. If the cotton fibres be then removed and examined microscopically with an inch object-glass, they will be found covered with crystals of uric acid, if this agent be unduly present in the serum. The crystals form on the thread somewhat like the masses of sugar-candy on string. Hence this process is termed " the uric acid thread experiment."

† *The Nature and Treatment of Gout and Rheumatic Gout.* Second Edition. p. 333. London, 1863.

them will not fail to find out, in a very short time, particularly in London practice, that they have sacrificed their best resource in the cure, namely, the strength of the patient; and have made a lengthened and distressing case, where they meant to make a short and brilliant cure."*　Although, however, depletion is in every way contra-indicated, yet this physician states that he has often found a very small bloodletting (three to six ounces) productive of the greatest good by relieving the overloaded heart and congested vessels; but he never makes use of this remedy where the constitution is impaired or defective.　Leeches are some-times applied to gouty joints; though for my own part I confess that I have very rarely seen any benefit result from the practice.

Laxatives must almost always be employed; not violent, but mild warm aperients, such as aloes, senna, rhubarb, jalap, &c.　A mixture of equal parts of the compound infusion of gentian and infusion of senna (the compound gentian mixture of the London Pharmacopœia) will agree well; as will Pullna water, or any one of the preparations to be found under the heads of F. 144, 145, 146, 148, 149, 151, &c.　Anthony White, who had much expe-rience in the treatment of this disease, maintained that the liver was the organ in which the poison of gout got elaborated; and hence he believed that the physician's chief object should be to restore the natural functions of this gland, as indicated by a copious discharge of bile through the bowels.　He relied almost exclusively on the use of a pill made of one grain each of calomel, colchicum, aloes, and ipecacuanha; which at first was given six times a day, and afterwards every eight or twelve or twenty-four hours, accord-ing to circumstances.　But though this eminent surgeon's patho-logy was wrong, yet it is certain his remedies often did good; and consequently where there is hepatic congestion, with urine free from albumen, his pill may be prescribed.　When, however, the kidneys are affected, no preparation of mercury should be given; for not only will small doses of this metal be apt to produce severe saliva-tion, but they seriously impoverish the already deteriorated blood.

With regard to *diuretics* and *diaphoretics* there can be no doubt they often afford great relief.　Hence we should give the acetate, citrate, or bicarbonate of potash; we can administer some pre-paration of opium; and often we may employ the hot air or the vapour bath with advantage.　But in all cases, speaking generally, with these remedies we must combine *colchicum*; since there are many reasons for believing that this drug may be regarded as a specific for the gouty paroxysm.　It ought not to be administered until the bowels have been well opened; and it must be given not (as often recommended) so as to gripe and purge, but in small quantities, easily borne without pain or inconvenience.　At the commencement, one full dose should be exhibited—such as from

* *On Gout: its History, its Causes, and its Cure.*　Fourth Edition, p. 307. London, 1860.

two to three grains of the acetic extract; and then ten or fifteen minims of the wine of colchicum, or of the tincture of the seeds, three times a day, in Vichy water, or with sedatives and alkalies, or with iodide of potassium, will often suffice (F. 31, 46, 212, 351,352).

Narcotics generally do harm by diminishing the secretions, though they cannot be withheld where the pain is very great. Henbane is less efficacious than opium, but it will also prove less injurious by not interfering with the secretion of bile. A combination of opium and belladonna (F. 344), or of morphia and chloroform and Indian hemp (F. 317), can be recommended. Eight or ten grains of the extract of hyoscyamus, or one fluid drachm of the tincture, are the smallest doses from which any appreciable effect of this drug can be expected.*

With regard to *general rules* it is to be noticed, that the patient should be confined to his bed, at all events for the first few days. The affected limb must be kept elevated and warm. The painful part ought to be covered with cotton wool and oiled silk; or else with an anodyne lotion (F. 265, 267, 297); or with a poultice on which some extract of belladonna has been freely spread, or some tincture of opium sprinkled. It is only in cases of chronic gout that small blisters can be of any service. If the foregoing local remedies give but little relief, they will do no harm; which is more than can be said of cold applications. Several cases are known where death has occurred in a few hours from patients plunging their feet into cold water, with the idea of cutting short the fit. And lastly, during the early stages the diet should be light; consisting chiefly of milk, arrowroot, tapioca, tea, &c. Diluents may be taken freely with considerable advantage; none being better than barley or toast or plain water, or Seltzer or soda or Vichy water. Much mischief results from allowing animal food too soon. But when the fever has sensibly diminished, and the powers of digestion are strong enough, beef tea, white fish, poultry, and mutton may be gradually allowed; with perhaps one glass of good sherry or a tablespoonful of whisky well diluted.

The most important question still remains,—*How are we to prevent the return of gout?* Clearly, by enforcing the observance

---

* Many patients have told me that they have benefited by the use of the anti-gout liquid and pills of Dr. Laville. From an analysis, the *liquid* would appear to owe its properties to the active principle of colocynth, quinine, and cinchonine, with unimportant salts of lime. It is used at any period of the attack; a teaspoonful being taken in sugared water or tea, and repeated in six or seven hours if the pain continue or the bowels be not moved. Then twenty-four hours are to elapse before the next dose; when half the quantity may be employed daily for two or three times, unless the bowels are irritable. The *pills* consist of a peculiar extract called physalin (obtained from the Physalis Alkekengi, or winter cherry, a perennial herbaceous plant belonging to the natural order Solanaceæ), and of silicate of soda. They are employed to remove all traces of the disease, as well as to prevent future attacks. Of an alterative nature, one is taken at the commencement of a meal once or twice a day; sometimes being continued thus for many weeks.

of a well-regulated diet ; by exchanging a life of indolence for one of bodily activity ; by adopting early and regular hours ; by avoiding too great sexual indulgence, as well as by omitting all severe mental application ; and by the aid of medicine. Moderate exercise in the pure air ; warm, tepid, or sea water baths ; and the fostering of a tranquil disposition,—these are remedies not to be despised. Starving the disease will not cure it. An animal and vegetable diet should be used ; the point being to take care, that both as regards quantity and quality, the stomach can digest, and can consequently extract healthy chyle from, the materials put into it. Salt meats have only the recommendation mentioned by Montaigne's friend,—"that he must needs have something to quarrel with in the extremity of his pain, and that he fancied that railing at and cursing, one while the Bologna sausages, and at another the dried tongues and the hams, was some mitigation to his torments." Ale, porter, port wine, sherry, marsala, madeira, are certainly injurious ; but whisky or gin and water may sometimes be allowed. It is very probable, also, that a moderate quantity of some light wines—such as claret, hock, chablis, dry champagne, &c.—will prove of occasional service rather than otherwise. The best medicines are an antacid purgative at intervals, and some of the neutral salts frequently used. The citrate or tartrate of potash, or the phosphate of soda, are valuable remedies, taken in very small doses, in half a pint of water, once or twice a day ; or one or two bottles of Vichy water, or soda or potash water, can be drunk in the twenty-four hours ; or a tumblerful of a weak infusion of the leaves of the Fraxinus Excelsior or common ash (one ounce of the leaves infused in a pint and a half of water) may be taken on an empty stomach, night and morning. During the last four or five years Dr. Garrod has made many trials of *carbonate of lithia* as an internal remedy, both in cases of the uric acid diathesis connected with gravel, and in chronic gout (F. 64). When given internally, in doses of from three to six grains dissolved in plenty of simple water, or of aërated water, and repeated two or three times a day, in patients voiding uric acid gravel, it causes the deposits to become less, or even to cease altogether. If a large amount of alkali be desirable, the carbonate of lithia may be prescribed in combination with the carbonate or citrate of potash. My own experience with this remedy has not been small ; but it is difficult to say much either for or against, its employment.

In *chronic gout* the blood is to be purified and kept pure. With this object we must regulate the diet, and prevent indigestion ; maintain the proper action of the bowels and skin ; and trust to such remedies as colchicum, alkalies, iodide of potassium, chlorate of potash, &c. Guaiacum is now and then recommended, though it is not deserving of the slightest confidence. The supply of animal food is to be limited ; but white fish, milk, and eggs prove beneficial. Malt liquors and port wine must be strictly forbidden ;

even a little dry sherry or brandy and water being scarcely permissible. In weakly subjects, when the disease lingers about the system, mild vegetable tonics—such as quassia, calumba, gentian, or bark, do much good. The efficacy of quinine (except in combination with colchicum) is doubtful; and if from an anæmic condition iron be indicated, only small doses of some mild preparation ought to be employed (F. 394, 403, 404, &c.). The alterative and tonic effects of arsenic have led me sometimes to use this metal with benefit; administering it either alone, or with colchicum, or the iodide of potassium, or steel (F. 52, 399, 402).

As a rule, the collections of chalk-stones should not be opened; unless from their size the skin is about to ulcerate. If the knife be used, the smallest opening which will permit of the escape of the creamy fluid ought to be made; otherwise an obstinate sore may result. Mr. Spencer Wells states that these accumulations can be often dispersed by the administration of the iodide of potassium, which possesses the power of dissolving urate of soda; while local friction with the same salt or with the iodide of ammonium (F. 280) will often do good.

For attacks of *irregular* or *misplaced gout*, salines and colchicum are generally needed; while we should try to bring the disease to the extremities by mustard pediluvia, &c. With regard to *retrocedent gout* we must especially avoid cold, as this is often the cause of the mischief. Antispasmodics are the remedies which give most relief; chloroform, ether, ammonia, and brandy being often needed. If the stomach be affected, vomiting does good; and afterwards a sinapism or turpentine stupe should be applied over the epigastrium. Warmth or counter-irritation ought also to be employed to the joints, so as to bring back the inflammation.

After an attack of gout in any shape a wise patient will take a thorough holiday. A visit to some of the mineral waters—to Bath (F. 460), Buxton (F. 464), Cheltenham (F. 461), Harrogate (F. 466), or Leamington (F. 463); or for a greater, and therefore perhaps better change, to Wiesbaden (F. 489), Vichy (F. 479), Carlsbad (F. 496), or Aix-la-Chapelle (F. 483), will be productive of the greatest benefit. The mineral waters of any of these springs may be employed; always provided the patient has no symptom of any impending attack, nor any disease of the kidneys or of the heart. But I believe that these remedies are chiefly of use in so far as they improve the general health; though it is said, that an annual residence at Vichy for three weeks, will keep many a gouty man free from his enemy for the rest of the year.

XXII. RHEUMATISM.

Rheumatism [Ρευματισμὸς = a flux or looseness; ῥευματίζομαι = to be affected with looseness, from ῥεῦμα = a humour floating in the body causing disease] is one of the most common, painful, and severe diseases of this country. It arises from some unknown abnormal condition of the blood. The action of the poison is not limited to any one texture or organ ; although it particularly affects the white fibrous tissue which enters into the formation of the aponeurotic sheaths and fasciæ, ligaments and tendons, as well as the fibro-serous membranes. Consequently the parts most frequently involved are the joints and surrounding structures, with the pericardium and endocardium. There are two very distinct forms of rheumatism, the acute and chronic.

1. ACUTE RHEUMATISM.—Acute rheumatism, or rheumatic fever, is a disease characterised by fever, profuse acid sweats, and inflammation of the fibrous tissues surrounding one or several of the large joints. It is especially formidable from the suffering it causes, from the intensity of the fever, and from the damage which is so frequently produced by it to the heart. When the febrile action is very slight, and the inflammation of a moderate or mild character, the disease is generally spoken of as sub-acute rheumatism.

Symptoms.—The earliest symptoms of acute rheumatism are mostly restlessness and fever ; succeeded at the end of some twenty-four or thirty-six hours by stiffness with aching pain in the limbs and joints. These indications of coming mischief usually follow exposure to cold and damp, and similar depressing influences. The pain quickly increases ; and in a very short time is accompanied by swelling and great tenderness of one or more of the large joints, together with high fever and much constitutional disturbance. When the disease is established, the patient presents a pitiable spectacle of helpless suffering. He is very restless, yet dare not or even cannot move : the pain in the affected joints is so agonizing, that the weight of the bed-clothes can barely be borne. The face is flushed, hot, and moist. The skin is generally bathed in sweat ; which has a very disagreeable acid or sour odour, and which reddens litmus paper. The temperature in the axilla varies, at different times in the day, perhaps from 100° Fahr. to 102° or 103°. Where it rises as high as 105° the danger is decidedly very great ; while in cases about to end fatally it has reached even to 109° and even 110°. The pulse is frequent and large, hard and quick ; but it continues regular in uncomplicated cases. The thirst is extreme, and often insatiable. There is usually constipation, but occasionally the bowels are much relaxed. The tongue is moist, but white and thickly furred ; while the saliva is acid. The urine is high coloured, scanty, of high specific gravity, very acid, with perhaps scarcely a trace of chlorine, and loaded with uric acid, or more frequently with urates. It has lately been shown that the deposits formerly regarded as consisting of urate of ammonia have a variable composition ; being made up of the urates or lithates of lime, potash, and soda.* Relapses are very common. A chemical analysis of the blood shows the presence of a superabundance of fibrin (hyperinosis), with a deficient amount of salts and red corpuscles.

A remarkable feature in this disease is the great tendency to metastasis. Thus, the inflammation may suddenly leave one joint and appear in another, and then in a third, afterwards jumping back again to its original seat. But the most serious change is when it shifts its place, or extends, to the membranes of the heart. This it is most likely to do in severe cases, when we may suppose the blood to be loaded with the materies morbi; in young persons; and when the irritability of the heart is great, as it is after bleeding and excessive prostration. Since, however, rheumatic pericarditis and rheumatic endocarditis do not differ from simple inflammation of the pericardium or heart—except perhaps in being less fatal, I shall defer further notice of the signs of these affections until treating of the diseases of the heart generally. Here it need only be urged, that as these complications are much to be feared, the existence or absence of a friction sound, or of an endocardial murmur, should be determined once or twice daily by a careful examination. Occasionally, the cardiac affection precedes the articular, even by a few days. Moreover, in addition to pericarditis and endocarditis, carditis or inflammation of the walls of the heart will possibly set in; or small vegetations or fibrinous concretions can occasionally be produced on the valves or lining membrane independently of inflammation.

Rheumatic fever may also, but more rarely, be complicated with bronchitis, pleurisy, pneumonia, or even with inflammation of the brain or its membranes; while very rarely the local effects are such as to lead to disorganization of one or more of the affected joints. An attack now and then follows scarlet fever. Moreover, we sometimes meet with cases, especially where the heart has become implicated, in which irregular choreal movements come on during the progress of the disease. This complication is most likely to arise when the patient has become much depressed, and when therefore the irritability of the nervous system is increased.

Whenever rheumatic fever is uncomplicated, its average duration under proper treatment is from twelve or sixteen to twenty-five or thirty days. In those cases which end fatally, death is almost always due to the cardiac inflammation. According to the reports of the Registrar-General the deaths from "rheumatism" in England, during the year 1866, were $\frac{\text{Males } 1186}{\text{Females } 1152} = 2338$. Taking the returns for the last ten years, this number may be said to be about the average. And considering that these figures apply to the direct

* Urine containing an excess of urates may be distinguished by its high colour, increased density, and turbid appearance when cold—somewhat resembling pea-soup. On applying heat to a portion in a test-tube, it becomes bright and clear. Examined by the microscope, an abundant amorphous material is seen.

mortality of the disease, they are larger than might be expected. What the indirect fatality may be we have no means of learning. When recovery takes place after the heart has been affected, the patient has very often a sad time in store for him,—future bad health, palpitation on any excitement, attacks of dyspnœa, incapacity for any exertion, and dropsy. By far the greater number of cases of acute rheumatism occur in persons between fifteen and fifty years of age, this disease being equally rare in the very young and very old. Undoubtedly it is sometimes hereditary. Damp and variable weather will be found to have a greater influence in causing acute rheumatism, than either extreme cold or heat.

Pathology.—Dr. Prout first suggested that the presence of a superabundance of lactic acid in the system was the cause of rheumatic fever ; a view which has been since entertained by many authors. Dr. Richardson (following the example of Mr. John Simon and Dr. Brinton) has made an interesting series of experiments ; from which he infers that " lactic acid has the power, when existing in an animal body in excess, of producing a class of symptoms attaching themselves mainly to the fibro-serous textures, and which, regarded in all points of view, are essentially the symptoms of acute rheumatic inflammation."* Thus, he injected into the peritoneum of a healthy cat, seven drachms of a solution of lactic acid mixed with eight of water. Two hours after the operation the action of the heart became irregular ; in four hours more the animal was left for the night ; and in the morning it was found dead. The inspection showed no peritoneal mischief ; but there was the most marked endocarditis of the left cavities of the heart. The mitral valve, thickened and inflamed, had become coated on its free borders with firm fibrinous deposit. The whole endocardial surface of the ventricle was intensely vascular. Upon repeating the experiment on a dog, the inspection revealed the most striking pathological signs of endocarditis. The tricuspid valve was inflamed and swollen to twice its ordinary size. The aortic valve, swollen and inflamed, was coated on its free border with fibrinous beads. The endocardial surface was generally red from vascularity. The pericardium was dry and injected. As before, the peritoneum escaped injury. The joints were not attacked, but there was distinct sclerotitis in the left eye. Again, in a third instance not only did endocarditis result, but there was well-marked vascularity of the sclerotic, and various joints were affected ; while there was metastasis, now one joint suffering, then another, and again the heart. As Dr. Richardson remarks, it has yet to be learned by experiment whether acids of an analogous character to the lactic— such as formic, acetic, lithic, and butyric, are capable of producing the same results.

In rheumatic endocarditis, the left side of the heart only is affected as a general rule. Hence, Dr. Richardson infers that the

* *The Cause of the Coagulation of the Blood*, p. 389. London, 1858.

chemical change whereby the morbid matter of acute rheumatism is produced, is completed in the pulmonic circuit; that in the respiratory act the *acid* quality of the poison is produced; that thus formed, the poison is carried by the arterial circulation to be disposed of by decomposition, or elimination, or both; and that it does not return as an acid by the veins, but simply as a product which admits of re-transformation in the pulmonic circuit into the acid state.

Regarding the origin of the lactic acid, Dr. Headland suggests that ordinarily the starch of the food is first converted into this agent, which then combines with oxygen to form carbonic acid and water, in which state it is excreted by the lungs; but that under conditions unfavourable to this oxidation, the lactic acid accumulates in the system.

Treatment.—A vast number of different plans have been recommended. And considering that this disease has a strong tendency to terminate favourably, it is not surprising that each authority can adduce numerous successful cases in proof of the efficacy of the drugs he employs.

Remembering the high fever and severe pain which accompany acute rheumatism, it can readily be anticipated that *venesection* has long been advocated. But most physicians are now agreed that bloodletting will merely give temporary relief, at the expense of future suffering; while recollecting also that it increases the irritability of the heart, and consequently predisposes to rheumatic inflammation of this organ, I should, as a rule, never resort to it. The use of large *blisters*, applied completely round the limb and close to the affected joints, has been strongly advocated by Dr. Herbert Davies; their application being followed by the employment of large linseed poultices to promote the discharge of serum. No medicines are to be given. If the evidence of patients is of any value, this practice must be considered as a very successful one. Moreover, I know of one or two medical men, who, having had personal experience of it, are almost enthusiastic in their praises. According to their testimony, the speedy relief to pain is most marked; while the duration of the attack is greatly shortened. *Saline purgatives* (F. 141, 144, 152, 165, 169), given so as to obtain one free evacuation daily, will be beneficial; especially after the bowels have been well acted on by a large dose of calomel and jalap (F. 140). *Opiates* in full doses are frequently necessary to relieve the pain, and to allay the general irritability. They will also help to encourage sweating, and thus aid nature in eliminating the poison by the skin. Two grains of extract of opium, with one-third of a grain of extract of belladonna, may be given every night; and unless the skin acts freely, five grains of the compound ipecacuanha powder every four or six hours will do good. The efficacy of the latter will be increased if the nitrate of potash be substituted for the sulphate in making it (F. 213). *Quinine* in large doses has been used by some physicians, but I am not in a position to speak of its effects. In combination with iodide of potassium (two grains of quinine to four or five of the iodide, repeated thrice daily) it is sometimes useful at a late stage of the disease. The *American Hellebore* (F. 321) is spoken highly of, as an arterial sedative; and has been employed in acute rheumatism with advantage. The *Nitrate of Potash* is said by Dr. Basham to be the most efficacious remedy with which he is acquainted. Its action is thus explained:—The blood in acute rheumatism contains excess of fibrin and diminution of salts; it has, moreover, an increased tendency to the formation of exudatory products, the most dangerous of which occur in the heart and on its valves. As the nitrate of potash is known to have the property of preventing the separation of fibrin from the blood, it is rational to infer that it will prevent exudatory formations which consist of fibrin. Clinical observation, it is said, proves this view to be correct. The treatment adopted by Dr. Basham is to give a solution of nitre, ad libitum, to allay thirst; and also to apply it externally to the joints. Patients will sometimes take 480 grains in twenty-four hours. This remedy is preferred to the alkaline carbonates from being less liable to cause gastric derangements. And then, *Lemon-juice*, in two or three ounce doses, repeated three or four times a day, has been recommended by Dr. Owen Rees; who considers that the citric acid undergoes changes in the stomach, supplying oxygen to such elements as tend to produce uric acid, and inducing thereby the formation of urea and carbonic acid instead. The result of its use, however, has not been such as to make me recommend it; for I have not only found it fail to do as much good as other remedies in the few instances in which I have tried it, but more than once alarming depression has been caused.

The treatment which I believe to be the best, under ordinary circumstances, remains for consideration. Essentially, the plan is the same as that advised by Dr. Garrod, Dr. Fuller, &c. It consists in relieving the pain by opium and belladonna, while the alkalies and their salts are freely administered to correct the abnormal condition of the blood and excretions. Thus, from twenty to sixty grains of the bicarbonate of soda or potash can well be given every three or four hours, in half a bottle of soda water, or in an effervescing citrate of ammonia or potash draught; continuing it regularly until the articular affection and febrile disturbance are very much lessened, till the pulse is reduced, and the urine rendered alkaline. If the patient be robust, and the urine continues much loaded with urates, ten minims of the wine of colchicum should be added to each draught. Or if the disease remain stationary in one or two joints, from three to five grains of iodide of potassium may be advantageously administered with each dose. So also the hot air or vapour bath can be simultaneously employed, if the perspiration be scanty; though the necessity for such baths is quite exceptional. During convalescence, few medi-cines will do so much good as bark and ammonia (F. 371) ; with subsequently some mild preparation of steel (F. 403). Cod liver oil is often of service directly the acute symptoms subside, and some-times even before they do so.

The *diet* must at first be low, consisting of slops, arrowroot, mutton broth, &c. Directly there are signs of depression, good beef tea, raw eggs in tea, milk and lime water (F. 14), or prepared milk (F. 15) may be administered ; with, if necessary, ammonia and spirit of chloroform in soda water. Light puddings, potatoes, and white fish should be allowed as soon as the appetite returns, and the stomach appears capable of digesting them ; while mutton, poultry, game, and beef ought not to be given until convalescence is thoroughly established. During the early stages, when there is much thirst, a refreshing saline drink (F. 355, 356, 360) will be beneficial ; or plenty of soda or potash water, or good lemonade may be allowed. Sugar is bad for the dyspeptic, the gouty, and the rheumatic : since it is transformed into fat, lactic acid, and other substances which readily disagree with the organs of diges-tion. Malt liquors and most kinds of wine are equally injurious. Moreover perfect rest must in every case be enjoined, and all sources of mental anxiety should if possible be removed.

With regard to *local remedies* it is to be remembered that great relief is often experienced from wrapping the affected joints in cotton wool and oiled silk, by which a sort of local vapour bath is formed. So, when the wrists or ankles are chiefly affected, I have seen benefit arise from frequently soaking them in a hot alkaline bath ; or from fomenting them with water to which a mixture of the bicarbonate of soda and opium has been freely added. Where the acute symptoms have partially subsided, small blisters, the size of a penny piece, may be advantageously applied ; or the swollen joints can be painted with iodine (F. 205), and then covered with wool. In every case it will be far better for the patient to sleep between blankets, rather than to have linen or calico sheets ; inas-much as the latter soon get damp and cold from the perspiration.

Supposing any of the signs of cardiac affection (such as violent and irregular action of the heart, præcordial pain, enlargement of the normal area of dulness, friction sounds or bruits, dyspnœa, and fever) manifest themselves, what is to be done ? Most authors say, apply leeches over the region of the heart or resort to general bleeding, and quickly get the system under the influence of mer-cury. If the remarks which have been made in the section on inflam-mation, however, are true, no such remedies will be necessary. Believing them to be correct, I consider that it is much better merely to get freedom from pain by full doses of opium, to apply hot moist linseed or mustard poultices over the cardiac region, and to continue the bicarbonate of soda or potash draughts. Where the action of the skin appears at all insufficient, the vapour bath should be employed. Perfect rest and abstinence are also needed ; but the practitioner must not be over-cautious in allowing good soups and broths, milk and raw eggs, orange juice and cod liver oil, as soon as the powers of life appear to be failing. I have now been able fully to carry out this plan in many severe cases of rheumatic pericarditis ; and the comparatively rapid recovery of these patients, together with the general train of symptoms during the treatment, has convinced me that it is to be strongly recommended. Should effusion take place into the pericardium, the application of a blister, or of a succession of blisters, will possibly do good; and perhaps diuretics, with the iodide of potassium, may in certain instances be beneficial.

2. CHRONIC RHEUMATISM.—This is sometimes the sequel of rheumatic fever, but more frequently I believe a separate constitutional affection, coming on quite independently of any previous acute attack. During the decline of life it is common ; not very many old people being altogether ignorant of its symptoms. A peculiar form is apt to complicate, or to follow, gonorrhœa : hence one variety of this disease has been termed *gonorrhœal* rheumatism.

The fibrous textures around the joints, or the fibrous envelopes of the nerves, or the aponeurotic sheaths of the muscles, the fasciæ and tendons, or the periosteum, are the parts that suffer in chronic rheumatism. Whichever tissue may be affected, there is, at first, only slight constitutional disturbance ; but the sufferer is constantly annoyed, and his existence at length made miserable with wearying pains, causing him to be restless at night, and destroying all comfort during the day. In some instances, the pains are worse at night, being aggravated by the warmth of the bed ; with others, warmth affords the greatest relief : the former is usually the case when the blood is circulating a poisonous material through the system, as in venereal rheumatism, or in that due to derangement of the digestive organs and secretions ; the latter, in rheumatism of an erratic kind, dependent on exposure to damp and cold, &c.

There are two or three different *forms* of chronic rheumatism. Thus, rheumatic inflammation of the lumbar fascia is termed *lumbago ;* the pain being referred to the fleshy mass of muscles on one or both sides of the loins, being very severe, and being increased by every movement of the back. *Stiff* or *wry neck* is another variety, generally due to sitting in a draught. To relax the painful muscles the patient inclines his head to the affected side ; and as the muscles soon become rigid, the proper position is not regained without a sharp twinge. *Synovial rheumatism* is that kind in which the morbid action especially favours the thin and delicate membrane covering the articular extremities of the bones ; thus causing an excessive formation of viscid and glairy fluid in the closed synovial sacs. It affects most frequently the knee-joint, the synovial membrane of this part being the largest in the body. In *sciatica* the suffering is due to disease affecting the neurilemma of the sciatic nerve ; but it will be more correct to treat of this kind in describing the forms of neuralgia, than in the present section.   When the inter-costal muscles, or the fibrous fasciæ lining the chest, are affected, the disease is often called *pleurodynia*.   The " stitch" which follows a deep inspiration must not be mistaken for the lancinating pain of pleurisy.   And lastly, in *rheumatic ophthalmia* there is acute inflam-mation of the sclerotic ; which is always attended with some amount of fever and constitutional disturbance, as well as with more or less severe nocturnal pains about the orbit and temple.

The *diagnosis* of chronic rheumatism is generally easy.   There are, however, certain painful muscular affections which sometimes simulate it.   These pains (technically *myalgia*) are familiar to us all as "soreness and stiffness," following upon some extraordinary exer-tion, but they are not always as readily recognised when they occur during convalescence from any long illness.   Yet it is clear, that the mere sitting upright in a chair, without any support for the head or arms, may be as fatiguing to some of the muscles (the trapezius amongst others) of an invalid, as the attempt to ascend Mont Blanc would prove to an ordinary gentleman only accustomed to a daily desultory saunter through the London parks.   Muscular pains of this nature are not uncommon also, in persons suffering from general debility.   They have their seat in the fleshy parts of muscles, in their tendinous prolongations, or in the fibrous aponeuroses. Dr. Inman of Liverpool, in a pamphlet on this subject, states that they are usually described as hot or burning; they are absent on rising in the morning, and increase with fatigue ; the pain is referred to some muscle or its tendon, and is relieved by relaxing or supporting this muscle; the pulse is generally weak and fast, but is unaffected by the pain ; and the patient frequently suffers from cramps.   Now the diagnosis is important.   For if we hesitate to administer ferruginous tonics and nourishing diet, or to afford proper rest and support to the weak muscles until they regain their tone, we shall fail to give any relief to the poor sufferer : who will either be haunted continually by the idea that he bears about him some incurable disease, or more wisely—in his justifiable contempt for medicine, will hasten to try the good diet and pure air of some hydropathic establishment, where he will certainly get well " after being given over by the faculty."

Another disorder which has sometimes been mistaken for chronic rheumatism is *acute mollities ossium*.   The latter usually commences with weakness, weariness, and pains in the limbs.   But in this disease of the bones the suffering is much more severe, and more lasting ; while, after a time, the softening of the osseous tissue and the accumulation of fatty matter in the Haversian canals leads to deformity.   The urine also is generally loaded with phosphate of lime.   When mollities ossium occurs during pregnancy, the deformity of the pelvis which may ensue from the bulging inwards

of its sides by the pressure of the thigh bones against the aceta-
bula, has necessitated the performance of the Cæsarean section.
This disease occurs in the middle period of life and is usually fatal
in from twelve to twenty-four months.

In the *treatment* of chronic rheumatism it is always necessary
to attend to the general health, as by improving this the disease will
generally be materially mitigated. Care must be taken that the
function of digestion is performed naturally; while sleep ought to
be afforded by sedatives, if necessary. There are several special
remedies which give relief, one of the best being the iodide of
potassium with tincture of serpentary or with bark (F. 31). If the
secretions are very acid, bicarbonate of potash should be combined
with it. Cod liver oil (F. 389) is very valuable in the great majority
of cases. Quinine, with or without belladonna, (F. 45, 379, 383);
iodide of iron (F. 32); ammonia and bark (F. 68, 371); oil of
turpentine (F. 50); colchicum (F. 46); sarsaparilla; perchloride
of mercury or corrosive sublimate (F. 27); the red iodide of mercury (F. 54); arsenic (F. 52); aconite (F. 330); guaiacum and
sulphur (F. 43); sulphate of soda and sulphur (F. 148); and
chloride of ammonium or sal ammoniac (F. 60),—all have their
advocates. The tincture of actea racemosa in half drachm doses,
three or four times daily, produces slight narcotic and eliminative
effects. It will often cure lumbago, as well as pains in the back
due to an irritable condition of the uterus with great rapidity (F.
320). When the symptoms are very chronic, the cold sulphurous
waters of Harrogate (F. 466), or the hot sulphur springs of Aix-
la-Chapelle (F. 483), may be resorted to; or sea air and warm
salt water baths can be employed in this country. Sometimes the
alkaline waters of Vichy (F. 479) do good; or, if there is constipation in addition to rheumatism, the antacid springs at Carlsbad
(F. 496) can be advantageously visited. The latter, however, take
a longer time to act on the system than the former.

Hot water, or hot air, or vapour baths (either plain, or alkaline, or medicated with sulphur) are often remarkably serviceable in
this disease, especially when the pains are severe (F. 121, 125, 130).
During the intervals of the attack, the tepid salt water sponge or
plunge bath should be regularly employed every morning with a
flesh brush, coarse towel, &c.

Local applications to the painful parts, such as blisters (F. 208),
iodine paint (F. 205), belladonna and aconite liniment (F. 281),
chloroform and opium liniment (F. 282), or an ointment of veratria
(F. 304), often give relief. Subcutaneous injections of atropine
and morphia (F. 314) are very valuable. In lumbago, a large
belladonna plaster, or the emplastrum ferri, or the emplastrum
calefaciens, applied over the whole loins, will be productive of
great comfort. The old woman's remedy of ironing the part, a
piece of brown paper being placed between the hot iron and the
skin, deserves mention. For rheumatism especially affecting the

tendinous portions of the muscles we may recommend the external application of sulphur—either powdered or as an ointment, with bandages of new flannel; the latter being again covered with oiled silk, to increase the warmth and obviate any disagreeable smell. Some patients merely dust the inside of their stockings with sublimed sulphur, when the legs or feet are the affected parts. Where the pains are decidedly relieved by heat, acupuncture is said always to give ease, and often to effect a cure; but I have had no experience in its use. All sufferers from chronic rheumatism should wear flannel; while they must beware of exposure to damp and cold. They ought also to be careful in their diet, and should particularly avoid beer and heating wines; as I am convinced that many paroxysms of this disease are brought on through disorders of the digestive organs. Ventnor (F. 434), Hastings (F. 432), Rome (F. 447), and Nice (F. 443), are good winter stations for rheumatic patients who can afford to leave their homes.

XXIII. CHRONIC OSTEO-ARTHRITIS.

Chronic Osteo-arthritis [from 'Οστέον = a bone + ἄρθρον = a joint, terminal -itis = inflammation] is the designation adopted by the Royal College of Physicians of London, in the "Provisional Nomenclature," for the disease generally known as *rheumatoid arthritis*, or *chronic rheumatic arthritis*, or *rheumatic gout*.

It has been a matter of some controversy whether gout and rheumatism can ever be present at the same time, in the same individual. Or, to put the matter more clearly and in a simpler form,—Is there any disease which may be regarded as a compound of these two affections? Dr. Garrod has long maintained, that such a state as the term rheumatic gout implies is never seen; and this opinion is now almost undisputed. The disease to which this name has been applied will best be described as a chronic inflammatory affection of the joints, not unlike gout in a few of its characters, somewhat resembling rheumatism in other points, but differing essentially from both.

Chronic osteo-arthritis, or rheumatoid arthritis ['Ρεῦμα = a humour floating in the body causing disease + εἶδος = appearance; and ἄρθρον = a joint, terminal -itis], is commonly one of the most troublesome and obstinate affections which the practitioner can have to treat. Young and old, rich and poor, the careless and the cautious, equally suffer from this disorder. Women are attacked more frequently than men; possibly because they are more liable to have the general health depressed by menorrhagia or some other irregularity of the uterine functions, or to get ill from causes connected with parturition. In the cases I have seen, there has been no history of hereditary predisposition. This disease attacks either the large or small joints, or the temporo-maxillary articulations, or the articular processes of the vertebræ—especially of the cervical region ; but the hip, shoulder, elbow or knee, and hands are probably the most favourite seats of the morbid action. It may also be a constitutional, or simply a local disorder. Thus Dr. Robert Adams remarks that,—" when we observe it affecting all the joints in the same individual on both sides symmetrically, we may feel assured that the chronic articular affection in such a case has proceeded from some deep constitutional taint. In the majority of such cases we shall, I believe, discover that the general chronic affection has been immediately preceded by an attack of rheumatic fever, from the lingering remains of which the chronic rheumatic arthritis had evidently sprung."* On the other hand, as a local disease it may arise from accident or from the over-use of some particular joint, when it will of course be limited to this part. In the examples which have come under my own care, the affection has certainly appeared to be constitutional ; and it has seemed to me that mal-assimilation has generally been at the root of it. Some of the most annoying cases, moreover, which I have met with, have occurred in women at the critical period of life ; though I have also seen it in girls at puberty, in connexion with disordered uterine functions, and in men at different ages.

The *symptoms* consist chiefly of pain, swelling, contraction, and stiffness of the affected joints. In acute cases, the disease may come on abruptly with considerable fever and general disturbance ; but much more frequently the affection is of a subacute or chronic character, commencing with languor, general irritability, restlessness, loss of appetite, and vitiated secretions. The joints then become stiff and painful, while effusion into the synovial membranes causes them to appear swollen and distended ; and if the hips, knees, or ankles be the parts affected, there is more or less lameness. On placing a hand at each side of the joint, fluctuation can sometimes be detected ; or if we grasp the part, a distinct kind of crepitus may often be felt. A peculiar crackling of the joints on movement is also appreciable to the patient. When the disease is of long continuance a degree of rigidity may occur from the thickening of all the articular textures, equal to that produced by bony anchylosis ; or the joint will even become quite disorganized from a gradual wasting of the cartilages. Then in addition to the foregoing, the articulations become more or less deformed ; there are frequently painful spasms in the muscles of the affected limbs ; there is great mental depression, and general lassitude ; dyspepsia, with acidity of the stomach and flatulence, is an exceptional occurrence ; the rest at night is disturbed, and every change in the weather is felt ; while owing to the languid circulation the patient suffers much from cold

* *A Treatise on Rheumatic Gout ; or, Chronic Rheumatic Arthritis of all the Joints*, p. 6. London, 1857.

extremities. Neither the heart nor the pericardium ever becomes affected. The complaint always lasts for several months, and very frequently for years.

With regard to the *morbid anatomy* of rheumatoid arthritis, the following points are worthy of notice. If the disease be in an early stage, the synovial membranes are found thickened and distended with a quantity of synovial fluid; while internally the hypertrophied synovial fimbriæ can be distinguished as vascular tufts. In a more advanced state the capsular membranes are seen to be of increased density; the articular cartilages are more or less absorbed; while the exposed surfaces of the bones either present an ivory-like appearance from the friction they have undergone, or the fine cancelli are laid bare. The heads of the bones are generally enlarged in an irregular way owing to new ossific deposit. Not unfrequently the joints contain numerous small cartilaginous or bony foreign bodies, either loose, or attached by little pedicles to the articular surfaces.

If mention be made of the *pathology* of this disease, it is only to show what the affection is not. Dr. Todd believed that this rheumatic affection of the joints might be most correctly described as an abnormal nutrition, occasioned by the presence of a " peculiar matter" in the nutrient fluid; affording certain points of resemblance to simple chronic inflammation, yet differing from it in a marked manner. What this " peculiar matter" in the nutrient fluid may be, we do not know; but it is certain that it is not uric acid, and there is no reason to believe that it is lactic acid.

The *treatment* is often very unsatisfactory, and always tedious. The general health must be attended to; while in women, any uterine disturbance that may be present is to be relieved. A generous diet, with animal food, ought to be allowed. Hungarian and Greek wines, claret, good sherry, brandy and water, whisky, and dry cider or bitter ale will not usually prove injurious. Sugar, pastry, pickles, and cheese, however, had best be forbidden. Walking exercise is often impossible; but the patient should be taken out in a carriage or chair as often as the weather will permit. Warm clothing is necessary. Then mild aperients, especially the sulphate of soda and sulphur (F. 148, 153); cod liver oil; warm douches over the affected joints; and simple water, or vapour, or hot air baths with gentle friction, may be used in all cases. It is of the greatest importance to maintain a healthy action of the skin, and sometimes particular benefit seems to arise from sulphur or alkaline baths (F. 121, 125). In cases unattended by acute exacerbations M. Gueneau de Mussy recommends arsenical baths. To commence with, about fifteen grains of arseniate of soda, with a quarter of a pound of carbonate of soda, are added to thirty gallons of hot water; the bath at first being employed every second day, and afterwards daily, with an occasional interval. Although slight diarrhœa, temporary excitement, and insomnia sometimes result, yet more often there is merely progressive improvement ; the suppleness of the joints, and the power of motion increasing after each bath. From my own observation I can speak highly of these baths, when they are used as a subordinate part of the treatment. Theoretically it might be expected that they would prove valuable. For indeed arsenic is most beneficial in many of these cases, and from no other special remedy have I seen an equal amount of good result. This metal may either be given alone ; or with quinine, iron, syrup of iodide of iron, iodide of potassium, bromide of potassium, liquor potassæ, taraxacum, or colchicum, (F. 52, 381, &c.) Each of these drugs has also been separately lauded by different writers (F. 31, 32, 46, 379). In women all the preparations of iodine and bromine are to be avoided where there is any tendency to menorrhagia, since they will certainly increase the flow. If the gums be pale and spongy, lemon juice does good ; or the mineral acids (F. 376, 378) are occasionally to be recommended. I have seen guaiacum, given either with ammonia or sulphur or sarsaparilla, do neither good nor harm : it is a remedy from which nothing can be expected in the majority of cases. I have occasionally been pleased with bark and aconite and serpentaria (F. 374) ; and where the skin is inactive and the nervous system depressed, twenty minims of the tincture of arnica montana thrice daily, combined with other remedies, has seemed worth trying. Some practitioners recommend the repeated application of leeches to the affected part, but they must be used cautiously if at all. For my own part, I much distrust their utility. Blisters will possibly do good ; the officinal liquor epispasticus being a convenient application where it is desired to produce vesication. I am fond of strapping the joint with the iodide of potassium or the mercurial plaster spread on chamois leather ; a proceeding which may be occasionally varied by covering the part with sulphur ointment and applying a flannel bandage, or by using a lotion made of equal parts of glycerine and tincture of iodine and tincture of aconite and tincture of opium. To keep the affected articulations motionless by the application of splints, is to run the risk of causing stiff joints ; an evil not counterbalanced by any great advantage.*

* The steady perseverance required to effect a cure in these cases is well illustrated by the following history :—4 *July* 1859. Mrs. H., 46 years of age. Married. Has had eight children, the last being five years old. Catamenia becoming irregular : during the preceding few months, the intervals have often been six weeks. Came under my care with chronic rheumatoid arthritis on the above date. This disease has been coming on very gradually for about ten or twelve months. Without exaggeration it may be said that every joint in the body is more or less affected. Cannot walk or stand ; is unable to cut her food or to do any needlework ; and is conscious that she will soon be incapable of making the slightest movement, since the difficulty and pain of now doing so are very great. Further particulars are unnecessary. Suffice it to say, that with the exception of two short intervals (when owing to the influence of her friends she was persuaded first to try the Bath waters, and afterwards a course of homœopathic globules), she continued under my care until the 27 *May* 1867 ; on which day she was allowed to give up all treatment, her cure being ap-

Other means failing, recourse must be had to the internal and external use of the Harrogate (F. 466), Buxton (F. 464), or Bath waters (F. 460), at home ; or to the springs of Aix-la-Chapelle (F. 483), Wiesbaden (F. 489), Baden-Baden (F. 492), Carlsbad (F. 496), or Vichy (F. 479), abroad. After the employment of either of these saline waters, a course at Schwalbach (F. 488), or at Spa (F. 467), will probably be desirable.

XXIV. OBESITY.

The over-accumulation of fat under the integuments, and around some of the viscera, constitutes obesity [from *Obesus* = fat or gross].　By some authors it is spoken of as polysarcia [Πολὺς = much + σὰρξ = flesh].　The term "corpulency" may perhaps be retained for those cases where the amount of fat is not sufficient to constitute a disease.

A moderate amount of fat is a sign of good health ; and physiologists generally allow that the adipose tissue ought to form about the twentieth part of the weight of man, and the sixteenth of woman.　Independently of the importance of fat, as a non-conducting substance, in impeding the too rapid escape of animal heat, it may also be regarded as a store of material to compensate for waste of tissue under sickness or other circumstances entailing temporary abstinence from food.　Nevertheless in excess this substance not only becomes burdensome and unsightly, but a real and serious evil.　It is hardly necessary to give any description of obesity, since it is a condition recognisable at first sight.　Yet it must be remembered that a man may be large, having the muscular system well developed, and the fat proportionately increased, without being obese.　" This corpulency, or obesity," says Cullen, " is in very different degrees in different persons, and is often considerable without being considered as a disease. There is, however, a certain degree of it, which will be generally allowed to be a disease ; as, for example, when it renders persons, from a difficult respiration, uneasy in themselves, and, from the

parently permanent. From being a helpless cripple, she has by very slow degrees become able to walk freely and naturally. The remedies to which I believe she owes her recovery are,—A warm water sponge bath, with friction and the use of plenty of soap, every night. Flannel under-clothing. Cod liver oil. A diet into the composition of which milk and raw eggs largely entered. An aperient mixture, twice or thrice a week, of sulphate of soda and sulphur.　A night draught containing ether, Indian hemp, and morphia.　With a mixture, thrice daily, consisting of quinine, phosphoric acid, tincture of perchloride of iron, chloride of arsenic, and some bitter infusion.　Of all these remedies, I attach the most importance perhaps to the arsenic.　And it is worthy of observation that this drug was taken twice or thrice daily for nearly eight years with the greatest advantage.　When it was displaced by the trip to Bath, and afterwards by the globules, she was so sensible that ground was being lost, that I do not think she remained out of my hands for more than eight weeks in all.　When last heard of in May 1868, Mrs. H. was continuing well.

inability of exercise, unfit for discharging the duties of life to others."* The *accumulation* of fat must not be confounded with the *degeneration* of muscle and other tissues into this substance.

The obese condition may be partial, or more or less complete. Of *partial* obesity we have examples in fatty tumours; and in that condition popularly spoken of as "pot-belly," from the enlargement of the omentum with fat. This structure has been known to weigh as much as 30 lbs., from excessive adipose deposit. In *complete* obesity we find the fat accumulated under the integuments (especially of the abdominal walls), between the muscles, upon the heart beneath the pericardium, in the mesentery and omentum, around the kidneys, in the mediastinum, and around the mammæ as well as about the nates of women.

Obesity is not peculiar to any particular period of life. The young, the middle-aged, and the old may suffer from it. Females, however, are more predisposed to this condition than males; and they appear more especially liable to it after the cessation of menstruation. Women, too, who have never borne children seem to be more frequently affected than such as have had several pregnancies. And I believe it will generally be found that in fat women the menstrual flow is more scanty and irregular, than it is in those whose organs are not so encumbered.

The *causes* of obesity are numerous. It is often hereditary or constitutional, the inclination being derived from either parent. This tendency is seen not only in individuals but in nations: *e.g.*, the Dutch are as stout, as the Americans are proverbially thin. Over-feeding will induce fat, and so will the habit of taking too much fluid. The obese are not always great eaters: but they invariably drink a great deal, even though it be only water. Farinaceous and vegetable foods are fattening, and saccharine matters are especially so. The instance of the slaves in Italy, who got fat during the grape and fig season, has been quoted by Galen. In sugar-growing countries the negroes and cattle employed on the plantations grow remarkably stout while the cane is being gathered and the sugar extracted. During this harvest the saccharine juices are freely consumed; but when the season is over, the superabundant adipose tissue is gradually lost. And then amongst other causes we must reckon insufficient exercise, long continued prosperity and ease of mind, indulgence in too much sleep, and an absence of the sexual appetite. Eunuchs are generally described as being flabby and fat; whilst amongst the lower animals, fattening is readily produced after the removal of the testicles or ovaries. The way in which the same fact can be made to tell in favour of two opposing theories is curiously illustrated by two writers on this subject. Thus, Wadd cites the butchers as examples of corpulence, alleging that their excellent condition is due to animal food. He speaks particularly of the advantages of the "butcher's steak;"

* *First Lines of the Practice of Physic*, vol. iv. p. 219. Edinburgh, 1784.

and does not believe that these men and their wives owe their good looks to " the effluvia of the meat."* Dancel also speaks of the frequency with which the members of the same class become obese; but he says it is because the butchers eat meat and plenty of vegetables, while their wives generally prefer vegetables to animal food. He has no faith in the opinion that their embonpoint has some connexion with the atmosphere of nutritive animal odours in which they live.†

Fats are obtained abundantly from both the animal and vegetable kingdoms. Their predominating elements are carbon and hydrogen. They never contain nitrogen, except as an accidental ingredient. They are made up of three closely allied bodies; viz., stearin [from στέαρ = suet], margarin [from its lustrous appearance, μάργαρον = a pearl], and olein [oleum = oil] which is fluid. When fatty matters are heated with the hydrated alkalies, they undergo saponification, during which process a viscid sweet fluid— glycerine [γλυκὺς = sweet]—is yielded. Now several physiological studies lead to the conclusion that oils and fats may not only be formed in the system from food which contains it ready prepared, but also from the chemical transformation of starch or sugar. Many experiments have been performed on geese, ducks, and pigs, which have proved that these animals accumulate much more fat than could be accounted for by that present in the food. M. Flourens had the bears at the Jardin des Plantes fed exclusively on bread, and they became excessively fat. Magendie, in making experiments on the forage of horses, found that these animals constantly returned more fat in their excrements than their food contained. And several authors have shown that bees form wax, which strictly belongs to the group of fats, when fed exclusively on purified sugar. If with foods of this nature the animals be subjected to a warm atmosphere and allowed but little room for movement, the adipose tissue rapidly gets increased. At Strasburg, the place of all others most noted for its pâtés de foie gras, the geese are fatted by shutting them up in coops within a room heated to a very high temperature, and stuffing them constantly with food. Here all the conditions for insuring obesity are resorted to—viz. external heat, obscurity, inactivity, and the cramming of the animals with nourishment. A still greater refinement for pandering to the appetite is resorted to by the Italians, who appear particularly to relish the fat of the ortolan. To procure this in perfection, the natural habits of the bird were watched; and it having been proved that food is only taken at the rising of the sun, cunning men have arranged that this luminary shall rise much more frequently than

* Cursory Remarks on Corpulence; or Obesity considered as a Disease. Third Edition, p. 81. London, 1816.
† Traité Théorique et pratique de l'Obésité, p. 84. Paris, 1863. This physician's first treatise on the subject—Préceptes fondé sur la Chimie organique pour diminuer l'Embonpoint sans altérer la Santé—was published in 1849.

nature has ordained. To effect this, the ortolans are placed in a dark, and warm chamber, which has but one aperture in the wall. Food being scattered over the floor, a lantern is placed at a certain hour in the opening; and the birds, misled by the dim light, believing that the sun is about to shed its rays upon them, at once consume their rations. The meal finished, the lantern withdrawn, and more nutriment scattered about, the ortolans fall asleep, as in duty bound; though probably not without a feeling of surprise at the shortness of their day. Two or three hours having elapsed, and digestion being completed, the lantern is again made to throw its light into the apartment. The rising sun recalls the birds to the necessity of again feeding; and of again sleeping as they become enveloped in darkness. Thus this process is repeated several times in the twenty-four hours; until, at the end of two or three days, the ortolan becomes a delicious little ball of fat, ready to minister to the palate of the gourmand.

The *consequences* of obesity are often more serious than is generally believed. To put aside many minor inconveniences (which, however, may be sufficiently annoying to make the sufferer desirous of reducing his weight, even at a little risk to his health) it may be taken as a general rule that obesity does not conduce to strength or to longevity. The functions of various important organs being constantly impeded must cause many distressing disorders. Falstaff, whose "pelly was all putter" as the Welsh parson said, suffered more from his ridiculous figure than from any real evil. The chief fear of this "huge hill of flesh" seems to have been that they might "melt him out of his fat drop by drop, and liquor fishermen's boots" with him. Daniel Lambert at one time weighed 52 st. 12 lbs., or 740 lbs.; and he died suddenly in 1809, in his fortieth year. Bright, a grocer at Maldon in Essex, who had attained to 616 lbs. at his death, and the capacity of whose waistcoat was said to be such that it could enclose seven ordinary persons, only lived to be twenty-nine. Palmer, the landlord of the Golden Lion at Brompton, in Kent, weighed 25 st. It is said, that coming to London to see Lambert he was so affected at the greater grossness of his more corpulent rival that the irrepressible envy caused his death. Whatever the truth may be, he certainly died three weeks after his visit to the metropolis. John Love (an apprentice of Ryland, the celebrated engraver who was executed for forgery) became so emaciated through grief at his master's fate, that his friends thought he was becoming consumptive. A physician recommended an abundance of nutritious food; under the influence of which he soon became as heavy and corpulent as he had previously been slender. He died, "suffocated by fat," in his fortieth year, his weight being 26 st. or 364 lbs. Dr. F. Dancel in his excellent work (p. 26) already referred to quotes from the *Javannach-News* for 1853, the following:—There lived, eighteen miles from Batavia, a young man who weighed 565 lbs. (40 st. 5 lbs.) when he was twenty-two years of age.   His size continued to increase until a little over 600 lbs. (42 st. 12 lbs.).   He was comfortable and took care of a plantation.   At the end of four weeks he began to increase again in weight, at first to the extent of 1¼ lbs. daily, and then of 2 lbs.   In the last week he died suddenly in his chair, suffocated by fat.   Three days before his death he weighed 643 lbs. (45 st. 13 lbs.)

As a rule, to which every one can call to mind exceptions, excessive corpulence diminishes both bodily and mental activity. One of the most anomalous cases is mentioned by Maccary, who states that he met at Pavia the most enormously fat man he ever saw, but who nevertheless was a dancer, and was exceedingly agile and graceful in his movements.   Yet generally obesity is accompanied with diminished vital power; there are disturbances of the organs of respiration, circulation, and digestion; the blood is proportionately deficient in quantity or quality; the muscles are weak and have but little firmness; while the countenance is bloated and sallow.   And although the disposition is often sanguine, so that the sufferer continues lively and cheerful, and has the happy habit of looking at the best side of everything, yet active mental occupation is generally as uncongenial as repose and idleness are in harmony with the inclinations.   Lord Chesterfield is no great authority, but he mixed much with men; and in his opinion fat and stupidity were such inseparable companions, that he was accustomed to say they might be used as convertible terms.*

The *treatment* of obesity would now seem to rest upon a more sure basis than it has hitherto done, the investigations pursued by Dr. Dancel having been mainly instrumental in leading to this result.   As a proof of the truth of this remark we may look back for a moment to the curative agents formerly in use.   Thus, we find a tolerable list of remedies in the pages of Maccary,† which includes —bleeding from the arm or jugular vein; leeches to the anus; dry cupping; prolonged blistering; vegetable diet with vinegar; acids, except nitric and phosphoric; hot baths; salt water baths; baths of Aix, Spa, Forges, Rouen, and Acqui; occasional starvation; decoction of guaiacum and sassafras; scarifications; salivation; the induction of grief and anxiety; purgatives; issues; pricking the flesh with needles; walking with naked feet; and removal of exuberant fatty tissue with the scalpel.   Since this

* Lord Byron undervalued David Hume, denying his claim to genius on account of his bulk, and calling him, from the Heroic Epistle—"The fattest hog in Epicurus' sty."   Another of this extraordinary man's allegations was, that "fat is an oily dropsy." To stave off its visitation, he frequently chewed tobacco in lieu of dinner, alleging that it absorbed the gastric juice of the stomach, and prevented hunger.   *Rejected Adresses.* By James and Horace Smith. Twenty-fourth Edition.   Note to p. 13.   London, 1855.—Somewhat in the same strain Mirabeau said, alluding to a very corpulent man, that he had only been created to show to what an extent the human skin could be stretched without bursting.

† *Traité sur la Polysarcie.*   Paris, 1811.

ridiculous catalogue was published, Turkish baths, sea voyages, very little sleep, emetics, digitalis, soap (a relative of Mr. Wadd's ordered a quarter of a hundredweight of Castile soap for his own private eating), salt, mercury to salivation, the inhalation of oxygen gas, anti-corpulent belts worn round the stomach day and night, quinine, purgatives, diuretics, the extract of the fucus vesiculosus, and preparations of bromine or of iodine have been freely tried. Dr. Thomas King Chambers, believing that the chemical affinity of alkalies for fat points them out as appropriate alteratives in this complaint, has recommended liquor potassæ, in half drachm or drachm doses, thrice daily. The medicine is taken in milk and water; since milk covers the taste better than anything else, while the efficacy of the potash is not endangered because a part of it is saponified. Dr. Chambers of course regulates the diet, interdicting fat, oil, and butter; while he recommends very light meals off substances that can be quickly digested. The patient is also to devote many hours daily to walking or riding. Moreover, he may employ cold salt water baths, or vapour baths, with friction to the skin.*   But all these plans, however perseveringly carried out, fail to accomplish the object desired; and the same must be said of simple sobriety in eating and drinking.†   For it must be remembered that as physicians we are called upon not only to prevent the increase of fat, but to diminish the redundant quantity which has already been formed, without lessening the normal vigour of the system. The question is, can this be done ?

* *Corpulence; or, Excess of Fat in the Human Body.* London, 1850.
† The inutility of a diet restricted to slops is well shown in the following case, related by Wardell. The subject of the history was a female patient at the Edinburgh Royal Infirmary. She was forty years of age, of short stature, and so obese as from the first to make her case an alarming one. The features were grown up with fat, so that the eyes looked small and sunken. Even walking up and down the ward was attended with difficulty, the exertion giving rise to great embarrassment of breathing. "The appetite was preternaturally large; somnolency so persistent, that whenever left but a few minutes to herself, she dozed over into slumber. There was a torpor of mind, an aversion to all exercise, a listless apathetic state, which so characterize this curious disease. She was ordered a diet not more nourishing than allowed to the fever patients, consisting chiefly of panado and slops, yet the polysarcia progressed, and after being some time an inmate in the hospital she died, with comatose symptoms."—*Remarks on Obesity.* p. 11. London, 1849. Reprinted from the *London Medical Gazette.*
Wadd has also told us that "among the Asiatics, there is a sect of Brahmins who pride themselves on their extreme corpulency. Their diet consists of farinaceous vegetables, milk, sugar, sweetmeats, and ghee. They look upon corpulency as proof of opulence; and many arrive at a great degree of obesity, without tasting anything that has ever lived."—*Opus jam citat.* p. 80.
Dr. Fothergill stated that a strict vegetable diet produces exuberant fat more certainly than other means. And Mr. Moore mentions the case of an enormously fat woman who exhibited herself at some house in the Strand in 1851. Upon questioning her and the exhibitor, he found that they were both rigid vegetarians, and were not a little proud of belonging to this sect.—*Corpulency, i.e. Fat, or Embonpoint, in Excess.* Fourth Edition, p. 14. London, 1860.

Now I believe that obesity may safely be diminished; and that we are indebted for our power to do so to the light which has been shed by physiological chemistry on the production of fat in the body, and our knowledge of the influence of respiration in removing carbon from the blood. The researches of Dr. Dancel have also served to reduce all this to a system, as well as to direct attention to it. But it is only fair to allow, while giving every credit to this physician, that something is due to Mr. Banting for bringing the subject before the public in a plain and sensible manner.* In the month of August 1862, this gentleman was 66 years of age, 5 ft. 5 in. in stature, and 14 st. 3 lbs. (202 lbs.) in weight. He could not stoop to tie his shoe, was unable to attend to the little offices humanity requires, was compelled to go downstairs slowly backwards to avoid the jar of increased weight on the knee and ankle joints, and was made to puff and blow with every slight exertion. After trying many remedies (including fifty Turkish baths, with gallons of physic) without the slightest benefit, he consulted Mr. William Harvey for deafness. Mr. Harvey, believing that obesity was the source of the mischief, cut off the supply of bread, butter, milk, sugar, beer, soup, potatoes, and beans. In their place he ordered the following diet, which I venture to briefly criticise in the hope of improving the lesson :—

Breakfast. Four or five ounces of beef, mutton, kidneys, broiled fish, bacon, or cold meat (except pork); a large cup of tea without milk or sugar, a little biscuit or one ounce of dry toast. [Brown bread, or crust off the common household loaf, might have been allowed.]

Dinner. Five or six ounces of any fish except salmon [it would have been as well also to have forbidden herrings and eels], any meat except pork, any vegetable except potato, one ounce of dry toast, fruit out of a pudding, any kind of poultry or game, and two or three glasses of good claret, sherry, or Madeira. Champagne, port, and beer forbidden.

Tea. Two or three ounces of fruit, a rusk or two, and a cup of tea without milk or sugar. [Coffee might have been permitted.]

Supper. Three or four ounces of meat or fish, and a glass or two of claret.

For *nightcap*, if required, a tumblerful of grog (gin, whisky, or brandy, without sugar) or a glass or two of claret or sherry. [Like other nightcaps, this was certainly unnecessary.]

At the same time a draught containing a drachm of the aromatic spirits of ammonia, with ten grains of carbonate of magnesia, was given once or twice a daily, on an empty stomach. The result of this treatment was a gradual reduction of 46 lbs. in weight; with better health at the end of several weeks, than had been enjoyed for the previous twenty years.

The explanation of all this is very simple. Food, as has been already mentioned, consists of azotised or nitrogenous, and non-nitrogenous principles. The *former* (the nutritive or plastic class)

---

* *Letter on Corpulence, addressed to the Public.* Third Edition. London, 1864.

includes all fibrous and albuminous matters, such as animal food; these matters aiding the formation of blood and muscle, but not entering into the composition of adipose tissue. The *latter* (the calorifacient or respiratory class) consists of oily and fatty materials; with sugar, gum, starch, and vegetable acids, all of which contain carbon and hydrogen, the elements of fat. Man undoubtedly requires a mixed diet: that is to say, nitrogenous food is needed for the formation or renewal of the tissues and other nitrogenous parts of the body; while the respiratory food is required for the production of the fatty components of the body, and as affording materials for respiration and the production of heat. Hence it is clear, that while we may limit the non-azotised substances, they must not be altogether cut off. Moreover, it is of practical importance to remember that the elements which are chemically convertible into fat are rendered more fattening if alcoholic liquids be added to them in the stomach; probably because of the power which stimulants possess of lessening or delaying the destructive metamorphosis. It may be said that a diet such as Mr. Harvey recommended is calculated to induce the uric acid diathesis with gout. The only answer is that this occurrence seems provided against by the draught of ammonia and magnesia. Moreover, as a matter of experience, this gentleman tells me he has not found any indication of gout to follow his treatment; and, in cases which I have successfully treated according to his rules, not the slightest symptom of the kind has occurred. But even should an attack of gout result, it is really a disease of minor importance compared to obesity, except as a confirmed affection.

Two points only remain for consideration. One is that every patient under treatment for this morbid state should be regularly weighed, while the condition of his health is to be carefully watched. Particularly, heed is to be taken that the appetite does not fail, the power of digestion fall off, constipation take place, the action of the heart become enfeebled, or the blood get impoverished. As a rule, the diminution in gravity should not be allowed to progress more rapidly than at the rate of one pound a week; and it ought not to be carried to too great an extent. In a previous section (p. 154), as well as subsequently in the remarks on Phthisis, the reader will find tables of the normal weight in proportion to the age and stature; which tables may form rough guides for the practitioner, serving to show him the extent to which redundant fat may be safely reduced.

And lastly, on the part of both physician and patient, firmness of purpose and steady perseverance will be needed. The former, however, must be careful not to hold the reins with too tight a hand. Frequently, he will have to pour balm upon the irritable feelings of the man who, on this as on a few other occasions, may think he is paying too dearly for the relief of his disease. We cannot affect to feel any surprise at the querulousness of Charles Lamb, when he asks in one of his letters to Wordsworth,—"What have I gained by health? Intolerable dulness. What by early hours and moderate meals? A total blank." Shall we therefore be surprised when those who consult us are not altogether as tractable as could be wished? And when a sociable citizen finds, that to lose some pounds of superfluous fat he is obliged forcibly to mortify his tastes, as well as to alter the mode of living to which he has for years habituated himself, is it to be wondered at that such a one should often politely thank us for our advice, but still prefer to let his palate and stomach deal with him as they think fit.

PART II.

FEVERS.

FEVER [from *Ferveo* = to burn], or Pyrexia [Πῦρ = fire + ἔχω = to hold], is to be defined as a grave morbid condition caused by the action of a poison on the blood, and through this on every tissue of the body. Consequent upon this action there is a preliminary stage of languor and weakness, defective appetite and nausea, frontal headache and pains about the loins and limbs, with some degree of chilliness or shivering; this being succeeded by the confirmed stage in which we find preternatural heat of body, increased waste of tissue, acceleration of pulse with derangements of the capillary circulation, great muscular debility, and disturbance of most of the functions. Owing to the derangements of innervation and circulation and secretion which are set up, an accumulation of effete products takes place in the blood. The concluding phenomena are those of crisis and elimination.

Much has been written on the classification of the *idiopathic* or *essential* fevers (so-called to distinguish them from *symptomatic* fever, or that abnormal state which accompanies many different diseases as one of their phenomena), each author having some favourite arrangement which does not always simplify the subject. In order to be as clear as possible, I shall consider the different varieties of fever according to the following plan :—

 I. Continued Fevers.
 1. *Simple Continued Fever.*
 2. *Typhus Fever.*
 3. *Enteric* or *Typhoid Fever.*
 4. *Cerebro-Spinal Fever.*
 5. *Relapsing* or *Famine Fever.*
 II. Intermittent Fever, or Ague.
 III. Remittent Fever.
 IV. Yellow Fever.
 V. Eruptive Fevers.
 1. *Small-pox*, or *Variola.*
 2. *Cow-pox*, or *Vaccinia.*
 3. *Chicken-pox*, or *Varicella.*
 4. *Measles*, or *Morbilli.*
 5. *Scarlet Fever*, or *Scarlatina.*
 6. *Dengue.*
 7. *Erysipelas.*
 8. *Plague*, or *Pestis.*

Two of the Continued fevers resemble the Eruptive in being infectious or contagious—these terms being regarded as synonymous, in having a peculiar eruption on the skin, and in the fact that one attack generally confers immunity from any subsequent assault of the same disease. Thus typhus affords protection from typhus for the future, but not from enteric fever; just as the susceptibility to small-pox is exhausted by an attack of this disease, though the system may still be affected by measles, or scarlet fever, &c. Each type of fever has its own special cause. At least three varieties of continued fever have their origin in known and preventible causes; in this respect resembling intermittent fever, and differing from the so-called eruptive fevers. And then, fevers run a regular definite course, and have a certain duration : each may be said to have a self-limited career.

I. CONTINUED FEVER.

Continued Fever is so termed from the fact that it pursues its course without any well-marked remissions.

The cause of fever is the contamination of the blood by some morbific agent. When this change (the nature of which is unknown) has proceeded to a certain extent, the researches of Dr. Parkes teach us that the nervous system, or rather that part especially connected with nutrition and organic contractility, begins to suffer alterations in composition. The muscles, and probably some of the organs, deprived more or less of nervous influence, begin to disintegrate, this disintegration producing undue heat; the condition of the vagus and vaso-motor nerves induces increased action of the heart and dilatation of the vessels ; the contaminated blood is still further deteriorated by receiving the rapidly-disintegrating tissues, by the continued action of the morbid agent, as well as by the functions of the lungs and liver and spleen &c., being impeded ; while, since no food is taken, the various alkaline and neutral salts are no longer received into the system.

There are five varieties of Continued fevers :—1. *Simple continued fever*, including *febricula*, which is non-contagious, and arises from over-fatigue, errors in diet, and exposure to the sun's rays. 2. *Typhus*, which is infectious, occurs among the poor, and is due to some poison generated by famine and destitution, as well as by overcrowding in prisons and workhouses, or even ill-ventilated rooms. 3. *Enteric, typhoid*, or *pythogenic fever*, met with equally amongst rich and poor, generated by the putrid emanations from decaying animal matter, most prevalent in autumn, and which is infectious though less so than typhus. 4. *Cerebro-spinal fever*, a malignant epidemic disease attended with lesions of the membranes and surfaces of the great nervous centres ; and which, of late years, has mostly occurred where numbers of persons have been congregated together. And 5, *Relapsing* or *famine fever*, which is very contagious, and is probably produced by famine alone.

To show the relative prevalence of the four principal forms, it may be mentioned, that during the ten years ending with December 1857, there were admitted into the London Fever Hospital 6628 cases of fever; of which 861 were Febricula, 3506 Typhus, 1820 Enteric, and 441 Relapsing fever. With the exception of the years 1850 and 1851 there was a preponderance of typhus; but in one of these two years, the typhoid cases, and in the other the relapsing, were in excess. There seems to be a comparative immunity from typhus during certain years in London; as may be shown by the returns for 1858 and 1859, in which years there were admitted into the hospital only 63 examples of typhus against 356 of typhoid fever. Now again, the typhus cases are largely in excess. Taking the three years 1864, 65, 66 the numbers with typhus have been 2497, 1961, and 1735; while the examples of enteric fever were 252, 520, and 575. Moreover, in neither of these years was there a single instance of relapsing fever; although in 1851 there were more cases of this kind than of any other.

According to the Reports of the Registrar-General, the deaths from all forms of continued fever, in England, during the ten years from 1857 to 1866, both inclusive, were 182,210. Hitherto, the different species have not been distinguished in the Returns.

1. SIMPLE CONTINUED FEVER.—This variety of fever, where it runs an uncomplicated course, is always a mild disease; having a variable duration of from one to ten days. When lasting only for a day or two it is spoken of as *ephemeral* [from ‘Επὶ = through + ἡμέρα = a day] fever. *Febricula* [dim. of *Febris* = a fever] is an appropriate name as denoting its comparatively trifling character.

Simple fever commences for the most part without any warning; the patient being suddenly seized with lassitude, disinclination for bodily or mental exertion, loss of appetite, sickness, frontal headache, dull aching of back and limbs, coldness of the surface—especially of the back, and often shivering. At the end of a few hours, in most cases, the chilliness passes off, and the skin becomes dry and hot. There is no characteristic eruption: a crop of herpes perhaps appears on the lips. The pulse is then found frequent, large, and hard—perhaps 120 or 130 in a minute. There is increased headache and restlessness; a dry and furred tongue, with urgent thirst, as well as constipation. The urine is scanty and high coloured. Moreover, the patient usually complains of pains in his limbs, or of a feeling of soreness over his body; he rapidly emaciates; his countenance becomes pale and haggard; he wanders in his talk, or even has slight delirium; and he seems very seriously ill to his friends. An exacerbation or aggravation of all the symptoms frequently occurs towards night; with a slight remission at the approach of morning, when sleep is often obtained. These symptoms usually continue for three or four days, although exceptionally they are prolonged for two or even three weeks. But in the common run of cases, it happens on the fourth day, sometimes on the fifth or sixth, that the tongue becomes moist; the skin gets less harsh and dry; the headache and pains in the limbs abate; and then a profuse sweating follows. This sweat proves the natural crisis or termination of the disease. It leaves the patient languid and exhausted; but with a pulse of the natural standard, and a complete freedom from the fever. Where perspiration does not occur, a critical bæmorrhage from the nose, or rectum, or uterus, may set in; or there will perhaps be an attack of diarrhœa; or an eruption of herpes breaks out on the face; or there may be an increased action of the kidneys, the urine becoming loaded with urates. Convalescence gradually and steadily takes place, some weeks perhaps elapsing before the patient thoroughly regains his flesh and strength.

Simple fever is very seldom attended with any danger; and inasmuch as it is not due to any specific poison, is non-infectious. Nosologists have divided it into different classes, according as one particular organ has been more affected than another; so that in some books we find unnecessary distinctions into brain, catarrhal, gastric, mesenteric, and bilious fevers. Dr. Murchison says, that from his own observations in India and Burmah, he is convinced "that the Common Continued Fever, the Ardent Fever, and the Sun Fever of the tropics, are nothing more than severe forms of the Simple Fever or Febricula of Britain."* The disease as seen in India, occurs chiefly among recruits newly arrived, rather than in disciplined soldiers. It usually comes on directly after exposure to the sun's rays, in the hot dry season (March, April, and May), when the thermometer ranges from 92° to 114° Fahr. The prominent symptoms enumerated by Dr. Murchison are chilliness, perhaps with nausea and vomiting. A pulse of 100 to 120; a burning skin, flushed face, and intense headache; great thirst; restlessness and sleeplessness; and scanty dark urine, of low sp. grav., containing crystals of uric acid. About the fifth day there is often delirium; followed by unconsciousness, contracted pupils, and perhaps coma. Death may happen from coma or collapse. With favourable cases, between the sixth and ninth days, there is a free perspiration, a fall in the pulse, increased secretion of urine loaded with urates, and convalescence.

All fevers seem disposed to run a certain course, and to terminate naturally in the re-establishment of health when uninterfered with by art. But, as in the treatment of other disease, there are certain general objects, called the *indications of cure*, which must

* *A Treatise on the Continued Fevers of Great Britain*, p. 598. London, 1862.

be kept in view. In fever these indications are:—(1) To moderate, where necessary, the violence of arterial excitement by saline laxatives, rest in bed, and low diet. (2) To support the powers of the system as soon as they begin to flag. (3) To obviate local inflammations and congestions. And (4), to relieve any urgent symptoms as they arise. It was well observed by Pitcairn—"I do not like fever-curers. You may *guide* a fever; you cannot *cure* it. What would you think of a pilot who attempted to quell a storm? Either position is equally absurd. In the storm you steer the ship as well as you can; and in a fever you can only employ patience and judicious measures to meet the difficulties of the case." What these *judicious measures* really consist of the reader will be able to deduce from the remarks on the treatment of typhus.

For the ardent fever of India and other tropical countries, emetics, purgatives, diaphoretics, low diet, and tepid sponging are employed. With some plethoric subjects, venesection, leeches to the temples, cold applications to the head, cold affusion, as well as the administration of tartar emetic, have been required. When the urgent symptoms are removed, quinine should be given.

2. TYPHUS FEVER.—The prominent symptoms of typhus are an increase in the temperature of the body, an unduly abundant excretion of urea and carbonic acid by the kidneys and lungs, the eruption of a mulberry rash, and a state of utter helplessness and prostration. This form of fever* is eminently infectious; it often prevails epidemically, during seasons of general scarcity, attacking individuals of both sexes and all ages; and it is the accompaniment of destitution, being generated in over-crowded and ill-ventilated dwellings. Its duration is from fourteen to twenty-one days.

Causes.—A predisposition to typhus may be engendered by all depressing bodily and mental influences. Intemperance, bad or insufficient food, over-fatigue, fear and mental anxiety, diarrhœa and lowering diseases generally, prevent the system from resisting the contagion. Over-crowding of dwelling houses—that general unhealthy condition engendered by the accumulation of a number of individuals in unventilated houses or rooms, technically known as *ochlesis*, is a most important cause. Where houses are so huddled together that free currents of air cannot pass through them, and where the ill-fed inhabitants fail to pay any attention to domestic or personal cleanliness, there typhus will revel. Whether, intense crowd-poisoning may be alone sufficient to generate the toxic material of typhus is doubted by some authorities;

* Prior to 1759 the disease was known as Putrid, Pestilential, Malignant, Jail, Ship, Camp, or Hospital Fever. Sauvages then described it under the name of Typhus. This word is derived from Τῦφος = smoke; an expression employed by Hippocrates to denote a lethargic disease, in which the patient is suddenly deprived of his senses, as if thunderstruck. In the present day, typhus is often popularly spoken of as *Brain fever*.

although a mass of evidence in favour of this view has been adduced.

Symptoms.—After the reception of the fever-poison there is commonly a period of *incubation*, during which the patient perhaps complains of slight chilliness, nausea, pain in the back, loss of appetite, thirst, languor, and headache. The duration of this precursory stage varies; but it is usually short—from one or two to twelve days, and it ends suddenly in an attack of shivering quickly followed by the symptoms which are common to many acute affections. These are chiefly increased headache, dryness with heat of skin, thirst, a heavy dull look, constipation, frequent soft pulse, dry tongue, stupor, prostration, and muscular pains; while towards the evening of each day there is aggravated irritability and restlessness, causing a wakeful night. The evening temperature as taken by the thermometer in the axilla is often rather lower than that of the morning : the mercury will perhaps reach 105° by 8 a.m. on the third day. The mulberry typhus rash (sometimes called a *morbiliform* eruption, from its resemblance to the efflorescence of measles) appears between the fourth and seventh days from the commencement of the disorder. It consists of irregular spots, of a dusky or mulberry hue, disappearing on pressure, and feeling as if slightly raised above the skin. These spots may be few and single, or numerous and large owing to the coalescence of several, or they may be pale and produce merely a mottled appearance; while their number and depth of colour will be found to be in proportion to the severity of the attack. They are most commonly first seen on the abdomen, and then on the chest and extremities; in a day or two they become of a brick-dust colour, and only slightly fade on pressure; while each patch of eruption remains permanent till the end of the fever. This eruption is often accompanied by, or becomes converted into, petechiæ. It is very rarely indeed absent in adults; but in children, particularly in mild cases, it will perhaps be present in only three cases out of four.

During the first week the patient generally complains much of headache and noises in the ears; while subsequently there may be deafness. The conjunctivæ are found injected : when delirium sets in the pupils are often contracted, and insensible to light. The sense of taste is impaired, as is also that of smell; there is loss of appetite, but no symptom of intestinal irritation, no flatulence, no diarrhœa; while the tongue, which at first is pale and soft and tremulous and notched by the teeth, becomes brown and dry, and in grave cases almost black and covered with offensive bloody sordes. In most instances there is more or less wakefulness, particularly at night. Perhaps the sufferer sleeps, however, though when he awakes he declares he has not closed his eyes. Now and then, especially about the ninth or tenth day, there is profound somnolence, which may end in fatal coma. Or there may be that condition described as coma-vigil by Sir William Jenner; in which the patient lies with his eyes wide open, evidently awake, but indifferent or insensible to all going on around him. This state may last from one to four days, when it is almost invariably terminated by death.

The urine is often diminished in quantity, and is of high specific gravity; while it contains an increased amount of urea and uric acid and pigments. The chlorides are much diminished. Now and then there is albuminuria; and occasionally a complete suppression, with convulsions and fatal uræmia. Care must always be taken not to mistake retention for suppression. If no urine be passed, or if it be found constantly leaking away, a catheter should at once be introduced. A constant dribbling of urine is the most certain symptom of an overloaded bladder. The weakness which affects the muscular system, almost from the first, is very remarkable; the prostration gradually increasing, until those who have been strong and robust become so powerless that they cannot turn in bed or raise a limb. The countenance is of a dusky tint, the gaze dull and vacant, while the features get wasted and pinched to an extreme degree. The breath may have an ammoniacal odour. Muscular twitchings of the face and hands are not uncommon; or there may be some irritation of the diaphragm causing troublesome hiccup.

Delirium is seldom present before the end of the first week, and the way in which it then comes on is worthy of notice. The patient from being perfectly rational passes through every grade of delirium, perhaps in the course of two or three hours, to the most wild and furious perversion of mind. At first there is merely "wandering," and the sufferer is conscious every two or three minutes that he is talking nonsense. Then there is confusion of ideas with vague rambling talk, from which he can be roused. This is followed by illusions, especially of the senses of hearing and vision; while soon every function of the mind becomes disordered by unreal images and aberrant trains of thought, which cannot be corrected by any external impressions. These ravings, however, are usually remembered, and the sufferer is able to explain the reasons for his shrieks and violence. He recollects, for instance, that he was confined in some dungeon, or was pursued by enemies bent on murdering him. He visited distant countries to seek concealment, but in vain. His foes were at hand; he would not yield, however, without a struggle. And then he raved, sprang from the bed, and attempted to reach the door or window to fly from his tormentors. In a case of erysipelas with great prostration, which I well remember nursing through a long night, the delirium was of the same character as occurs in typhus. The patient every few minutes became furious, shouting out " Police," "The villains are coming," " Help," &c., at the same time attempting to jump out of bed. It afterwards appeared that he was being made an example of for his sins; that strong men took and forced him into a brass box the size of an orange; and that then he was carried to a height and hurled down. As he escaped from the broken cage he became somewhat calmer, asked for drink, and said it was dreadful torture; until suddenly starting again, with a wild look he would cry out, at the top of his voice, " There, look,—they are coming. Police," and so on. Sometimes this delirium ends in coma; but in favourable cases it gradually passes off in two or three days, the patient enjoys a long quiet sleep, and then begins to recover his memory as well as the other mental powers.

With regard to the condition of the heart, Dr. Stokes points out that it is liable, in common with other organs, to suffer from organic and functional alteration; in one set of cases there being excitement of the heart, while in another class we may find depression, but neither of these results being due to inflammation.   A progressive loss of impulse as well as of the systolic sound, a slow pulse, sighing respiration and a tendency to syncope, are the principal indications of the depressed state of the heart; this depression being generally due to a softened state of the walls of the ventricles, especially on the left side, though undoubtedly the heart may be found simply weakened without softening.   Conversely, a strong and jerking impulse, with distinctness of both sounds, indicates the excited condition; in which, however, the pulse will be found feeble and the extremities cold, while occasionally there is loss or diminution of the second sound.   The production of a murmur, in connexion either with the excited or depressed state of the heart, is of rare occurrence.

The observations which have been made with the sphygmograph by Marey, Wolff, Anstie, Sanderson, Foster, and others have proved that remarkable changes occur in the pulse during the course of febrile diseases.   The pulse-curve in health has a tricotous form;* but in fever this curve has a tendency to become dicrotous or even monocrotous.   According to Wolff,† these changes are chiefly effected by the deepening of the aortic notch. When this notch has not sunk to the level of the curve-basis, and has not quite swallowed up the first secondary wave though it has annihilated the second and slightly retarded the dicrotism, the pulse is said to be hypo-dicrotous.   With this, the temperature of the body seldom exceeds 100° Fahr.   When the notch sinks to the level of the curve-basis, the first secondary wave having almost disappeared while the dicrotism is still more retarded, the pulse is called dicrotous.   The rate of the pulse is then about 100, and the temperature 103°.   If the aortic notch sinks below the level of the curve-basis and the dicrotism appears partly blended with the line of ascent of the next pulsation, the pulse is called hyper-dicrotous.   The temperature is generally above 104°.   Where this hyper-dicrotous pulse changes into the monocrotous form at an

* See the remarks on the Sphygmograph in the description of the Valvular Diseases of the Heart, Part V., Section 27.

† Quoted from an excellent review of recent works on the Sphygmograph in the *British and Foreign Medico-Chirurgical Review*. No. 83, p. 15. London, July 1868.

advanced stage of fever, death is almost sure to follow. Another grave sign is irregularity in the pulse curve ; while an undulatory irregularity is of still more serious import, since it shows that the force of the ventricle is momentarily changing. Although the arterial tension is low in fever, yet with a heart acting well the pulse-trace will show a vertical line of ascent with a sharp summit ; but when the heart's action fails, then the ascension line is short and non-vertical with a square summit. Finally, it has been shown by Anstie that the administration of alcohol in the low stage of fevers, and other acute diseases, when a stimulant is really required, increases the arterial tension—it shallows the depth of the dicrotic notch, and lessens the frequency of the pulse. On the other hand, where the alcohol acts injuriously as a narcotic, it lowers the arterial pressure—increases the dicrotism and quickens the pulse-rate. Moreover, while the summits of the pulse trace are pointed and the curves of good height, there is not much cause for anxiety ; but directly the apices are softly rounded and the curves small, with the fever still high, prompt and liberal stimulation is needed to assist the failing heart.

The lungs are apt to become secondarily affected ; and the danger of the fever will thus be increased by the occurrence of acute bronchitis, or pleurisy, or pneumonia. The latter may run on to pulmonary gangrene, which is almost always fatal. Congestion and œdema of the lungs are not uncommon. In a few instances there has also been inflammation of the larynx and pharynx ; and in a still smaller number of cases, inflammation of the brain or its membranes. Amongst other occasional complications must be mentioned diarrhœa, obstinate sickness, swellings and suppurations of the parotid or submaxillary glands, erysipelas, pyæmia, convulsions, and gangrene of the toes or feet.

The approach of convalescence is in the majority of cases somewhat sudden ; being indicated by a diminution in the nervous symptoms, by the eruption completely fading away, by the tongue getting cleaner, and by the partial return of the muscular power ; while the pulse also beats more quietly and with less rapidity, the temperature falls, the appetite improves, and the patient sleeps at night. The amendment generally begins between the tenth and sixteenth days—most frequently on the thirteenth or fourteenth ; and only occasionally is preceded by some *crisis,* such as a prolonged sleep, or copious sweating, or an attack of diarrhœa, or the deposit of a large quantity of urates in the urine.

Prognosis.—Amongst unfavourable symptoms may be noticed:— A presentiment of death. A pulse above 120, particularly if this rate be present at an early stage ; absence of cardiac impulse with an inaudible systolic sound ; and excited action of the heart, with a feeble pulse at the wrist. A morning temperature of 106°, especially if this be maintained after the ninth day ; or a temperature below 98° with a rapid pulse. The presence of pulmonary complications.   Sleeplessness, with delirium : coma-vigil : great contraction of the pupil, and squinting.   Extreme prostration, muscular tremor, and hiccup.   A brown, hard, tremulous tongue. Great lividity of the surface, with abundant eruption.   And albuminuria, or especially suppression of urine.

Where the disease proves fatal, it usually does so between the twelfth and twentieth days.   And then death is immediately preceded by very great prostration, retention or suppression of urine, involuntary defecation, the formation of bed-sores, an undulatory pulse of 160 or even more, subsultus tendinum or involuntary muscular twitchings, convulsions, lividity of countenance, very rapid breathing, coma-vigil and syncope, or somnolence passing into stupor and coma.   According to Dr. Murchison, one person out of every five attacked by typhus dies.   Out of 4787 cases admitted into the London Fever Hospital during 14½ years (from 1848 until June 1862), there were 1000 deaths; making a mortality of 1 in 4·78.   Many of the cases, however, were moribund on admission.   The greater the age of the patient, the greater the danger : the mortality in youth is very small.

Diagnosis.—A great deal has been written as to the identity or non-identity of typhus or typhoid fever; and the subject is sufficiently important to demand considerable attention.*   Until about the year 1840 these fevers were generally confounded together, and regarded as merely two stages of the same affection ; being frequently described as typhus, or low nervous, or jail, or hospital, or camp, or malignant fever.   There appear very good grounds for believing, however, that they are essentially distinct diseases, —as distinct as small-pox and measles ; being attended by different important symptoms, and being due to different blood-poisons. They commence much in the same way, and at first present the same features, as simple fever ; while, like it, they occasionally become complicated with inflammation of the brain or its membranes, with bronchial congestion, or even with pneumonia.   But

* Dr. Murchison strongly and very properly insists that, in many points of view, the recognition of the several species of Continued Fever is highly important.   For example, there can be no doubt that true typhus is a more contagious affection than enteric fever.   Consequently, while cases of the latter may, perhaps, be distributed with impunity among the patients of a general hospital, it seems highly probable that it would be most unwise to allow of such an arrangement with regard to typhus patients.   Then, again, the use of bloodletting has been recommended in fever, owing to the reduced mortality said to result from this remedy.   But on examining the facts upon which this statement is advanced, it is found that the patients treated by bleeding were in all probability suffering from relapsing fever, the fatality of which is extremely small compared with that of typhus and enteric fevers.   And further, on studying the causes of continued fever in a sanitary point of view, while we find some observers arguing that this disorder results only from putrid emanations there are others who teach that destitution is its great source, and that putrid emanations are perfectly innocuous. We have here the old fable of the gold and silver shield, the opposing parties having drawn their conclusions from observing different diseases.—See a review of the works of Murchison and Tweedie on Fever, by the author, in *The Lancet*, 7 February 1863.

they differ from *febricula* thus :—Instead of early terminating by a critical sweating, the symptoms in typhus and typhoid fever increase in severity ; the febrile action becomes much more intense ; in each case the pulse gets more frequent, weaker, and more compressible ; the tongue grows drier and browner ; certain eruptions show themselves on the skin ; more sordes, and of a darker colour, accumulate on the teeth and lips ; the hands are moved restlessly to and fro ;* the fæces are often passed involuntarily ; bed-sores are produced, unless great care is paid to keeping the patient clean and dry, &c. ; delirium ensues ; there is great prostration of the vital powers ; and often a strong tendency is manifested to death by exhaustion or coma.

The way in which typhus and enteric or typhoid fever are to be distinguished from each other may be best shown by a comparison of their most prominent symptoms. Thus (1) in *typhus*, the eruption consists of a mulberry rash, coming out between the fourth and seventh days, and lasting until the termination of the disease ; the general hue of the skin being at the same time dusky and mottled. In *enteric* or *typhoid fever* the eruption is formed of rose spots ; appearing upon the thorax, back, and abdomen between the seventh and fourteenth days ; being thinly scattered, so that the spots often require to be carefully looked for, and even then probably are not found in at least ten or twelve per cent. of the cases ; and then in two or three days fading and giving way in one place to a new and equally sparing crop on another part. (2) In *typhus*, diarrhœa seldom occurs unless a large quantity of liquid food has been taken, and hæmorrhage from the bowels never. With *typhoid*, diarrhœa is very common, and there is hæmorrhage from the bowels in about one case out of every three. In an excellent monograph on these fevers, by Sir William Jenner, published in 1850, this gentleman shows that in all the fatal cases of *typhoid fever* which he examined, the agminated glands or Peyer's patches, situated in the ileum, were found ulcerated ; the ulcerations increasing in extent as they reached the ilio-cæcal valve. In a few instances, also, the solitary glands were ulcerated ; and one-eighth of the cases recorded died from extension of the ulceration, with perforation of the intestine. As regards the cases of *typhus*, ulceration did not exist in a single instance. (3) In *typhus*, the pulse and temperature rise steadily (the former to about 120 and the latter to 105°) until about the third day, when they remain stationary for a few days, and then begin to fall about the ninth day. With *typhoid* there is no uniformity, the pulse and temperature rising and falling independently of each other ; though

---

* These movements of the hands were well described by Hippocrates more than 2000 years ago :—" I have made these observations upon the movements of the hands. In acute fevers, in peripneumonias, in phrenitis, and in headaches, the hands moved to and fro before the face, hunting through the void, as if gathering bits of straw, picking at the coverlet, or tearing objects from the wall, are all so many bad and deadly symptoms."—*The Book of Prognostics.*

both generally remain high (with the exception of a few days at the beginning of the second week) to the fifteenth day. In *typhus*, the evening temperature is often slightly lower than that of the morning : in *typhoid* there is usually quite the reverse. (4) *Typhus* is a very rare disease among the better classes (making the exception of the visiting clergy, medical men, and students) ; whereas *typhoid fever* is if anything more common among the rich than the poor. Again, *typhus* may occur at any age, while *typhoid fever* rarely attacks person after forty, and is most common in youth ; the former is slightly less dangerous than the latter ; and then relapses do not occur in *typhus*, while they occasionally happen in *typhoid*. (5) Both diseases are contagious, but each propagates itself, and not the other : an attack of the one does not act as a preventive to infection by the other at any future period. (6) In *typhus*, the duration of the symptoms is from fourteen to twenty-one days ; whereas in *typhoid* it is seldom less than from twenty-two to thirty days. Moreover, in the former the danger increases until the end of the second week, when the disease reaches its maximum ; whereas in the latter the maximum is not attained for at least a week longer. In either case it occasionally happens that the patient falls a victim to the disease at the very onset ; knocked down and killed at once, as it were, by the virulence of the poison. Speaking generally, Dr. Murchison shows that the rate of mortality from continued fever, during a series of years, has differed but little in the various hospitals of England and Scotland, being about one in eight. The fatal cases in typhus and typhoid are one in between five and six ; whereas in relapsing fever they only average about one in forty.*

There have been some very few cases in which both typhus and typhoid fever have existed together in the same individual ; a circumstance that is no more remarkable than the co-existence of typhus and erysipelas, or of measles and small-pox.

Morbid Anatomy.—A case of typhus may run its course and

* It is very difficult to draw correct conclusions as to the value of any particular form of treatment from a comparison of the mortality at various hospitals. Even in the same institution the physician or surgeon of greatest repute may have a larger proportion of fatal cases than his less celebrated colleague. The beds of the latter are filled with ordinary cases from the out-patient room : those of the former receive confirmed invalids from all parts of the country,—often sufferers coming as a forlorn hope, having been deemed incurable by others. With regard to fever, Dr. Murchison shows that the per-centage of deaths at King's College Hospital between 1840 and 1858 was high. But one circumstance of importance is to be noticed,—viz., that in this small institution very bad cases were frequently admitted to the exclusion of others. Thus, when I was House-Physician in 1847, it often happened that there were only two or three empty beds out of the sixty devoted to medical patients, although some eight or ten applicants for admission presented themselves. In selecting from this number, but one rule guided me, and it was to choose the most severe forms of disease. And, moreover, rather than send away any very bad case, an extra bed would often be put up. Clearly, under such circumstances, the death-rate must appear greater than where all comers can be received for treatment.

end fatally, without leaving any traces of its existence. In the majority of instances there is nothing more than slight congestion of the mucous surfaces of different organs.

When the case has been complicated with secondary affections, we of course look to the structures which have suffered. The brain is seldom altered; but there may be engorgement of the sinuses, or congestion of the cerebral substance. The pia mater is occasionally loaded with blood, and sometimes there has been found slight hæmorrhage into the cavity of the arachnoid. The effects of inflammation will, perhaps, be discovered in some part of the respiratory apparatus; while occasionally the muscular substance of the heart is found soft, so that it is easily torn. The condition of the alimentary canal is normal; the liver is healthy; while in about half the cases the spleen is softened, and in a smaller proportion is likewise enlarged.

The blood contains a deficient amount of fibrin; and according to most authorities the blood cells have a great tendency to liquefy. Dr. Richardson says that in a case of typhus which he examined during life, the presence of ammonia in excess in the body was indicated by prominent signs. The chief of these were that the breath was so markedly ammoniacal that it coated acidified glass with crystals of the chloride of ammonium, and restored the blue colour to reddened litmus; the blood-corpuscles were misshapen, agglomerated, and partially dissolved, precisely as they are found when weak solutions of the alkali are added to healthy blood; while the symptoms were also those of alkaline poisoning. The foregoing tests are more delicate than that of holding a glass rod moistened with dilute hydrochloric acid before the mouth; though if when this is used, there is distinct evidence of white fumes, it is sufficient to prove that the amount of ammonia expired is beyond the normal proportion.

Treatment.—To prevent the generation of the typhus poison the poor should be supplied with wholesome food, while they must be housed in properly ventilated dwellings. The first requisite is not always possible; but man can live with a comparatively small amount of food, though to secure health an uninterrupted supply of pure air is necessary. We read with horror such stories as those of the Black Hole in Calcutta and of the Westminster Round House; but the effects of over-crowding among the poor are just as destructive though less speedily so.* In the common lodging-houses of the

* It was on the 21st June 1756 that the Black Hole in Calcutta was the scene of suffering alluded to. The night was close and sultry; and at eight o'clock 146 human beings, the majority Europeans, were placed in a dungeon 18 feet by 14. There were only two small windows, looking to the west, strongly barred with iron, from which those confined could scarcely receive any circulation of fresh air. In a few minutes every prisoner fell into a profuse perspiration, causing great thirst. Before nine o'clock every one's thirst was intolerable and respiration difficult. In the ravings for water and the attempts to get the little which was brought, some were trampled to death. Be-

metropolis the police can enforce an allowance of 250 cubic feet of space for each inmate.   Insufficient as this is, the regulation is evaded.   In workhouses, the minimum space of 300 cubic feet is required for each bed, in wards occupied through the night only by healthy adults or children.   The soldier, in barracks, has allotted to him a space of 600 cubic feet ; 1200 being allowed in military hospitals.

fore eleven o'clock one-third were dead.   By half-past eleven most of the living were delirious.   At six o'clock the next morning the prison was opened : only 23 were alive : and several of these died afterwards from fever. —The event is graphically described by Mr. Holwell, one of the survivors, in the *Annual Register for* 1758.   Second Edition, p. 278.   London, 1761.

In the year 1742, the high constable and others of Westminster, committed to the Round House several persons whom they found in the street.   Twenty-eight were sent to that of St. Martin, the keeper forcing them into a place called the Hole, not above six feet square, and with the ceiling scarce five feet ten inches high.   He paid no regard to their cries of murder; so that four women were suffocated, one of whom was big with child.   The keeper was afterwards found guilty of wilful murder and transported.—*The Principles of Forensic Medicine.*   By John Gordon Smith, M.D.   Third Edition, p. 221.   London, 1827.

Of course it will be said that such atrocities as those committed by Surajut Dowla and the keeper of the Round House could not take place in the present day.   Perhaps not.   But before we boast of our civilization it would be as well to look at the metropolitan dwellings of the working and dangerous classes in Bethnal-green, Spitalfields, Saffron-hill, the Coal-yard, Great Wyld-street, Dudley-street, &c.   The admirable way in which the guardians of the poor save the pockets of the ratepayers, and generate crime and fever and death, would satisfy the most ultra-disciple of Malthus.   This is what Mr. Godwin saw in a cellar-dwelling at Bethnal-green :—"Through the narrow space of the window that is left open there came a glimmering light, which fell upon two figures on a broken truckle, seemingly naked, with the exception of some black rags passed across the middle of the bodies ; but the greater part of the room, small as it is, was in total darkness.   In this profound depth our sagacious guide, Mr. Price, thought that there were more figures visible; and on asking if any were there, a female voice replied, 'Yes; here are two of us. Mother is out.'   And gradually, as the eye became accustomed to the gloom, two other figures were to be seen lying in a corner upon rags.   This was between twelve and one o'clock in the day.   We were not disposed to look further into this mystery ; but it was evident that one of the unfortunates was resting close to the damp and poisonous wall.   Neither words nor drawing can convey a complete idea of this den, and its thick and polluted atmosphere.   Instead of being filled with the pure life-giving air which is needful for human existence, it seemed occupied by something which might be moved and weighed.   The height of the room, all of which is below the surface, is not quite six feet.   The window would not open ; the ceiling was ready to fall ; and the walls, so far as the light showed, were damp and mildewed. The lodgers here were a widow and her four children ; one a girl of twenty years of age, another girl eighteen, a boy of fourteen, and a boy of twelve."— *Another Blow for Life*, p. 14.   London, 1864.

And we are told nothing can be done for evils similar to the foregoing,— they are as unavoidable as the authorities in the days of Howard believed the generation of jail fever to be.   There is a " Law of suffering," it is argued. Some of our fellow-creatures must be allowed to rot in the wealthiest city of the world ; though we complacently guard them from " spiritual destitution," and freely afford them the opportunity of praying for deliverance "from plague, pestilence, and famine."

Every hospital, workhouse, lodging-house, &c., should be thoroughly cleansed, and the walls lime-washed, at the least, once a year ; and of course much oftener if any cases of fever have been in them.   The propagation of the poison is to be checked by disinfecting the clothes, bedding, sponges and towels, excretions and vomited matters, &c., of every typhus patient (F. 74, 75) ; by not allowing him to be taken to the hospital in a street cab or omnibus ; and by the greatest attention to personal cleanliness. The room in which a case has been treated ought not to be reinhabited until it has been thoroughly purified with chlorine or sulphurous acid gas, been white-washed or repapered, and been left with the doors and windows widely open for many days.

The curative treatment consists of the following measures. When it is possible the practitioner should choose for his patient a large, well-ventilated apartment ; which ought to be free from bed and window curtains, carpets, and superfluous furniture.   The windows had better be open : in cold weather it suffices to have them down at the top for a couple of inches. Chloride of lime (F. 75), or a weak solution of chloride of zinc (F. 79) may be used as a disinfectant.   Iodine (F. 81) is valuable for the same purpose ; so is carbolic acid ; and particularly so is sulphurous acid gas (F. 74).   A fire in the room acts as a ventilator. All unnecessary intercourse between the patient and his friends, as well as between the nurses and domestics or residents, should be forbidden ; the apartment ought to be kept quiet, neither whispering nor rustling dresses being allowed ; while care must be taken to select one or two cheerful and experienced nurses, since much depends upon their fidelity and competency.

If the patient be treated in an hospital, the ward ought to be so arranged that each inmate may have from 1500 to 2000 cubic feet of air space ; the beds are to be six feet distant from one another ; and there is to be such ventilation as will at least insure from 30 to 40 cubic feet of fresh air to every sufferer for every minute in the twenty-four hours.

During the early stages, and throughout the whole course of mild cases, it is particularly necessary to beware of doing too much—of interfering too actively with the natural progress of the disease.   It ought to be remembered that we are able to treat but cannot cure these maladies, any more than we can cure small-pox or measles ; and therefore our aim must be to keep the patient alive until the fever poison has expended itself.   In opposition to this opinion, however, I must mention that Dr. Goolden, Physician to St. Thomas's Hospital, has informed me that, after more than ten years' experience, he regards quinine in large doses as almost a specific for cutting short cases of typhus and typhoid fever.   He gives ten grains in solution, with a few drops of diluted sulphuric acid, every two hours, until an effect is produced—*i.e.*, until either the fever is lessened, or cinchonism is induced ; and he has thus continued it for three days.   He has also assured me that it may be given even if there be diarrhœa with bloody stools ; that he has never seen it do harm ; and that it has saved hopeless cases. Quinine when thus administered acts on the nervous system and on the heart as a depressant; hence the patient's powers must be supported with beef tea, and wine or brandy.*

When the patient is seen early, it may perhaps be advantageous to commence the treatment by the administration of an emetic; the ipecacuanha wine in doses of one ounce, with plenty of warm water, or the powdered ipecacuanha with ammonia (F. 233), being preferable to antimony. At the same time a single dose of some mild purgative, to clear the intestines, will generally be useful. Then, the dilute phosphoric or hydrochloric acids, or the aromatic sulphuric acid, in doses of twenty or thirty minims every four or six hours, freely diluted, may be administered with benefit. There are many advantages in giving them as the daily drink (F. 357, 358, 359). If it be true that the blood contains an excess of ammonia, these acids must act as valuable alteratives. All other medicines had better be avoided. Certainly it is seldom wise to prescribe the carbonate of ammonia ; which, though useful as a stimulant, is likely to be injurious owing to its alkaline property altering the blood for the worse. Moreover, this salt sometimes seems to increase the perspirations, and to set up diarrhœa. At this stage the patient's uneasy sensations will be much soothed by sponging the surface of the body with cold or tepid water two or three times in the day. Dr. Armitage speaks highly of the use of cold affusion, especially where there is a tendency to stupor, or where the delirium threatens to merge into coma. Sinapisms, or flying blisters, over the pneumogastric in the neck, are also worth trying under such circumstances. When there is a great degree of irritability, the warm bath at 93° to 95° Fahr., prolonged for three-quarters of an hour, may be very useful. In cases where the acid drink is not prescribed a free supply of toast water, barley water, plain water, lemonade, or raspberry-vinegar and water ought to be allowed. Ice is always very refreshing. The diet should be restricted to milk, farinaceous food, and thin broth well salted. Tea and coffee are probably useful in aiding the elimination of urea from the blood.

Directly the powers of life begin to fail—as soon as there is a signal loss of strength, a dark-brown tongue, a frequent feeble pulse, or an abruptness and weakness of the first or systolic sound of the heart, then a stimulating plan of treatment should be commenced. This consists in ordering strong beef or chicken tea, with carlowitz or claret or tokay, or the brandy and egg mixture of the British Pharmacopœia, or brandy. The last is, in my opinion, the agent

* Dr. Dundas of Liverpool has also given evidence in favour of Dr. Goolden's views in his Essay on Fever, *Medical Times*, October 1851. On the other hand it has been shown, by a large number of eminent authorities, that quinine thus administered not only fails to arrest the disease, but often does much mischief. I confess to being sceptical as to its proving at all serviceable.

generally to be preferred. It should be given in such quantities as the extent of prostration demands. One teaspoonful, or one dessert-spoonful, or one tablespoonful, may be administered in water or milk or beef tea, every two hours, or every hour, or even in bad cases each half-hour; the effect produced being closely watched, and the repetition of the dose guided by such effect, remembering that severe febrile symptoms do not contra-indicate it. Where the utility of this or any other stimulant can be measured by the sphygmograph, so much the better. But independently of this valuable though not always handy instrument, we may be certain that a right course is being pursued, if, after a few doses, the pulse becomes less frequent and softer and more equal; and if the anxiety of countenance be lessened, if the evidence of flagging be more indistinct, and if the trembling of the hands diminishes. Extra precaution is needed in the use of alcohol when the urine is scanty or albuminous; or when there is violent delirium, with throbbing pains in the head. A few doses, however, will show whether the delirium is increased or diminished by its use, and thus form a guide for the practitioner. Dr. Todd was in the habit of teaching that, to a certain extent, we may learn if we are administering more alcohol than is required by noticing the state of the breath. Thus, supposing the breath to be saturated with the smell of alcohol when twenty or thirty minutes have elapsed since the exhibition of the last dose, then it is probable that the stimulant is being pushed too far, and that it is exerting an injurious narcotic action. Under such circumstances the alcoholic remedies ought to be at once diminished. On the contrary, if we can reasonably believe that benefit is arising from their employment, then care must be taken to regulate the dose and the intervals which may be allowed between each administration. Supposing the frequent exhibition of the stimulant to be called for, explicit directions are to be given not to allow the patient to sleep too long without it. Nurses and friends are naturally unwilling to rouse a patient who may have previously been without sleep for days, to give him his nourishment; but unless they do so at each appointed hour, he is not unlikely to awake and pass into a state of fatal collapse.

Where there is much general irritability and sleeplessness, without any lung complication preventing the due aëration of the blood, a well-timed dose of opium will work wonders; it being better to give about half a grain of the extract every three hours until the patient is calmed, than to administer a single large dose. Frequently I combine it with henbane. Sometimes, this drug alone has seemed sufficiently soothing, but it will be useless to give less than eighty or one hundred minims of a good tincture. Where the sense of hearing is very sharp, Sir Dominic Corrigan recommends stuffing the ears with wool. If there be much headache, or injected conjunctivæ, or active delirium, the opium should be guarded with a small dose of ipecacuanha, or perhaps even of tartar emetic, as recommended by Dr. Graves.   Some cold lotion, or a bladder containing ice, may also be cautiously applied to the scalp ; cold affusion over the head can be tried ; or, if we fear any cerebral effusion, small blisters may be put on to the temples.

The secondary affections which occasionally arise are not to be looked upon as contra-indicating the use of stimulants.   The true test for their need is still the force of the circulation.   I am sure that I have seen fever prove fatal, because the practitioner has thought that pneumonia was present, and has been consequently afraid to administer wine or brandy.   But while giving stimulants in these pulmonary disorders, we ought also to apply turpentine stupes to the chest, or sinapisms, or plain linseed poultices.   The softening and fatty degeneration of the muscular fibres of the heart which may occur, show how important it is not to neglect the use of nourishment.   Then, in every instance, whether the fever be running a regular or complicated course, the skin over the hips and sacrum and other prominent parts of the body should be frequently looked to ; so that if there is found any redness or tenderness, we may at once order a water-bed.   After the first three or four days the patient is not to be allowed to use the night-stool, or to get out of bed ; but is to be provided with a bed-pan, containing some of Condy's antiseptic fluid (F. 78).   The bladder ought also to be daily examined, lest there be retention of urine.   If there be suppression, citrate of potash will sometimes encourage the action of the kidneys.   Under this management, the patient often remains in a very precarious state for several days.   But so long as life endures, so long may a favourable turn be hoped for.   Frequently, just as the relatives are despairing the patient all at once begins to mend, gaining power and sleeping much as he improves. A course of the mineral acids and bark (F. 376), or of quinine and steel (F. 380), with a gradual return to solid food, will ultimately complete the cure.

3. ENTERIC FEVER.—Enteric or typhoid fever is an endemic, slightly infectious disease ; which is most prevalent in autumn, and is generated by putrefying animal matter.   The effluvia from foul drains, or the contamination of drinking water by the decomposing sewage making its way into the wells, are the frequent sources of this disorder.   Where the simplest sanitary laws are grossly neglected, there enteric fever will revel.   It attacks rich and poor indiscriminately ; but the latter, in their small homes, are less able than the former to avoid the injurious influences which flow from local nuisances, and the distribution of polluted water. This fever is not particularly a disease of early youth and adolescence ; though more common then than at a greater age.

Enteric (long known as *typhoid*) fever has been described under many names ; such as *abdominal typhus, ileo-typhus, febris putrida, gastro-bilious fever, febris gastrica, febris mesenterica maligna, night-*

soil fever, infantile remittent fever, and *typhia*.   In some parts of
America it is known as the *autumnal* or *fall fever*.   In the present
day many writers justly object to the appellation Typhoid; since,
in the first place, this term literally means "like Typhus" [Τύφος
= stupor + εἶδος = appearance], and the disease is essentially different ; while, secondly, the word is often used as an adjective, to
designate a set of symptoms which come on in the course of many
acute diseases, whence there arises confusion.   It has therefore
been proposed to call it *Enteric fever* ["Εντερον = an intestine] ; a
term which seems about to be adopted by general consent, although
it is rather undesirable to affix a name derived from the abdominal
lesion, as such may lead to the supposition that the intestinal ulceration is the cause, instead of the result, of the fever.   It was on this
ground that Dr. Murchison, looking to the origin of the affection, suggested the appellation of *Pythogenic fever*,—πύθογενης, from
πύθων(πύθομαι = *putresco*) + γεννάω,—literally, "born of putridity."

 Causes.—Dr. William Budd has urged with great force that
the poison of typhoid fever, instead of originating in decomposing
sewage, is merely transmitted by it, being derived from the infectious stools of an individual affected with fever.   The contagious
matter cast off by the intestine may communicate the fever to
other persons in two principal ways,—either by contaminating
drinking water, or by infecting the air.   In opposition to this illusive
hypothesis, Dr. Murchison states that,—(1) There are many facts
which show that enteric fever often arises from bad drainage, independently of any transmission from the sick.   The danger ensues
when the drain becomes choked up ; when the sewage stagnates
and ferments ; and when the transmission of a poison from any
distant locality is impeded, if not completely arrested.   (2) There
are numerous instances of enteric fever appearing in houses having
no communication by drains with any other dwelling : *e.g.* isolated
country houses.   (3) There is no evidence that the stools of enteric
fever are of such a virulent nature as has been stated.   The attendants on the sick are rarely attacked.   Pigs suffer from enteric
fever ; yet a pig fed for six weeks on the excreta of typhoid fever
patients, got very fat and continued well.   (4) The fact that the
prevalence of the disease is influenced by temperature is opposed
to the idea that it depends on a specific poison derived from the
sick ; but is readily accounted for on the supposition that the
poison is generated by fermentation or decomposition.*

 Allowing therefore that the disease is probably generated spontaneously by the decomposition of fæcal matter, we should expect
to find it most prevalent after the long heat of summer.   And
such is really the case ; for this fever is most common during the
autumn and early winter months, subsiding as great cold sets in.
Inasmuch, too, as it is not dependent on over-crowding, so the

* "On the Causes of Continued Fevers."   *The London Medical Review*,
p. 505.   April 1863.

rich and poor suffer equally from it.   Enteric fever proved fatal
to Prince Albert, on the twenty-first day from the time of seizure,
on the 14 December 1861.   The disease may be carried by the
infected into healthy localities ; but it is very much less contagious
than typhus and relapsing fever.   The infantile remittent fever of
England is, as will be presently mentioned, merely enteric fever,
somewhat modified by the tender age of the sufferer.

   Symptoms.—The attack may occur immediately on exposure to
the poison, especially where the latter is concentrated, beginning
with vomiting and purging ; so that such cases have given rise to
a suspicion of poisoning by one of the irritants, or narcotico-irri-
tants.   In most instances, however, there is a period of incubation ;
which, according to Dr. W. Budd, varies from ten to fourteen
days.   Then the disease usually sets in slowly and insidiously : the
sufferer feels languid and uneasy without being exactly able to
define the nature of his sensations, his bowels are probably inclined
to act more freely than customary and the stools are pale, while
there is a sense of anxiety, with fatigue and aching about the body.
In the course of a day or two (or in exceptional cases not until the
lapse of several days) he has chills, headache, intolerance of light,
thirst, complete loss of appetite, a tongue red at the tip but elsewhere coated with a creamy fur, and pains in his limbs ; followed
by a sense of weakness, a rather frequent dicrotous pulse, tenderness about the abdomen on pressure, a tendency to sickness and
diarrhœa, more or less wakefulness, and a disinclination to sit up.
At night there is great heat of skin (even to 104°) and restlessness ;
while the bed is complained of as being hot and uncomfortable,
change of posture gives no relief, and the patient is tormented by a
fierce thirst which nothing seems to assuage.   The expression of the
countenance now gets altered ; being either very languid and pale,
or marked with a circumscribed flush on each cheek.   The eyes
have a sunken appearance.   The urine is diminished in quantity,
high coloured, and acid ; having an increased amount of urea and
uric acid, while the chloride of sodium is lessened perhaps to a
trace.   At times, a little albumen may be present.   Now and then
there is retention of urine, requiring the use of the catheter.
There is great loss of strength.   The fever assumes a hectic character, and runs high towards the evening.   In severe cases the
pulse rises above 120, and gets feeble and irregular ; the respiration begins to be rather hurried, and the breath offensive—
perhaps ammoniacal ; the lips become parched and cracked, and
the tongue dry and brown or red and glazed ; there is great
depression ; and withal considerable abdominal tenderness, especially near the right iliac fossa.

   These symptoms either continue somewhat stationary, or slowly
become aggravated ; until at the commencement of the second week
the characteristic eruption generally begins to show itself on the
chest or abdomen, in the shape of rose-coloured papules.   These spots
hardly exceed a line in diameter, they are few in number, are cir-

cular, disappear temporarily on pressure, and fade away in two or three days to be replaced by a fresh crop; this latter going through the same course, and so on again and again until the end of the fever. They are seldom accompanied by true petechiæ. Although the rose-coloured rash is never met with in any other cases, yet it is certain that typhoid fever may sometimes run its career without our being able to discover a single spot. Dr. Tweedie thinks that in ten or twelve per cent. the rash will be absent. Occasionally, sudamina also appear about the end of the second week on the neck, chest, abdomen, or inguinal regions; while the temperature lessens, and at different times of the day the skin is found covered with sweat.

Amongst the other symptoms which may be present after the middle of the second week, we frequently have mental confusion and somnolence; these being followed by delirium, at first slight, but soon getting violent. Perhaps too, there are spasmodic con-tractions of many of the muscles, and hiccup; tinnitus aurium, or deafness; muscular pains with debility; a pinched or attenuated state of the features, with occasional hectic flushes on the cheeks; and bed-sores over the sacrum. There will be likewise increasing, and often extreme, loss of flesh and strength; a tongue which is of a dirty brown colour, and dry and fissured, these cracks being painful and often bleeding slightly; dilatation of the pupils, unless there be great stupor, when they are contracted as in typhus; and occasional attacks of epistaxis. The belly is found enlarged, and resonant on percussion; while careful pressure in the right iliac fossa usually produces pain and causes gurgling. At a later stage, meteorism or considerable tympanites, from the accumulation of air in the colon, may give rise to much distress, and require to be relieved by the passage of a long stomach-pump tube. There is sometimes nausea and sickness. As a rule there is diarrhœa; which generally increases towards the end of the second week, so that there may then be eight or ten stools a day, some of them containing blood and others having the appearance and consistency of pea-soup. These stools are remarkable in being alkaline (in-stead of acid, as healthy ones are), of a peculiarly offensive and putrid character, and for containing a large quantity of ammoniaco-magnesian phosphates with little shreds of sloughs. As the diar-rhœa sets in, the pulse increases in frequency—often to between 130 and 140; while the evening temperature of the skin again rises, to the height even of 105° or a little more. Occasionally we have also serious attacks of hæmorrhage from the ulcerated patches in the ileum and cæcum; one of which losses may either produce fatal syn-cope, or so depress the patient that he has no power left to bear up against the continuance of the disease. Another great danger to be feared is the extension of the ulceration till the coats of the bowel are perforated; an occurrence which may take place and cause fatal peritonitis at an advanced stage of the fever, or even just as we have reason to hope that convalescence is setting in. This chance of rupture must also be remembered by the physician on examining the abdomen by palpation; while it ought certainly to forbid the employment of purgatives after the lapse of the first two or three days from the setting-in of the disease. The symptoms of intestinal perforation are well and curtly laid down by Louis, who says that "if in the course of a severe or slight typhoid affection, or even under unexpected circumstances, the disease having been latent to that moment, there supervene suddenly, in a patient with diarrhœa, abdominal pain aggravated on pressure, altered expression of the features, and more or less quickly nausea and vomiting, there must be perforation of the small intestine." In the event of this occurring, the case is not to be given up as absolutely hopeless. Once in a way the exhibition of full doses of opium, with the administration of nourishment by enemata only, may rescue a patient from what looks like certain death.

There are yet more perils which jeopardize life. Thus, as in typhus, we may have to deal with one or other of the varieties of cerebral disturbance; or with congestion of the kidneys, impeding the elimination of urea and leading to convulsions; or with an attack of erysipelas; or a pulmonary affection may be set up, such as bronchial catarrh, congestion of the lungs, pleurisy with effusion, and pneumonia. Occasionally, suppuration has occurred; one or more large abscesses forming in the muscular tissue, or in a joint, or even in an internal organ. In a few instances, gangrene of some portion of the body—as of the penis, vulva, or one of the extremities has happened; this result being possibly due to obstruction of the chief vessel of the part by a thrombus or clot. But independently of any of these complications the disease may destroy life from the simple exhaustion which it induces, though this occurrence is rare. When this fever occurs during pregnancy, abortion mostly takes place: sometimes the expulsion of the fœtus is followed by fatal prostration, especially if there be flooding.

Enteric fever is often prolonged to the thirtieth day, and in some instances is followed by a relapse. The termination is usually by insensible resolution; though now and then a critical diarrhœa, or sweating, or both combined, or bilious vomiting, has been observed. Slight desquamation of the cuticle, particularly of that covering the abdomen, may succeed the disappearance of the febrile phenomena. During convalescence—as happens also after relapsing fever, a venous murmur in the neck may not unfrequently be heard; while on absculting the heart an inorganic systolic bruit can often be detected, having the soft blowing character generally observed in anæmic murmurs. Dr. Stokes states, that it usually disappears or diminishes on the patient assuming the erect position; while it is quickly cured when tonics and suitable nourishment can be borne. I am inclined to believe, however, that enteric fever may occasionally produce permanent valvular disease; while I have seen cases where fatty degeneration of the muscular fibres of the heart has appeared to have its origin in an attack of this disease some years previously to the cardiac mischief getting sufficiently troublesome to attract attention.

Morbid Anatomy.—It is only necessary to allude, under this head, to those alterations which are found in the ileum, probably as the *result* of the fever poison ; since they constitute the true pathological peculiarities of enteric fever. We may find, it is true, congestion of the brain or its membranes, or ulceration of the œsophagus, or softening or ulceration of the mucous membrane of the stomach, or an augmentation of the volume of the liver with a diminution of its consistence, or enlargement and softening of the spleen ; but then these changes are in no way to be regarded as essential elements of enteric fever.   The two lesions which may be said to be invariably present, are certain changes in Peyer's patches, and in the corresponding glands of the mesentery. The *alterations in the agminated glands or Peyer's patches* are the most marked in the groups of glands which are nearest the ileo-cæcal valve. Where the case has terminated fatally at an early stage, we may merely detect a swollen condition of the mucous membrane over the diseased patch ; or we shall, perhaps, find the typhoid deposit more or less copiously effused into the solitary glands, as well as into the tissue of Peyer's patches.   But death generally happens at a later period—towards the end of the third or beginning of the fourth week, and then we observe that the patches have undergone ulceration ; the fever product having been transformed into a brownish slough, which has become detached, and has left a cavity or ulcer of a size varying from a pea to a florin. Perhaps one or more of these ulcers, instead of cicatrizing, will have been the immediate cause of death ; owing to their extension until perforation has happened and allowed the escape of the intestinal contents into the peritoneum.   The *mesenteric glands* in the neighbourhood of the patches are very generally enlarged and softened ; and occasionally they have been seen in this condition when the intestinal lesion has only been very slight.

Prognosis.—The most unfavourable symptoms are hæmorrhage, persistent diarrhœa, a very frequent pulse, and great heat of skin. Continuous delirium with muscular twitchings, or lively jactitation, forbode an unfavourable termination.

When death occurs it usually happens between the twentieth and thirtieth day.   The most frequent cause of a fatal termination is perforation of the bowel ; hæmorrhage standing next.   Cerebral and pulmonary complications also tend to swell the mortality.

A lessening of the temperature of the skin, provided it does not fall below 97°, and a copious eruption of sudamina over the chest, are among the most certain forerunners of recovery.

Treatment.—The prevention of this disease is to be accomplished by good drainage.   If an old cesspool be found in or under any house, the inhabitants of the latter should leave while the contents of the privy are being carted away.   Water contaminated by leakage from a sewer is poisonous.   To guard against the transmission of the fever, the patient's excreta should be passed into a bed-pan containing Condy's Fluid (F. 74).

The curative measures are in most respects the same as those required in typhus; but there are two or three exceptional points which require notice. When the disease is seen at its commencement emetics do good; and we may prescribe an ounce of ipecacuanha wine every eighteen or twenty-four hours for the first three days. Aperients, however, should seldom be given, as the bowels will most probably act spontaneously; but if they do not do so, a dessertspoonful of castor oil, or a wineglassful of fluid magnesia, or a simple enema may be administered.

With regard to the intestinal irritation and continued diarrhœa, no remedies are so useful as bismuth, catechu, rhatany, logwood, &c., in combination with small doses of opium (F. 97, 105, 108, 112). Sulphate of copper and opium (F. 106) often answer admirably; while a pill of these materials will help also to check the hæmorrhage which is so apt to happen. Enemata of ten or fifteen minims of the liquid extract of opium, in two ounces of mucilage of starch, often give much relief; or when there is much tympanites, a few minims of turpentine and opium, or of solution of morphia with bismuth (F. 113) are useful. Suppose there are symptoms indicative of irritation from the retention of offensive secretions, these matters ought to be gently got rid of by enemata of warm water; which will not only serve to wash out the rectum, but also to excite the peristaltic action of the coats of the bowel by which the contents of the upper parts of the gut will be urged onward. When peritonitis is actually present; or when in conjunction with abdominal tenderness and increased frequency of pulse, there is a sudden rise in the temperature of the body to 105° or even more, showing a strong tendency to abdominal inflammation: then, in either case, opium is the remedy. The best preparation is the extract, in small pills, in doses sufficient to annul pain and tenderness. Simultaneously, the belly is to be covered with the extracts of belladonna and poppies (F. 297) and a light linseed poultice, or with poppy fomentation flannels. If there be hæmorrhage from the bowels, we must carefully apply cold over the abdomen, and administer gallic acid with opium (F. 103). The ammonia iron-alum (F. 116) is also an excellent styptic. Ice to suck is useful. In such instances the patient ought to be assiduously watched by his medical attendant; while wine or brandy is to be administered in exact proportion to the demand for stimulants by the system. The skill of the physician is shown by his commencing the remedy at the proper time, and administering it to the requisite amount: but this power can only be acquired by assiduous study at the bedside.

During convalescence greater care will be required than after other forms of continued fever; since any irritation applied to a cicatrizing ulcer in the ileum will possibly affect it unfavourably, and re-excite that morbid action which may end in perforation. Milk and raw eggs, as well as cod liver oil, are invaluable. Six ounces of port wine or good claret, or two ounces of brandy, should be allowed daily until the pulse has fallen below 100.　Tonics are to be carefully given; none being more suitable in the commencement than some preparation of bark.　The return to a generous diet must be very gradual; beginning with puddings of ground rice and milk, and progressing to white fish and chicken panada and mutton.　But it cannot be too strongly insisted on, that no solid food is to be allowed until the diarrhœa has ceased, the tongue become clean and moist, the pulse got soft, and till all feverish excitement has vanished; until which time, also, the patient should neither be allowed to leave his bed, nor even to sit up much in it.

I know of no place better than the present for making a few observations on enteric or typhoid fever as it occurs in children; remarks on this disease being the more needful, inasmuch as confusion has arisen from improperly naming it INFANTILE REMITTENT FEVER.　Discarding this term, it is to be noticed that enteric fever happens during childhood in two degrees; *i.e.*, in a mild and in a severe form.　The cases which terminate fatally are few in number, and usually belong to the second class.　Dangerous complications, however, may occasionally happen during the progress of the less severe variety.

In cases of the first, or the *mild* kind, the disease comes on very gradually.　Generally, the earliest symptoms that attract attention are loss of appetite, great thirst, and mental depression, so that the child is no longer lively and cheerful.　During the day also, it is listless and indolent and peevish; while though drowsy towards the evening, yet its nights are restless and there is a want of sound refreshing sleep.　When these indications of ill health have persisted for a few days, it is noticed that the skin is hot; at some hours of the day being dry, at others covered with perspiration. The breath is very unpleasant.　The bowels are generally loose, the evacuations being unhealthy and offensive; although sometimes there is obstinate constipation.　At the beginning of the second week the symptoms increase.　The child passes very bad nights; screams, moans, grates its teeth, and starts in its sleep; suffers much from thirst, and occasionally from sickness and vomiting; and perhaps has slight delirium.　There is exacerbation of the fever towards the evening, with remission as the morning approaches: occasionally there is a second though less severe exacerbation about eleven o'clock in the morning.　In mild cases there is seldom a rash: if any appear, it will be at this time in the form of the rose spots—so characteristic of enteric fever.　The skin of the lips, face, nose, and fingers becomes dry and rough; and the child is constantly picking it.　There is marked loss of flesh, anorexia, and great debility.　Towards the end of the second, or the beginning of the third week, the symptoms begin to abate; and then day by day the child improves in health.　Nevertheless, some little time often elapses before convalescence is completely established.

With the second, or *severe* form of fever, the symptoms just enumerated commence more suddenly and are more strongly marked. There is vomiting, great drowsiness, and sometimes slight rigors ; the countenance looks heavy ; and the mind wanders at night, so that the child sits up or tries to get out of bed, does not know its nurse, and looks about the room in a strange frightened manner. The skin is very hot and dry : the pulse gets very frequent. From the sixth to the tenth day a very scanty eruption of rose spots makes its appearance upon the back, thorax, or abdomen. As the disease progresses, the restlessness and delirium become aggravated ; the tongue is dry, brown, and glazed : the abdomen is found tumid and tender ; while the respiration is accelerated, and there may be cough, with a feeling of oppression at the chest. There is generally diarrhœa ; the urine is scanty and high coloured ; and perhaps the evacuations are passed unconsciously. By the end of the second week, the patient is reduced to the most emaciated and helpless state ; until, when apparently in the worst possible condition, slight signs of amendment show themselves. Day by day the improvement increases, and at the end of several weeks health is restored.

Supposing the disease should terminate in death, the prominent post-mortem appearances will consist probably of slight congestion of the cerebral membranes, engorgement of the lungs, softening of the spleen, enlargement of the mesenteric glands, and more positively of tumefaction and ulceration of the agminated glands or Peyer's patches.

This fever has to be managed on the same principles as those laid down for guiding the adult through an attack. Medicines are to be avoided as much as possible ; none in fact being required unless there be much pain, or excessive diarrhœa, or hæmorrhage. Milk freely given proves very serviceable ; while raw eggs, strong beef tea, cod liver oil, and perhaps wine will also be required. During convalescence, sea-air has a valuable influence.

4. CEREBRO-SPINAL FEVER.—Although for the last sixty years small epidemics of cerebro-spinal fever have occurred at different parts of Europe and America, yet our knowledge of the disease is recent and incomplete. Partly on this account, and partly because this fever is sometimes masked by a variety of symptoms, it is difficult to define it briefly. I would, however, attempt to describe it as,—A malignant epidemic fever, attended with lesions of the great nerve centres (the brain and spinal cord) and chiefly of their surfaces and membranes. Eruptions of various kinds, not uncommonly of a purpuric character, are present in about half the cases. There is acute headache, vomiting, contraction of the muscles of the back of the neck with exquisite pain, tenderness of the spine and limbs, and violent delirium. The disease attacks more males than females, more young persons under 14 than adults, and more frequently prevails during winter and spring than in summer. Possibly it is slightly contagious, though

the evidence on this head fails to convince me that it is so.   The duration is variable, — perhaps from two to seven days on an average.   Relapses are frequent.   The mortality varies from 25 to 80 per cent.

The synonyms of this fever are numerous.   The principal are,— *Malignant purpuric fever, malignant purple fever, epidemic cerebro-spinal meningitis, cerebro-spinal typhus, neuro-purpuric fever,* and *spotted fever.*   By the French it is known as *Fièvre cérébro-spinale,* and *Fièvre purpurée maligne;* by the Germans, as *Epidemische meningitis;* and by the Italians, as *Febbre cerebro-spinale.*

Causes.—On this head there is little to say beyond this,—that all attempts to explain the origin of the various epidemics, or to bring them within the circle of those laws which apply generally to diseases of the zymotic class have failed.   Most of the epidemics have occurred in the cold seasons of the year; but there have been many during the warm months, especially in France and Sweden. Still it must be allowed that the developement of the disease is favoured by cold.   The inhabitants of high and low districts, of salubrious and insalubrious localities, of ill and well drained towns have suffered alike from cerebro-spinal fever.   It has generally been remarked that males are more prone to this disease than females;   while vigorous youths have been attacked in greater proportion than those advanced in life.   Vieusseux, in giving the first authentic history of an epidemic of this fever which occurred at Geneva in 1805, says that it attacked people of every rank at once; the poor and rich, the inhabitants of dirty and crowded rooms in unhealthy districts, as well as the residents in great houses where well-aired chambers had but a single occupant.* The experience of recent years has shown that cerebro-spinal fever is especially apt to break out in establishments where numbers of people are congregated together, as in barracks and workhouses and prisons.   But even here the disease shows a peculiarity; since it attacks soldiers in a larger proportion than paupers or convicts. There is a great difference of opinion as to whether the disease is

---

* The epidemic described by Bascombe as occurring about the close of 1802, in the small Franconian town of Roettingen, situated on the river Tauber and surrounded by mountains, seems to have been of the nature of cerebro-spinal fever.   After a very hot and dry summer, there were thick fogs and incessant heavy rains during November.   Towards the end of this month—"an extremely fatal disease broke out, which was without example in the memory of its oldest inhabitants, it being totally unknown to them previously.   The young and strong were suddenly seized with pain and anguish at the heart, with violent palpitations, and lacerating pains in the nape of the neck: profuse, sour, ill-smelling perspiration broke out over the entire body; and a suffering, as though a violent rheumatic fever had seized on the tendinous expansions, accompanied this terrible malady: in the worst cases a spasmodic trembling ensued, the patient fainted, the limbs became rigid, and death closed the scene, frequently within twenty-four hours from the commencement of the attack."—*A History of Epidemic Pestilences from the earliest ages,* 1495 *years before the birth of our Saviour to* 1848, p. 147. By Edward Bascombe, M.D.   London, 1851.

communicable by the sick to the healthy. The evidence, especially that derived from the French military experience, in favour of its being slightly infectious, seems somewhat difficult to combat. The members of the Massachusetts Medical Society were "very generally agreed," however, as to its non-infectious character; and they report that out of 268 cases in which the question was asked as to the origin through contagion, the replies were in the negative so far as 252 were concerned.

Symptoms.—This fever assumes such a multiplicity of disguises that it has been divided by different writers into several classes. But however varied the symptoms, the disease is essentially one. Just as confusion would arise in the description of enteric fever if one set of observers paid attention chiefly to the general fever, while another class only regarded the diarrhœa and other intestinal symptoms, so it has happened with cerebro-spinal fever. In enteric fever we have a blood disease with intestinal lesions: in cerebro-spinal fever there is a blood disease with lesions of the great nervous centres or their membranes. With both enteric and cerebro-spinal fever life may be destroyed in less than eighteen or twenty-four hours by the force of the blood-poison—probably by necræmia or dissolution of the blood; although in both fevers the disease is usually of a milder type, in the one case accompanied with symptoms of intestinal inflammation and ulceration, in the other with symptoms of inflammation of the cerebro-spinal axis or its membranes.

The symptoms by which cerebro-spinal fever almost invariably manifests itself are chilliness or actual shivering, giddiness, severe headache, and irrepressible vomiting; these being quickly followed by feverishness, a sense of mental and bodily prostration, and sharp pains with stiffness in the muscles of the back of the neck. And these different symptoms usually come on suddenly in the midst of apparent health; so that sometimes the sick man can scarcely be persuaded that he has not been wilfully poisoned. This opinion gets confirmed also, if—as may happen, the symptoms succeed each other with such rapidity that in an hour or rather more the patient has become very seriously ill. Often, however, there are premonitory indications of illness which are neglected; and the effects of the fever show themselves more gradually through a space of one or two days. Certainly, the closer their sequence on each other, the greater will be the severity of the attack. In any case, the disease produces results which assume an alarming aspect more or less speedily. Neuralgic pains, with tenderness of the affected parts, give rise to hideous cries. The headache becomes incessant and most distressing; the countenance gets livid or pale, anxious and pinched; and there is miserable restlessness, with some mental confusion. The tongue, pulse, and temperature of the body are scarcely affected at this stage. The bowels may be constipated or loose; but the former state is that mostly observed. The cramps and muscular agitation seem to dart all over the body. At the upper part of the spine, and in the tissues at the nape of the neck, there is severe aching ; while the muscles there are frequently contracted, drawing the head backwards and fixing it rigidly. Deglutition is difficult. Trismus is common; with convulsive and uncontrollable muscular contractions at different parts of the body, as in tetanus. Hallucinations and delirium set in early, sometimes proving violent within the first twenty-four hours. Through the night the patient seems to doze, dream, and wander ; starting up every few minutes in a kind of wild maniacal excitement, as the racking cramps rouse him into a state of semi-consciousness.

While time advances—as the fifth or sixth day is reached, the pulse increases in frequency ; the eyes get bloodshot, and the pupils are often contracted or irregular ; the corneæ and retinæ perhaps become inflamed ; the tongue becomes dry and shining, or brown and covered with sordes ; while the temperature in the axilla may be found as high as 102° Fahr. An eruption generally appears on the skin ; consisting either of patches of herpes about the face or lips, or of a rash like that of measles or roseola or typhus, or of petechiæ, or of extensive purple ecchymoses. Meantime, the progress of the disease about the nervous centres is lessening the sufferer's consciousness ; the heavy stupor which sets in being attended with great loss of power, tremulousness, imperfect vision, deafness, relaxation of the sphincters, and an inability to swallow. With the failing circulation and innervation, the respiratory movements get embarrassed. The urine may be retained only, or there may be suppression : sometimes it is found loaded with albumen. The prostration becomes excessive. Frequently the exhausted and emaciated frame seems hardly to be the seat of life ; so deep is the coma, and so complete are the paralysis and anæsthesia. In other instances, the characteristic features of tetanus predominate over all others almost till the last ; the countenance having the horrid grin of lock-jaw, while the contraction of the muscles of the back is keeping up a state of rigid opisthotonos.

Where the disease is not of such an abrupt or explosive form (*méningite foudroyante*) that death occurs at the onset from collapse, the unfavourable cases may run on for five or six or eight days before life is destroyed. Of fatal cases, it is probable that seventy-five per cent. die before the close of the tenth day. The most dangerous time is from the second to the fifth day. Where the symptoms are less grave, the progress towards recovery is almost sure to be slow. There is a liability to relapse : at any moment the primary symptoms may return and prove fatal. The stage of convalescence too is apt to be interrupted by such secondary diseases as pericarditis, pleurisy, bronchitis, pneumonia, enteritis, abdominal neuralgia, sero-purulent effusions into the joints, persistent headache, bed-sores, various forms of ophthalmia, and inflammation with ulceration of one or both auditory canals. In a few

instances there have been fits of epilepsy. The muscular paralysis frequently continues for a time, but ultimately passes
off; and so with the nervous exhaustion and mental disturbance,
the intelligence very seldom being permanently damaged. Exceptions to this last remark have been met with, however, especially
amongst young children; many of whom have been left idiotic, or
blind, or deaf, or deaf and dumb for life.

Diagnosis.—The diseases with which this fever has been most
frequently confounded are typhus and enteric fever, idiopathic
tetanus, sporadic spinal meningitis, and malignant measles.

A brief recapitulation of the most important symptoms will aid
the practitioner in his attempt to form a correct opinion. The
most prominent and constant phenomena are the following :—
Headache, which comes on very early and suddenly, is very severe,
and is either paroxysmal or persistent to the end. *Vertigo,* often
accompanied with faintness and dimness of sight on the patient
trying to assume the erect posture. *Prostration,* so great and so
rapid as to form a striking feature. *Delirium,* varying from
transient wandering to violent mania. *Coma,* a sign of most unfavourable import when deep. *Cutaneous hyperæsthesia,* so that the
patients feel sore and ache all over, and groan or struggle when
moved. *Darting pains in the limbs and spine,* sometimes compared
to shocks of electricity, and causing faintness and sickness.
Neuralgia, especially of the bowels, so marked in some epidemics
that the disease has been popularly known as bellyache. *Tetanic
spasms,* the result of the spinal lesions, and of variable severity
according to the extent of the changes in the cord and its membranes. *Paralysis,* usually partial. The muscles of deglutition
are perhaps those most frequently affected. The power of motion
is generally regained at the end of a few weeks, as the process of
absorption removes some exudation which has caused pressure on
the nerves at their origin. *Vomiting,* which is irrepressible; and as
in all cases of cerebral sickness continues whether there be anything in the stomach to be ejected, or not Rarely, the matters
thrown up contain altered blood : green bilious fluids are more
frequently seen. *Constipation* is not constant, but it is often present as in other cerebral affections. *Cutaneous eruptions* are more
common in some epidemics than others; while of the different
kinds of eruption, labial herpes and petechiæ have been seen more
frequently than purpuric spots or large ecchymoses. Neither
increased heat of skin, nor *frequency of pulse,* nor *difficult respiration,*
nor *albuminuria,* nor *swelling of the parotid or submaxillary glands,* nor
strabismus, nor *lesions of the organs of sight or hearing* can be called
prominent symptoms of this fever, though they may be present.

Prognosis.—The death-rate in different epidemics has varied
between wide extremes. Under any circumstances the disease is
a very dangerous one; and therefore it is fortunate that it does
not prevail in large epidemics. M. Boudin has collected the

statistics of thirteen epidemics, in which there was a total of 1304 patients with 809 deaths. During the winter of 1863—64 the American army suffered much from this disease, the deaths being 70 per cent. of those attacked. The epidemic which prevailed about Dantzic (province of West Prussia) in the commencement of 1865 was very fatal. The mortality at the Hardwicke Hospital in Dublin, in 1866, was not less than 80 per cent.

The mortality seems to be greater in those under 14 years of age, than in such as are between 14 and 35. After this latter year, the danger is much increased. When life is prolonged beyond the fourth day from the commencement of the attack, the gravity of the prognosis lessens. Still it is not to be forgotten that fatal relapses have occurred during convalescence. The most unfavourable symptoms are a preternaturally slow pulse; rigid retraction of the head; general convulsions; incontinence of urine; albuminuria; coldness of the skin, with a diffused purplish hue; indifference as to the issue; paralysis of the muscles of deglutition; dilatation and insensibility of the pupils; and especially deep coma. Recovery after violent delirium is not uncommon; but when the patient has become profoundly comatose, there is scarcely any hope. All complications greatly aggravate the danger; those which especially do so being pericarditis, pneumonia, pulmonary collapse from obstruction of one or more bronchi, the formation of large bullæ with gangrenous spots, obstinate vomiting, and profuse diarrhœa.

Duration.—Life has been destroyed by this disease in less than five hours. Dr. Mapother has quoted a case in which death occurred in four hours and forty-five minutes from perfect health. Probably one-third of all the fatal cases have not had a longer duration than forty-eight hours, if so long. In many instances death has occurred between the fifth and eighth days. On the other hand, patients have lived five or six weeks and then died just as recovery seemed probable. Some epidemics have been more rapidly fatal than others. When the acute symptoms have subsided, there is still a certain amount of danger from intense exhaustion during the tedious and irregular convalescence which frequently follows. Neuralgia, headache, dyspepsia, palpitation of the heart, stiffness of the neck, &c. will often retard the patient's progress. Relapses too are not uncommon. In favourable cases, a period varying from fourteen days to six months may elapse between the day of attack and that of complete recovery.

Morbid Anatomy.—The essential lesions are characteristic, and are always present save in the explosive (foudroyante) form of the disease. They consist of hyperæmia of the membranes of the brain and spinal cord, gelatinous or purulent exudations, and certain changes in the intimate composition of parts of the nervous centres. On opening the skull and the spinal canal, the dura mater is seen congested; while the sinuses are full of soft black coagula. The vessels of the arachnoid are found distended with blood, and the membrane itself opaque and thickened. The pia mater is not only congested, but its meshes are also infiltrated with a purulent exudation. The amount of this exudation, and the extent to which it is diffused, vary in different cases. The arachnoid cavity and the cerebral ventricles often contain a notable amount of serum. Several deposits of lymph or of pus, more or less extensive, have been found at different parts of the surface of the brain, on the medulla oblongata, on the inferior portion of the cerebellum, and on the spinal cord.

The substance of parts of the brain, especially the surface, is frequently softened; and the spinal marrow has now and then been seen reduced to a mere pulp. Sometimes there are accumulations of pus at the base of the cerebrum and cerebellum, as well as in the spinal canal.

Treatment.—The three remedies which have hitherto been most largely used, and which have only served to lessen the patient's chances of recovery, are bleeding, purging, and calomel. The application of cold to the head and spine, by means of ice or freezing mixtures in India-rubber bags, has appeared to be of service and is deserving of further trial. The cautious subcutaneous injection of morphia with atropine (F. 314) into the nape of the neck seems to me to be promising. Morphia alone has been employed very frequently, and has certainly relieved the neuralgic pains and spasms without doing any mischief; but I am not aware that the combination of the two drugs, as suggested, has been tried.

The complications and sequelæ of the disease must be treated on the usual principles. Quinine, belladonna, bromide of potassium, and iodide of potassium appear to be the medicines which have been most frequently required.

The regimen should be the same as in other severe fevers. Ice, iced drinks, soda water, cold tea, &c., to relieve the thirst ought to be freely allowed; milk and nourishing broths, raw eggs and cod liver oil, will prove serviceable if they can be taken; while stimulants are to be avoided until absolutely demanded by the flagging circulation. Where the vomiting is such that nothing can be retained on the stomach, attempts are to be made to combat the prostration by nutrient enemata (F. 21). Although it is doubtful if the fever be communicable from one person to another, yet it will be as well to recommend disinfection and isolation.

5. RELAPSING FEVER.—The names of *relapsing*, or *famine*, or *recurrent fever* have been bestowed upon this infectious disease, owing to the fact that at a certain period of the convalescence there is a relapse of all the symptoms. Epidemics of it have been recognised, during seasons of famine and destitution, since 1739; and have been described under the various names of *five-day fever, seven-day fever, bilious remittent fever, recurrent fever, mild yellow fever, synocha, Irish famine fever,* and *typhinia* (Farr).

This disease is more common in Ireland and Scotland than in England. In the latter country, the Irish poor are the chief sufferers from it. Persons of both sexes and all ages are attacked. The poison may remain latent in the system for from two to four days, or its effects can be manifested immediately. It is less infectious than typhus. One seizure does not insure immunity from a subsequent attack.

The *symptoms* commence abruptly with rigors, frontal headache, muscular pains, and depression. Soon, febrile reaction sets in; and we find great heat of skin, anxiety of countenance, intolerance of light and sound, a white tongue, and a full rapid pulse. Complaint is made of urgent thirst; and often there is pain at the epigastrium, with vomiting of a bitter bilious fluid. In some cases, there is a great desire for food, but usually the appetite fails. When night comes on the symptoms become aggravated; giving rise to much irritability with sleeplessness, and occasionally to delirium. As the disorder advances there is also constipation, scanty high-coloured urine, sometimes jaundice, and increasing prostration; though there is never any characteristic eruption. True petechiæ and spots of purpura may form, as may also sudamina at the period of crisis. The pulse is frequent (perhaps 140 in the minute), the temperature in the axilla may be as high as 105° or even one or two degrees above this, the pains in the back and limbs are severe, and there is much distress and restlessness; while occasionally complications occur, such as parotitis. But just as matters seem to be assuming a very threatening aspect, on about the fifth or seventh day, a profuse perspiration breaks out over the whole body, the fever disappears, the pulse falls to its normal standard, the appetite returns, the urine increases in quantity, and the patient is left almost free from the disease, though weak. The convalescent, of course, fancies that his troubles are over, and that tonics and nourishment will soon restore him. The apyretic interval, however, is short; for about the fourteenth day from the commencement of the disorder, or the seventh from the critical sweating, there is an abrupt relapse with a repetition of all the symptoms. Generally upon the third or fourth day perspiration again sets in, and for a second time is followed by complete relief. The debility is often considerable; while the return to perfect health is somewhat slow, especially in the aged and such as were previously in a bad condition. Moreover, it is not very rare that a second or third relapse takes place.

Troublesome *sequelæ* sometimes greatly retard recovery; such as muscular weakness, rheumatic pains in the limbs and joints, œdema of the legs and feet, bronchitis and pneumonia, suppuration of one or more enlarged lymphatic glands, boils, or ophthalmia. When relapsing fever occurs in pregnant women it has a greater tendency than many acute disorders to cause abortion or premature labour: the fœtus is usually dead. The disease is seldom fatal; although sometimes death takes place during the progress of the fever from sudden syncope, and occasionally more slowly from uræmic poisoning. During an epidemic of this fever which prevailed at St. Petersburgh in the winter of 1864-5 the cases admitted into the civil and military hospitals numbered 7625, of which 836 died. This mortality was much above the average. No special lesion can be detected upon making a post-mortem examination; but often the liver is discovered to be enlarged from congestion, and still more frequently the spleen is found considerably increased in size.

The *treatment* is very simple. Gentle aperients will at first be required where there is evidence of intestinal atony, or of the retention of fetid secretions. Then we should order refrigerating drinks, a farinaceous diet, milk, and perfect repose. Where there is much irritability and pain, opiates are useful; while if the prostration be great, wine and nourishment will be needed. Sponging the body twice or thrice in the twenty-four hours, with vinegar and water, or tepid water, does good. The jaundice is best treated with the nitro-hydrochloric acid (F. 378). The headache can sometimes be relieved by dry cupping to the nape of the neck, by frequently repeated doses of nitrate of potash—which also keeps up the action of the kidneys, and by allowing the patient to drink freely of tea or coffee. Quinine has been frequently given in the hope of preventing the relapse; but neither this drug, nor any other, appears to have exerted a beneficial influence in this respect.

II. INTERMITTENT FEVER, OR AGUE.

Intermittent [from *Intermitto* = to give over for a time] *Fever*, or *Paludal* [*Palus* = a fen or marsh] *Fever*, or *Periodic Fever*, or *Ague* [perhaps from the Fr. *Aigu* = sharp], is a disease chiefly due to marshy miasms; in which the febrile phenomena occur in paroxysms, are ushered in by rigors, and end in critical sweats. During the intermission or apyrexial period there is good health; but at the end of a definite interval the phenomena are repeated, and this happens again and again until a cure is effected. In England, during 1866, the deaths of $\frac{\text{Males 64}}{\text{Females 71}}$ = 135 persons were registered as due to ague and its complications. This number is about 30 below the annual average, taking the total (1642) for the ten years 1857—66.*

* Two hundred years ago, when the soil round London was neither drained nor cultivated, and when the marshes of Cambridgeshire and Lincolnshire were covered during some months of every year by immense clouds of cranes (Macaulay), ague was a most fatal disease in England. The tertian form was the cause of death to James I., in London, in March 1625. When told by his courtiers that "An ague in the spring is physic for a king," James answered that the proverb only applied to a *young* king.—Oliver Cromwell died from ague at Somerset House, in 1658, after disregarding the ad-

Varieties.—There are three species of intermittent fever or ague, viz., the *Quotidian, Tertian,* and *Quartan* type. Of these the tertian is the most common in this country, and the quotidian in India. When the paroxysm occurs every day, it is called quotidian ague; when every other day, tertian, though secundan would be more appropriate; and when it is absent for two whole days, and then recurs, quartan. In the first species the interval is twenty-four hours; in the second, forty-eight; in the third, seventy-two. The time between the commencement of one paroxysm and the beginning of the next is termed the *interval;* while that between the termination of one paroxysm and the commencement of the next—the period of apyrexia, is called the *intermission.* In quotidians the paroxysm occurs, for the most part, in the morning; in tertians, at noon; in quartans, during the afternoon. The first variety is most common in the spring; the second, in the spring and autumn; the third, in the autumn. Quotidian and tertian agues are much more frequent than quartan.

Irregular types of intermittent fever are sometimes observed; such as the double quotidian in which there are two paroxysms daily, the double tertian, double quartan, &c. In the regular forms the paroxysm usually recurs at about the same hour of the day; though as the poison gets eliminated or neutralized the time is postponed for two or three hours prior to the final cessation of the attack.

Causes.—The predisposing causes of ague are fatigue, travelling, restlessness, exhaustion, mental depression, improper or insufficient food, intemperance, exposure to night air, and the circumstance of once having suffered from it. It is worth remembering that malarious districts are most dangerous at night, and that this poison lies low; or, as Sir Thomas Watson says, "loves the ground." Dr. Macculloch observes that it is a common remark in many parts of Italy, that as long as the labourers are in the erect posture, they incur little danger; but that the fever attacks those who sit or lie on the ground.*

The exciting cause consists of certain emanations or invisible effluvia from the surface of the earth, known as malaria. These effluvia or miasms emanate chiefly from marshy lands; but their

vice of his physicians. "I tell you," he cried, with characteristic confidence to the latter,—"I tell you I shall not die of this distemper: I am well assured of my recovery. It is promised by the Lord, not only to my supplications, but to those of men who hold a stricter commerce and more intimate correspondence with Him. Ye may have skill in your profession: but nature can do more than all the physicians in the world, and God is far above nature." (Hume).—The minute description given by Robinson Crusoe of his attack of ague has excited every boy. Defoe must have narrowly watched this disease, even if he had no experience of it in his own person. The latter supposition is not improbable; for the fen district in Suffolk was of large extent when he retired to this county, in August 1704, on his liberation from Newgate. *Robinson Crusoe* was not published until 1719.

* *An Essay on Malaria, &c.,* p. 268. London, 1827.

s 2

nature is still a mystery, for though chemists have analysed the air
of malarious districts they have not been able to detect any peculiar
poisonous principle. As cultivation of the soil and drainage are carried
out, so malarious diseases disappear. The general belief, that malaria
is produced by decomposing animal and particularly vegetable matter, is probably true ; the air being more noxious where both matters
are undergoing decay, than where vegetable matter alone is doing
so. At all events, it is found in the tropics that malarious diseases
are most common in the season succeeding the cessation of the
rains, when the temperature is high ; and in parts where the surrounding country abounds in dense jungle and low swamps, and
where insects and reptiles are abundant.

Poisoning by malaria is most apt to occur between sunset and
sunrise. The young, unhealthy, over-fatigued, and such individuals as are exhausted from want of food or sleep, are the most
susceptible. The form of disease which arises from exposure to
malaria varies according to the constitutional predisposition of the
individual ; that which will produce ague in one person, perhaps
giving rise to remittent fever or to dysentery in another. Moreover, if the poison be insufficient to excite any of the recognised
forms of miasmatic disease, it can yet impress a paroxysmal type
upon any intercurrent disorder; or it may simply lower the
general health, causing anæmia and weakness and sallowness of
the complexion—a condition known as the malarial cachexia. So
again, when the poison has been imbibed, it may remain latent in
the system for from six to twenty days, and possibly even for a
few months ; a point necessary to remember in the diagnosis of
obscure cases where the ague fit is not well developed.

Symptoms.—The disease either sets in suddenly, or the symptoms
will come on gradually with a feeling of general indisposition,
which at the end of a few days culminates in a regular paroxysm.
An ague-fit is composed of three stages—the cold, hot, and sweating. The *cold* stage is ushered in with feelings of languor and
chilliness ; though the heat of the body, as ascertained by a thermometer in the axilla, is really increased, and gradually rises
through this and the succeeding period. Then sensations as of
streams of cold water running down the back are complained of,
together with shivering; the skin is shrivelled and the papillæ
rendered prominent (goose skin or cutis anserina) from the contraction of microscopical muscles called the arrectores pilorum ;
while the teeth chatter, the nails turn blue, and the whole frame
is shaken. All this time the temperature is at least 101° or 102°
Fahr. and perhaps 105° or 106°. There is exhaustion ; often
urgent thirst ; the countenance appears anxious, the features
shrunk and pale, and the eyes dull and hollow ; the pulse is
quickened ; the respiration hurried and oppressed ; and there is a
peculiar mental irritability. The duration of this stage varies
from half an hour to three or four hours ; and is gradually suc-

ceeded by the *hot* stage, which is one of reaction.   The surface of the body then becomes dry and intensely hot; the temperature being raised considerably above the natural standard (up to 107°), while Dr. Mackintosh says that he has known it to be as high as 110° even with patients in Great Britain.   The mouth is parched, and there is excessive thirst; a frequent bounding pulse, with a painful sense of fulness in the head; and great restlessness, general uneasiness, with sometimes delirium.   This condition continues rarely less than three or more than twelve hours, and then follows the *sweating* stage; commencing with a gentle moisture, which appears first on the forehead and breast, increases, and gradually extends over the whole body.   The pulse and breathing now become natural; the temperature of the body falls to the normal standard; the headache, heat of skin, and thirst abate; and all the distressing symptoms are relieved, so that the patient, if the case be recent, often thinks himself restored to perfect health.   Occasionally, however, and especially in tropical climates, this stage ends in great exhaustion; so that the free use of some alcoholic stimulant is required to prevent fatal collapse.

The water, urea, uric acid, and chloride of sodium of the urine are all suddenly increased during the cold and hot stages; the quantity of each of these constituents diminishing as the sweating sets in.   The urine occasionally contains albumen and renal casts during the fit.

Effects.—Disease of the *spleen* is a very frequent concomitant or result of intermittent fever.   This gland is found enlarged, sometimes to a great extent, and occasionally indurated; in which condition it is popularly spoken of as *ague cake.*   Some authors say that the spleen may be found invariably to enlarge during the cold stage; owing to the blood being driven from the surface of the body to the viscera, but especially to this organ.   The enlargement subsides during the intermission, but not completely; so that after each attack the size of the gland is a little greater than it was previously.   In like manner, morbid changes occur in the *liver;* giving rise to depraved secretions and disturbance of all the digestive organs, and in a few cases to persistent enlargement and induration.   The *kidney* is sometimes permanently affected in consequence of ague; chronic Bright's disease resulting.   Intermittent hæmaturia may occur many months after exposure to the influence of malaria, and prove obstinate.

In protracted cases *complications* are not unlikely to arise; and the brain, or the lungs, or the stomach and bowels, occasionally become the seats of inflammatory action.   Death from uncomplicated ague is probably never seen in this country.

Treatment.—When the patient is obliged to remain in a malarious district, the difficulty of curing ague will be very much increased.   The diet should be good and nourishing, with a regulated supply of stimulants, from the first; unless there is evident derange-

ment of the alvine secretions, and then we had better commence
with beef tea, milk, arrowroot, &c. In the cold stage, warm diluent
drinks, such as barley water, weak tea, or weak negus, or white-wine
whey may be freely allowed; while the application of external
warmth is to be assiduously employed, by means of thick clothing,
hot bottles to the feet, and hot water or hot air baths. The latter
can be easily prepared by means of a long wicker-work cradle,
closed at one end with a board. This is laid over the patient and
covered with blankets : a curved tin tube is then passed through a
hole in the centre of the board, the other end of the tube, expanded
into a bell-shape, looking downwards, and having the flame of a
spirit-lamp placed beneath it, so that the air under the wicker-work
soon becomes very hot. An opiate given a little before the cold
stage is often beneficial. During the hot stage an opposite plan
should be pursued; ice and cooling drinks being then required,
while the surface of the body is to be sponged with tepid or cold
water. When the hot has subsided into the sweating stage, the
action of the skin ought to be encouraged by tepid drinks.

A dose of some rather active purgative can often be advantageously given at the outset; none being better than four or six
grains of calomel with the same of rhubarb, followed by a draught
of the compound mixture of senna. The bowels having been emptied, the use of one of the two specific remedies for ague—bark or
arsenic—may be commenced. The best plan, as a rule, is to give
from three to five grains of the sulphate of quinine dissolved in the
acid infusion of roses, every four or six or eight hours, during the
intermission; taking care to continue its use, in lessened doses,
for some short time after an apparent cure has been effected.
The subcutaneous injection of this salt (F. 379) has been recommended; and it is said that four grains so employed are equal in
power to four times the quantity taken by the mouth. In Indian
intermittents the exhibition, during the sweating stage, of quinine
in a dose of twenty or thirty grains, instead of smaller portions
frequently repeated, has been strongly advocated. These quantities are generally well borne unless there is extraordinary exhaustion, when they might be dangerous; cinchonism (as indicated
by tinnitus aurium and headache) being less readily produced in
ague than in other affections. According to Ranke, quinine
diminishes the quantity of uric acid in the urine.

If it be desirable, on account of its cheapness, to employ
arsenic, it must be remembered that large doses will be needed
(F. 52). Dr. Morehead calculates that half a grain of arsenic
acid—one drachm of the liquor arsenicalis—is equivalent in power
to fifteen grains of quinine; but as such a dose of arsenic can
hardly be given without some risk, he has suggested that it is
better to prevent the expected fit by quinine, and then trust to
moderate doses of arsenic to complete the cure. The combination of quinine and arsenic in moderate doses can be strongly

recommended, especially when the symptoms become chronic. The salt of the willow bark (salicine) has been recommended as a substitute for quinine; but it is by no means as efficacious. In cases of enlargement of the spleen, great benefit will be derived from a combination of quinine and sulphate of iron, perseveringly used (F. 380); or perhaps from the bromide of potassium (F. 42). Cod liver oil may also be recommended. Inunction over the splenic region with the ointment of red iodide of mercury proves very useful, especially in chronic cases.

While treating the complications we must carefully avoid depletion. Quinine is still the remedy to trust to, the dose being large in proportion to the urgency of the symptoms. In tropical countries it sometimes happens that a patient is not seen until he is delirious or comatose; but even then a dose of twenty or thirty grains of quinine, will probably restore consciousness and health. If troublesome vomiting prevent the retention of the remedies, a large blister should be applied over the stomach; while an enema of quinine and infusion of coffee is to be administered. In all cases, when the disease threatens to become chronic, change of climate is an absolute necessity. A sea voyage does great good.

For temporary residents in malarious districts it will be found that a nutritious diet, warm and dry clothing, with a due amount of repose, are valuable prophylactics. Still it may be as well, in order to give complete immunity, to administer from two to six grains of quinine daily to each individual exposed to the unhealthy influence of the soil. Soldiers and sailors &c. will take this drug willingly if it be mixed with orange wine, or with spirit and water.

Brass-Founders' Ague.—A peculiar form of intermittent fever, which affects brass-founders and other workmen exposed to the fumes of deflagrating zinc, has been noticed by Mr. Thackrah and more fully described by Dr. Greenhow. All that Mr. Thackrah says, is this:—"The brass-melters of Birmingham state their liability also to an intermittent fever, which they term the brass-ague, and which attacks them from once a month to once a year, and leaves them in a state of great debility. As a preventive, they are in the habit of taking emetics. They are often intemperate."* Dr. Greenhow's observations show that the symptoms have some resemblance to an imperfect fit of ague; but the paroxysms occur irregularly. The attack commences with malaise, and a feeling of constriction or tightness of chest, occasionally accompanied by nausea. These phenomena always happen during the after-part of a day spent in the casting-shop; and are followed in the evening or at bedtime by shivering, sometimes succeeded by an indistinct hot stage, but always by profuse sweating. The sooner the latter follows the setting in of the cold stage, the shorter and milder is

* *The Effects of Arts, Trades, and Professions, and of Civic States and Habits of Living, on Health and Longevity.* Second Edition, p. 101. London, 1832.

the attack and the less likely is the caster to be incapacitated for work on the following day. Headache and vomiting frequently accompany the paroxysm, which at the worst is only ephemeral; but the attacks are sometimes of frequent occurrence. Persons who have but lately adopted the calling, or who only work at it occasionally, and regular brass-founders who have been absent from work for a few days, are more liable to suffer from this disease than those who are employed at it continually. The men themselves attribute it to inhaling the fumes of deflagrating zinc or "spelter," and their opinion is probably correct. For, on the one hand, several other classes of operatives are habitually exposed while at work to conditions exactly similar to those of the brass-founders, except the liability to inhale the fumes of zinc, and yet do not suffer from this ailment; and, on the other hand, brass-founders suffer from it in almost exact proportion to their liability to inhale these fumes. A belief prevails that milk has a strong prophylactic and curative influence, and hence many of the workmen habitually drink it. The occasional use of emetics has a tendency to prevent the disease.*

III. REMITTENT FEVER.

This disease may be described as a non-infectious fever, attended with distinct exacerbations and remissions [*Remitto* = to remit, or abate]. It presents a cold, a hot, and a sweating stage; the hot being more marked than either of the others.

Causes.—The causes of remittent fever are the same as those of the disease described just previously, and hence we might appropriately speak of it under the designation of *miasmatic* or *malarial remittent fever*. The symptoms also bear a resemblance to those of intermittent fever; with this notable difference, however, that in the intervals there is no complete apyrexial period—no cessation of the fever, but simply an abatement or diminution. The period of remission varies from six to twelve or fourteen hours; at the end of which time the feverish excitement increases, the exacerbation being often preceded by chilliness and rigors.

This form of fever will be found to vary much in severity, according to the nature of the climate in which the poison is generated. The autumnal remittents of countries like England and France are comparatively mild; whereas the endemic remittents of tropical climates are often very severe and fatal. Moreover, the locality where the fever prevails seems often to impress some peculiarity upon it, especially as regards the nature of the complications which arise; and hence we find remittent fever described under the names of the *Walcheren fever*, the *Mediterranean fever*, the *Jungle* or *Hill fever* of the East Indies, *Bengal*

* "On Brass-Founders' Ague." *Transactions of the Royal Medical and Chirurgical Society*, vol. xlv. p. 177. London, 1862.

fever, the *Bilious remittent* of the West Indies, *Sierra Leone fever*, *African fever*, &c.

Symptoms.—The paroxysm of remittent fever commences usually with chilliness, a sense of oppression about the epigastrium, lassitude, mental depression, a feeling of cold down the back, and headache. To these sensations soon succeed febrile symptoms, constituting the hot stage. The prominent phenomena then consist of flushing of the face with great heat of skin, a temperature of 105° being often attained ; severe headache and giddiness, often accompanied by mental confusion or even delirium ; a frequent (perhaps 120) and full pulse ; a dry and furred tongue ; nausea and vomiting—generally of bilious matter ; a sense of pain at the epigastrium, and tenderness on pressure ; with signs of pulmonary congestion such as dyspnœa, a feeling of oppression at the chest, cough, and a livid colour of the countenance. The urine is often scanty, high coloured, and loaded with urates ; but it is passed in increased quantities during the remissions. There is very seldom any albumen present.

The remissions usually occur in the morning, and have a duration ordinarily of eight or twelve hours. The principal exacerbation generally takes place towards the evening, and continues for the greater part of the night ; though sometimes the paroxysm lasts for twenty-four, or even thirty-six hours. The disease will run on for about seven or fourteen or twenty-one days, unless shortened by proper treatment. It may terminate rather abruptly in an attack of sweating ; or its symptoms will occasionally merge into those of low fever. The period of convalescence is usually short, except some organic mischief has occurred. In the latter case, considerable time may elapse before a restoration to health is effected ; the debility being kept up by night sweats, sleeplessness, dyspepsia, hypochondriasis, neuralgia, jaundice, and even dropsy.

In tropical climates remittent fever proves more dangerous than in milder latitudes. This arises either from the general severity of the symptoms and the high degree of febrile reaction ; or because there is a depressed condition of the vascular and nervous systems, with defective secretions ; or it is owing to the sudden setting in of great exhaustion towards the close of an exacerbation, which exhaustion has a great tendency to end in fatal collapse ; or, lastly, the increased danger is in consequence of the disease being complicated with convulsions, or with delirium passing into drowsiness and coma, or with great gastric irritability, or with bronchitis and pneumonia, or with hepatitis and jaundice.

Treatment.—The principal indications to be followed ought to be the same as are demanded in the treatment of ague, if the supposition that both are due to malaria be correct. At the same time it is to be remembered that, as the febrile exacerbation is of much longer duration in remittent than in intermittent fever, so there is a greater fear in the first of internal organs being damaged, and ultimately of more severe depression ensuing. Our object will therefore be to shorten the period of the exacerbation, and lengthen that of the remission. This we attempt to do by saline and effervescing draughts (F. 348, 349, 355); cold drinks, such as iced water, lemonade, cold tea, cream of tartar, &c. (F. 356, 360); an aperient (F. 139, 144, 165, 169) if the bowels are confined; an emetic of ipecacuanha (one scruple of the powder, or an ounce of the wine) if there be nausea without vomiting, which is seldom the case; and frequent tepid sponging (F. 138) of the whole surface of the body. Immediately remission takes place, a dose of quinine, varying from two to six grains, should be exhibited, and repeated every third or fourth hour; taking care to omit this remedy directly the hot stage again sets in. At the next remission we once more resort to the bark, and so on until it seems certain that the febrile phenomena have permanently disappeared. Where the bowels are sluggish, one or two of the doses of quinine can be combined with either a drachm of the wine of aloes, or with one hundred and twenty grains of sulphate of magnesia; or, in the event of the stomach being irritable, with an effervescing draught; or, if there be diarrhœa or restlessness, with half a grain of morphia.

In tropical climates the complications of remittent fever must be treated very cautiously. Where there is much cerebral derangement, an active purgative, with the constant application of cold to the head, or the occasional use of cold affusion may prove very beneficial, in addition to the remedies already mentioned; while if there be great drowsiness during the remission, a blister should be applied to the nape of the neck. On the contrary, the low delirium with drowsiness from exhaustion demands the free use of stimulants and nourishment. When the stomach is irritable, or when there is jaundice, the application of sinapisms, or iodine liniment, or turpentine stupes, or of a blister to the epigastrium will give relief; while we may allow ice to be freely taken. If there be congestion of any internal organs, the wet sheet packing (F. 136) proves one of the best remedies by producing free action of the skin. In all cases quinine is to be given during the intermissions. Bleeding has been recommended by some authorities where there are symptoms of cerebral or abdominal oppression; but although the views as to its value are very contradictory, yet depletion would seem only to give temporary relief, while subsequently it produces alarming depression. And lastly, supposing there seems reason to fear the occurrence of any permanent structural disease, the patient must be sent to a temperate region free from malaria.

IV. YELLOW FEVER.

This remarkable disease may be described as an acute malignant epidemic fever. That it is infectious seems now to be generally admitted. As a rule, one attack gives exemption from a subsequent seizure. Ushered in with chilliness and languor, its prominent characters are,—pain about the loins and severe headache, a greenish-yellow hue of the skin, more or less delirium, sometimes watchfulness, sometimes a tendency to stupor, a liability to suppression of úrine, uneasiness about the epigastrium, and black vomit. From this latter symptom the term *hæmogastric* fever has been applied [Αἷμα = blood + γαστήρ = the stomach]. There are exacerbations and remissions, but they are so connected that the disease resembles a continued fever.

Yellow fever is a disease of warm climates; an average temperature for some weeks of at least 72° Fahr. being necessary for its production. The specific poison of this disease is said to be destroyed by a temperature of 32° Fahr. on the one hand, or of 212° on the other; though neither temperature has any effect in arresting the fever in the system. Yellow fever is not of infrequent occurrence in cities on the borders of low marshy plains; while it may be said to be habitually present in the sea-port towns of the West India Islands, in Africa, the southern parts of Spain, and some parts of the coasts of North and South America. It has been described under the various names of *bulam fever, mal de Siam, typhus icterodes, febris flava, black vomit,* &c. Like all other fevers, it occurs in different degrees of severity. At one time it attacks only a few individuals sporadically, at another period it prevails epidemically; its outbreaks are generally preceded by some unusual meteorological conditions; and while it may cause the greatest devastation in low grounds, the inhabitants of elevated regions enjoy almost complete immunity from its effects. I believe it is correct to say, that yellow fever has only once or twice occurred at a greater elevation than 2500 feet above the level of the sea.

Symptoms.—An attack of this fever oftens sets in abruptly, perhaps in the middle of the night. Occasionally, for two or three days before the seizure there is languor, loss of appetite, giddiness, frontal headache, and mental depression. Sometimes the disease commences with coldness of the surface, or even distinct rigors; followed by fever which lasts for several hours. In another class of cases, there is prostration from the first, without febrile reaction; stupor, coma, and convulsions soon following.

Where there is decided fever, it generally becomes aggravated towards night; the temperature of the skin sometimes rising as high as 105° or even to 107° Fahr. The pulse moreover gets frequent, the mouth parched and dry, the eyes congested and painful, and the face flushed. Distressing headache, perhaps confined to one temple, is very common. There are pains in the back and limbs, as well as in the large joints. Irritability of the stomach is usually present; together with tenderness on pressure, a sense of tightness about the præcordia, and nausea which is followed after a few hours by constant vomiting and retching. There is thirst, with a desire for cold drinks. The urine is diminished in quantity, and of a dark red colour : it is usually albuminous. Generally there is constipation, or if any stools be passed they are found free from bile. Distressing restlessness, mental anxiety, sleeplessness, and perhaps active delirium tend to show the force of the disease.

At the end of the second or third day, the severity of the symptoms greatly diminishes. The patient feels much relieved; while the face gets slightly jaundiced, the skin becomes moist, and there are copious bilious stools. In favourable cases, convalescence is firmly established. More frequently the improvement is of short duration. After some twenty-four hours, the epigastric tenderness is aggravated; the jaundice increasing and spreading over the body. There is a tendency to stupor; the pulse becomes feeble, irregular, and slow—perhaps as low as thirty beats in the minute; the tongue gets foul and dry; the respiration is embarrassed; and hiccup, thirst, nausea and vomiting, &c. are constant. Unless the symptoms remit, grumous blood is vomited —black vomit. The urine is suppressed or simply retained; the skin becomes of a dark-brown hue; dark-coloured blood is effused in patches under the skin, or exudes from the nose, gums, tongue, stomach, anus, vagina, &c.; and most offensive tarry-looking stools are passed. There are now all the features of a most malignant fever: an almost imperceptible pulse; slow or stertorous breathing; involuntary evacuations; difficulty of deglutition and articulation; suppressed or bloody urine; with formation of buboes or patches of gangrene. Death takes place, preceded by coma or convulsions; or the patient retains consciousness to the close.

Two or three of the foregoing symptoms may be deemed of particular importance. Thus, the appearances presented by the tongue at different stages, are very variable; this organ being usually furred, sometimes flabby and white and indented by the teeth, at other times dry and brown. The matters vomited are at first white, slimy, and tasteless; but soon they assume the appearance of coffee-grounds, owing to blood being effused into the stomach, where it is acted upon by the acid contents of this viscus. This altered blood is the essential element of the so-called black vomit. Then, the dejections likewise have a tarry appearance, from admixture with blood. There is frequently more or less complete suppression of urine; or this secretion may be smoky-looking, and loaded with albumen and casts of tubes. A copious and natural renal secretion is a most favourable sign. The fever in women always causes the catamenia to appear— or at all events produces uterine or vaginal hæmorrhage, even if the normal menstrual period has only just ceased.

Prognosis.—The usual duration of the fever is from three to seven or even nine days; though in some severe cases the patient is at once "knocked down" by the poison, and dies in a state of collapse at the end of a few hours. When the sixth day elapses without the occurrence of black vomit or suppression of urine, there is great hope of recovery; but if all other symptoms are absent, and only one of these present, our prognosis must be very unfavourable. The occurrence of black watery and shreddy stools, is also indicative of great danger ; and so is severe lumbar pain. If the pupils be widely dilated, cerebral complications are to be feared. The mortality seems to be at least 1 in 3. At Lisbon, in 1857, the fatal cases in the unhealthy quarters of the city were nearly forty-three per cent. But occasionally epidemics of a much milder character have occurred in the West Indies and America. Death usually occurs from exhaustion, or uræmic poisoning, or apoplexy.

Morbid Anatomy.—The special poison of yellow fever appears particularly to affect the *liver ;* and Professor A. Clarke, of New York, has suggested that the change so constantly observed in this organ, in fatal cases, is an acute fatty degeneration. Dr. La Roche confirms this opinion ; for he says that in all the examinations made during the epidemic of 1853 at the Pennsylvania Hospital, this change in the liver was discovered.*

Various changes have been found in the *blood.* The most frequent are,—a yellowness of the serum ; an appreciable unpleasant odour ; an acid reaction ; a deficiency of fibrin ; an excess of urea ; and a disintegration of the red corpuscles. The *kidneys* are usually congested ; a minute examination showing the tubes choked with fibrinous casts, fat cells, and blood corpuscles. The *tissues of the body* generally, and those of the *heart* to perhaps a marked extent, are pale and flabby and abnormally friable. Lastly, the *stomach* and *intestines* usually contain black vomit ; while the mucous membrane is sometimes here and there detached from the subjacent tissues.

Treatment.—The indications presented by the fever are to be observed. The disease cannot be cured, but the patient may be guided through it. Hence, it will be better to follow Dr. La Roche's advice, and treat the urgent symptoms as they happen ; leaving the rest to the reparative powers of the system. Removal from the infected locality is not only a valuable prophylactic measure, but where it can be had recourse to in affected cases, the change is often followed by marked amelioration of the symptoms. Nothing so soon and so thoroughly arrests yellow fever on board ship, as running into a cold latitude. Where this cannot be done, the greatest attention should be paid to cleanliness ; both by the free use of disinfectants, and by pumping out foul bilge water, &c.

From the commencement of the disease until convalescence is firmly established, the patient had better strictly maintain the recumbent posture. His bed ought to be placed in the centre of a well-ventilated room. The diet must be very simple ; consisting of barley water, arrowroot, milk and lime water, cold tea, ice and iced water, lemonade, broth, beef tea, &c. Purgatives are at first almost universally employed ; podophyllum, calomel, and sulphate

---

* *Yellow Fever considered in its Historical, Pathological, Etiological, and Therapeutical Relations,* vol. i. p. 404. Philadelphia, 1855.

of magnesia with jalap or senna being the favourite drugs of this class. Sometimes they are combined with large doses of quinine. Bark or quinine can also be administered after the bowels have acted; or the tincture of perchloride of iron with a mineral acid may be tried, or the nitro-hydrochloric acid well diluted. A few drops of chloroform can be given four or five times in the twenty-four hours, if there is pain or restlessness or severe vomiting; or, in extreme cases of suffering, about one-fourth of a grain of morphia with the same quantity of extract of belladonna may be prescribed, provided the urine be copious and free from albumen. Turpentine, owing to its action on the skin and kidneys, is thought useful by many observers: if tried, it should be administered in small doses—min. 20 to 60, frequently repeated, almost from the commencement of the attack. It seems to me highly probable, however, that some preparation of oxygen (F. 370) would prove more serviceable. The prolonged use of the warm bath, or wrapping the patient in the wet sheet, may occasionally be advisable. Blisters or sinapisms to the nucha, calves of the legs, &c., are recommended to relieve headache and pain; as well as to stimulate the system in cases of collapse. Cold applications to the head are useful. M. Guyon states that the intense cephalalgia may be relieved by compressing the temporal arteries; which can be done effectually with a semicircular curved band of steel, having a pad at each end like that of a common truss.

A word or two of caution is necessary as to the selection of stimulants. And, in the first place, we should carefully avoid giving ammonia; for Dr. Blair particularly notices the ammoniacal state of the blood, breath, and vomited matters. In some cases, this observer says that the blood was found as fluid as port wine, the corpuscles being all dissolved; while it was strongly ammoniacal. Secondly, of all alcoholic stimulants champagne or sparkling moselle will be found the most grateful. Any kind of wine or spirit, however, may prove very injurious where the action of the kidneys is embarrassed. The congestion of these organs will be increased; death probably following from suppression of urine, though the patient be drenched with brandy.

About the year 1448, when Venice was the great emporium of Eastern trade, quarantine regulations appear to have been first promulgated. Since then, they have prevailed in most countries. At the present day, able men have advocated their abolition on the grounds, that while they are injurious to commerce and very vexatious to travellers, they do not prevent the spread of epidemic disease. For it has been shown that yellow fever is local or endemic in its origin; while there is no evidence that it has been imported, save in one or two exceptional instances. In fact many epidemics have been stayed by removing the sick from the infected locality, and dispersing them through healthy districts. One circumstance has, however, been pointed out, that " besides the common external localizing causes, there is one constitutional predisposing cause of paramount importance, namely, non-acclimatization—that is, the state of the system produced by residence in a cold climate ; in other words, European blood exposed to the action of tropical heat ; the practical lesson being that the utmost care should be taken to prevent individuals or bodies of men, recently arrived within the yellow fever zone, from going into a district in which the disease actually exists or has recently been present."*   It may be hoped from all the foregoing that the day is not very distant when sanitary works will be substituted for quarantine restrictions.

V. ERUPTIVE FEVERS.

The eruptive fevers may be regarded as continued fevers, having an eruption superadded.   The chief are—*small-pox, cowpox, chicken-pox, measles*, and *scarlet fever ;* to which it is convenient to add *dengue, erysipelas*, and *plague.*

The principal diseases of this class have these common characters :—A variable amount of time elapses between the reception of the poison and the setting in of the symptoms, called the period of incubation.   They are preceded by rigors, and are accompanied by a fever which runs a defined course.   They are attended by an eruption, which goes through a regular series of changes.   They for the most part affect every individual once, and once only, during life.   Lastly, they arise from a specific contagious poison.   Of all the eruptive fevers scarlatina is probably that which most frequently affects the system a second time.

The mortality from these fevers in England, in different years, varies considerably.   To exhibit the contrast, as well as to show how each year is distinguished by the occurrence of some one or two master epidemics, the death from eight of the principal zymotic [Ζυμόω = to ferment] diseases may be thus arranged:—

	1860.	1861.	1862.	1863.	1864.	1865.	1866.
The Estimated Population	19,902,713	20,119,314	20,336,467	20,554,137	20,772,308	20,990,946	21,210,020
Deaths from all Causes	422,721	435,114	436,566	473,837	495,531	490,909	500,689
Measles	9,557	9,055	9,800	11,349	8,323	8,562	10,940
Scarlet Fever	9,681	9,077	14,834	30,475	29,700	17,700	11,685
Small-pox	2,749	1,320	1,628	5,964	7,684	6,411	3,029
Continued Fever	13,012	15,440	18,721	18,017	20,106	23,034	21,104
Diphtheria	5,212	4,517	4,903	6,507	5,464	4,145	3,000
Hooping-cough	8,555	12,309	12,272	11,275	8,570	8,647	15,764
Croup	4,380	4,397	5,667	6,957	6,777	5,921	5,168
Erysipelas	1,665	1,542	1,523	1,920	2,104	1,963	1,675

The following table shows the period of incubation, together with the date of eruption and time of its disappearance, in the four chief eruptive fevers :—

* *Second Report on Quarantine.* General Board of Health, p. 135. London, 1852.

Disease.	Period of Incubation.	Eruption appears.	Eruption fades.
Measles . . .	10 to 14 days.	On 4th day of fever, after 72 hours' illness.	On 7th day of fever.
Scarlet Fever	4 to 6 days.	On 2nd day of fever, after 24 hours' illness.	On 5th day of fever.
Small-pox . .	12 days.	On 3rd day of fever, after 48 hours' illness.	Scabs form on 9th or 10th day of fever, and fall off about the 14th.
Chicken-pox .	4 days.	On 2nd day of fever, or after 24 hours' illness.	Slight scabs form about 4th day of fever.

There is some doubt whether the features of a disease should be sketched, which presents many of the characters of measles and scarlet fever conjoined ; and which has been described as *Rubeola,* or *rubeola notha,* or *rötheln,* or *scarlatina morbillosa,* or a *hybrid of measles* and *scarlet fever.* I think, however, any special description unnecessary, because we all know that measles and scarlatina may exist in the body at the same time; and hence the affection is merely a compound of the two. There will be found the eruption and coryza of measles, with the inflammation of the fauces and submaxillary glands of scarlatina. As these inflammatory symptoms are usually the most urgent, this hybrid disease should be regarded with caution, so far as the prognosis is concerned ; while it must be treated according to the rules laid down in the section on Scarlet Fever. Care is particularly to be taken to maintain the functions of the skin. It may also be remembered that the use of colchicum has been strongly recommended. That rubeola is due to a specific poison, like each of the other eruptive fevers, has been suggested ; but I am not aware that this opinion has been substantiated.

Further, it is necessary to mention that measles may coexist with small-pox, or hooping cough, or chicken-pox, &c., as Mr. Marson has well shown.[*]

1. SMALL-POX.—Variola, or small-pox, is certainly the most remarkable of the eruptive fevers. It is due to the reception into the blood of a specific poison, which begins to give indications of its power about twelve days after absorption. In its entire course each case of variola [from *Varius* = spotted] goes through four stages—that of incubation, of primary fever, of eruption, and of secondary fever.

Small-pox may be defined as a continued and infectious and eruptive fever. The period of latency or incubation lasts twelve days,

[*] *Medico-Chirurgical Transactions,* vol. xxx. p. 129. London, 1847.

during which there are no symptoms of indisposition. Then the disease commences with shivering, fever, headache, vomiting, and well-marked muscular pains in the back. These symptoms are succeeded at the end of forty-eight hours, or the beginning of the third day, by an eruption of small red pimples; which in the course of a week inflame and suppurate and begin to scab. In many instances the disorder is accompanied by a similar affection of the mucous membrane of the nose and mouth and throat; in some, by swelling and inflammation of the subjacent connective tissue; and occasionally by marked irritation of the nervous system. With extreme rarity a few pustules are found on the ocular conjunctivæ, or on the margins of the eyelids. Pregnant women abort; or they are prematurely delivered, the fœtus more frequently being dead than not : the mother often does well. When the vomiting and pain of the back are violent, they are generally the precursors of a severe form of the disease.

The peculiar eruption of pimples or papulæ always begins to show itself on the commencement of the third day of the fever. It appears in the following order—first, on the face, the neck, and wrists; secondly, on the trunk; and lastly, on the lower extremities. The papulæ then gradually ripen into vesicles, and then into pustules; the suppuration being complete by the ninth day. About this time the pustules break, and crusts or scabs form. In four or five days more these scabs are falling off.

Now the severity of the disease almost always bears a direct relation to the quantity of the eruption. Where the pustules are few, they remain distinct and separate from each other; when very numerous, they run together, coalesce, and lose their regularly circumscribed circular form. We thus have a division of small-pox into two varieties—variola *discreta*, and variola *confluens*. The former is seldom attended with danger; the latter is never free from it. The eruption on the face may be of the confluent form, while it is scanty elsewhere; still the disease is of the confluent kind. Sometimes the pustules are so numerous that they touch each other, but nevertheless do not actually coalesce. The disease has then been said to be of the *cohering* or *semiconfluent* form.

In *variola discreta*, the eruption, in the words of Willan, is papular. On the third day a small vesicle, with a central depression, appears on each papula, containing some thin transparent lymph; around this an inflamed areola forms. About the fifth day of the eruption, or the eighth of the disease, the vesicles lose their central depression : they become turgid, and hemispheroidal. Suppuration has occurred, and the vesicles have become pustules containing yellowish matter. A peculiar disagreeable odour now begins to emanate from the patient, which once smelt cannot be forgotten; so that from it alone the disease might be diagnosed. About the eighth or ninth day a dark spot appears on the top of each pustule, the cuticle bursts, the matter oozes out, and the pustule dries into a scab. At the end of some ten days more the crusts fall off, leaving a purplish red stain, which slowly fades ; or where the pustule has gone so deep as to destroy a portion of the true skin, there will be found to result that permanent disfigurement—the so called pitting or pock-mark.

Variola confluens is usually ushered in by more distinct rigors and more violent fever than is the distinct variety. The eruption comes out earlier. The eyelids get tumid, so that by the fifth day the patient is often unable to see ; the tonsils and parotid glands become affected ; there is salivation also, or in children a vicarious diarrhœa with possibly convulsions ; and the limbs swell. The urine is diminished in quantity, while the urea and uric acid are increased ; and sometimes there is albumen for a few days, or even blood with renal casts. The vesicles on the face run together into one bleb, containing a thin brownish ichor ; while the face also becomes pale and doughy. The vesicles on the trunk and extremities, though often not confluent, have no areola and are pale. On the breaking of the pustules, large brown or black scabs are formed, exhaling great fetor ; while the pulse gets rapid, great debility sets in, and there is much restlessness. The mucous membranes become involved ; those of the nose, mouth, larynx, and trachea being the seat of an eruption. The tongue and palate become covered with small vesicles ; the throat is very sore ; there is difficulty of swallowing, with hoarseness and dyspnœa and cough ; while the glottis often becomes narrowed, and suffocation perhaps ensues. Delirium frequently occurs. When to the foregoing symptoms malignancy and putrescency are added, the disease becomes *malignant* small-pox ; a form which used to be described as the Black pock.

The greatest difference, however, between the distinct and confluent forms of the disease is in the *secondary fever ;* which, slightly marked in the first, is intense and perilous in the second. It sets in usually about the eleventh day of the disease, or the eighth of the eruption, and occasionally at once proves fatal ; the system appearing to be overwhelmed by the virulence of the seizure. During its course, various troublesome complications may arise ; such as erysipelas, swelling of the glands in the groin and axilla, abscesses, pyæmia, gangrene, phlebitis, pneumonia, pleurisy, bronchitis, dysentery or diarrhœa, conjunctivitis, ulceration through the cornea, suppuration of the ear, &c. Hence if the patient escape with his life, he may find himself permanently afflicted with blindness, deafness, or lameness.

When small-pox occurs after efficient vaccination, or after a previous attack of variola, the affection is spoken of as *modified* small-pox. *Varicelloid*, or *abortive* small-pox, is that form in which the eruption seems to stop in its vesicular stage ; most of the vesicles drying up, instead of going on to the formation of pustules.

There is no contagion so powerful or so certain as that of

small-pox. Clothes, bedding &c. used by patients in this disease, retain the power of infection for a long time unless they are thoroughly purified. One attack of this affection exhausts the susceptibility of the system to the future influence of the poison, as a general rule. This law is subject to very few exceptions, many of the recorded cases of recurrent small-pox not bearing a rigid investigation. It is sure to lead to error if the statements of patients on this head be trusted to. A great sensation was created in 1774, in France, by the death of Louis XV. from variola at the age of 64; it being generally believed that he had gone through the disease when he was 14 years old. From a careful inquiry, however, Dr. Gregory convinced himself that his Majesty never had small-pox in early life at all, but only varicella. The Small-pox and Vaccination Hospital was founded in 1746; and Mr. Marson has informed me (June 1864) that no instance had occurred of a patient being twice admitted, each time with variola.* Nevertheless it must not be thought that recurrent attacks never take place. I only wish to show that they are very uncommon. One gentleman, according to Dr. Gregory, said that he had met with between eighty and ninety examples in his own practice. This was clearly impossible. Even Dr. Jenner may have been mistaken in his allusion to "the lady of Mr. Gwinnett, who has had the small-pox *five* times."† But the most incredible case recorded is that of a surgeon of the South Gloucestershire Militia,

* The present building at Highgate was opened in 1850; since which time there have been four severe epidemics of small-pox in London. According to the medical report of this institution for the year 1866 it appears, that the first epidemic in 1851-2 gave to the hospital 1482 admissions; the second, that of 1854, 55, and 56 yielded 2321; the third, that of 1859-60 gave 2060; while the fourth, extending over 1863, 64, 65, and 66 contributed 5691 admissions. This last epidemic, judging from the admissions of patients into the hospital, commenced about November 1862, and began to decline soon after June 1863; but in the winter of 1864-5 it acquired increased violence, and in 1866 it had reached a higher degree of intensity. Of the 5691 patients brought to the institution during the epidemic of 1863-6 there were 1537 admitted in 1863; 836 in 1864; 1249 in 1865; and 2069 in 1866. Of the numbers admitted in 1866 there were 32 suffering from various forms of disease not small-pox; of the 2037 cases of small-pox 425 occurred in unvaccinated persons, and 1605 in persons who had been vaccinated. There were three cases which occurred after a previous attack of natural small-pox, two cases after inoculation, and two cases after vaccination and small-pox. The deaths in 1866 were 272, being in the proportion of 13 per cent. of the whole admissions. Of the 425 unvaccinated cases 152 died, being a mortality for this class of 35.7 per cent.; while of the 1605 persons who were vaccinated only 108, or 6.7 per cent., died. The average mortality in the hospital in the 16 years ending 31 December 1851, was at the rate of 21.38 per cent. per annum of the whole admissions; the death-rate in the unvaccinated being 35 per cent., and in the vaccinated, 6.76 per cent. The ratio of vaccinated cases to the whole admissions, during the same period, was 53 per cent., a proportion which has gone on progressively increasing.
† *The Life of Edward Jenner, M.D., &c.* By John Baron, M.D., vol. ii. p. 265. London, 1838.

who (according to Dr. Baron) was so wonderfully susceptible, that he took small-pox every time he attended a patient suffering from this disease.*

Variola occurring in persons unprotected by inoculation or vaccination is fatal on the average to one in every three; whilst in those attacked after efficient vaccination the mortality is very small—perhaps not as much as two or three per cent. The calculation has been made by the Registrar-General that the average number of deaths annually from small-pox, in London, during the years 1660-1679, were 357 to every 100,000 inhabitants; whereas in 1850 they were 42 for the same proportion. When the variolous matter is introduced into the skin by a few scratches—*inoculated small-pox*, the disease is in all respects of a remarkably mild nature. The practice of inoculation, introduced into this country by Lady Mary Wortley Montagu, is now illegal.†

* Quoted from Dr. W. Aitken's *Science and Practice of Medicine*. Second Edition, vol. i. p. 246. London, 1863.

† When and where *inoculation* originated is unknown. From time immemorial the Chinese have practised a method of "sowing or disseminating" the disease; which consists in introducing the scales of the eruption into the nostrils. At a very remote period, in Hindostan, a tribe of Brahmins resorted to it as a religious ceremony. A small incision was made, and cotton soaked in the virus applied to the wound. Offerings were devoted to the Goddess of Spots, to invoke her aid; this Divinity having first hinted at inoculation,— "the thought being much above the reach of human wisdom and foresight." But the merit of introducing the practice into this country, from Turkey, is due to Lady Mary Wortley Montagu. Writing from Adrianople, in April 1717, she observes,—"Every year thousands undergo this operation; and the French ambassador says pleasantly, that they take the small-pox here by way of diversion, as they take the waters in other countries. There is no example of any one that has died in it; and you may believe I am very well satisfied of the safety of the experiment, since I intend to try it on my dear little son. I am patriot enough to take pains to bring this useful invention into fashion in England." (*The Letters and Works of Lady Mary Wortley Montagu*. Third Edition, vol. i. p. 309. London, 1861.) The debt which our ancestors owed to this lady is not diminished by the fact that inoculation had been practised for very many years in South Wales, where it was known as "Buying the Small-Pox;" for this circumstance only became generally recognised as Lady Montagu's views engaged attention, and while she enjoyed the privilege of being the best abused person in England.

That the effects of inoculation were most remarkable is undoubted; though even to the present day, no satisfactory explanation has been given for the mildness of the disease when thus introduced into the system. The reports of the London Small-Pox Hospital for 1797, 1798, and 1799, show that among 5964 cases of inoculated small-pox, there were only 9 deaths, or 1 in 662; and this appears to have been the average mortality. There is also much evidence to lead to the belief that infection does not spread from an inoculated patient. Mr. Holwell, who inoculated multitudes in India, during a residence of thirty years, affirmed that "it never spreads the infection, as is commonly imagined in Europe." (Quoted from Dr. Chapman's *Lectures on the Eruptive Fevers, Hœmorrhages and Dropsies, and on Gout and Rheumatism*, p. 46. Philadelphia, 1844.)

With regard to this subject it is most interesting to notice, that a method which has proved of such value to mankind has been employed for the relief of

The "stamping out" in this country during 1866-67, of that fatal disease to cattle, the Rinderpest, has suggested to Sir James Y. Simpson the application of the same principle to the extirpation of small-pox in 1868. As the poleaxe was the leading measure required to blot out rinderpest, so *isolation* is to be the chief means employed to stamp out small-pox. Those affected with this disease must, in fact, be placed in strict quarantine, until they have completely passed through the disorder and lost all power of communicating it to others. That this might be effected without any extraordinary inconvenience can scarcely be doubted. Unlike the expulsion of the unclean leper from the camp under the Mosaic law, the necessary seclusion of the individual with small-pox would prove but of short duration. But it seems to me that were the proposal successfully carried out,—could we, for example, say on a certain day that there was not a single case of small-pox in Great Britain, yet our immunity would prove of short duration. Sir James Simpson mentions two cases which show how easily the disease is spread ; and though he suggests certain rules, according to which the occurrence of small-pox in any house should be at once notified

a disease in the sheep, corresponding to, but not identical with, human small-pox. In June 1862 a very severe outbreak of *Variola Ovina* occurred in a farm at Allington, in Wiltshire. The epidemic spread to eight or nine other farms, and was fatal to 800 sheep. When Professor Simonds was summoned to Allington in August, after 400 cases had occurred with nearly 200 deaths on this farm alone, he resolved " as the best means of saving the rest of the flock, and of putting a definite term to the outbreak," to inoculate the whole flock. This was done ; and in consequence, the disease appeared in the very mildest form in the majority of the cases.

A valuable report of experiments made under the direction of the Lords of the Privy Council, as to the influence of the vaccination of sheep in preventing sheep-pox, has been prepared (June 1864) by Mr. Marson and Professor Simonds. They state that sheep-pox is not known to have existed in England except on three occasions—in 1710-11, 1847-50, and 1862, and that it is always the result of infection. They find that vaccination cannot be relied upon as a preventive or mitigant, as the vaccine disease in these animals is but very imperfectly developed even in the most successful cases. But they consider that inoculation is a measure which, if rightly carried out, offers considerable advantages. It gives security against a natural attack, for as a rule, sheep-pox occurs but once. It limits the period of the existence of the disease in the flock, mitigates the severity of the malady, saves the lives of many sheep which would otherwise be sacrificed, and produces comparatively but little loss of condition. It controls the extension of the disease, as one confluent natural case does more to diffuse the poison than probably fifty ordinary inoculated cases would do. Lastly, the mortality of the inoculated disease, when compared with the natural, is on the average only as three per cent. in the one case, to fifty per cent. in the other.

The student who is desirous of investigating this subject more fully should refer to *The Address in Medicine*, by Dr. William Budd, in the *British Medical Journal*, p. 141, 8th August 1863; to *A Practical Treatise on Variola Ovina*, by James B. Simonds, Lecturer on Cattle Pathology at the Royal Veterinary College. London, 1848 ; and to the *Report of Experiments made under Direction of the Lords of the Council as to the Vaccination of Sheep, &c.* London, 1864.

to the authorities, yet I believe that the mischief would be accomplished before isolation could be had recourse to. Several years ago a beggar woman entered the town of Leith, carrying a child who was recovering from small-pox. She went to a low quarter of the town to find lodgings and there remained. Very soon the disease spread among the inhabitants, until a great number were attacked in all parts of the town, and ninety-nine perished by it. Again, a long time since (1818-19) a girl in travelling from York to Norwich, was exposed to small-pox at a market-town in the course of her journey. When she reached Norwich the disease appeared upon her. A druggist soon afterwards inoculated three children with variolous matter, and from these two causes a dreadful mortality was produced. About 3000 persons were attacked, and 530 died. Such histories as these could be easily multiplied. Granting, however, that it would not be impossible to draw a cordon round each patient known to have small-pox, and allowing for the sake of argument that we might seize and seclude every traveller arriving in this country undoubtedly affected with the disease, the question arises as to how we are to deal with those who have it without being aware of the fact? Sir James Simpson asserts, that " the disease does not mature into the stage of infection for some days after the eruption shows itself." If this were true, we should certainly have a manifest advantage in limiting the affection. But I cannot believe in the soundness of the remark. For according to Mr. Marson, who must be considered the highest authority on the subject now living, the disease is most likely communicable from the moment when the initiatory fever begins. It may be given by the breath of the patient before the eruption has appeared on the surface of the body. In proof of this, he mentions the following singular case :—A few years since, a lady while walking in Islington met a person with small-pox. Twelve days afterwards, the lady was taken ill : she was delirious for a few hours, but got well without the appearance of any eruption. A married sister, who had not been outside the house for three months because of her pregnancy, was seized with confluent small-pox twelve days after her sister's attack. My own experience on this question is also somewhat to the point. In the year 1848, I attended a poor woman in labour, who had been in a state of high fever during the preceding twenty-four hours. The infant was still-born and could not be resuscitated. On the day after her delivery, the skin of the face and arms became covered with an eruption of pimples, which appeared of a dark colour. There was delirium with great prostration ; and death occurred in a few hours (38 hours after birth of child). Exactly twelve days after the labour, the nurse of the patient was taken ill ; her disease proving to be an attack of distinct small-pox. I attended her until recovery was complete; and neither of us had any doubt but that the disease had been contracted at the labour. My own escape was probably due to the fact that I had suffered from small-pox two years previously.

Possibly many years hence, when wars and rumours of wars shall be unknown, and when the governments of different countries shall look upon the destruction of disease as a matter of primary importance, some attempt may be made on a large scale to stamp out several contagious disorders. But until this happy time arrives, and while the means of rapid transit from one country to another are constantly increasing, it would be hopeless to expect any permanent benefit from carrying out Sir James Simpson's proposal on such a small portion of the globe as is occupied by Great Britain.

The less drugs are used in the *treatment* of small-pox, the better ; inasmuch as they will neither shorten the disease, nor exert any favourable influence upon the eruption.* In the early stages, the patient should be kept quiet in bed, in a well-ventilated room free from carpets and curtains : iodine (F. 81), or sulphurous acid gas (F. 74), or carbolic acid, or some other disinfectant is to be employed. His diet should consist of arrowroot, gruel, weak beef tea, mutton or chicken broth, bread and milk, and tea with milk ; he should be allowed plenty of lemonade, barley water, plain water, raspberry-vinegar and water, soda water, or ice ; while ripe fruits, especially grapes and oranges, are unobjectionable. When the skin is very hot, tepid sponging will prove very refreshing, especially if its use be followed by a change of linen. Supposing that the bowels are confined, a few doses of some mild saline laxative (F. 139, 141, 148, 169, &c.) may be administered; if the throat be sore from the presence of many pustules, a gargle of tincture of myrrh in rose water can be ordered, or some black currant jelly will relieve the sense of dryness ; if there be diarrhœa, milk and rice, with some catechu and chalk mixture (F. 97), or bismuth and syrup of poppies (F. 112), will check it ; while when there is great irritability and nervousness, a dose of morphia and chloroform, or of opium and henbane (F. 315, 317, 325, or 340) at bedtime will do good. Where the maturation of the pustules goes on tardily, or imperfectly, good soups and cream and stimulants (wine or ether or ammonia) are indicated.

* "It is a melancholy reflection, but too true, that for many hundred years the efforts of physicians were rather exerted to thwart nature, and to add to the malignancy of the disease, than to aid her in her efforts. Blisters, heating alexipharmics, large bleedings, opiates, ointments, masks, and lotions to prevent pitting, were the great measures formerly pursued, not one of which can be recommended. What think you of a prince of the blood royal of England (John the son of Edward the Second) being treated for small-pox by being put into a bed surrounded with red hangings, covered with red blankets and a red counterpane, gargling his throat with mulberry wine, and sucking the red juice of pomegranates ? Yet this was the boasted prescription of John of Gaddesden, who took no small credit to himself for bringing his royal patient safely through the disease."—*Lectures on the Eruptive Fevers,* p. 78. By George Gregory, M.D. London, 1843.

A decoction of the root of the Sarracenia Purpurea, or pitcher-plant, has been extensively tried, owing to the statement of Dr. Chalmers Miles, that this remedy is regarded as a specific by certain tribes of Indians. But while we must acknowledge ourselves indebted to Dr. Miles for the trouble he has taken in investigating the supposed properties of this plant, yet it is to be feared that he has laboured in vain. It will suffice to give the experience of Mr. Marson, who employed it in fifteen severe cases at the Small-pox Hospital. The patients all died, as they would probably have done under any treatment. Mr. Marson remarks,—" I cannot say that the Sarracenia had any effect whatever. It did not save life ; it did not modify in the least the eruption ; it did not influence any of the secretions ; it did not increase the secretion of urine ; in only one instance it seemed to act on the bowels ; the seeming effect might, however, easily have been from other causes."*

In managing the *secondary fever*, the physician ought to keep the bowels gently open by mild laxatives; to administer sedatives if needful, once or twice a day ; and to support the system by a nourishing but digestible diet, such as strong beef tea, good soup, plenty of milk or cream, the whole of one or two raw eggs daily, &c. Stimulants (champagne or claret) are to be given in proportion to the weakness of the patient. Sloughy and gangrenous sores demand the liberal administration of quinine or bark and nitric acid, or of steel and cod liver oil ; of fresh-cooked animal food ; as well as of light bitter ale, or of wine, or even of brandy. When there is the least fear of the occurrence of ulceration on the back or nates, the patient should be placed on a water-bed, or on one of Hooper's large water-pillows. To relieve the intolerable itching, the pustules had better be frequently smeared with cold cream ; or they may be painted with a mixture of one drachm of the solution of subacetate of lead in seven drachms of almond oil, or with what often answers better—the officinal lime liniment. When the pustules have burst, some dry powder (as the oxide of zinc, or powdered starch) is frequently freely applied, to absorb the matter, and perhaps to prevent the pitting. For the latter purpose, moreover, the application of poultices, oils, ointments, collodion, and mercurial plasters, over the face and hands, has been recommended ; the object generally being to exclude air, lessen irritation, and to keep the tissues moist.

2. COW-POX.—Since the happy discovery of the protective influence of cow-pox or vaccinia by Jenner, towards the close of the eighteenth century, the fatality of small-pox has been very much diminished. And not only has the mortality been so considerably lessened, but the good looks of the people have been preserved by vaccination [*Vacca* = a cow]. "Unless the reader," says Dr.

* *British Medical Journal*, p. 22. London, 4 July 1863.

Andrew Wynter, "has scanned the long list of villanous portraits exhibited by the Hue and Cry in the old papers of the last portion of the seventeenth and first portion of the eighteenth centuries, he can form but a faint conception of the ravages committed by the small-pox upon the population. Every man seemed more or less to have been speckled with ' pock-holes ;' and the race must have presented one moving mass of pits and scars."[*] Vaccination was first performed in England in 1796, in America in 1799, and in France in 1800. It is now highly probable that efficient vaccination confers a degree of immunity against small-pox almost, if not quite, equal to that obtained by inoculation; while it is decidedly safer, much less disgusting, and does not tend to perpetuate a loathsome disease, as the practice of inoculation did. Moreover, when small-pox occurs in an individual who has been properly vaccinated, as it sometimes will, the disease always proves much milder and of shorter duration ; while it is usually unaccompanied by secondary fever. It is spoken of under these circumstances as *varioloid*, or *modified* small-pox. These facts receive a ready explanation at the hands of Mr. Ceely; for this gentleman has proved by experiments that vaccinia and variola are one and the same disease, the virus in the former having become modified by being passed through the system of the cow.

Vaccination is usually performed for the first time when the child is about four or six weeks old. It may, however, be practised on a healthy infant within a few hours of its birth ; if from the presence of an epidemic of small-pox it be thought desirable to shield it very early from the chance of variolous infection. The resulting phenomena are neither more nor less severe than are met with in children of more advanced age. Nevertheless, as a general rule it is better to postpone the operation until after the end of the first month ; chiefly because, under ordinary circumstances, there is no advantage in very early vaccination to compensate for the mental distress which it occasions to the mother. The fact is, that a feeling against early vaccination is rife in the public mind. Doubtless this is only a prejudice. At the same time it is a prejudice which I should advise the practitioner to respect, save under some special emergency.

When vaccine lymph has been successfully introduced beneath the cuticle of a healthy child, an elevation may be felt over the puncture on the second day, accompanied by slight redness ; on the fifth, a distinct vesicle is formed, having an elevated edge and depressed centre ; while on the eighth, it is of a pearl colour, and is distended with a clear lymph. This lymph consists of a transparent serum ; floating in which are leucocytes or bodies resembling the white corpuscles of the blood, and elementary granules of less definite structure. The vesicle is composed of a number of cells, by the walls and floor of which the lymph is secreted. An inflamed

* *Quarterly Review*, Article " Advertisements." London, July 1855.

ring or areola then begins to form round the base of the little tumour, and to increase during the two succeeding days; about the eleventh day it fades; and the vesicle, which has now burst and acquired a brown colour, gradually dries up, until by the end of the second week it has become converted into a hard and round scab. This falls off about the twenty-first day; leaving a circular, depressed, striated cicatrix, which is permanent in after life.

According to the official instructions issued to the public vaccinators in England, four or five separate punctures or scratches are to be made, "so as to produce four or five separate good-sized vesicles." The skin over the deltoid offers a good site. The first vaccination certainly affords protection for from seven to ten years, and perhaps for longer; but it is clearly a safe proceeding to revaccinate after this lapse of time.

The constitutional disturbance which accompanies vaccination is usually very slight. Between the sixth and ninth days there is a little febrile disturbance—vaccinal fever, accompanied by heat of skin and restlessness and acceleration of pulse. Eruptions of vaccine lichen or roseola sometimes appear, and may last for a week. Several interesting experiments made a few years ago by Dr. Gustav Wertheim of Vienna, tend to show that the frequency of the pulse is permanently increased by the process of vaccination. Thus, a man, aged thirty-eight, and a woman aged thirty-three, neither of whom had suffered from small-pox, were vaccinated for the first time; the pulse, in both cases, increased in frequency up to the sixth day after vaccination, when it began to decline; never declining—not at least for the four months during which the observations were continued—as low as it was before the introduction of the vaccine virus. For example, before vaccination, the man's pulse was on an average 66; afterwards the average was 78.

A popular belief has long existed that vaccination is occasionally the means of engrafting upon the constitution some impure disease. This opinion must no longer be ignored. As nothing is more common than to hear a mother assert in the hospital out-patient room,—"My child has never been well since he was vaccinated," so it is not surprising that a large number of the poor ignore the Act of Parliament rendering vaccination compulsory, and decline to submit their children to what they regard as a certain evil for the sake of a doubtful benefit. There can be no question that vaccination is often most carelessly and inefficiently performed. There is as little doubt but that in vaccinating we can not only introduce the cow-pox into the system, but by using a dirty lancet or foul lymph we may possibly induce that condition of blood-contamination known as pyæmia. And then, again, it is impossible to disbelieve the abundant evidence which now exists as to the fact of syphilis having been communicated by vaccination.

In 1856, Dr. Whitehead of Manchester wrote that he had " seen several instances of the transference of the syphilitic taint through the medium of vaccination."[*] This opinion, though almost unsupported at the time by the experience of others, is doubtless correct. Numerous facts which seem to corroborate it could be adduced; but it will probably suffice to mention one,— certainly a very startling instance. It occurred at Rivalta, a village in Piedmont, containing about two thousand inhabitants, where syphilis was said to be previously unknown. Here, on the 24 May 1861, a child eleven months old was vaccinated with a clean lancet from lymph out of a capillary tube. The infant was at the time apparently healthy; though it is probable that it had been infected two or three months previously with constitutional syphilis through being suckled on a few occasions by an unhealthy woman. From this child, on the 2nd June, forty-six children were vaccinated. And ten days subsequently one of these forty-six children furnished lymph for the vaccination of seventeen others. What is said to have followed has not been denied, and cannot be explained away. Within two months forty-six of the whole number of children were affected with a disease which was said to be syphilis by a commission of medical men appointed to examine the subject. Seven of the children died, the earliest death occurring three months after the vaccination. The first vaccinifer, after suffering from marasmus, alopecia, &c., recovered. The disease was also communicated by the children to twenty nurses or mothers; in three cases by the mothers to their husbands; and in three other cases by the children to their little playmates.[†] The only inference which it seems possible to draw from the foregoing is this :—That the lymph by which the first child was vaccinated was pure; but that the lymph taken away from it ten days subsequently, had become contaminated with syphilis. Hence, from this vaccinifer there was communicated the cow-pox; as well as, in a great majority of the cases, syphilis. The cow-pox appeared first and ran its natural course, because its period of incubation is only a few days. The syphilitic ulceration made its appearance on the inoculated part some time afterwards, and in due season was followed by secondary symptoms. The time of incubation in constitutional syphilis is from three to seven weeks.

But if the reader is still incredulous, and requires more confirmatory evidence, I would refer him to an admirable paper by Dr. Viennois.[‡] This gentleman, after a full and careful investi-

---

[*] *Papers relating to the History and Practice of Vaccination*, presented to the Board of Health by Mr. Simon, p. 114. London, 1857.

[†] The facts are given at great length by Dr. Giacinto Pacchiotti, Professor of Clinical Surgery at Turin, in his pamphlet, entitled *Sifilide trasmessa per Mezzo della Vaccinazione in Rivalta*, presso Acqui. Torino, 1862.

[‡] *Archives Générales de Médecine*, vol. i. p. 641; vol. ii. pp. 32, 297. Paris, 1860.

gation of the question, has come to the conclusion that if the lymph from a vaccine vesicle alone be inoculated, the cow-pox alone will be introduced; but if, in addition, the blood of a person with constitutional syphilis be also inoculated, then syphilis may likewise be communicated.

In a very small number of cases vaccination has been followed by erysipelas. Occasionally also, sloughing sores have been produced. Thus, in 1862 some lamentable results followed upon the vaccination of the soldiers of one division of the American Confederate Army. A few days after the insertion of the virus—in many cases within twenty-four hours, the seat of puncture became very much inflamed, with a deep inflammatory flush around it; the morbid action progressing until nearly the whole limb was affected. A pustule rapidly formed, which soon discharged an ichorous fluid; this fluid forming a dark mahogany-coloured scab in the course of forty-eight hours. This scab gradually increased in size until it was perhaps more than two inches in diameter; pus exuded from beneath it; and when it became detached a foul phagedenic ulcer was revealed, involving the subcutaneous connective tissue, and often exposing the muscular fibres beneath. As this ulcer spread the axillary glands enlarged, and sometimes freely suppurated; while wherever the ichorous pus from the ulcer touched the sound skin a similar pustule was formed.* The cause of these phenomena was doubtless the vitiated condition of the blood of the soldiers owing to their improper and spare diet, and their inability to attend to cleanliness. The disease resembled ecthyma, was of a scorbutic character, and was in no way due to any syphilitic virus.

Now what is to be learnt from these observations? Are they to shake our faith in the value of vaccination? Or are they to be set aside as being very exceptional cases? I believe that neither proceeding will follow; for the facts merely prove what has long been known, that vaccination, like every other operation on the human body, demands care and skill in its performance. The evils of pyæmia and phagedenic ulceration and syphilis which have ensued in certain cases have been due either to the use of a foul lancet, or of lymph which from remaining too long in the vesicle had begun to decay; or they may have arisen from employing lymph mixed with the blood of a diseased subject, or in consequence of the person vaccinated being in an unhealthy condition. The remedies are therefore very simple. Practitioners being forewarned will be forearmed. They must (1) be careful to employ a clean lancet. (2) The subject supplying the lymph must be healthy. (3) The subject to be vaccinated ought to be healthy, as a rule. And (4) clear pure lymph should be taken, on the eighth day, *un-*

* Report on Spurious Vaccination in the Confederate Army, by S. E. Habersham, M.D. &c. *Southern Medical and Surgical Journal,* vol. xxi. p. 1. Augusta, Georgia, 1866.

mixed with blood or pus or any other secretion. Let these rules be followed, and we shall hear no more of vaccino-syphilitic inoculation.

It only remains to say that vaccine lymph can be well preserved in hermetically sealed capillary tubes ; a plan of keeping the matter, in my opinion, much to be preferred to any other. If from any cause great economy has to be practised in using the lymph, it may be diluted with not more than ten times its weight of glycerine or water. But when possible, it is far better for the virus to be taken direct from a healthy child—arm-to-arm vaccination ; or even, if practicable, from the cow. The advantages of animal vaccination have been more generally recognised on the Continent than in this country : though it needs but little consideration to see that lymph taken from an animal vaccinifer is more likely to be active than that obtained by human transmission, while especially is it more certain to be pure. And as a result of practical experience it has been found, that in animal vaccination (from the calf to the human subject) the success is nearly universal ; the period of incubation is longer ; the pustules larger, and hence the local inflammation more severe ; while the general disturbance is more marked. Dairy-women are often infected from milking cows having the eruption of vaccinia on their teats.

According to the Act of Parliament—16 and 17 Victoria, cap. 100—which was passed in 1853, every infant is to be vaccinated within three calendar months from birth, unless its health renders the proceeding objectionable ; or unless the father and mother are dead, or ill, or unable to attend, when a month's grace is to be granted. In July 1855 another Bill was passed—18 and 19 Victoria—making it compulsory on all adults not protected by vaccination or an attack of small-pox, to undergo vaccination ; while the time for infants was limited to three months, under all circumstances. Again, in March 1856, it was enacted — 19 Victoria — that all children born after the 1st January 1857, should be vaccinated within four calendar months of birth. And then, finally, by 30 and 31 Victoria, an Act was passed on 12 August 1867, to consolidate and amend the laws relating to vaccination. By this bill, which came into operation on 1 January 1868, it is enacted that parts of certain preceding acts are repealed : that public vaccinators are to be appointed for different districts : that parents or guardians are to procure the vaccination of every child within three months of birth, unless the child is not in a fit and proper state of health for the operation : that parents neglecting to procure vaccination, or failing after vaccination to have the child inspected, may be fined twenty shillings : and that any person practising inoculation with variolous matter, or in any way wilfully producing small-pox in another individual, shall be liable to a month's imprisonment.

Hitherto it has been most unsatisfactory to find that the intentions of the legislature have been very imperfectly fulfilled,— so imperfectly, that according to Mr. Simon, "the public defences against small-pox are in great part insufficient and delusive."* It is, however, to be hoped that this slur upon our national character will no longer be allowed to exist. The fact would seem to be, that vaccination even as hitherto practised, has so far relieved the human race from such a malignant disease, that the public can form no adequate idea of the ravages which the latter committed when unfettered. And so, instead of showing any gratitude for the comparative immunity now enjoyed, there are some people who industriously endeavour to restore to us this loathsome disorder with all its original force; while others, who as legislators ought to know better, remove the London statue of Jenner from the locality where it might have inculcated a valuable lesson, to a secluded spot in which it is safe from the gaze of those who owe so much to the genius of the man it represents.

3. **CHICKEN-POX.**—Chicken-pox, or varicella, is a trifling complaint which is almost peculiar to infants and children under the age of twelve years, and which sometimes prevails as an epidemic. The disease completely runs through all its phases in six or seven days.

Varicella [the dim. of *Variola*] has some resemblance to modified small-pox; and there can be no doubt that in many of the cases which have been recorded of recurrent variola, one of the attacks has been simply chicken-pox. The two affections were formerly confounded together—prior to 1730; but no one in the present day doubts their non-identity. It is true that some confusion exists with regard to Professor Hebra's views; but this has chiefly arisen in consequence of his using the term varicella in a different sense to that with which we are accustomed to connect it in this country.

Chicken-pox may be said to consist of an eruption of small rose pimples, which appear at the end of twenty-four hours from the commencement of the mild initiatory fever. These pimples, on the second day, become converted into transparent vesicles surrounded by slight redness. The rash commences on the shoulders and back, and afterwards affects the scalp, but often spares the face; while about the fourth day the vesicles form small scabs, which rapidly desiccate. In a very few instances permanent " pitting " will possibly result. There is no constitutional disturbance of the least importance; and the accompanying pyrexia is slight throughout. There may be symptoms of catarrh. Dr. Gregory says that when the eruption is abundant, the body presents the appearance of having been exposed to a momentary shower of boiling water; each drop of which has caused a small blister.

Chicken-pox occurs but once to the same person; it has a short incubation, probably of four days; it is slightly infectious; and

* *Fifth Report of the Medical Officer of the Privy Council*, p. 6. Ordered by the House of Commons to be printed, 14 April 1863.

it requires no treatment beyond attention to the bowels, confinement to the bed-room, and restriction of the diet. When there is evidence of weakness during convalescence, proper nourishment with bark or quinine or small doses of steel will soon restore health and strength.

4. MEASLES.—Morbilli, or measles, may be described as a continued infectious fever; the result of the absorption of, and contamination of the blood by, a morbid poison. The disease is preceded by catarrh, accompanied by a crimson rash, and often attended or followed by inflammation of the mucous membrane of the organs of respiration. Severe epidemics of morbilli* occasionally prevail. As a rule, the susceptibility to this disease is destroyed by one attack. Some authors divide measles into two grades,—the *morbilli mitiores*, and the *morbilli graviores ;* but the latter only differs from the former in its greater severity, and in the fact that the eruption assumes a dark purple colour.

The length of incubation—or in other words, the time which elapses between the date of infection and the appearance of the disease is from ten to fourteen days. Sir Thomas Watson has known several instances in which it was exactly a fortnight. Occasionally, the patient suffers from languor, cough, and a sense of discomfort, during the breeding or incubative period.

The early *symptoms* of measles are lassitude, shivering, pyrexia, and catarrh ; the conjunctivæ, pituitary membrane, and mucous lining of the fauces and larynx and bronchi being much affected. Very soon there is swelling of the eyelids, with eyes suffused and watery and intolerant of light ; troublesome sneezing ; dry hacking cough, hoarseness, and severe dyspnœa ; drowsiness ; great heat of skin ; together with a frequent and hard pulse. Headache, and even pains in the back are sometimes complained of ; and there may be nausea with frequent attacks of retching, epistaxis, diarrhœa, deafness, prostration, confusion of intellect, &c. Actual delirium is rare. In young children especially, convulsions are not uncommon at the onset. Occasionally albuminuria is found. or the urine may contain blood : an abundance of urates is the most constant condition. The morbillous eruption comes out on the fourth day of the disease ; seldom doing so earlier, often being later. It consists of little circular dots, like flea-bites, which gradually coalesce into small blotches of a raspberry colour ; these presenting often a horseshoe shape, and being slightly raised above the surface of the-skin.

The rash appears first on the forehead and face, and gradually extends downwards. It begins to fade on the seventh day in the same order ; and is succeeded by slight desquamation of the cuticle, with considerable itching.

It is worthy of notice that the fever does not abate on the

---

* Morbilli, the dim. of *Morbus* = a disease. Μόρος βίον, the fate of life, *i.e.* death.

appearance of the eruption, as in small-pox ; nor does the severity of the attack at all depend upon the quantity of the rash. In many cases the patient is taken very ill, and abruptly so, on the first day of the fever. On the second and third he is better, so that the opinion of measles being the disorder is almost abandoned. But on the morning of the fourth day the lachrymation, nasal discharge, weakness, and fever, all again become aggravated ; while the rash is then seen to be commencing on the forehead. The sixth day is usually the worst. The contagion of measles is strong; but less powerful than that of variola. The disease is mostly seen in children.

The *prognosis* must depend upon the mildness or severity of the chest symptoms ; the complications most to be feared being croup, hooping cough, capillary bronchitis, collapse of the lung, pulmonary abscess, and pneumonia. Convulsions occurring towards the decline are of much more serious import than when they usher in the disease. Strumous children are comparatively unfavourable subjects for this as for other fevers. Among the children of the very poor, gangrenous stomatitis may occur; but fortunately this fearful complication is seldom met with. The diarrhœa, which often sets in as the rash declines, is for the most part beneficial.

The mortality is greater in large cities than in the country. And moreover, this disease is as fatal now as formerly. In the years 1660-79, the annual deaths from measles, in London, averaged 40 to 100,000 persons ; whereas in 1859 they were 47 to the same number. The fatality of measles is greater during the cold than the warm seasons of the year.

The *treatment* must not be too active ; and ought chiefly to be directed towards keeping the disease uncomplicated. Exposure to cold is to be carefully avoided. The patient should be confined to bed, in an apartment moderately warm. Putting the feet in hot water every evening is often beneficial. Milk diet, mucilaginous drinks, gentle aperients, and mild diaphoretics may be had recourse to. A draught, containing half a drachm of the liquor ammoniæ acetatis, ten or twenty drops of the spiritus ætheris nitrosi, and half an ounce of camphor water, may be given to a child six years old every four or six hours. The cough can often be relieved by a sinapism to the chest, and by very small doses of morphia.

The state of the three great cavities had better be carefully watched, especially towards the decline of the eruption. Should any head or chest or abdominal complications arise, they must be treated according to the rules which will be laid down in speaking of each affection. After the disease has subsided, the patient is to be warmly clad ; to be fed on easily digested nourishing food, and to have quinine and steel, with cod liver oil, if needed ; while he is not to be allowed to go out of doors too early. As one of the rare *sequelæ* of measles, paralysis may be mentioned. In the few cases which I have seen it has taken the form of paraplegia ; power being restored to the legs as the general nutrition has been improved by milk and animal food, cod liver oil with steel, and sea air. Friction of the spine and lower extremities, together with tepid salt water baths, may be recommended.

The inoculation of measles has occasionally been practised since 1758. The description of the results, however, is too contradictory to admit of any safe deduction. In this country it does not appear to have been resorted to subsequent to the commencement of the present century; and it would hardly be advisable to revive the proceeding now.

5. SCARLET FEVER.—This well-known disease may be defined as an infectious febrile affection, which manifests itself after a period of incubation of from four to six days. It is characterized by a scarlet efflorescence, of variable intensity, upon the skin and mucous membrane of the fauces and tonsils; the efflorescence commencing about the second day of the fever, and declining about the fifth. Scarlet fever, or scarlatina, is often accompanied by inflammation of the throat, and sometimes of the submaxillary glands. Like measles, it is essentially a disease of childhood; but it is more to be dreaded. As a rule, scarlet fever occurs only once during life. In the event of a second attack there is often no rash, little or no throat affection, and the disorder runs a favourable course. From my own personal experience, I can state that *scarlatina sine exanthemate* may be followed immediately by desquamation of the cuticle; and subsequently by renal congestion with albuminuria.

The scarlatinal poison is of a subtle nature, and does not appear to lose its power for some time. It attaches itself to bedding, carpets, clothes, &c.; or in other words it may be transmitted by fomites, as is proved by many medical men having carried the disease to their own families. The poison appears to be destroyed by a temperature of 205° F. The infecting power is probably greatest at the beginning of desquamation. In my opinion there is some relation between the severity of the disease in the recipient, and that in the individual yielding the poison. I know of cases somewhat like the following:—A servant girl at a small school at Hampstead paid a short visit one evening to a relative suffering from severe scarlet fever. In due time she was attacked with the disease, together with three of the pupils. All the five died. One of the boys was removed directly the first symptoms set in, and brought to a healthy locality in London. I saw him a few hours afterwards, and gave a very unfavourable prognosis; which was unfortunately justified, for he sank completely exhausted three days afterwards, in spite of the most careful nursing.

Attention has been of late directed to the circumstance that patients who have recently undergone a surgical operation, or who have wounded themselves accidentally, may suffer from a rash which cannot be distinguished from scarlatina, and which is followed by desquamation; although no history can be obtained of their having been exposed to infection. Dr. George May, of Reading, has reported* the case of a boy who suffered from a scarlet rash with fever, on the sixth day after receiving a scalp wound. The rash lasted a few days, was succeeded by complete desquamation, as well as by swelling of the glands on the left side of the neck. Yet the patient was believed to have previously suffered from scarlet fever; while there was no case of this disease in the village at the time of his illness, neither was any one else in the house affected by it. Dr. Wilks, Mr. Paget, and Mr. Hutchinson seem to have met with similar instances. It is, however, most probable that these were all examples of severe erythema, such as I have occasionally seen produced by the administration of belladonna, ôr of nux vomica. We certainly are without any evidence to show that a poison like that of scarlet fever can be generated by a surgical operation.

Varieties.—There are three varieties of this disorder. Scarlatina *simplex*, in which the skin is chiefly affected; scarlatina *anginosa*, in which both skin and throat are decidedly implicated; and scarlatina *maligna*, in which all the force of the disease seems to be expended upon the throat.

According to the researches of Dr. Fenwick it seems probable, that in all varieties a primary effect of the poison of scarlet fever is suddenly and violently to stimulate the natural cell growths of the various secreting organs. With regard to the stomach, the bloodvessels get congested, the epithelium is stripped from the tubes, and the tissues become softened. The tubes are found distended by granular and fatty matters, or by cells mixed with granules. Although it cannot be considered as proved at present, yet it is most likely, that after scarlet fever the epithelium of the stomach and intestines desquamates, just as this process takes place on the skin. The cells lining the tubules of the kidney are probably cast off in the same manner.

Scarlatina simplex, or *scarlatina sine anginá*, commences (after a latent period of from four to six days) with slight soreness about the throat, nausea or vomiting, chilliness soon succeeded by fever, lassitude, and headache. The pulse is frequent, the skin may have a temperature of 103° or 104°, deglutition is somewhat difficult, and there may be restlessness with wandering at night. Convulsions very rarely happen. The eruption appears on the second day, in the form of numberless bright red points; which show themselves first on the face and neck, then on the arms and abdomen, and lastly on the lower extremities. Sometimes the rash comes out so quickly, that in twenty-four hours from the first appearance it covers the whole body; though more commonly a day intervenes between each crop. On the limbs, but especially about the fingers, there is a diffused and continued efflorescence: upon the trunk the

* *British Medical Journal*, p. 428.   London, 8 October 1864.

rash is distributed in irregular patches. The eruption is of a bright scarlet colour, most distinct about the loins and the flexures of the joints. It very generally terminates by desquamation of the cuticle; which begins about the end of the fifth day upon those parts where the rash first appeared. On the face and trunk the desquamation is in the form of scurf; while on the hands and feet large flakes of cuticle are detached, so that sometimes a glove or slipper of scarf-skin comes away at once.

At the same time that the efflorescence has been spreading on the surface of the body, the mucous membrane of the mouth and fauces and nostrils, as well as of the gastro-intestinal canal, has also been affected. The tonsils are often congested and swollen, while the uvula is likewise seen to be œdematous. The tongue especially puts on an appearance characteristic of scarlatina. This organ, except at the tip and edges, is at first covered with a thick white fur, through which the red elongated papillæ project; but as this fur clears away, the whole tongue becomes clean and preternaturally red and of a strawberry appearance. The affection of the mucous membrane of the mouth, &c., terminates by resolution; with the disappearance of the rash the febrile symptoms subside; and the disease terminates at the end of eight or nine days, leaving the patient somewhat pulled down.

In this form, however mild the symptoms may be, as well as in the other varieties of scarlet fever, the urine should be frequently examined; more particularly as to its quantity, reaction, diminution of chlorides, and freedom from albumen. The latter abnormal ingredient is seldom met with before the sixth day, while it occurs most frequently towards the end of desquamation. The two great sources of danger in this disease are the more or less complete suppression of urine, with uræmia; and the deposition of fibrin in the right cavities of the heart.

Scarlatina anginosa is ushered in with more violent symptoms than the preceding. There is headache with some delirium, more pungent heat of the skin, troublesome vomiting, restlessness, and marked prostration. About the second day complaint is made of stiffness of the neck, uneasiness in the throat, hoarseness, and pain on swallowing. The fauces, palate, uvula, and tonsils get red and swollen; while the inflamed surfaces are found more or less covered with an exudation of coagulable lymph. As this inflammation goes on, all the febrile symptoms increase: the skin becomes very dry and hot. The temperature is 105°, or perhaps higher. The tonsils get gorged with blood; while foul and deep ulcers quickly form on them. The efflorescence does not observe the same regularity as in the simple form: it does not appear so early, is delayed to the third or fourth day, comes out in scattered patches on the chest and arms, and shows a tendency to vanish the day after its appearance and to reappear partially at uncertain times. With the fading of the eruption about the fifth or sixth day, the fever and

u 2

inflammation of the throat begin to abate; although the latter often remains sore, causing the act of deglutition to be painful and difficult, for a week or ten days after the disappearance of the rash. Occasionally this variety of scarlet fever assumes a still more aggravated form; being accompanied with an acrid discharge from the nostrils and ears, deafness, and inflammation of the parotid and cervical glands—sometimes going on to suppuration.

During the progress of the disease particular attention should be paid to the internal organs, since there is a great predisposition to inflammation of the serous and mucous membranes.

Scarlatina maligna, described by Cullen under the title of *Cynanche maligna*, differs but little in its symptoms, at first, from scarlatina anginosa. The fever, however, soon assumes a malignant or typhoid character; considerable cerebral disturbance being superadded to the affection of the fauces and skin. There is great irritability, restlessness, a feeble irregular pulse, oppressed respiration, obstruction of the fauces with viscid phlegm, occasionally diarrhœa, and generally delirium; the latter being sometimes of a violent, but usually of the low muttering kind. The tongue is dry and brown, tender and chapped; the lips, teeth, and gums are covered with sordes; and the breath is extremely fetid. The throat is not much swollen, but appears of a dusky red hue; while the velum, uvula, and tonsils are coated with dark incrustations, consisting of exudations of lymph. In some cases there is gangrenous inflammation of these parts, followed by sloughing. The cervical glands are often involved in the inflammation. The rash is exceedingly irregular as to the time of its appearance and duration; often coming out late, disappearing after a few hours, and being renewed several times during the progress of the disorder. It is at first of a pale hue, but soon becomes changed to a dark livid red; while petechiæ also often appear upon the skin.

In many instances this malignant form of scarlet fever terminates fatally on the third or fourth day. It is always a disease of such extreme danger that only patients with vigorous constitutions survive it: great hopes may be entertained, however, if the seventh day be passed.

Sequelæ.—Children who have suffered from scarlet fever are very liable to have their health permanently affected, and to become afflicted with some of the many forms of scrofula; especially strumous ulcers, ophthalmia, scrofulous enlargements of the cervical glands, abscesses in the ears, diseases of the scalp, &c. They also seem predisposed to suffer, either during the attack or shortly afterwards, from *acute rheumatism* and from *rheumatic pericarditis*.

The persistence of *otorrhœa*, or purulent discharges from one or both ears, for weeks after recovery from the fever should excite attention; since this affection not unfrequently proves the first step towards destruction of the membrana tympani, a loosening and expulsion of the ossicula auditûs, inflammation of the petrous portion of the temporal bone, and abscess of the brain. These successive phases of a troublesome disease may not be run through for ten or fourteen or twenty years; but it is not the less important to try and control the evil at the onset. The most hopeful plan for accomplishing this is to use astringent injections, to apply small flying blisters behind the affected ear, to administer steel and cod liver oil, to allow good nourishment, and to send the child to a bracing sea-side residence for a long time.

Not unfrequently, after the decline of the eruptive stage, a muco-purulent discharge takes place from the nares, and even from the mouth and fauces; while in a few instances an acrid secretion, similar in character, has flowed from the vagina in female children, and women. Considering how extensively the various mucous tracts are affected in this disease, it seems strange that *scarlatinal vaginitis* is not of more common occurrence. In one case (a girl twelve years of age) about which I was consulted, the nares, mouth, and pharynx were also affected; but the vaginal inflammation was the most obstinate, and persisted for a long time after convalescence had been firmly established. A cure was effected by the adoption of the plan of treatment just advised for obstinate otorrhœa, together with the local use of astringents. Dr. Robert Barnes and Dr. J. R. Cormack have noticed the occasional occurrence of this form of vaginitis;* though most authorities omit all mention of it.

Now and then, just as the patient is recovering from the fever, an important joint will become swollen and painful; the pulse increasing in frequency, a rigor occurring, and all that constitutional disturbance setting in which is usually indicative of the *formation of pus.* If the matter merely be developed in the connective tissue around the joint, the accident is of no great moment. On the abscess being opened all will go well, with care. But unfortunately suppuration within the joint is apt to take place; the inflammatory action starting at first in the synovial membrane, or quickly spreading to it from the outside. In either case, when pus is effused into the synovial cavity, all the structures entering into the formation of the joint begin to suffer. Erosions of the inter-articular cartilages take place; and are followed by more or less disorganization of the articular ends of the bones, alterations in the ligamentous structures, and ulcerations through the surrounding adipose and connective tissues. How to check such mischief is a very difficult question to answer satisfactorily. I know that it can be aggravated by bleeding, calomel, and antimony: by keeping the atmosphere of the sick room tainted, and allowing only a poor diet. The best remedies are probably soothing fomentations or linseed poultices; which can be put on while the part is kept perfectly quiet by means of a splint. This is to be applied gently, but so as to insure rest. Plenty of milk, raw eggs, and nourishing broths are to be the staple articles of diet. Pain ought to be moderated by sedatives. And then, as soon as

* *London Medical Gazette,* pp. 65 and 128. July and August 1850.

it is certain that pus exists, the surgeon will probably evacuate it by making a free incision in a depending position. Directly this is accomplished there will be an abatement of the urgent symptoms ; and then attempts can be made to lessen the permanent mischief as much as possible by having the joint fixed in moulded leather splints, by sending the patient to the coast, by giving him steel and cod liver oil, and by allowing the most nourishing food that the system can assimilate.

Another very serious sequel, and one which is more frequent than synovitis, is *anasarca*—serous infiltration of the subcutaneous connective tissue; this being often accompanied by dropsy of the larger serous cavities. It is apt to set in about the twenty-second day from the commencement of the fever. Now it is curious that this acute renal or scarlatinal dropsy is more frequent after a mild than after a severe attack of the fever; owing probably to the want of caution which is often observed in such cases during the period of desquamation. The patient gets exposed to cold, and immediately the escape of the fever-poison through the pores of the skin is checked ; which, as a consequence, is directed to the kidneys in larger quantities than they can bear, giving rise to *acute Bright's disease*. This renal affection has its origin from many causes (intemperance, cold, the cholera poison) besides the one we are considering ; but, however produced, its symptoms are the same. It commences usually with rigors or chilliness ; which are succeeded by feverish reaction, headache, restlessness, pain and tenderness in the loins, and often vomiting. The dropsy is an early symptom : the eyelids and face first become puffy, and then follows general swelling of the areolar tissue throughout the body, with effusion of fluid (which often contains urea) into one or more of the serous cavities. At the same time there is a frequent desire to pass urine ; though this is scanty, of a dark smoky colour, and on being tested by heat and nitric acid is found to be highly albuminous. Examined microscopically, it is seen to contain masses of coagulated fibrin, blood corpuscles, epithelial casts and cells, with occasionally crystals of uric acid. When the progress of the case is unfavourable, the secretion of urine gets nearly or completely suppressed ; death happening from convulsions or coma, the consequence of uræmic toxæmia, in some few days. Fortunately, a favourable termination is the rule ; and then the earliest signs of improvement are the disappearance of the dropsy, coincidently with an increase in the quantity of urine. It is not uncommon for a patient, during convalescence from acute desquamative nephritis, to pass from four to six pints of urine in the twenty-four hours ; the natural quantity averaging only from a pint and a half to two pints.*

* For the more full consideration of this renal affection, as well as for its treatment, &c., the reader must consult the Section on Acute Bright's Disease (Acute Albuminuria, Acute Desquamative Nephritis,&c.), in Part XI.; as well as the Sub-section on Uræmia, in Section I. of Part I.

Mortality.—In England in 1866, the deaths from scarlet fever were comparatively small, amounting only to 11,685; of which number 7719 or $\frac{3933\ males}{3786\ females}$ occurred in children under five years of age, while of these 690 were less than twelve months old. It is thus clear that young infants are not exempt from severe attacks of this disease as some authorities have asserted.

The fatality varies much in different epidemics. But speaking generally, the mortality would seem to be from 5 to 15 per cent. The most severe epidemics have generally occurred between the middle of the months of September and the commencement of December. Lastly, this fever occurs equally in both sexes.

Treatment.—The management of scarlatina yet remains to be considered The *simple form*, says Sydenham, is "fatal only through the officiousness of the doctor." It requires no treatment beyond confinement to the bedroom, a warm bath or two, proper clothing, an unstimulating diet, plenty of cold water acidulated with vinegar as a common drink, and attention to the bowels. Medical advice ought always to be sought, however, in these cases; since they are just those in which the most troublesome sequelæ are apt to occur.

.The patient should be separated from his family; but there will be little fear of the fever spreading through the house provided his room is kept efficiently ventilated, and his attendants are not allowed to mix with the other domestics. Fumigation with sulphurous acid gas (F. 74) is to be practised. Moreover, the danger of infection can scarcely be regarded as over until some few days after the termination of desquamation; while the sick-room is not again to be inhabited until it has been thoroughly purified.

By some practitioners the administration of ammonia, by others the use of acetic acid, is recommended in all cases of scarlet fever from the commencement. The chief value of these remedies seems to be, that they possess the property of keeping the fibrin of the blood fluid. The ammonia has appeared to me to prove most beneficial where there has been any tendency to depression; while the acid has been preferable when the employment of a cooling refrigerant drink has been indicated.

For *scarlatina anginosa* the treatment is often much the same as that for continued fever. Recourse is to be had to cold or tepid sponging with vinegar and water (F. 138), where there is great heat; emetics of ipecacuanha when the tongue is much coated, and when nausea and irritability of stomach exist; shaving the scalp and the application of cold lotions, where there is much delirium; and to the cautious administration of aperients when the bowels are confined. The frequent use of sulphurous acid to the throat, by means of a spray-producer as advised by Dr. James Dewar, is capable of giving great relief: in the same way, a solution of permanganate of potash does good. Iced soda water, lemonade, or saline effervescing medicines are grateful and cooling; or, where the pulse is feeble, good beef tea, milk and raw eggs, port wine and ammonia (F. 361, 371), may be beneficially ordered.

With *malignant scarlet fever*, a stimulating plan of treatment, such as that recommended in typhus, alone offers any chance of success. The vital powers are so prostrated by the deadly force of the poison, that unless we support them by the free administration of brandy or wine, quinine or ammonia and bark, they will fail altogether. Cold affusion (F. 134) does good where there is any tendency to coma. The gangrenous ulceration of the fauces, which often complicates this form, will be also best combated by the use of stimulants; as well as by the free local application of the carbolic acid or permanganate of potash or sulphurous acid spray (F. 262). Such fine medicated sprays are more easily used and more efficacious than all the gargles which can be thought of. Sucking ice or calf's-foot jelly gives temporary relief, at least. The chlorate of potash drink (F. 360) will be useful. Chlorine itself is used by some practitioners, who speak highly of its good effects, in even the worst cases (F. 77). Possibly some preparation of oxygen (F. 370) might be tried with advantage.

For *dropsy following scarlet fever* the compound jalap powder is an excellent remedy. Elaterium also often does great good; provided it be given early in the disease, and before the patient is very weak. Its effects must be carefully watched, however, as the severe purging and vomiting which it induces may give rise to great exhaustion. It can be given to children of ten years of age, in doses varying from the twelfth to the sixth of a grain; repeating it every two hours until its action is freely manifested. On the day following the exhibition of the purgative, the tincture of the perchloride of iron may be commenced, or the syrup of iodide of iron with cod liver oil. Digitalis, in combination with steel, is valuable. The diet should be very generous, without any stimulants. Warm baths are particularly useful, as is the vapour bath. After an attack of acute desquamative nephritis great care should be taken for a long time to clothe the patient warmly, with flannel next to the skin; to send him to the coast, if possible; to continue some preparation of steel until all symptoms of anæmia, as well as all traces of albuminuria, have subsided; and to feed him with wholesome food, containing plenty of fatty matters.

Belladonna, in very minute doses, has been recommended as a *prophylactic* against scarlatina. In an epidemic of this disease which occurred on board her Majesty's ships *Agamemnon* and *Odin* in 1853, the remedy was freely tried without the slightest benefit. Belladonna has also now been used by many practitioners, and found useless. It may be worth mentioning, that in using this drug for the relief of uterine and other diseases, I have sometimes found it produce an extensive erythematous rash bearing a close resemblance to the eruption of scarlet fever. The resemblance has been so close, and the accompanying heat of skin and general disturbance have been so great, that experienced practitioners have been misled and have formed a wrong diagnosis. To prevent any error it will suffice to see that the patient is taking belladonna; and to find that the symptoms rapidly subside on leaving off this drug and substituting for it a few doses of fluid magnesia with plenty of diluents.

6. DENGUE.—This affection, very rarely seen in Great Britain, is an epidemic, and perhaps infectious, fever; which is attended with an exanthematous eruption, severe headache, pain in one eyeball or behind one ear, and very distressing rheumatic or neuralgic pains in the limbs and joints. Sometimes the throat is inflamed, occasionally the testicles enlarge, and often the lymphatic glands of the neck and groin swell. . One attack affords subsequent protection. The disease often gives rise to severe symptoms, but seems to be seldom fatal. It lasts from eight or ten days, to five or six weeks: remissions and relapses are common. It is known as *Dengue,* a name of uncertain derivation; as *Dandy fever,* in the West Indies; as *Breakbone Fever,* in Philadelphia; and as *Scarlatina rheumatica, Eruptive articular fever, Eruptive rheumatic fever,* &c., in other countries.

An affection supposed to be dengue prevailed in Philadelphia in 1780. This fever was common in many parts of the East Indies, and especially in Calcutta, in 1824-25; in the West India Islands, in 1827-28; and during the same years in the Southern States of America, where it was also epidemic in 1847 and 1849. Again, in 1859-60, it became epidemic in Virginia; where it prevailed so universally that one practitioner alone (Dr. R. T. Lemmon) attended upwards of three hundred cases. Out of this number only ten died. Of these fatal cases, four were negroes over seventy years of age; one was a child, who was teething and had convulsions; two deaths were from tetanus; one from congestion of the lungs; one from epistaxis; and one from softening of the liver and stomach, with the symptoms of yellow fever.* As an illustration of the way in which all classes have been attacked in these epidemics it may be mentioned, that the editor of the *Southern Medical and Surgical Journal,* in his issue for December 1849, apologizes for typographical errors by saying,—"The editor, publisher, and printers are all suffering from *breakbone fever."* The population of the village of New Iberia, in Louisiana, did not exceed 250 in the year 1851. Yet, according to Dr. Duperier, in six weeks 210 of the residents had gone through an attack of this fever; while 40 of the inhabitants of the neighbourhood had also suffered from it.

The attack usually commences suddenly with vomiting, headache, and pains in the limbs. Sometimes there is chilliness, but distinct rigors are uncommon. The joints swell; beginning per-

* *The American Medical Times.* Vol. ii. p. 120. New York, 1861.

haps with one knee, or only with the small articulations of the hands and feet. Pain at the back of the neck, often starting from one mastoid process, is not uncommon. The headache is usually severe, and may be conjoined with pain in the eyeballs. The skin is hot and dry; all appetite is lost, while there is much thirst; the tongue is red; the bowels are torpid; and the pulse is small and feeble, sometimes being very rapid and sometimes remarkably infrequent. Violent cramps in the muscles of the extremities, abdomen, loins, or chest are not uncommon. The articular pains may be so severe that the slightest movement causes a sharp cry. The testicles and other glands swell. Perhaps about the end of the third day, it may be much earlier, there is a remission of the fever; the patient being left in a state of prostration. But on the fifth or sixth day the nausea and heat of skin and muscular pains return; and this time an eruption appears. This eruption is said by some observers to consist of a scarlet efflorescence, which commences on the palms of the hands and rapidly spreads over the body. But according to Dr. Lemmon, the character of the rash is not uniform; for in some of his cases it simulated scarlatina, in others chicken-pox, and in others herpes annularis. Then the symptoms gradually subside, unless there have been any complications,—such as pneumonia, bronchitis, jaundice, erysipelas, carbuncle, rheumatic ophthalmia, or tetanus. There may be general desquamation, but this is not constant. The disease always leaves the sufferer much weakened; while sometimes convalescents are annoyed with attacks of neuralgia and myalgia, necessitating the employment of quinine with large quantities of nourishment.

The remedies required in the management of a case of dengue are not numerous. The disease has a strong tendency to end favourably, after running a certain course which drugs cannot abridge; and consequently all that can be done by the physician is to guard against complications, and to relieve any urgent symptoms as they arise. Antacid purgatives will perhaps be useful, as may sudorifics; while the relief of pain by opium always proves grateful to the patient, without being provocative of any injurious consequences. Where profuse sweating sets in at the end of a few days, it is generally critical; and consequently should not be checked. During convalescence, bark or quinine, with milk and animal food, will best assist in making the recovery sure. Alcoholic stimulants have also been found beneficial.

7. ERYSIPELAS.—This is a specific disease (popularly called in Scotland the *Rose*, in this country *St. Anthony's fire*) characterized by a low form of fever, with a diffused and spreading inflammatory affection of the skin, and very commonly of the subcutaneous connective tissue.

Erysipelas [from 'Ερύω = to draw + πέλας = near—expressive of its tendency to spread; or, according to German lexicographers, from Ἐρυθρὸς = red + πελλος = livid—livid redness] is accompanied by the general phenomena of fever; while the affected structures all become of a deep red colour, hot, painful, and swollen. It is a miasmatic disease, due to the absorption of a specific poison. The miasm is most readily generated by the assembling together, in one ward, of patients with unhealthy discharges or secretions; especially if there be faulty ventilation, and a meagre employment of disinfectants.

No portion of the surface of the body is exempt from attacks of this disorder. But the integuments of the face and head are most commonly the seats of *idiopathic* erysipelas—that which arises from internal causes; while *traumatic* erysipelas, or such as follows wounds, commences at or around the seat of injury.

Idiopathic erysipelas resembles the other eruptive fevers; inasmuch as its phenomena are preceded by a period of incubation which varies from three to seven days, and are accompanied by fever and general constitutional disturbance. If often sets in with chilliness followed by distinct rigors; sore throat is an early and frequent accompaniment of it; occasionally the urine contains albumen, but the chlorides are always diminished; and disturbance of the cerebral functions, nausea, vomiting, and diarrhœa will often also be present. The delirium may be of that low, muttering kind frequently observed in fever; or the patient, especially if he be of intemperate habits, turns out noisy and violent. Then, on the second or third morning from the rigor, redness and swelling appear on some part of the skin; frequently on one side of the nose, spreading to the rest of the face, and often extending over the scalp, neck, and shoulders. The lips swell, the cheeks enlarge, the eyes become closed by their puffy lids, and all traces of the natural features are completely lost. The temperature of the body ranges between 99° and 105°; the pulse is frequent, 100 to 120; the lymphatic vessels and glands in the neighbourhood of the disease are apt to get inflamed; and the tongue will be found thickly furred, or dry and of a dark brown colour. After three or four days, the redness fades, the swelling subsides, and the cuticle desquamates. In most cases the inflammation is merely superficial, and the disorder is then spoken of as *simple* or *cutaneous* erysipelas; but occasionally it affects the subcutaneous connective tissue (*phlegmonous* or *cellulo-cutaneous* erysipelas) and is then apt to be followed by suppuration and sloughing, or even by gangrene.

Erysipelas now and then proves fatal, by the extension of the inflammation to the brain or its membranes, giving rise to effusion and coma. The same result may occur from the mucous membrane of the glottis becoming affected, so that the chink gets closed, and the patient dies unexpectedly from suffocation. In other cases, death is owing to the failure of the vital powers. The presence of albumen in the urine is unfavourable, especially if it be the result of pre-existing renal disease. Erysipelas occurring in cases of diabetes, gout, cancer, &c., is very dangerous.

Erysipelas can be generated by inattention to sanitary laws. It is infectious, and it spreads by fomites. One attack is no safeguard against subsequent seizures. A medical man should never visit a lying-in patient on the same day that he attends a case of this disease, without changing his clothes and using some disinfectant solution to his hands. The poison of erysipelas can undoubtedly give rise to puerperal fever. When erysipelas prevails epidemically, as it sometimes does, intemperance and insufficient food and foul air and trifling injuries favour its occurrence. If the disease breaks out in a hospital, the ward where it has appeared should be cleared out and thoroughly cleaned, to prevent the spread of the poison through the entire building.

The *mortality* from erysipelas in England averages about 1800 annually. It is remarkable that the figures fluctuate very slightly. Thus, for ten years (1857-1866) the highest number for any one year is 2104; while the lowest is 1523. Both sexes suffer equally.

The *treatment* must be conducted on the principle that it is more important to lead the disorder to a safe termination, than to try and cut it short by active remedies. At the commencement, the diet ought to be light; ice and cooling drinks may be freely given; while the patient must be confined to bed in a well-ventilated room. In the country, when the patients are young and vigorous, bleeding is commonly considered necessary : in London such practice would almost invariably be bad. The cases which have fallen under my own notice, have certainly been characterized by evidence of debility; and I have consequently followed the practice of those physicians who adopt a tonic mode of treatment as the great rule in idiopathic erysipelas. The late Dr. Robert Williams, of St. Thomas's Hospital, gave all his erysipelatous patients milk diet, sago, very gentle purgatives, and from four to six ounces of port wine daily, from the very first appearance of the disease, irrespective of the symptoms or the part affected. Speaking of the result he says, in his admirable work—"I have pursued this system for several years, and I hardly remember a case in which it has not been successful."* The carbonate of ammonia (F. 361, 371) will often prove an excellent substitute for wine. Bark or quinine can also be recommended.

In addition to the administration of wine, there are some cases where the tincture of perchloride of iron does great good. This medicine had better be commenced early; and the dose must vary from thirty or forty minims every four hours in mild cases, to half a drachm every hour in urgent instances. According to some writers, attacks of erysipelas which would probably run on for

* *Elements of Practical Medicine. Morbid Poisons,* vol. i. 284. London, 1836-39.

eight or ten days may be cured in three or four days by this preparation of iron. I have, moreover, found it answer better than ammonia where there has been albuminuria.

Of all the local applications which have been recommended, that which gives the most relief is the fomentation by flannels wrung out of a hot decoction of poppy-heads, assiduously applied. Flour freely dusted over the inflamed part has often a soothing cooling effect in mild cases; but it is apt to form a crust, which subsequently adheres to and greatly irritates the inflamed part. Some surgeons recommend painting the affected region with collodion; an agent which not only serves to protect the skin, but to contract the congested vessels. To check the extension of the inflammation, boundary lines may be drawn on the sound skin with tincture of iodine or the solid nitrate of silver.

With regard to the phlegmonous form of the disease, when suppuration has taken place and pus has become infiltrated through the areolar tissue, long and free incisions ought to be made to give it exit. Moreover, in these cases opiates, tonics, wine or brandy, and nourishing food, will have to be assiduously given.

For the cure of *infantile erysipelas*, the child's strength must be supported. If the mother's milk be deficient in quantity or quality, a vigorous wet-nurse should be obtained. Cordials—such as white wine whey, wine and water, &c., may be given to the youngest patient. In unhealthy children the slightest wound will possibly cause the development of this disease. Two infants are reported by the Registrar-General to have died in England, from erysipelas following vaccination, during 1861.

8. **THE PLAGUE.**—This most malignant disease, though generally classed among the exanthemata, is said to be, strictly speaking, a continued contagious fever, bearing a striking resemblance to severe typhus. Indeed, among those practitioners who have had the opportunity of observing both diseases, the opinion is almost unanimous that the plague of the torrid is the typhus of the temperate climate. And, moreover, that what proves now to be only an epidemic of typhus would, some two centuries back, have been the plague.

The plague is now a disease exclusively of Eastern occurrence. It is not seen in Europe in the present day, because the improved sanitary arrangements do not permit of typhus becoming intensified or fostered into plague. The sanitary condition of Egypt, however, is in many respects the same as it was a century ago. Dr. Mead, in assigning the reason why Cairo is the birthplace and cradle of the disorder, says—" Cairo is crowded with vast numbers of inhabitants, who live poorly, and nastily; the streets are narrow and close; the heat is stifling; a great canal passes through the city, which at the overflowing of the Nile is filled with water; on the decrease of the river this canal is usually dried up, and the people throw into it all manner of filth, carrion, and offal; the stench which arises from this and the mud together is intolerably offensive, and from this source the plague, constantly springing up every year, preys upon the inhabitants, and is stopped only by the return of the Nile, the overflowing of which washes away this load of filth. In Ethiopia the swarms of locusts are so prodigious that they sometimes cause a famine by devouring the fruits of the earth, and when they die create a pestilence by the putrefaction of their bodies. The effluvia which arise from this immense quantity of putrefying animal substance, combined with so much heat and moisture, continually generate the plague in its intensest form; and the Egyptians of old were so sensible how much the putrefaction of dead animals contributed towards breeding the plague, that they worshipped the bird ibis from the services that it did in devouring great numbers of serpents, which they observed injured by their stench when dead as much as by their bite when alive."*

The plague may be defined as a fatal contagious fever, which is due to the absorption of a poison that infects the blood. There is a period of incubation, probably varying from a few hours to three weeks. The force of the poison is chiefly exerted on the cervical, axillary, inguinal, and mesenteric glands, as is shown in the production of buboes; on the skin, causing carbuncles; and on the heart, liver, and spleen, giving rise to great congestion and softening. The disease produces at once great restlessness; extreme and rapidly increasing exhaustion; an indescribable feeling of oppression about the præcordia; fever of greater or less intensity; a peculiar rolling of the eyes; nausea and vomiting; emaciation; bleeding at the nose; swelling of the tongue; laborious breathing; darting pains in the axillæ and groins, with large buboes, carbuncles, &c.; constipation; and sometimes suppression of urine. The powers of life soon give way, and death either ensues without a struggle in two or three days, or is ushered in by an attack of convulsions. This intense form of the disease is generally observed at the commencement of an epidemic, when the deaths may be 90 per cent.; but after a time a milder (though still very dangerous) variety sets in. When recovery is going to take place, profuse sweats occur about the fifth day.

At the time this fearful pestilence (described as the *Black Death*, and the *Great Mortality*) desolated Europe, Asia, and Africa, in the fourteenth century, the mortality must have been immense; for it has been computed that Europe alone lost 25,000,000 of inhabitants by it. The last epidemic which raged in England—the "Great Plague"—was in 1665, the year preceding the great fire of London; when nearly one-third (68,596) of the population of the City perished from it. Supposing that this disease had occurred in London in 1859, when the population was 2,774,338, and had

* Quoted from the *Report on Quarantine.* General Board of Health, p. 37. London, 1840.

proved fatal in the same proportion, it would have been the cause of 600,000 deaths.

Most authorities now agree that the only place in which the plague originates is Egypt, from whence it is imported into other countries. To prevent the crew of a vessel with plague on board infecting the inhabitants of a tropical seaport town, recourse is still had to quarantine; which I believe is generally of not less than twenty-one days' duration.

One attack probably affords only slight security against another. When in attendance upon any case the practitioner had better carefully avoid all contact with the patient, or his clothes or bedding; while he should endeavour so to time his visits as not to pay them when exhausted from want of food or rest.

The principal remedies appear to consist of emetics, mild aperients, and diaphoretics. If employed, however, these agents should be used guardedly and with a skilful hand. Some authorities speak highly of the mineral acids; which on theoretical grounds would seem to be valuable. Quinine sometimes proves useful. Opium is often needed to allay irritation. Nourishment and stimulants are to be resorted to as if the case were one of severe typhus. Disinfectants should be systematically used, free ventilation ought to be enforced, and the patient must be kept scrupulously clean. Friction of the body with oil, has also been recommended as a preventive measure.

PART III.
VENEREAL DISEASES.

I. BALANITIS.

BALANITIS [from βάλανος = the glans penis; with the terminal -itis—from Ἵημί = to impel, and signifying inflammation when added to the Greek name of an organ], or *external clap*, or *gonorrhœa præputialis*, consists of inflammation, with redness and patches of excoriation, about the glans penis and internal surface of the prepuce. Some practitioners call the affection balanitis when only the glans is affected, and balano-posthitis [βάλανος, πόσθη = the skin covering the glans, and the terminal -itis], when it is complicated with inflammation of the lining of the prepuce. This refinement, however, can scarcely be necessary, as the two conditions are very rarely seen separate.

Causes.—The presence of the prepuce predisposes to this disease by keeping up the delicacy of the mucous covering of the glans, and by permitting retention of the sebaceous secretious from the numerous glandulæ odoriferæ about the corona. Balanitis is not met with in men who have been circumcised.

The exciting cause of the inflammation is the application of some irritant,—as menstrual blood, the muco-purulent secretion of vaginitis, the matter of gonorrhœa, or acrid leucorrhœal discharges. Inattention to cleanliness will alone induce it, however, without any sexual intercourse. Secondary syphilitic discharges from the uterus have the property of producing balanitis of a specific nature, which may be followed by thickening of the prepuce and constitutional infection. Mr. Langston Parker very properly insists, that in these cases a positive inoculation takes place; and he gives examples of its occurrence.

A similar affection to balanitis, due to causes of a like kind, will now and then arise in the female. *Vulvitis* is most frequently met with in women about eighteen or twenty years of age. It has, however, been observed in young children, from the irritation of teething or of worms; or it sometimes sets in during the progress of one of the eruptive fevers (particularly scarlatina), especially where there has been a dread of cleanliness.

Symptoms.—Heat and itching, with a muco-purulent discharge, are the first indications. On denuding the glans, its surface (as well as that of the prepuce) will be found coated with discharge, or covered here and there with flakes of curd-like matter; beneath which are patches of redness and occasionally of excoriation. There is seldom any pain in passing water.

Sometimes the prepuce becomes œdematous; and either from this cause, or because the orifice is naturally very contracted, it may be impossible to draw the foreskin back over the glans. This condition is known as *phymosis;* and so long as it exists the practitioner should give a guarded opinion as to the nature of the discharge, since the long narrow prepuce will perhaps be concealing a chancre. Moreover, a similar condition of the foreskin has sometimes led to the formation of an abscess, and even to gangrene. Occasionally simple balanitis gives rise to a sympathetic *bubo;* which, however, very rarely suppurates. Balanitis may also be complicated with gonorrhœa.

Treatment.—Simple balanitis is readily removed by cleanliness, a light touch with lunar caustic, or the application of any astringent wash. Painting the parts with the solution of subacetate of lead, or with a solution of nitrate of silver (two or three grains to half an ounce of distilled water), or the injection under the foreskin of an alum wash, often suffices. Sometimes the mere washing and drying of the part, twice in the twenty-four hours, with the application of a fine layer of cotton wool between the glans and prepuce will quickly effect a cure.

Where the disease has induced phymosis, cold bread and water poultices should be applied, or the penis can advantageously be enveloped in lint kept wet with the dilute solution of subacetate of lead. Such remedies will soon remove all swelling and permit of retraction of the foreskin. But when this condition is congenital, and the muco-purulent discharge continues in spite of the proper use of injections, it will be desirable to perform circumcision; or if this be objected to, the prepuce ought to be slit up. Where, however, there is an insuperable dread of any operation, the opening of the foreskin may be stretched by introducing and separating the blades of a fine pair of dressing forceps, or by using a sponge-tent (F. 426) for a few hours. As soon as the glans has been uncovered and the remedy applied, the foreskin should always be drawn forwards again; since, if this be neglected, paraphymosis will probably ensue, the constriction leading to great swelling with pain about the glans.

II. GONORRHŒA.

Gonorrhœa [from Γονὴ = the semen + ῥέω – to flow, hence improperly applied to the disease under consideration], or *blennorrhagia* [βλέννα = mucus or slime + ῥήγνυμι = to burst forth], or *blennorrhœa* [βλίννα + ῥέω], or vulgarly the *clap*, is a specific inflammation, more or less acute, of one or more parts of the genito-urinary passages, accompanied by a discharge. It demands notice under three heads :—As it occurs in an acute form in the male, in a chronic form (gleet), and as it affects the female.

1. GONORRHŒA IN THE MALE.—This disease is an inflammation (a specific urethritis) of the mucous membrane lining the urethra,—generally of the anterior portion ; and it is accompanied by the flow of a highly contagious purulent or mucopurulent fluid.

Gonorrhœa has been recognised as an " uncleanness" from the earliest times. It was in reference to this disorder (as we learn from the 15th chapter of Leviticus) that Moses and Aaron were commanded to speak to the children of Israel—" When any man hath a running issue out of his flesh, because of his issue he is unclean."

Causes.—The common cause is the application of gonorrhœal matter during sexual intercourse. Although the existence of this animal poison has only been inferred from the effects, yet there can be but little doubt that there is such a poison of a special nature ; and that it does not arise simply from indiscriminate sexual intercourse. Though at first the morbid material seems to produce only a local disease, yet it certainly infects the system, manifesting its power particularly on the fibrous tissues ; for only on this supposition can the occurrence of such a disease as gonorrhœal rheumatism be explained.

At the same time it must be remembered that the application of many different kinds of irritants will produce a disease closely resembling the clap. These non-specific inflammations are attended with a muco-purulent discharge ; but the latter is perhaps, as a general rule, thinner and less abundant than that which is poured out in true gonorrhœa. They may arise from connexion with a woman who is free from any specific disease. A female suffering from severe leucorrhœa, inflammation of the vagina, simple excoriation of the lips of the uterus, or from malignant ulceration of the cervix, can communicate a discharge having the characters of a gonorrhœa. She may do the same if too indolent to wash herself, or if she permit intercourse during menstruation. And if suffering from an acrid purulent discharge, owing to constitutional syphilis affecting the uterus, she is very likely to irritate, and perhaps to inoculate, whoever has connexion with her. Moreover, it is not unlikely that unduly frequent intercourse, between parties quite healthy, may beget simple inflammation. While it is quite possible for a prostitute to have true gonorrhœal matter left in her vagina that will infect her next visitor, but which exerts no unfavourable influence upon the insensible mucous membrane of her own genital organs.

A spurious gonorrhœa now and then arises without any sexual congress.   Thus, it is sometimes met with in young children, owing to the irritation of worms in the rectum or of teething.   So it can be induced in adults by masturbation, habitual costiveness, the immoderate use of alcoholic stimulants, or by calculi in the bladder or ureters.   I have even heard a credulous surgeon suggest that making water in the cold night air might induce urethritis, just as exposure to wet may cause common catarrh.

Symptoms.—Between the date of exposure to the source of contagion and the appearance of the symptoms, there is an interval varying from twenty-four hours to five or six days.   Probably three days may be taken as the average time of incubation.   The affection then begins with heat and itching about the glans, a puffiness and redness of the urethral orifice, and shortly afterwards a kind of sanious or glairy discharge.   The latter soon increases in quantity, becomes muco-purulent, and has a greenish or yellowish tinge.   On passing water a burning pain or scalding is experienced, this symptom being most acute in first attacks.   And then there may be pain in the groins, a thickening with tenderness of the urethra, tenesmus, irritability of the bladder, as well as a sense of weight and dragging in the testicles ; while occasionally there is feverishness, with more or less severe constitutional disturbance.

When the disease is located in the fossa navicularis (that portion of the urethra within the glans penis) the pain of micturition is confined to this part, and the discharge is comparatively small in quantity ; when in the spongy portion, extending from the glans to the bulb, chordee is frequent, and the discharge abundant ; when the bulbous portion is affected, there is pain in the perineum, chordee, and considerable irritability of the bladder ; while where the membranous part has to bear the brunt of the disease there is most severe pain in the perineum, a frequent desire to micturate, tenesmus, and perhaps swelling of the prostate and testicles.   In all cases the rule is, that the symptoms diminish between the tenth and twentieth days ; while shortly afterwards the inflammation either subsides entirely, or it takes on a chronic character, and a gleet becomes established.

Diagnosis.—The only disease with which it is important that a gonorrhœa should not be confounded, is a primary sore in the urethra.   In the latter, the ulcer will frequently be visible on everting the edges of the urethra ; while the discharge is found to be small in quantity, sanious, and bloody.   On examining the urethra, a circumscribed and painful induration can generally be felt.

Complications.—The most frequent is *chordee*, in which there is erection with a bending of the penis into the form of a bow.   This annoying condition is said to be due to inflammation of the corpus spongiosum, impeding expansion of its erectile tissue ; but the explanation is not very satisfactory.   Voluptuous dreams, warmth,

x 2

highly spiced or seasoned food, and alcoholic stimulants are likely to excite it.   When the chordee is severe, it may cause rupture of one or more small vessels, so that *hæmorrhage from the urethra* results. *Balanitis,* perhaps with œdema of the prepuce, may occur from the irritation of the discharge ; this being most common when there is phymosis.   *Sympathetic bubo* will perhaps take place ; the inguinal glands, however, rarely suppurating.   An *abscess* occasionally forms, either in the urethra, or in the perineum,—perhaps owing to in-flammation of Cowper's glands.   *Prostatitis* and *cystitis* are now and then induced, very probably in consequence of an extension (not a metastasis) of the inflammatory action.   So, in the same way, *epididymitis* is not unfrequently set up ; the inflammation being confined to the epididymis, though the whole testicle looks swollen, perhaps from an accumulation of serum in the tunica vagi-nalis.   And lastly *gonorrhœal rheumatism*—sometimes accompanied by *gonorrhœal ophthalmia,* may supervene ; setting in either during the acute stage, or in the decline of the disease, or after the discharge has ceased.   With regard to gonorrhœal conjunctivitis being always the result of the direct application of the virus to the mucous covering of the eyeball, I can only say that I am very sceptical.   That this kind of ophthalmia is sometimes constitu-tional, like the rheumatism, I am strongly inclined to believe.

Treatment.—In the choice of remedies something must depend upon the stage at which the disorder is seen.   But the object of the practitioner should always be to stop permanently the dis-charge,—which indeed is synonymous with effecting a cure.

No one remedy can be strongly recommended—there is no specific.   On the other hand, a caution is necessary with regard to two drugs, which are still very frequently employed, are generally inefficient, are very nauseous, and which often do much mischief to the stomach.   These medicines are balsam of copaiba and cubeb pepper.   Without saying that they are never to be prescribed, yet I would guard their administration with so many " ifs," as almost to amount to a prohibition.   Thus, if the disease be in an early stage, and the inflammatory symptoms urgent, they are inadmis-sible ; if there is constitutional disturbance, they are to be avoided ; and so also, if the bladder be irritable, if there be chordee, if there be a sense of dragging weight in the testicles, if there be a ten-dency to skin eruptions, or if nausea is readily induced.   With regard to the use of antimony, mercury, and turpentine, nothing need be said ; inasmuch as no educated practitioner would now think of attempting to subdue a gonorrhœa by them.

There are some few cases where, if the disease be seen almost at the outset, it may be checked by what is called the *abortive* treatment.   This consists essentially in the injection, by the prac-titioner, directly after the patient has passed water, of a strong solu-tion of nitrate of silver (from 5 to 10 grains in one ounce of distilled water) ; the tube of the syringe being formed of silver electro-

gilded, and having a length of an inch and a half.   Directly after
the injection, an active purgative is to be taken; there is to be
complete rest for the day; and all stimulating food and drink
must be strictly avoided.   After each micturition the patient may
employ an injection of one drachm of the solution of subacetate of
lead, or five grains of sulphate of zinc, to three ounces of water.
If there be much pain, the penis should be perseveringly bathed
with hot water; while a suppository of two grains of opium can
be introduced into the rectum, after the bowels have acted freely.
Supposing this treatment to be successful, the discharge will be
found very much diminished in quantity and consistence at the
end of twenty-four or thirty-six hours; and then a cure can possibly be effected in two or three days more by continuing the use
of the lead or zinc injections (gradually increasing the intervals
between each use of the syringe), by a diet free from stimulants,
and by the avoidance of much exercise.   Now this plan of treatment has not merely the disadvantage of being applicable only at
the commencement of the disease, but it is liable to lead to most
serious results.   In some cases it has induced very violent inflammation of the urethra, ending in abscess, or in stricture; it has
caused severe testitis; while in a few instances it has even produced
peritonitis.   Hence it will only be advisable to resort to the
abortive treatment under exceptional circumstances, and when a
rapid cure is demanded at all hazard; while it should never be
practised without warning the patient of the risk he is incurring,
and the necessity for his strict attention to the rules laid down.

For the ordinary class of cases the remedies which promise most
are,—aperients, a careful unstimulating diet, as much rest as
attention to business will allow, and mild injections.   While
using the latter, one of the potash salts had better be given.   Mr.
Milton speaks strongly of the efficacy of a draught made with fifty
grains of acetate of potash, thirty minims of spirit of nitrous ether,
and one ounce of water; which is to be taken twice or thrice daily.
If the pain be considerable, warm baths will afford much relief.
The best aperients are jalap, compound scammony powder, the
rhubarb and henbane pill, or the effervescent citro-tartrate of soda.
In the shape of food, white fish, mutton, vegetables, eggs, tea, and
milk may be allowed; but we ought to forbid all salt meats, soups,
"made dishes," pastry, cheese, coffee, beer, and spirits.   It is
sometimes impossible for the patient to avoid taking wine; and a
little sherry, or claret, with water or soda water, will form the least
injurious beverage of the kind.   Tobacco, whether smoked or used
as snuff, may possibly not prove injurious, but it certainly will not
assist the cure.   As regards the injection, some prefer the sulphate
of zinc or copper, some the chloride of zinc, some the nitrate of
silver or alum, &c.   But that which has appeared to me to be
generally the most useful is made with one fluid drachm of the
solution of subacetate of lead to four ounces of water: and this

should be employed every eight or twelve hours. ‧ When it appears to lose its effect, as it will do in a few days, the sulphate of zinc (two grains to the ounce of water), or the nitrate of silver (one grain to the ounce) ought to be substituted.

To prevent erections and chordee, a combination of camphor and belladonna will be found valuable. Five grains of the former, with half or two-thirds of a grain of the latter, in a pill at bed-time, will generally succeed; especially if the patient sleep on a mattress, without too much covering. To hinder his lying on his back, a reel for cotton can be fastened over the spine by means of a tape. To guard against the occurrence of testitis, a suspensory bandage should be worn; more particularly if the patient is obliged to walk much. For the scalding, bathing the penis with water as hot as can be borne, and drinking freely of weak tea or plain water may be recommended. Hæmorrhage from the urethra will easily be checked by the application of cold, or of two or three grains of tannic acid in a little cocoa butter, or by pressure. If there be retention of urine, a catheter had better not be used until a hot bath and a dose of opium have failed to remove the obstruction. And then any other complications which may arise must be remedied according to the rules which ordinarily guide the practitioner in the management of rheumatism, ophthalmia, testitis, prostatitis, &c.

The practitioner is occasionally asked how the danger of contagion may be obviated? There are perhaps some who would refuse to answer the question, or would reply in the words of John Sintelaer,—"The only preservative against catching the venereal, is to keep the finger out of the red-hot frying-pan." But it seems better to admit that there is no specific for this purpose; and that the only precautions which can be taken are, not to prolong the congress, to pass water immediately afterwards, and to bathe the penis thoroughly.

2. CHRONIC GONORRHŒA, OR GLEET.—This disease consists of a mild chronic inflammation of some portion of the urethra. It is attended with a slight discharge; but is unaccompanied by scalding or pain during micturition. It is not unfrequently the sequel to an acute attack of gonorrhœa.

A gleet may depend upon many circumstances, but in a large number of cases it would seem that the urethra is appreciably affected. In other words, on passing a bougie one or more portions of the mucous membrane of this canal will be found irritable and somewhat contracted, perhaps in a condition resembling that observed in granular conjunctivitis; or there may be detected a permanent stricture, from thickening of the mucous membrane or from the effusion of coagulable lymph into the connective tissue around the urethra. Irritation of the prostate, or of the neck of the bladder, will perhaps be the cause of the discharge in another class of cases;* while it can also be kept up by constitutional debility arising from debauchery and malpractices. The discharge is generally transparent, and of a mucous character; but on a minute examination it will be seen to contain pus corpuscles with scales of epithelium. Where there is irritation of the prostate or of the neck of the bladder, the patient will be troubled with oft-repeated calls to pass water; while the urine will be found on standing to deposit more or less tenacious mucus. Pain in the perineum is frequently complained of, sometimes with irritation at the end of the penis.

Unless properly treated, a gleet or blennorrhœa may continue for many months; occasionally ceasing for a few days, and then returning again and again, much to the patient's disgust. It is therefore important to discover the cause of the discharge, as only on the removal of this can a permanent cure be looked for. In all cases a temperate mode of life is necessary, and care should be taken that the digestive organs act efficiently. Then, if there be an organic stricture, this must be dilated; the discharge generally ceasing as the effused lymph becomes absorbed. If patches of the urethra are contracted and over-sensitive, the use of a bougie smeared with some astringent ointment, twice or thrice a week, will be needed. The nature of the ointment should vary with the irritability of the urethra, as it is necessary to cause moderate smarting. Equal parts of the mercurial and compound subacetate of lead ointments may suffice; or the ointment of nitrate of mercury, diluted with from two to eight parts of lard, will often be better; or the spermaceti ointment, with from twenty to sixty grains of nitrate of silver to the ounce, is occasionally needed. The bougie ought generally to be allowed to remain in the urethra for from ten to forty minutes. In very obstinate cases, the solid nitrate of silver, applied by means of Lallemand's porte caustique, can be recommended. Moreover, it is sometimes advisable, while the medicated bougie is being thus employed by the practitioner, for the patient to use an injection night and morning, of subacetate of lead (twenty or thirty minims of the officinal solution to the ounce of water), or of chloride of zinc (one or two grains to the ounce).

Where there is irritation about the prostate or neck of the bladder, bougies and astringent injections will only increase the mischief. The treatment then resolves itself into the removal of this irritation; the best remedies being warm baths, opium and belladonna suppositories at night (F. 340), and frequent doses of the officinal infusion of bearberry (uva ursi), or of buchu, or of decoction of pareira. In certain troublesome cases the iodide of potassium (F. 31) has given relief more speedily than other remedies; while, sometimes, painting the under surface of the urethra and the perineum with tincture of iodine proves useful. By Mr. Milton and some practitioners, blisters to the perineum and penis seem to be justly regarded as valuable applications.

For cases where the gleet is kept up by constitutional debility, tonics will be required. An excellent mixture can be made with phosphoric acid, nux vomica, and bark (F. 376); or gallic acid (F. 103,) or the ammonia iron-alum (F. 116), or steel and cantharides (F. 400) may be ordered. There is one disadvantage, however, in ferruginous tonics which is generally overlooked, viz. that they are apt to induce a desire for sexual intercourse; this drawback being scarcely removed by the fact that obstinate gleets have sometimes been cured by connexion. It is no doubt true that the thin mucous discharge of a gleet is harmless to a healthy female; but it must be remembered that any excess in spiced food, wine, &c. may quickly render the secretion purulent, and then there is at least a possibility of infection. Lastly, it must be mentioned, that when a gleet continues obstinate in an individual of a strumous constitution, cod liver oil, sea bathing, and a nourishing diet will be required; that when the system is gouty, colchicum can be given with benefit; and that in the rheumatic, iodide of potassium may effect a cure. At the same time that such remedies are being employed, astringent injections will be found useful auxiliaries.

3. GONORRHŒA IN THE FEMALE.—This disease is of a somewhat different character to gonorrhœa as it occurs in man. It consists of acute or chronic inflammation of the vulva, or urethra, or vagina, or canal of the cervix uteri; and it is accompanied by a more or less copious muco-purulent discharge. But neither in the actual condition of the parts, nor in the symptoms, do we find anything by which positively to distinguish an inflammation due to ordinary causes common to the most chaste female, from that which is produced by the specific discharge of a clap. Yet it is impossible to doubt that women do suffer from true gonorrhœa. Dr. Henry Bennet, while expressing his belief in the existence of a contagious and a non-contagious form of vaginitis, says,—" I am bound to confess that the only difference that I can see between the two is, that vaginitis apparently contracted by contagion— or blennorrhagia—appears to be more acute than ordinary vaginitis, that there is a greater quantity of pus secreted, greater redness, congestion, and swelling of the mucous membrane, that the inflammatory action has a greater tendency to spread to the urethra, and that it is very much more intractable to treatment. These conditions, merely implying degrees of inflammatory violence, do not evidently constitute a distinction as to morbific characteristics. It is, however, I repeat, a remarkable fact, that simple vaginitis in the immoral portion of the population should usually assume the severer form of the disease, and be readily communicated; whereas with the moral part of the community it should usually affect the milder form and be seldom communicated."* My own experience

_____
* A Practical Treatise on Inflammation of the Uterus, &c. Fourth Edition, p. 229. London, 1861.

quite confirms this opinion, and is perhaps the more valuable because it has been drawn from a different class of patients to that seen by Dr. Bennet. For whereas he has had great opportunities of observing uterine and vaginal disease in the higher classes of society, my views have been derived from a very large practice amongst hospital patients. And this may certainly be said, that I have never yet seen any woman suffering from such a train of symptoms that I could go into a court of law and assert that she was affected with gonorrhœa, in the meaning commonly attached to this term. There have undoubtedly been many instances where I have thought such was the case,—where there has existed a discharge from the meatus urinarius and vagina, of a thick muco-purulent matter; but a very different conclusion might have been come to by an *intelligent* jury, had I been submitted to a sharp cross-examination.

This subject will again be brought under the reader's notice in the section on the Diseases of the Female Genital Organs. But it may here be mentioned that when, in my practice, the diagnosis has been—a specific gonorrhœa, the treatment has been as follows. In the acute stage, prolonged hot hip-baths; with the injection of large quantities of warm water every eight or twelve hours, by means of a syphon syringe. Mild aperients, rest, and low diet have also been needed. If there have been an abscess in either labium, as is not uncommonly the case, it has been opened. Directly the symptoms have moderated, astringent injections (F. 425) have been freely employed; and then when the discharge, in diminished quantity, has constituted the sole remaining symptom, a medicated pessary (one containing tannin or acetate of lead, see F. 423) has been used every night, or for two or three nights in the week. The cervix uteri has also been examined by the speculum, and any inflammatory or excoriated patch freely touched with nitrate of silver. It need scarcely be added that until an apparently complete cure has been effected, sexual intercourse has been strictly prohibited; for where this rule has been disregarded, the treatment has proved of little value.

III. NON-SPECIFIC EXCORIATIONS, VEGETATIONS, &c.

To prevent mistakes in the diagnosis and treatment of venereal diseases, it is necessary to give a brief description of certain non-specific affections, which sometimes follow sexual intercourse, and hence are apt to be regarded with suspicion by the public. The affections thus grouped together are,—vegetations, excoriations, herpes præputialis, and eczema.

1. **VEGETATIONS, OR WARTS.**—These growths consist of hypertrophied papillæ covered with epithelium. They form around

the corona glandis and on the frænum; either as the result of balanitis or of gonorrhœa, or independently of these diseases from not attending to cleanliness.   They also occur in females, owing to any irritating discharge; and are found in clusters about the perineum, the vaginal labia, &c.   They must not be confounded with mucous tubercles or condylomata; which are formed of raised patches of skin, are of a flattened irregular shape, red and moist on the surface, and are generally covered with a dirty-white secretion. These condylomata are usually accompanied also by other secondary symptoms, or even by primary sores.

The *treatment* of warts is simple.   Occasionally great cleanliness and the use of an astringent wash will cure them, when they are small.   Frequently they are dry and horny; but if any moisture exudes from their surfaces it will be well to cover them with a fine layer of cotton wool, or to dust them with the oxide of zinc. When these means fail or are not applicable, the growths should be removed with the curved scissors, so as not merely to cut away the projecting portions, but the whole of the enlarged papillæ. Any bleeding which results can be checked by cold, or by pressing a pellet of cotton wool on the cut surface, or by applying a drop of the solution of perchloride of iron.   Sometimes, however, this treatment will be thought too violent, and then the solid nitrate of silver must be rubbed into the structure, the surrounding parts being covered with olive oil; or in the same way we may use the glacial acetic acid, or the dried sulphate of zinc, or the acid solution of nitrate of mercury, or the glycerine of carbolic acid. Without subsequent ablution once or twice daily, the vegetations will probably be reproduced.

2. EXCORIATIONS &c.—An abrasion of the epithelium or epidermis is often met with as the result of sexual intercourse. There is no ulceration; but we find either an excoriation, or a slight rent or tear near the frænum.   Men with a delicate skin and a long narrow prepuce, sometimes suffer in this way after every connexion. Free ablution with tepid or cold water will soon give relief; but a permanent cure can occasionally only be effected by circumcision. If, by chance, an abrasion should fail to heal, the general health will probably be found depressed; and then a mild astringent wash had better be ordered, while bark with some mineral acid is given internally.   It must be remembered that an excoriation, at the time of its occurrence or subsequently, may have become inoculated with chancre-virus.   There will be some difficulty in deciding whether this has happened, at all events until after the lapse of thirty-six or forty-eight hours from the occurrence.

Where there is a preternaturally short frænum I have sometimes seen this structure partially torn through, causing pain and occasionally troublesome hæmorrhage.   The best plan is to divide the frænum completely.   If the artery bleed much, its orifice can usually be obliterated by sharply nipping the end of the vessel with a pair of forceps ; but this failing, a ligature should be applied.

3. **HERPES PRÆPUTIALIS.**—Clusters of herpetic vesicles frequently form on the integument of the prepuce ; being accompanied with troublesome itching and more or less burning pain. The vesicles either desiccate, or their heads are rubbed off ;. and then a thin crust remains, which in two or three days falls away, leaving a red unbroken surface. Herpetic eruptions are rather more troublesome when situated on the inner surface of the prepuce. The milky-looking contents of the vesicles become purulent about the third day ; while the cells coalesce into a slight ulcer, which will possibly assume a very suspicious appearance, if it be improperly irritated with caustic.

The usual history of these cases is that the patient, after dining out, has had intercourse with a loose woman. The itching and heat soon remind him of his indiscretion, and he hurries off to his physician. Probably the dinner has had more to do with his complaint than the subsequent weakness. However this may be, a seidlitz powder, or a dose of the solution of carbonate of magnesia will do good; while the rash runs its course and soon gets well.

4. **ECZEMA.**—This disease will be more completely treated of in a subsequent page. Nevertheless it may be mentioned here, that it sometimes occurs on the glans, or inner surface of the prepuce, or low down on the penis, or on the scrotum, from inattention to the proper use of water. It is not uncommon in prostitutes, the rash being generally situated about the labia and perineum.

The minute papules or vesicles are attended with itching, heat, and redness ; and then the sero-purulent exudation forms small scales, with cracks in them. Sometimes, the scratching resorted to for relieving the itching caused by the pediculus pubis or crab-louse (for an account of which see the section on Diseases of the Appendages of the Skin), produces scabs which may be mistaken for eczema. An examination of the part with a lens will readily expose the blunder.

Bathing and washing the eczematous patches with the diluted solution of subacetate of lead will generally effect a cure. But if the eruption be chronic, a mild course of arsenic may very likely be needed.

IV. PRIMARY SYPHILIS.

Primary syphilis* occurs as a specific ulcer or chancre, the ulcer appearing on the part to which the virus has been directly

* Several derivations have been given of the word syphilis ; but, as Dr. Mayne states, none seems better than that of Blancardus—Σύν = together + φιλέω = to love.

applied. According to many surgeons there must be some abrasion or breach of surface for inoculation to take place; while others believe that the mere application of the poison to the delicate mucous membrane of the sexual organs will suffice. In the present day all practitioners allow that gonorrhœa and syphilis are essentially distinct diseases, due to poisons altogether different in their nature. Time never yet matured a clap to pox, though Pope says it will at last do so. Whether there are also varieties of the syphilitic virus has been strongly contested; the question as to the unity or duality of the poison having led to the expression of many opinions, without producing any convincing argument decisive of the question. Certainly, and this is the really important point, there are two distinct classes of venereal sores, viz., the infecting and the non-infecting. In the former class there is only the true syphilitic or hard chancre; in the latter, we find the soft chancre, with the phagedænic, and the gangrenous sores. Thus, four kinds of ulcers may result from impure sexual intercourse. Occasionally these varieties of action succeed each other,—that is to say the patient receives the virus of both the infecting and non-infecting sores, both of which may show themselves together in the same part, one before the other, conformably with the fact that the first-named have a somewhat long period of incubation. According to Mr. Henry Lee,*—

The first form of ulcer is the *indurated, hard, Hunterian, infecting,* or *true chancre.* The ulcer yields only an insignificant quantity of discharge, made up of molecular débris without any pus. It is accompanied by the adhesive inflammation; " and produces a peculiar chronic enlargement of the inguinal glands, which does not involve the skin or the cellular membrane. This variety is followed by secondary symptoms; and requires both in its primary and secondary forms, mercurial treatment." It is an exceptional occurrence for this disease to happen twice in the same individual.

The second, is the *simple, soft, non-indurated chancre.* It is accompanied by suppurative inflammation. The secretion from the sore contains pus cells. It does not necessarily affect the inguinal glands, and is a local disease which is neither accompanied nor followed by secondary symptoms. Hence only local treatment is needed. When a bubo forms it will be of the suppurating kind, and not indurated as happens with the infecting sore.

The third, is the *phagedænic sore.* It is accompanied by ulcerative inflammation. " It produces suppuration, generally of one inguinal gland only, which yields an inoculable secretion. It is not followed by constitutional syphilis, and may be treated by local means."

The fourth, is the *sloughing sore,* or *gangrenous phagedæna.* It

* *A System of Surgery.* Edited by T. Holmes, M.A., &c. Vol. i. p. 461. London, 1860.

" is accompanied by mortification. It does not affect the inguinal glands, is not followed by constitutional infection, and requires only local treatment."

The fact must not be forgotten that primary venereal sores sometimes have their seat in the urethra, when the discharge is apt to be mistaken for that of a gonorrhœa. Hence (as before advised), in all cases of the latter disease the urethra should be pressed between the fingers so as to detect any induration, if an ulcer be present ; while the lips of the meatus also ought to be separated, so that if a sore exist it may be properly treated.

Chancres in the female are most commonly situated on the labia majora, on the nymphæ, on the walls of the vagina, or in the folds about the clitoris. In very rare cases they have been found on the lips of the uterus, or even just within the canal of the cervix uteri. Speaking generally, these ulcers give rise to less local distress than is the case with the opposite sex ; so that where there is a neglect of personal cleanliness, their presence may be overlooked for several days. And it is an important point to recollect, that the infecting chancre in women is seldom accompanied with induration.

1. THE INDURATED CHANCRE.—If we take a typical example of the *indurated, Hunterian, true*, or *infecting chancre* we shall find that this disease consists of a superficial circumscribed abrasion or sore, situated on an indurated base. The loss of substance is slight. The surface appears glossy, or as if covered with a thin coating of gum. There is no inflammatory areola, but the edges terminate abruptly ; so that the sore looks somewhat cup-shaped, from the elevation of its margin.

The disease does not generally commence until several days have elapsed from the date of exposure to infection. Some authorities deny, while others assert (and I agree with them) that there is a period of incubation, varying from a fortnight to four or even six weeks. During this interval nothing suspicious may be observed : still, the poison unseen is in action. Then, a small red pimple appears ; or a slight abrasion or fissure assumes an unhealthy appearance ; or an indurated tubercle is found without loss of tissue. Generally the cuticle very soon gives way, and a circular excavated sore results. This gradually extends for a few days, successive fine layers of the surface perishing and being thrown off. The secretion from it is small in quantity, consisting of a little serum and lymph-globules, with epithelial débris ; but the character of this discharge is readily altered, and the amount increased, by the application of caustic or any irritant.

The characteristic feature of these sores is the induration of their margins and bases, from the adhesive inflammation giving rise to effusion of lymph. Sometimes this induration is superficial, and not thicker than a piece of parchment ; but, as Mr. Lee points out, it is only entirely absent when the sore has its seat on the upper and central portion of the glans penis. In this case the sore is more like an abrasion than an ulcer; and "although it does not become indurated itself, it may be followed by induration of neighbouring parts, which have not themselves ulcerated." Most commonly the infecting chancre is solitary; two or more distinct sores occurring simultaneously on the same patient not being met with more frequently than in one case out of five or six.

When the disease has arrived at the stage of induration—in other words, when the system has become appreciably altered by the specific action of the virus, the patient cannot be inoculated with the secretion from his sore. Out of 99 cases of indurated chancre in which inoculation was attempted by Ricord, a characteristic pustule was only produced once. And even in this case inoculation was performed at an early period, while the chancre was increasing in size.

As the specific induration of the chancre appears, the absorbent glands in direct connexion with the lymphatics of the part become affected. It is an exceptional occurrence for only one inguinal gland to suffer. Generally two or more become indurated; being felt under the skin, like foreign bodies, the size of almond-shells. Hence Mr. H. Lee describes these tumours as *amygdaloid indolent buboes*. They are very chronic, painless, and hard; this hardness remaining even after all induration about the original sore has disappeared,—until indeed the disease is thoroughly cured. They only suppurate if accidentally irritated to the extent of producing inflammation; thus differing widely from the bubo which accompanies the non-infecting chancre.

Cases of a mixed form of chancre are occasionally met with. In these there has been a twofold inoculation. Thus it has been shown experimentally by M. Lindwurm that if the secretion from an infecting sore be inoculated on a soft chancre, this latter will become an indurated sore, and will be followed by secondary symptoms.

In the *treatment* of infecting chancre it must be remembered that we have a constitutional affection to deal with. We ought carefully to distinguish between effecting an apparent and a perfect cure; only resting satisfied with the latter, so that the general system may not subsequently suffer. If any blood-contamination be left, plastic matter will afterwards be effused upon the iris, or on the bones, or in the muscles or areolar tissue, or in the substance of internal organs, giving rise to what are known as secondary and tertiary symptoms.

Local applications are of comparatively little use. The healing of the sore may perhaps be facilitated by using mercurial ointment to it, or by dressing it with black wash—calomel combined with a little mucilage and lime water. Supposing the part to which the syphilitic virus has been applied can be destroyed with caustic within a few hours (some say "four days") from the application of the poison —before there has been time for systemic contamination, then a permanent cure may be effected by such treatment ; but the opportunity of doing this is very rarely offered to the practitioner. As soon as there is induration, it is certain that the virus has become disseminated. Then constitutional remedies are needed, and must be persevered with until all hardness at the seat of inoculation or of the inguinal glands has entirely disappeared. To avoid useless repetition, these remedies will be treated of in the section on Constitutional Syphilis; but it may be mentioned that I believe mercury to be the only agent which has the power of completely destroying the syphilitic virus. And were I asked to give any proof of the truth of this view, I would point to those cases of constitutional syphilis which we meet with in married women. A female so affected may conceive again and again, and as often as she does so the gestation ends in abortion or in the birth of a dead child. She takes drugs of every kind, except that one especially needed, without the slightest benefit. But let her, and the husband if necessary, undergo a judicious mercurial course, and the most direct evidence will be afforded that the real antidote or remedy has been employed. To my mind it appears, that the cure of ague by quinine is not more certain than that of true syphilis by mercury.

2. THE NON-INDURATED CHANCRE.—This variety of venereal disease, much more common than the infecting chancre, consists of a suppurating sore ; which is known as a *simple, soft*, or *non-indurated chancre*. As it is often produced by the inoculation of an abrasion or fissure, so it does not generally commence with a pimple or pustule. There is only a very short period of incubation. Within three days at the outside of the inoculation, the symptoms show themselves. Frequently, when the patient first comes under observation, there are two or more circular sores ; these ulcers having spongy bases, and well-defined edges, which look as sharp as if portions of the healthy tissue had been punched out. The ulcer gradually extends for a time ; its surface gets covered with indolent granulations ; and the comparatively abundant secretion from it becomes purulent, within five or six days from the time of contagion. This secretion is auto-inoculable. The absorbent vessels and glands do not necessarily become affected ; but if lymphatic absorption does occur, then a suppurating bubo will follow. This variety of chancre is a local disease, which will heal spontaneously in from three to six weeks. It frequently leaves a scar but no induration.

When the disease extends below the mucous membrane so as to involve the connective tissue, it spreads more rapidly, and the inflammation causes a certain amount of induration. But even here, the purulent discharge will suffice to distinguish this *phlegmonoid suppurating sore* from the infecting chancre. On minutely examining the secretion it will be found to consist of well-formed pus globules.

If the sore be seen within five days from the application of the poison, effective cauterization will cure it.   For this purpose, nitrate of silver will hardly suffice, since it is too irritating without being sufficiently destructive.   The affected part must be destroyed with nitric acid, or potassa fusa, or with the acid solution of nitrate of mercury ; great care being taken to limit the action of these powerful escharotics.   In other cases, simple dressing of the sore with an astringent lotion may hasten cicatrization.   If there be a suppurating bubo, it should be freely opened.   At the same time, quinine with ferruginous tonics, nourishing food, and exercise in the open air will prove useful.

3. THE PHAGEDÆNIC SORE.—In this form of venereal inflammation we generally find a small and irritable and ragged ulcer, secreting unhealthy pus.   Its peculiar character is the tendency it has to spread irregularly.   When it extends from several points, in the form of portions of circles, it is known as the *serpiginous* chancre.   Whether it spreads in this manner or simply in a circular form, an inguinal gland soon becomes swollen and very tender, so that the patient walks somewhat lamely ; there is generally a rigor, with constitutional disturbance ; and relief is ·not obtained until after suppuration has taken place, and the pus been discharged. The destruction of the affected gland and the skin over it, gives rise to a troublesome unhealthy ulcer in the groin.   In some instances a venereal sore is phagedænic from the commencement ; while in others this eroding character is engrafted, as it were, upon one of the other varieties.   The secretion from such a sore is inoculable upon the patient.

The *treatment* of these cases will have to be mostly palliative. Fomentations and poultices, with full doses of opium internally, are generally very beneficial.   As a rule, caustics and irritants are hurtful.   In one very obstinate case of serpiginous chancre which was under my care, all remedies were useless until they were employed in conjunction with mercurial fumigation (F. 131). Where there is general debility, bark and nitric acid, or some ferruginous tonic with quinine, will be indicated.   If there be much inflammatory action, large doses of iodide of potassium with sarsaparilla can usually control it.   Cod liver oil is serviceable.   The patient had better keep his bed.   The diet ought to be nourishing, without stimulants.

4. THE SLOUGHING SORE.—In these cases we have a venereal sore in combination with destructive gangrenous inflammation.   Hence the disease is known as the *sloughing sore,* or *gangrenous phagedæna.*   Sometimes the death of the tissue to which the virus has been applied is so complete that the poison is destroyed by the same action, as if by a powerful caustic ; so that when the slough is cast off a simple sore alone remains.   The general health is always impaired, and occasionally

to a very marked degree. Although this variety of sore is so severe that now and then the whole prepuce gets destroyed, with perhaps even a portion of the glans, yet when cicatrization commences it generally goes on quickly. The inguinal glands do not become affected, neither do secondary symptoms follow.

The *treatment* is much the same as that required in the phagedænic chancre. Stimulants and very nourishing food will be needed; while the pain must be relieved by large doses of opium. The use of mercury is inadmissible. The patient ought to be confined to bed in a well-ventilated room.

When this disease occurs in poor enfeebled prostitutes, it sometimes proves very severe. The whole of the labia and nymphæ may slough away, and death ensue—perhaps from hæmorrhage. Happily, such cases are very rarely met with in the present day.

V. BUBO.

A bubo consists either of a simple or of a specific inflammatory enlargement of a lymphatic vessel, or of one of the glands in connexion with such vessel. The superficial glands are alone affected,—those directly connected with the seat of irritation by the lymphatic vessels. The poison, when there is one, seems to be arrested in these glands, and does not pass to the deeper series. Women very rarely suffer from this affection.

There are several varieties of bubo :—

1. *Simple Sympathetic Bubo.*—Whatever causes lymphatic irritation can give rise to simple inflammatory adenitis. Hence it may occur in balanitis, or in gonorrhœa, or from the irritation of any kind of sore on the penis, or merely from excessive sexual intercourse. Perhaps strumous subjects are more liable to this bubo than others. Frequently, not only the gland itself but the lymphatic vessel leading to it is found enlarged and indurated, feeling like a piece of whipcord. The inflammation may end in resolution; or by its severity suppuration may be established. In the latter case, a simple abscess results; the pus from which is healthy and free from any specific quality. After its evacuation, healing is seldom long delayed. The great object of *treatment* must be to obtain resolution, and perfect rest is more likely to accomplish this than anything else. Warm bathing will be useful. Tonics and cod liver oil can often be advantageously prescribed. When suppuration does take place a free opening ought to be made at the lowest part of the bubo, in order to avoid the burrowing of the pus in the surrounding connective tissue.

2. *Primary Bubo.*—In this case a bubo is said to form from the direct absorption of syphilitic matter, without the occurrence of any chancre or sore on the penis. The pus produced by the sup-

puration of a gland so affected will give rise to venereal sores when inoculation with it is practised. This *bubon d'emblée*, as it is designated by the French surgeons who first described it, is so rarely met with that many practitioners of experience doubt its existence.

3. *Amygdaloid Indolent Bubo.*—This form of bubo has been already described in the section on Infecting Sores. It generally comes on simultaneously with the occurrence of induration in the chancre; and as the latter is indolent, so are the buboes which almost necessarily accompany it. Suppuration only occurs from some accidental cause; but should it take place the pus is not inoculable upon the patient. Usually the whole chain of superficial glands, in the groin corresponding to the side of the penis on which the sore is seated, is indurated. These buboes are the least painful and troublesome locally, but the most important as regards the patient's general health; since they are a proof of constitutional infection.

4. *Virulent, or Inoculable Bubo.*—The absorption of the venereal virus from a soft, or from a phagedænic chancre, produces this variety of bubo. In the greater number of cases it happens towards the end of the second week from the first appearance of the disease. The poison will not only affect the first gland to which it is conveyed, but in its passage may also inoculate the lymphatic vessel. The gland, and perhaps the vessel, then suppurate; while when the abscess opens, we find its walls forming a venereal sore, the pus from which is auto-inoculable.

The attempt to prevent suppuration will be useless. As soon as pus has formed it should be evacuated by a free incision. If the skin be thin and undermined, it may be sometimes better to make an opening by means of potassa fusa rather than by the knife. Subsequently, soothing dressings, and frequent syringing with warm water, will usually be more useful than severer measures. If any sinuses form, they are to be laid open. Quinine and iron, good nourishing food, and pure air, will be needful.

VI. CONSTITUTIONAL SYPHILIS.

There is probably no poison which has a more powerful yet insidious influence in deteriorating the constitution than the syphilitic. And not only does it render the sufferer a confirmed invalid for a long time, but it slowly works its dire effects upon several of the most important tissues of the body. Many cases of chronic ill-health are due to it; while it is often the cause of obscure diseases of the vital organs, affections of the bones, rebellious ulcers of the cutaneous or mucous surfaces, troublesome skin eruptions, headaches and neuralgic pains, impotence or sterility, abortion, and the death of the fœtus in utero.

When syphilis became distinctly recognised in Europe about

1483, we learn from the description of the symptoms that the disease was more severe and ran a more rapid course than it does in the present day. This, however, need not have been owing to a greater virulence of the poison; but was probably due to the more free use of intoxicating drinks, inattention to cleanliness, delay in seeking advice, and to the treatment being ill-understood.

It was probably in the last century that the phenomena of syphilis were first artificially divided into different stages,—viz. the primary, the secondary, and the tertiary. The primary symptoms are due to the application of the venereal poison by sexual intercourse or by inoculation, and they have already been treated of. The constitutional or secondary symptoms are the result of the indurated or infecting chancre. They may make their appearance in the course of two or three weeks, or not for several months, after the healing of the primary sore; being due to the tainting of the blood by the syphilitic virus. The longer the duration has been of the primary infecting sore, and the more marked the induration with which it has been attended, the greater will be the severity of the secondary symptoms. Moreover, the worse the general health at the time of contracting the primary ulcer, the greater the risk to the constitution subsequently.

There is every reason to believe that constitutional syphilis can be communicated from an infected to a healthy person directly—*i.e.*, without the intervention of primary disease, more especially where there is frequent contact between the two parties.* Secondary skin diseases and condylomata may be so communicated from the husband to the wife; the seminal fluid of a tainted man deposited in the vagina of a healthy woman acting thus, without pregnancy occurring; or the husband being constitutionally affected may taint the ovum, and through the latter the mother will get infected. It also seems proved (see the section on Cow-pox, p. 283) that the poison of syphilis may be introduced into the system

---

* The non-contagion of secondary syphilitic affections was long maintained by M. Ricord—following the opinion of John Hunter. It was more correctly taught at an earlier period, however, that the contagion of secondaries is a fact. Old Daniel Turner quaintly says,—" And this I intend shall suffice for its *Chronology* or Time, the *Topology* or Place, and the *Histriography* or Account of the disease in general; which, with some other writers thereon, we shall now define, *A venomous or Contagious distemper, for the most part contracted by impure Coition, at least some contact of the Genitals of both Sexes, or some other lewd and filthy Dalliance between each other that way tending.* I said *for the most part*, because it is beyond Controversy, the Infection is also communicated by other ways, as from Pocky Parents, by Inheritance; by sucking an infected Nurse, to the Child; suckling a diseased Child, to the Nurse; lying also in Bed with the Diseased, without any Carnal Familiarity; by which, though it may be possible for strong and vigorous Bodies to escape, yet are the tender ones, especially of little Infants, very likely to be contaminated, as I have more Reason to believe than by bare Imagination."—*Syphilis; a Practical Dissertation on the Venereal Disease.* By Daniel Turner. p. 10. London, 1717.

by practising vaccination with impure lymph.   Tertiary symptoms generally appear at a long period after the primary disease, and usually some time after the secondary phenomena have disappeared. The diseases which have been termed tertiary are commonly deep-seated affections of the skin, as tubercles; morbid actions in the bones, as periostitis, exostosis, caries, and necrosis; and destructive disorders connected with the production of gummata in important internal organs.   Possibly the children of parents suffering from tertiary symptoms are predisposed to scrofula, or pulmonary consumption, or tabes mesenterica, or hydrocephalus.

Symptoms.—Constitutional syphilis usually manifests itself in the beginning by a considerable amount of general systemic disturbance.   We find fever, mental depression, lassitude, pains in the limbs and joints, severe headache, and sleeplessness; while the skin assumes a sallow hue.   Nocturnal exacerbation of this syphilitic fever and these pains is common.   There may be dyspnœa, palpitation, œdema of the feet, and a cardiac bruit,—all the result of anæmia.   Then unmistakeable evidence is afforded by the production of well-marked cutaneous diseases; by ulcers on the skin; by warts, and condylomata or mucous tubercles; by tumours of the skin and subcutaneous areolar tissue; by partial or total alopecia or baldness, with loss of the eyebrows and eyelashes; by syphilitic iritis; by inflammation and ulceration about the roots of the nails; by superficial ulcerations on the tongue, lips, and pillars of the fauces; by ulceration of the larynx; by enlargement and induration of the testicle—syphilitic sarcocele; by diseases of the periosteum and bones; and, in a few instances, and as late tertiary symptoms, by diseases of the brain, spinal cord, lungs, heart, liver, spleen, &c.

The *syphilodermata* or *syphilitic cutaneous affections* are of various kinds; for they may belong to either of the orders exanthemata, vesiculæ, pustulæ, papulæ, squamæ, or tubercula.   Probably of all the syphilides the squamous or scaly diseases are the most common; the eruption appearing in patches, being of a reddish coppery colour, having the scurf renewed as fast as it is shed, often showing a tendency to excoriate or ulcerate, and being attended with fever or some constitutional disturbance.   The syphilitic tubercle varies in size from a pea to a pigeon's egg, is of a polished brown hue, is very prone to ulcerate, and most frequently has its seat on the chest or face or abdomen.   Small groups of tubercles sometimes attack the nose, the forehead, or the tongue; usually terminating in the formation of inveterate ulcers.   The syphilitic maculæ or stains may be of a brown or dirty yellow colour, and as they often prove incurable it is fortunate that they are of little consequence.   It is surprising how frequently chloasma is erroneously set down as one of the results of syphilis, being confounded with these maculæ.

Speaking very generally, the syphilodermata are obstinate: many of them will persist for years, unless properly treated.   They give rise to less heat and irritation than non-specific cutaneous rashes.   Mixed forms of eruption are often present at one time, especially at early periods of the disease ; pimples, pustules, scabs, and scales, running into each other on the surface of the same bearer.   The skin is seldom affected without other indications of syphilitic infection being present ; such as a thinning of the hair, alterations in the voice, ulcers on the tongue, redness about the fauces, nocturnal pains in the limbs, substernal tenderness, muscular or osseous nodes, mucous tubercles, syphilitic sarcocele, iritis, &c.   And lastly, the diagnosis will sometimes be aided by the effect of remedies ; mercury and iodine proving much more valuable in the syphilitic than in the non-specific eruptions.

Condylomata or *mucous tubercles* either occur as small rounded tubercular elevations of the integument, or as large irregular and indurated patches owing to the coalescence of several tubercles. With women, particularly, they are often amongst the earliest of the constitutional affections ; appearing on the labia, perineum, and about the anus.   In men they form chiefly on the scrotum, around the anus, on the nates, thighs, prepuce, &c.   Sometimes the elevated patches are of a whitish colour, looking as if nitrate of silver had just been rubbed over their surface ; while in other cases they are copper-coloured, and exhale an acrid fetid discharge.

These indurated tubercles may appear on individuals who have never had any primary sore.   For example, a man who has suffered from an infecting chancre and been apparently cured, gets married. A few months afterwards, his wife exhibits numerous condylomata, swellings of the glands in the groin, superficial ulcerations about the fauces, and subsequently a secondary eruption.   Yet the husband has had no fresh disease.   Unfortunately, his constitution has never been freed from the poison engrafted prior to marriage.

Secondary syphilitic affections of the uterus are by no means uncommon.   They may either prevent conception ; or, failing to have this effect, they will probably be the source of infection to the embryo.   In these cases, the vaginal portion of the uterus is found enlarged and tender ; the lips are indurated ; there are often one or more patches of excoriation around the os, of such extent now and then as to be mistaken for the ulceration of cancer ; and there is a constant tenacious muco-purulent discharge from the uterine cavity.   When the throat or the skin is likewise affected, the diagnosis will be much facilitated.   These symptoms are rebellious, and only removed with difficulty ; a combination of local with constitutional treatment being required.

Syphilitic tumours of the skin and subcutaneous connective tissue generally appear long after the healing of the primary sore.   They may have their seat on any part of the body, the forearm and outer part of the leg being the regions in which I have most often met with them.   If their resolution is not effected in the earlier stages, they gradually soften and ulcerate ; or if in ignorance of their true nature they be lanced, or if attempts be made at their excision, the most foul and painful and inveterate sores will be produced.

Inflammation of the iris originating in syphilis is often associated with other forms of secondary disease, especially with one of the syphilodermata. In tertiary affections this modification of iritis has a tendency to become chronic : relapses are very common. The chief features which it presents are these :—The affected iris loses its natural brilliancy, while the pupil has a dull, and perhaps irregular, appearance. There is a rapid effusion of lymph on the iris, especially at the edges of the pupil, in the form of reddish-yellow nodules, which are sometimes so large as nearly to close the pupil ; or the lymph may be spread over the area of the pupil as a film, which gradually increases in thickness. Blue irides assume a greenish tint, owing to the presence of yellow albumen in the aqueous humour. The cornea will either remain transparent, or become hazy throughout its lower half from the presence of numerous minute spots. There is a vascular zone in the sclerotic, but the diffused redness of the eyeball characteristic of rheumatic iritis is wanting. There is but little pain or intolerance of light, compared with what happens in other forms of iritis. One or both eyes may be affected ; but in cases of relapse the right and left eyes are often attacked alternately.

Loss of hair from syphilitic poisoning seldom occurs without other symptoms. It may take place not only on the head (*alopecia* or *baldness*), but will now and then affect the eyebrows, eyelashes, whiskers, &c. This result is frequently combined with the excessive formation of scurf upon the scalp. In such cases too, atrophy of the finger nails, with a crumbling of their edges, is not uncommon. At times we find the patient suffering from onychia ; or there sets in some chronic inflammatory action (psoriasis) about the roots of the nails, so that these structures become thick and furrowed, crack or break easily, and even fall off. Cases of syphilitic whitlow are not very common.

The *syphilitic ulcers of the fauces, tonsils, and pharynx* are in many instances excavated, covered by an ash-coloured slough, and surrounded by a livid unhealthy appearance of the mucous membrane. Occasionally they slough, and extend rapidly ; they cause but little pain, and no great difficulty of deglutition ; and they are always attended with more or less constitutional disturbance. *Ulcerations of the nostrils* are also not uncommonly the only symptoms of the general infection of the system. They give rise to offensive and profuse discharges, with a marked alteration in the voice ; and, if not checked, to disease of the cartilages or nasal bones. *Deep fissures, ulcerations, and fungoid vegetations upon the tongue* may owe their origin to the poison of syphilis, or to the abuse of mercury. In the former case there will generally be found other symptoms of this disease ; while, in the latter, the submaxillary glands are frequently also swollen and tender. The venereal ulcer which shows itself at the side of the tongue is callous to the touch, is made painful by stimulating food or drink, is hard, is often covered with a slight dirty-yellow secretion, and looks as if a portion of tissue had been punched out. The smooth bald patch sometimes met with on the same organ is believed by certain authorities to be always venereal. Dr. Colles states, as a remarkable fact, that syphilitic ulcers invariably occur on the upper lip, while cancer as invariably invades the lower.

The partial enlargements of the bones called *nodes*, arise only when the system has been much affected by the poison of syphilis: they are the result of effusion between the periosteum and bone, and are perhaps caused by superficial inflammation of the osseous tissue. A careful examination of the sternum, and especially of the lower half, will sometimes detect a tender spot, technically known as *substernal tenderness*. In many of these cases some of the superficial inguinal glands will also be found enlarged, hard, and painless; or even one or more of the posterior cervical glands may be swollen and indurated. All the syphilitic affections of the periosteum and bones are attended with wearying pains; which latter are increased by warmth, are aggravated at night, and are relieved by iodide of potassium. This agent, however, seldom effects a permanent cure; mercury in some form (best by the vapour bath, F. 131) being required to prevent a relapse.

Indurations of limited portions of a muscle are now and then met with, feeling very much like distinct tumours. These *muscular nodes* or *gummata* have been mistaken for cancerous growths; and under this impression surgeons have occasionally attempted their extirpation. M. Ricord and others have recorded the histories of cases where nodes of this kind have been found in the walls of the heart.

With regard to the other internal organs most liable to suffer from the syphilitic poison we must remember the liver, the brain and dura mater, the spinal cord and nerves, the lungs, and the testicle. Independently of the special syphilitic diseases of these viscera, the bad health which the poison gives rise to acts from time to like many other cachectic conditions, and helps to set up that kind of tissue metamorphosis known as the amyloid or albuminous degeneration. The peculiarity of the syphilitic poison consists in the proneness to form a new fibro-plastic material in different parts of the body; this material being either thrown out in masses or gummata, or else infiltrated through the tissues. These conditions are well seen in the *liver*. Thus, according to Dr. Wilks, there are three varieties of the syphilitic liver. The first is that in which the whole gland is infiltrated by a new fibre-tissue, producing general hardening and enlargement: it is mostly seen in young children who have died of hereditary syphilis. In the second, a new material deposited in the course of the portal vessels has produced a contraction resembling that of cirrhosis. It may cause dropsy; while it is often associated with lardaceous degeneration. The third kind is that in which the organ is pervaded by distinct nodules of new formation. These masses are seen scattered through the gland; while they vary in size from that of a pea to a walnut. So again in the *lungs*, the syphilitic affection occurs under the form of nodules or gummata, or as a diffused or interstitial material. Dr. Wilks states that in several cases where marked syphilitic disease has existed elsewhere in the body, the lungs have presented that condition known as fibroid disease—described by some as chronic pneumonia. This gentleman also expresses his belief that phthisis is a common consequence of syphilis; not by the production of tubercle, nor by the formation of distinct gummata, but by the interstitial fibroid change which eventually disorganizes so that the patient presents the ordinary physical signs of consumption. And lastly, in the *brain* itself, or on its membranes, gummatous nodules are found, either in connexion with, or independently of, syphilitic inflammation of the cranial bones. Cerebral softening, and other lesions of the brain substance, are not uncommon in cases where the symptoms of constitutional syphilis have extended over some years. Amongst other terminations, hemiplegia, paraplegia, and epileptiform convulsions are not so very rare. It is in these instances of brain lesion that Virchow has observed aneurismal dilatations and other morbid conditions of the large bloodvessels.

Diagnosis.—The longer the interval which elapses between the primary disease and the appearance of the secondary symptoms, the greater will be the difficulty of diagnosis. It may be of assistance to remember that syphilitic cutaneous affections generally occur in connexion with various forms of ulceration about the soft palate and fauces; and that the skin disease repeatedly assumes a dusky copper colour. Sometimes the sub-occipital lymphatic glands are enlarged in these cases. Of symptoms which exist singly, syphilitic sarcocele is the most common; while it is also, as a rule, one of the latest exhibitions of the disease. The syphilitic tubercle of the face, when ulcerated, is not unfrequently mistaken for lupus; but it may be distinguished by its greater depth, the sharpness of its edges, and its dusky brownish colour. The history of the case can perhaps be made to throw light upon its nature; but a truthful report is not always to be obtained. When the patient is a married man, the health of his wife and children will form a guide in enabling us to arrive at a correct diagnosis.

Many cutaneous diseases have been erroneously referred to the poison of syphilis, and much unhappiness thereby produced. Suicide has even been attempted under the distress thus engendered; as will be shown in the section on Syphiliphobia.

Prognosis.—Constitutional syphilis, if neglected, is most likely ultimately to destroy life. It may do so directly by inducing some affection of the larynx, nervous system, liver, spleen, kidneys, or intestines; but very often it acts indirectly by bringing out latent tubercular disease, or it can directly produce pulmonary consumption. Certain authorities state that a perfect cure is never effected; but in patients under forty, at all events, complete recovery generally follows well-directed treatment. I am rather sceptical of cases getting well when left alone; but there are writers who think the disease may wear itself out.

In many cases of constitutional syphilis the symptoms are relieved by remedies, without a radical cure being effected. Periods of latency then occur, during which the patient appears well; but even after a long time the poison can be roused into activity again and again, and especially by causes which depress the powers of life. Moreover, during the period of latency the individual may beget a tainted child.

Treatment.—Directly the constitutional affection clearly manifests itself, attempts should be made to effect a cure. With women, pregnancy forms no bar to the treatment; since abortion is much more likely to follow from the disease, than from the remedies.

The therapeutical agents required in the treatment are not very numerous, but they demand great caution and discernment in their application. The *diet* should usually be light and nutritious. White fish and meat may be allowed; cream, milk, and raw eggs are excellent articles; but with the exception of a little claret or of sherry and water, stimulants are commonly to be forbidden. Warm *clothing* is requisite; and generally flannel ought to be worn next the skin during the day. *Cold* and *damp* are injurious. Consequently, although confinement to the house is very seldom necessary, yet care is to be taken to avoid exposure to wet or to the night air. In all cases the use of *warm water* or *vapour* or *Turkish baths*, once or twice a week, will prove of great service; and, provided they do not induce debility, cannot be productive of any mischief. *Opium*, also, will be needed where there is much pain, or when there is an inability to sleep at night, or when there is general irritability; and it may be given to the extent of three or four grains in the twenty-four hours. The extract is the preparation which I usually prefer; its efficacy being increased by combination with small doses of extract of belladonna, or full doses of henbane. But the essential remedy, and that which is absolutely necessary to effect a permanent cure, is *mercury*. " Nothing," says John Hunter, " can show more the ungrateful or unsettled mind of man than his treatment of this medicine. If there is such a thing as a specific, mercury is one for the venereal disease in two of its forms."* There are two principal ways in which this mineral may be introduced into the system—viz., either by the stomach or by the skin. In the former case, we administer a solid or liquid preparation, such as blue pill, calomel, or the solution of corrosive sublimate; in the latter we resort to inunction with the mercurial ointment, or we use the mercurial vapour bath. In my own prac-

* *The Works of John Hunter*. Palmer's Edition, vol. ii. p. 427. London, 1835.

tice recourse is always had either to inunction or the bath. Both methods I believe to be equally efficacious; but whereas one plan is dirty and disagreeable, the other is cleanly and pleasant. If it be thought preferable to trust to inunction, from the eighth to the fourth of an ounce of the mercurial ointment should be thoroughly rubbed into the body (the inside of the thighs is a convenient part) every night at bed-time, until the gums are slightly touched. This proceeding is particularly valuable in the treatment of young children; sixty grains of the ointment being spread on a flannel roller, which is then wound round the body. When mercurial fumigation is employed, the bath (F. 131) ought to be used at first every night, and then for two or three nights a week. By such baths I have frequently cured cases which have resisted all other plans of treatment. In many chronic examples the solution of perchloride of mercury (F. 27) repeated for many weeks, proves very useful. For the squamous cutaneous diseases, the green iodide of mercury (F. 53), or the red iodide of mercury (F. 54), can be advantageously used; especially if the mercurial vapour bath be employed at the same time. The subcutaneous and muscular tumours will generally be dispersed by the green iodide of mercury, the mercurial vapour, blisters, and pressure with the mercurial plaster.

Amongst other remedies which deserve a brief notice, mention should be made of *Donovan's triple solution* (F. 51), which will often cure the squamous cutaneous diseases; the *iodide of potassium* (F. 31), which is invaluable when the bones are affected, if the mercurial vapour be gently used at the same time; the *iodide of sodium* (F. 39); and of the *iodide of iron* (F. 32), which is particularly valuable in advanced stages of the disease, or in weak anæmic subjects. The influence of setons and repeated issues in preventing the localization of the disease in important internal organs has not yet been ascertained. In epilepsy due to this affection, however, setons and blisters to the back of the neck have been thought to keep off the attacks.

In all forms of late or so-called tertiary syphilis, when the patient's constitution will generally be found broken down, we must try and effect a cure by nourishing food, cod liver oil, opium, large doses of iodide of potassium, and the calomel vapour bath. Such cases, however, are very intractable.

These remarks would be incomplete without a notice of the treatment of this affection by *syphilization*. A few years only have elapsed since Auzias Turenne, in performing some experiments on animals with the poison of syphilis, ascertained that each succeeding chancre produced by inoculation became less and less, until a period arrived when no sore of any kind could be produced by the application of the venereal virus. From this the inference was drawn that, by prolonged inoculation with the syphilitic poison, a constitutional state was produced in which the system proved to be no longer capable of being affected by syphilis; just as happens, mutatis mutandis, in inoculation for small-pox.   Hence, to obtain perfect syphilization or immunity, an individual must undergo constitutional syphilis; but he must be forced rapidly through this state by repeated inoculations, in order that his organization may not be injured.   This practice has found, and in all probability will find, but little favour in our country; although recently in France and Germany and Italy attention has been paid to it, and curious phenomena brought to light.   Amongst other syphilographers who have made essays in this line of treatment, Sperino, Physician to the Venereal Hospital of Turin, has distinguished himself.   This gentleman published in 1853 a detailed account of 96 cases of syphilization; of which 53 were examples of aggravated primary syphilis, and 43 of severe constitutional disease.   Of the primary cases 50 were cured, 2 failed, and 1 was treated by other means in addition to syphilization: of the 43 with constitutional syphilis, 26 were treated by syphilization alone, 25 of these being cured; 17 were treated by syphilization, with mercury and iodine. Sperino inoculates for from 6 to 10 chancres at each sitting; and allows about three or four days to elapse between each operation. By continued inoculation the ulcers become less and less until no effect is produced; but the individual is still susceptible, though in a less degree, to another kind of matter, again to a third, and so on until at last no effect is produced by any syphilitic poison. It is strange that the general health does not suffer,—indeed it improves during the process of inoculation.   The time required to produce immunity varies; in one case it was obtained after 71 chancres, but this number seems to be much smaller than usual; for in most instances upwards of 300 were produced, the treatment lasting for nine or twelve or twenty months and more.   The majority of Sperino's patients were prostitutes, and they submitted themselves most readily to the treatment.   It may be practised at any age.   To obtain a complete cure when the patient has previously been mercurialized, the use of iodine has often to be combined with syphilization.   Dr. Boeck asserted in 1858, in consequence of results he had obtained from syphilization alone in those who had not been previously mercurialized, that *in no disease have we a more certain method of cure*.   The disadvantage of the method is its offensive nature, and the length of time necessary for effectually carrying it out: but then, on the other hand, the immunity produced is thought probably to last for life.

In conclusion it must be allowed that if syphilization be capable of effecting all the good that its supporters assert, we have still something to learn as to the varieties and effects of the syphilitic poison.   For these gentlemen deny that the cure is due to the lapse of time, or to the production of simple suppurating sores which act on the principle of depuration.   Some authorities get rid of the difficulty by throwing doubts upon the nature of the virus used for inoculation. Mr. Henry Lee is of opinion that the matter employed in these cases was obtained from the soft non-infecting sore, since Boeck states that the best kind is that derived from a chancre attended by a suppurating bubo ; while the phenomena of the artificial disease, excited by inoculation, are characteristic of the soft and not of the hard chancre. Supposing this view to be true, syphilization is only an " inoffensive playing with soft chancres." But its correctness has been denied, and amongst others by one of M. Boeck's friends, M. Bidenkap ; who asserts that the virus of the infecting chancre has been constantly used for curative syphilization in the Hospital of Christiana. He does not say, however, that indurated sores result,—a circumstance which seems impossible when the system is contaminated.

VII. INFANTILE SYPHILIS.

Syphilis in the infant may be hereditary or acquired. *Hereditary* syphilis happens thus :—The mother during pregnancy suffers from constitutional syphilis ; and she either supplies a vitiated ovum, or her blood contaminates the nutritive elements furnished to the fœtus during intra-uterine life. Or the taint is derived entirely from the diseased semen of the father ; the mother having been and continuing healthy, unless she becomes infected by the poisoned fœtus. Or again, both parents may be suffering from constitutional syphilis at the time of fecundation, in which case there is a very slight chance of the offspring escaping. In *acquired* syphilis the delicate infant's body gets infected by inoculable matter on the mother's genitals at the time of birth ; or its system suffers from sucking at the breast of a syphilitic nurse ;* or else ino-

* This mode of infection was early recognised. The following curious history shows very clearly the evil results which follow from the employment of an unhealthy nurse :—" An honest citizen saith he granted his most chaste wife, that she should nurse the childe which she was lately delivered of, if she would keepe a nurse to be partaker of the travell and paines : the nurse that she tooke by chance, was infected with *Lues Venerea*, therefore she did presently infect the foster childe, and he the mother, and she the husband, and he two children which he had daily at his table and bed, not knowing of that poison which he did nourish in his own body and intrals. But when the mother considered and perceived, that her childe did not prosper or profit by the nourishment, but continually cried and waxed wayward, desired me to tell her the cause of that disease, neither was it any hard matter to doe, for his body was full of the small-pocks, whelkes, and venereous pustules: and the brests of the nurses and mother being looked on, were eroded with virulent ulcers: and the body of the father and his two sonnes, the one about three yeares, and the other foure yeares of age, were infected with the like pustules and swellings that the childe had : therefore I shewed them that they were all infected with *Lues Venerea*, whose beginnings, and as it were provocations, were spred abroad by the nurse that was hired, by her maligne infection. I cured them all, and by the helpe of God, brought them to health, except the sucking childe, which died in the cure : and the nurse being called before the

culation occurs from the use of impure lymph at vaccination. The disease in two of these forms of acquired syphilis may manifest itself by a primary sore, resembling a chancre in the adult. But such cases must be very rare, as I have never yet seen an instance of it; whereas examples of constitutional syphilis in nurslings are daily met with in hospital practice.

Symptoms.—For the first two or three weeks after birth, the infant may be apparently healthy; or, as rarely happens, it will be born with its skin of a dull colour, and having its features contracted, so that it looks like a little old man. Supposing when it comes into the world there are no manifestations of disease, yet often within the month symptoms of coryza gradually set in; attended with a peculiar snuffling during breathing, hard cough, slight difficulty in sucking, and dryness of the lips and mouth. The skin soon gets harsh and dry, the voice shrill and hoarse (it has been compared to the squeaking of a penny trumpet), the mucous membrane of the mouth and throat becomes affected with superficial ulcerations, and an erythematous blush appears upon the soles of the feet and palms of the hands. The nails also crack or split in many cases. When the disease runs on unchecked, large patches of the skin assume a light-brown colour; the epidermis exfoliates; and the parts around the mouth, nostrils, buttocks, anus, and flexures of the joints become copper-coloured and fissured and excoriated. The eyes are either specially affected, or they may simply get weak, while the margins of the eyelids are sore. The hair gets dry and thin, or it falls off. Moreover, the child becomes irritable, cries almost constantly, wastes rapidly, and daily grows weaker; while it often has sickness and diarrhœa.

There are certain special diseases to which syphilitic children are liable, and which therefore demand attention. Amongst these may be mentioned *disease of the liver.* According to Diday, where the lesion has reached its maximum the gland is hypertrophied, hard and globular. It is resistent to pressure; and when cut into, it creaks slightly under the scalpel. Its appearance is peculiar; for there is seen on a yellowish ground, a layer of white opaque granules, like grains of semola. This fibro-plastic matter obliterates the capillaries, and diminishes the calibre of even the larger vessels; it compresses the hepatic cells; and hence there is an arrest of the secretion of bile.* I am not aware that encysted

magistrates, was punished in prison, and whipped closely, and had been publikely whipped through all the streets of the citie, if it had not been for the honors of that unfortunate family."—*A Profitable and Necessarie Book of Observations for all those that are burned with the Flame of Gunpowder, &c.* By William Clowes. p. 152. London, 1637.

* The syphilitic nature of the hepatic affection in the following cases is perhaps not quite certain, but it seems sufficiently probable to render it worthy of notice. On the 26 February 1862, I saw, in consultation with Mr. Holding, an infant ten days old suffering from jaundice. The liver appeared increased in size, and seemed more dense than was natural. A healthy wet-nurse was ordered to be procured, and the infant was put in a weak nitro-

gummy tumours, of a cheesy consistence and appearance, have been found in the livers of new born children. Such growths in adults are always syphilitic.

Our knowledge of the *syphilitic pulmonary affections* is scanty. A form of lobular pneumonia, due to indurations of the parenchyma of the lung, has been described by Depaul. The indurated nodules soften, cavities form in their centres, and thus collections of purulent fluid take place. They are generally found developed at birth, and they early lead to a fatal termination. Syphilitic abscesses may form in the thymus gland, as well as in the lungs.

Syphilitic iritis in infants is very uncommon. In 23 cases collected by Mr. Hutchinson, the average age at which it began was 5¼ months. When it occurs we shall generally find other symptoms of inherited syphilis,—such as copper-coloured eruptions, mucous tubercles about the genitals, aphthæ, and the snuffles. According to Mr. Dixon the lymph which is effused does not assume the form of tubercular masses on the edge of the pupil, as in the adult; but either fills the area of the pupil as a pale yellow or reddish semi-fluid mass, or sinks down to the bottom of the anterior chamber, like ordinary hypopyon. The pupil is irregular, and the iris discoloured. This disease is to be treated by mercurial inunction, good pure milk, beef tea, and cod liver oil if necessary. Dilatation of the pupil ought to be kept up by the daily use of atropine drops or paper.

Chronic interstitial keratitis—often called strumous corneitis—has been especially studied by Mr. Hutchinson. From his researches it seems proved that this is essentially an heredito-syphilitic disease, often accompanied or preceded by iritis. It appears between 5 and 18 years of age. At the commencement there is a diffused haziness near the centre of the cornea of one eye, without ulceration, and with very slight evidence of the congestion of any tunic. There is, however, always some irritability of the eye, with dim sight. On careful examination, dots of haze (" microscopic

hydrochloric acid bath, night and morning. Five days afterwards death took place. The mother of this child was thirty-seven years of age and healthy, though far from strong. The father appeared well, but had lost his hair. The mother had been pregnant eleven times. The first child died when fifteen months old: the second is living, and is twelve years old; the third is living, and is ten years old: then there were two abortions; and subsequently six children were successively born, who were apparently healthy at birth, but who in a few days became affected with fatal jaundice. The yellow tinge was not generally well-marked. My opinion was that after the delivery of the third child, the husband suffered from constitutional syphilis, which had left a slight taint; and that his infants had waxy or albuminoid disease of the liver, from the effect of this poison.

At the end of August 1863 the mother applied to me, being about five months advanced in her twelfth pregnancy. I at once put her upon a course of corrosive sublimate; and this medicine was continued until 29 December, when I delivered her of a fine healthy girl. About ten days afterwards the infant had a slight attack of jaundice, which however passed off completely: on the 22 October 1864 she remained strong and well.

masses of fog") are perceptible in the structure of the cornea; which dots increase until the whole transparent tissue, except a band near its margin, has become as opaque as ground glass. Now, there is a zone of sclerotic congestion; with intolerance of light, and pain round the orbit. After six or eight weeks the other cornea gets attacked. Then follows a period in which there is nearly complete blindness, but after this the eye first affected begins to clear. During the course of a year a surprising degree of improvement will probably take place. In milder cases, and under suitable treatment, the duration may be much less and the restoration to transparency complete; although in many instances patches of haze remain for years, if not for life. Where the best recoveries have been obtained, the eye usually remains somewhat damaged as to vision, and often a degree of abnormal expansion of the cornea is apparent. The subjects of this disease almost always present a very peculiar physiognomy; of which a coarse flabby skin, pits and scars on the face and forehead, cicatrices of old fissures at the angles of the mouth, a sunken bridge to the nose, and a set of permanent teeth peculiar for their smallness and bad colour *and the vertically notched edges of the central upper incisors*, are the most striking characters. Moreover, in many cases one or more of the following suspicious forms of disease have either been coincident with it, or have occurred previously; viz.—ulcerated lupus, nodes on the long bones, psoriasis about the face, otorrhœa, chronic enlargement and subsequent atrophy of the tonsils, ulcers in the throat, a thickened condition of the parts under the tongue, and chronic engorgements of the lymphatic glands.

Deafness is not very infrequent in the subjects of inherited syphilis. It is usually partial. The sense of hearing fails, without any local cause being apparent.

Amongst other marks of the heredito-syphilitic diathesis, the condition of *the permanent teeth* is deserving of attention. According to Mr. Hutchinson the peculiarities they present are the most reliable amongst the objective symptoms, if the patient be of age to show them. This gentleman says,—"Although the temporary teeth often, indeed usually, present some peculiarities in syphilitic children, of which a trained observer may avail himself, yet they show nothing which is pathognomonic, and nothing which I dare describe as worthy of general reliance. The *central upper incisors of the second set are the test teeth*, and the surgeon not thoroughly conversant with the various and very common forms of dental malformation will avoid much risk of error if he restrict his attention to this pair. In syphilitic patients these teeth are usually short and narrow, with a broad vertical notch in their edges, and their corners rounded off. Horizontal notches or furrows are often seen, but they as a rule have nothing to do with syphilis. If the question be put, Are teeth of the type described pathognomonic of hereditary taint? I answer unreservedly, that when well characterized, I believe they are. I have met with many cases in which the type in question was so slightly marked that it served only to suggest suspicion, and by no means to remove doubt, but I have never seen it well characterized without having reason to believe that the inference to which it pointed was well founded."*

Prognosis.—The duration of the disease varies. Death may occur at an early period ; but under efficient treatment, recovery, or apparent recovery, usually takes place speedily. When a child survives the first year, the danger to life is very much lessened. In some few instances death occurs suddenly,—perhaps just as the disease appears to have yielded to the remedies.

Treatment.—Supposing the mother to present any symptom of syphilitic disease, she ought not to be allowed to suckle her infant for a single meal. A vigorous healthy wet-nurse will have to be procured, or the child must be carefully brought up by hand. The latter is the only alternative when the infant is already suffering, lest the nurse herself become diseased. For although Ricord and others deny the possibility of this occurrence, yet I cannot but think there is more risk than a healthy woman should be allowed to incur. At all events, no nurse ought to be employed under these circumstances without warning her, in the presence of both parents, of the chance she runs of infection.

Then, as a general rule, directly symptoms show themselves in the child, mercury, in some form or other, is the remedy to be resorted to. It has been recommended to cure the infant through the medium of the mother, by getting her system under the influence of mercury ; but this practice is too uncertain to be depended upon, and is unjustifiable if the parent have no symptoms demanding a mercurial course. The best plan is either to administer the hydrargyrum cum cretâ, or to apply the mercurial ointment, as long since recommended by Sir Benjamin Brodie. To an infant six weeks old, one grain of grey powder with two or three of the aromatic chalk powder, may be given twice or thrice in the day until all the symptoms cease : or should this medicine gripe and purge, or appear inefficient, as it frequently will, the mercurial ointment is to be used. This is easily applied by spreading sixty grains, or a little more, on the end of a small flannel roller, and then winding the band round the infant's abdomen or knee, repeating the application daily. The movements of the child produce the necessary friction ; and the cuticle being thin, the mercury speedily enters the system. " Very few of those children ultimately recover in whom the mercury has been given internally ; but I have not seen a single case in which the other method of treatment—mercurial inunction—has failed."† Without believing in the absolute correctness of the inference to be drawn from this

* *A Clinical Memoir on Certain Diseases of the Eye and Ear, consequent on Inherited Syphilis,* p. 204. London, 1863.

† Sir Benjamin Brodie's *Lectures on Pathology and Surgery,* p. 245. London, 1846.

sentence, I still think more highly of inunction than of any other procedure.

When the use of mercury appears objectionable, the iodide of potassium in half-grain, or the chlorate of potash in two or three grain doses, repeated every six hours, may be tried. The latter salt, with a few drops of tincture of bark, has often appeared serviceable in cases attended with great feebleness.

The local treatment for the excoriations consists in great attention to cleanliness, and the application of the oxide of zinc ointment; or a cerate composed of sixty grains of the unguentum hydrargyri nitratis to one ounce of lard may be employed. The child should be put in a warm bath at least once a day.

VIII. SYPHILIPHOBIA.

Syphiliphobia [from *Syphilis* + φοϐέω = to dread], or Monomania Syphilitica, may be described as a morbid or hypochondriacal fear of syphilis, producing imaginary symptoms of the disease. And inasmuch as it is one of those nervous disorders which cause much unhappiness, and by which the advertising quacks thrive, it demands a short notice.

All classes of society may suffer from this affection,—the rich and poor, those without occupation and the busy workman. In men the symptoms are very much allied to such as are presented in fictitious cases of spermatorrhœa or of impotence. The amount of mental torture which the patients undergo is often sufficient to impair the general health; and then this impairment is regarded as a convincing proof that the system is contaminated. The symptoms are also further aggravated by the sufferer perusing works on diseases of the generative organs, and perhaps by visiting filthy and indecent museums. At times the distress has been so great and continuous, that the victim has committed suicide to escape from his imaginary evil. Men, in most respects shrewd and sensible, become almost fatuous about their health under the influence of this syphiliphobia. But some of the most troublesome cases which have fallen under my notice have been in women. A lady was long under my care, whose condition in May 1864 became really serious. About ten years previously, when abroad with her husband, the latter contracted a gonorrhœa. This he appears to have communicated to his wife, for she suffered from an abundant purulent discharge with burning pain during micturition. She was told that her sufferings were due to the venereal disease, and that it must have been contracted by sitting on a dirty water-closet. Although she seems to have been thoroughly cured in a few weeks, and soon to have dismissed the subject from her mind, yet about the beginning of 1862, when her health began to fail, she unfortunately recollected the attack.   Living near the banks of a river, in a very dull locality, she suffered from ennui and rheumatism ; and then the one idea constantly presented to her mind was, that the venereal poison had attacked her bones.   She was unwilling to reside away from her home during the damp foggy months of the year, and hence would not listen to the suggestion that her house was unhealthily situated.   And though after each interview with me she appeared convinced that her opinions on the subject were erroneous, yet a night's rest sufficed to banish the recollection of all she had been told, and the delusion became as strong as before. I am glad to add that she subsequently recovered ; appearing quite well and happy when last seen towards the close of 1867.

In the management of these cases it has to be remembered that the patient experiences much mental distress.   This suffering is not to be lightly treated. The practitioner must exhibit considerable tact and great patience ; he should show that he really feels an interest in the case ; while instead of roughly controverting the delusion, he must gain the patient's confidence, and gently endeavour to prove the non-existence of disease.   As regards drugs, the remedies which I have found most efficacious are the various preparations of zinc, and small doses of strychnia or nux vomica (F. 407, 409, 411).   But sometimes ferruginous tonics (F. 380, 392, 408) appear to be necessary ; sometimes the mineral acids (F. 376) — perhaps with cod liver oil ; and sometimes the hypophosphite of soda with bark (F. 419).   In all cases a good nourishing diet should be ordered ; while tepid or cold baths (especially sea-bathing) had better be recommended, together with free exercise in the open air.

PART IV.

DISEASES OF THE NERVOUS SYSTEM.

THE nervous system may be said to consist of two portions,—the cerebro-spinal and the sympathetic. The former is composed of the brain and spinal cord, with the sensory and motor nerves proceeding from them; and it constitutes Bichat's nervous system of animal life. The latter, or the sympathetic or ganglionic portion, consists of a series of ganglia, arranged on either side of the whole length of the vertebral column; these ganglia being united by interconnecting nervous strands or prolongations, communicating with all the other nerves of the body, and supplying branches to the thoracic and abdominal and pelvic viscera as well as to the coats of bloodvessels. It forms Bichat's nervous system of organic life.

Both portions are made up of grey or vesicular neurine, and white or tubular neurine. In the vesicular substance, which contains nerve cells in countless numbers, impressions are received and stored up; while from it we say that nervous force originates. The tubular or fibrous matter conveys impressions from without to the ganglia, and transmits impressions from the latter to organs or tissues where it is distributed. Hence, without any apparent difference in the structure of nerve-fibres, we find variety of function; one distinct set of fibres (centripetal, or afferent, or sensitive nerves) conveying impressions from the periphery to the centre; while another set (centrifugal, efferent, or motor nerves) conducts central impressions to the muscles.

The purposes served in the economy by the different nervous centres may be thus roughly sketched. Suppose that it were possible experimentally to destroy the whole sympathetic nerve, the consequence would be an immediate cessation of the action of the heart, bloodvessels, lungs, abdominal and pelvic viscera, &c. In the same way, destruction of the spinal cord would put an end to all power of movement and to sensibility. And so again, if the brain alone could be removed, every part of the body might remain sound but all manifestations of mind would cease,—sensation, emotion, volition, and intelligence would be abolished.

z 2

The sagacity of an animal is in accordance with the amount of vesicular matter in the brain; this being abundant in proportion to the number and depth and complexity of the convolutions. The brain being the material organ of the mind, the manner in which the mental faculties become affected in disease gives us some clue to the precise situation of the abnormal force.   Thus, there is disordered mental power at an early period, when the morbid action commences in the membranes of the brain, proceeding from without inwards; while this symptom is delayed in the case of tumours originating in the tubular neurine, the growth proceeding from the centre towards the circumference.   In the one case the vesicular matter is early implicated: in the other, it only becomes so at an advanced period.   Furthermore, chronic affections of the vesicular matter of the cerebral hemispheres induce insanity; while acute disorders cause maniacal delirium. Where the central ganglia are likewise diseased, there will be found paralysis with mental derangement.

The nervous ganglia require a certain amount of repose, together with a due supply of pure arterial blood, for their nutrition and healthy action.   Venous or impoverished blood, no less than blood contaminated with certain drugs or poisoned by bile or urea, will blunt the intellectual faculties as well as indispose for muscular action, in proportion to the amount of deterioration.   When the oxidizing power of the blood is artificially increased, or where the blood is sent to the nervous centres in too great a quantity, an increase of mental and muscular power may be manifested; but such increase being accompanied by undue waste must lead to rapid exhaustion.   The products of decay are removed through the urine; the urea, chlorine, phosphoric and sulphuric acids being augmented in quantity when there is increased mental exertion.   Both tea and coffee are excitants of the brain and nervous system, while they retard the decay of tissue and hence diminish the urinary constituents just mentioned.*   Dr. Hammond, after experimenting upon himself with alcohol and tobacco, concludes that these agents increase the weight of the body by retarding the metamorphosis of the old tissues, promoting the formation of new, and limiting the consumption of fat.†

The average weight of the adult male brain (cerebrum, cerebellum, pons Varolii, and medulla oblongata) is 48 or 49 ounces avoirdupois.   That of the female organ is some 4 or 5 ounces less.

---

* Sydney Smith wondered what the world would do without tea? How would it exist? One evening he said,—" I am glad I was not born before tea. I can drink any quantity when I have not tasted wine; otherwise I am haunted by blue-devils by day, and dragons by night. If you want to improve your understanding, drink coffee. Sir James Mackintosh used to say, he believed the difference between one man and another was produced by the quantity of coffee he drank."—*A Memoir of the Reverend Sydney Smith.* By Lady Holland, vol. i. p. 383.   London, 1855.

† *Physiological Memoirs,* p. 55.   Philadelphia, 1863.

Insanity sometimes diminishes, sometimes increases, the brain-weight. Below a particular limit, an intelligent brain is not found. M. Broca has fixed this limit at 37 oz. for the male brain, and 32 oz. for that of the female. According to Professor Welcker 63·5 oz. is the greatest attainable weight of brain within a skull not pathologically enlarged. Cuvier had a brain of 64·5 oz., but Dr. Thurnam remarks that this celebrated man is said to have suffered from hydrocephalus when young. Dr. Abercrombie's brain was 63 oz., and Spurzheim's 55·06. The average specific gravity is 1·036. The composition of nervous material is roughly shown in the following table by L'Heritier :—

Analysis of the Brain at different Periods of Life.

	Infants.	Youths.	Adults.	Aged.	Idiots.
Water	827·90	742·60	725·10	738·50	709·30
Albumen	70·00	102·00	94·00	86·50	84·00
Fat	34·50	53·00	61·00	43·20	50·00
Osmazome and salts .	59·60	85·90	101·90	121·80	148·20
Phosphorus	8·00	16·50	18·00	10·00	8·50
	1000·00	1000·00	1000·00	1000·00	1000·00

During the last year or two (1867-68) an advance has been made towards facilitating the diagnosis of diseases of the cerebro-spinal system by the use of the ophthalmoscope ; so that it would seem far from improbable, that in time the physician may be as much indebted to Helmholtz for his invention as is the ophthal-mologist. The occurrence of symptomatic lesions about the fundus of the eye is found to be the rule, rather than the excep-tion, in affections of the nervous system. At present our know-ledge of these lesions is imperfect ; but too much importance can scarcely be attached to marked alterations in the size or course of the large retinal arteries and veins, the condition of the vessels of the choroid, the state of the cream-coloured optic nerve (the optic disc or papilla of some authors), and the presence of even very small extravasations of blood or of morbid growths or of pigment de-posits. In many examples of Bright's disease, with imperfect vision, yellowish-white deposits of a fatty nature have been found sprinkled over the retina. Syphilitic inflammation of the textures within the cranium may be accompanied by a similar affection of the retina ; the latter being left with irregular white patches scat-tered over its surface, while the optic nerve is also obscured by a layer of lymph. In these cases, irregular deposits of black pigment are likewise often seen distributed among the opaque portions of the retina ; although such pigmentous deposits may also occur as the sequel of any kind of chronic inflammation.

According to M. Bouchut most of the diseases of the brain and spinal cord are accompanied by optic neuritis, retinitis, inflammation of the choroid, or atrophy of the optic nerve. The coincidence of optic neuritis with organic injuries of the nervous system is explained by the anatomical connexions of the eye with the brain and spinal cord. Where disease or injury of the cerebro-spinal system causes some impediment to the cerebral circulation, there hyperæmia of the retina and optic disc will be the consequence. Let those portions of the brain in connexion with the optic thalami, the corpora geniculata, or the corpora quadrigemina become the seat of acute or chronic inflammation, and the morbid process can readily extend to the eye by following the course of the optic tract and nerve. M. Bouchut also shows how other ophthalmoscopic appearances may facilitate the diagnosis. Thus, in optic neuritis and retinitis caused by acute or chronic diseases of the nervous system, the inflammatory action is generally observed equally in both eyes; whereas in injuries of the brain or its membranes, the optic neuritis is most marked within the eye corresponding to the affected hemisphere. Lastly, when together with changes in the optic nerve and retina we have impairment of sensibility and motion and intellect, the existence of organic disease of the encephalon is invariably indicated.

On making examinations of nervous tissue after death considerable care is necessary to prevent morbid changes from being overlooked. The various essays of Lockhart Clarke have shown, as might be expected, that structures which would be regarded as healthy on an ordinary examination, may yet be proved to be very unsound by a minute examination of the properly prepared tissue. To thoroughly investigate the state of the nervous centres, they ought to be removed from the body as soon after death as possible. Then, having been viewed with a lens, incisions should be made according to some pre-arranged system; small portions being removed for examination, while fresh, under the microscope. The nature of the lesion being thus learnt, the morbid parts are to be steeped for three or four weeks in weak solutions of chromic acid; so that after hardening, thin sections may be cut, which can be moistened with glycerine and examined by the microscope.* The strength of the chromic acid solution recommended by Lockhart Clarke varies for different parts of the cerebro-spinal centres. Thus, for the convolutions of the cerebral hemispheres and cerebellum, the proportions are 1 of crystallized acid to 400 of water; while for the pons Varolii, medulla oblongata, and spinal cord, 1 of acid is required to 300 or even 200 of water. Of course, the cases

---

* Full directions for making and preserving these sections, as well as for rendering them permanently transparent, are to be found in a paper entitled, —" Further Researches on the Grey Substance of the Spinal Cord." By J. Lockhart Clarke, F.R.S., &c. *Philosophical Transactions of the Royal Society of London.* Vol. cxlix. p. 458. London, 1860.

which have been thus investigated are comparatively few. But as until the last few years portions of the nervous centres appearing healthy to the naked eye have been set down as natural, it follows that the reports of such autopsies are quite useless. For just as many diseases which our forefathers regarded as functional are now known to be the results of well-recognised organic changes, so it is probable that by and by alterations of brain-matter will be made conspicuous (as in cases of insanity) where at present our blindness prevents us from distinguishing anything abnormal.

I. INFLAMMATION OF THE BRAIN.

Our knowledge of the effects of inflammation of the parts within the cranium [the *Encephalon*, from ἐν = in + κεφαλή = the head] is scarcely sufficiently perfect to enable us to point out with certainty the symptoms which indicate inflammation of the substance of the brain—*cerebritis*, as distinguished from that of the membranes or *meningitis*. Fortunately the distinction (desirable as it must be to frame a perfect diagnosis) is not of much practical importance; for if we allow that in a very few cases cerebritis occurs simply, or that meningitis happens alone, still it is certain that in the majority of instances the two affections are combined.

Before treating of this combination (*encephalitis*), however, a few words may be said as to what little we do know with regard to the diagnosis of meningeal from cerebral inflammation.

1. SIMPLE MENINGITIS.—Inflammation of the membranes of the brain, or meningitis [from Μῆνιγξ = a membrane, with the terminal -*itis*] sometimes arises without any apparent cause; or it can be produced by a fall or blow, or by disease of the ear or nose, or by exposure to the sun. The poison of syphilis or rheumatism can also induce meningitis; and so may the deposit of tubercle, as will be shown presently. Inflammation of the dura mater seldom occurs save as the consequence of blows or wounds, or of some disease of the bones of the skull. In treating of meningitis it is usual to distinguish between inflammation of the dura mater, and that of the arachnoid and pia mater.

Speaking generally, the chief *symptoms* of meningitis are fever, acute pain in the head, irritability with early and violent delirium, frequent flushing of the face followed by pallor, hard pulse, muscular twitchings, prostration, and drowsiness with coma.

Taking a typical example of *inflammation of the arachnoid and pia mater over the convexity of the brain*, there will be noticed first a rigor, or instead (especially in children) a convulsion. The skin then becomes hot and dry, the countenance expressive of anxiety and suffering, and the bowels get confined; while there is intense pain in the head, which is increased by every sound or movement. The temperature is elevated, but not so high as in many kinds of fever, seldom reaching 102°. The face is alternately flushed and pallid : the conjunctivæ are injected, while the eyes are suffused and staring. Where it has been possible to use the ophthalmoscope the existence of optic neuritis and retinitis has been shown. The delirium sets in early, the patient being noisy and very violent. There is great restlessness, muscular twitching, and sometimes strabismus. Vomiting is such a constant and important feature, that it will be again referred to. The symptoms now noticed generally last from three to four days; when the fever lessens, the pulse flags, the tongue gets brown and dry, the excitement diminishes, and the delirium is apt to pass into coma. In a few days more, the prostration has become extreme; and the symptoms get to resemble those presented in the last stage of typhus. When the disease ends favourably, the improvement is usually very gradual; being unattended by any critical sweat or looseness of the bowels.

Before proceeding, it will be better to fulfil the promise just made of further noticing the sickness which occurs in cerebral diseases. Every one knows that headache from gastric disturbance is as common as vomiting from cerebral derangement. A sick headache, *i.e.* retching with distressing pain in the head, is the especial symptom of stomach derangement (gastric catarrh). In children, obstinate vomiting is particularly indicative of brain disease. The peculiarities which distinguish gastric or hepatic from cerebral sickness, may be thus arranged to aid our diagnosis :—

Gastric or Hepatic Vomiting.	*Cerebral Vomiting.*
1. The nausea is relieved, at all events temporarily, by the discharge. It returns directly food is taken.	1. Little or no nausea, and the vomiting continues in spite of the discharge of contents of stomach.
2. There is tenderness over the liver and stomach. Pressure induces the inclination to retch.	2. No tenderness over liver or stomach. Pressure borne without inconvenience.
3. The pulse is frequent and weak.	3. The pulse is infrequent and hard.
4. Tongue furred; breath offensive; conjunctivæ often yellowish; and headache secondary as to time.	4. Tongue clean ; breath sweet ; conjunctivæ colourless or injected ; and headache primary.
5. Griping abdominal pain, diarrhœa, and clay-coloured stools.	5. Generally, obstinate constipation.
6. Retching, and increased salivation.	6. Stomach emptied without effort; no salivation,
7. Sickness lessened by counter-irritation to epigastrium only.	7. Sickness lessened by counter-irritation to nape of neck only.
8. Complete disgust for food.	8. No disgust for food : perhaps the reverse.

The statements in these columns must of course be taken with some qualification. Speaking generally, they are correct. On the one side, the vomiting depends upon derangement of the liver or of the gastro-intestinal canal; on the other, it is owing to increased sensorial or reflex action. I would only add, as a caution, that

vomiting due to increased reflective mobility is not always caused
by cerebral disease. Thus, it occurs during pregnancy, as well as
in certain uterine and ovarian disorders. Moreover, the most severe
case of constant vomiting which has ever fallen under my notice
was due to a slight ring of cancerous deposit around the œsophagus,
nearly an inch above its termination in the cardiac orifice of the
stomach. In this instance the morbid product seemed to act upon
the stomach by reflex action, for the disease was so inconsiderable
in amount that it could not directly interfere with the normal
functions of this viscus. In the sickness of pregnancy, as well as
in cases resembling that just mentioned, there are no symptoms
of gastric or hepatic derangement.

In *meningitis confined to the base* (frequently due to tuberculosis)
the diagnosis is very difficult. Andral* relates the particulars of
two fatal instances where the symptoms were very dissimilar. In
one there was delirium at the commencement; with great fever, contracted pupils, raving, frequent pulse, teeth clenched as in trismus,
and a retraction of the head. The tongue was natural. The
patient seemed as if in profound sleep; while as the coma got more
profound, the respiration became embarrassed, and death occurred
as in apoplexy. On examination the entire lower surface of the
cerebral hemisphere was found covered by a thick layer of pus
contained in the pia mater.—The second example presented at
first pain in the temples, vomiting, constipation, symptoms of wry-
neck, loss of appetite, and a desire for rest. When seen a few
days afterwards the face was pale and dejected, and the look vacant :
the eyes were sensible to strong light. The intelligence was clear, with
the pulse and skin normal. The headache seemed the only important
symptom ; and it was unrelieved by bleeding, leeches, and blisters to
the leg. Coma gradually set in, became profound, and ended in death.
Up to the termination the pulse continued natural, and only at the
last was respiration disturbed. At the autopsy the upper part of
the brain and meninges proved to be healthy ; but the lower surface
of the pia mater was infiltrated with a purulent layer from seven to
eight lines in thickness.

A peculiar modification of meningitis occasionally sets in during
the progress of acute rheumatism. The invasion is sudden, is accompanied with great fear of approaching death, is followed by
delirium, and often ends fatally—sometimes very rapidly so. It
is a question whether the attack is due to a metastasis of the rheumatism from the joints to the brain, to rheumatic meningitis, to
the employment of bleeding, or to the use of large doses of quinine
(such as are especially used in France) for combating the rheumatic
fever.† The post mortem appearances are very variable ; the

* *The Clinique Médicale.* Spillan's Translation, p. 16. London, 1836.
† As typical of this kind of treatment, the following case of death from
supposed *cerebral rheumatism* may be mentioned :—A robust man, a hard
drinker, was admitted into the Hôtel Dieu, under Professor Trousseau's care,
on account of a severe attack of rheumatic fever. He had already suffered

membranes of the brain being sometimes found healthy, sometimes congested, sometimes with sub-arachnoid serous effusions, while very rarely pus has been discovered over the hemispheres.

Meningitis, as a result of constitutional syphilis is not so infrequent as might be imagined. The dura mater is more frequently affected than the arachnoid and pia mater. Lymph is generally effused; and the membranes usually become adherent. Small gummatous deposits are now and then found embedded in the meninges; sometimes being in connexion with nodes on the cranial bones. The chief symptoms produced by these deposits as well as by the inflammatory action, are mental depression or irritability, and sometimes sickness; with severe headache, which becomes especially aggravated at night. Giddiness, convulsions, paralysis, epilepsy, &c. have been observed. The appearance of the patient and his previous history will help the diagnosis. Iodide of potassium (F. 31) is the remedy; but the cure may perhaps be expedited by the simultaneous use of calomel vapour baths, or of mercurial inunction. Sleep is to be afforded at night by opium.

Inflammation of the dura mater is generally the result of violence, or of tertiary syphilis, or of disease of the bones of the skull— particularly of the petrous portion of the temporal bone or of the ethmoid. Specimens of syphilitic caries of the frontal bone are to be seen in every hospital museum. With children, chronic affections of the ear and nose, which are often long regarded as trifling, sometimes terminate fatally by a rapid extension of the morbid action to the dura mater. In an instance of this kind about which I was consulted at the last moment, the acute symptoms came on so insidiously that no danger was apprehended until the child suddenly became comatose. In fact, up to the time that the latter occurrence supervened, nothing was complained of but headache and a desire for repose; the pulse continuing natural until death,

similarly on three occasions; and in consequence there was a double lesion of the ventriculo-aortic orifice, adherent pericardium, and a large heart. On the day of his admission (the twelfth of the disease) several joints were affected, and it was predicated that the attack would prove severe and prolonged. Twenty grains of sulphate of quinine were given: the praecordial region was cupped in six different places. The following day the quinine was increased to two scruples, this dose being repeated on the third day. On the fourth day, thirty grains were taken. The dose for the fifth and sixth days is not mentioned. On the evening of the latter, the pain in the joints had considerably diminished; and the patient was much pleased at his condition. An hour after expressing this pleasure he said he could not see, called out "thief," rushed from his bed and fell down. He struggled with two attendants while being assisted to bed, dropped back, and died. All took place in less than fifteen minutes. At the autopsy nothing was revealed to account for the result. The brain was remarkably healthy, but there was injection of the pia mater covering it. The cardiac lesions were those already mentioned. There was no effusion into the affected joints, nor were the synovial membranes injected. The whole history of this case is detailed in Professor Trousseau's *Lectures on Clinical Medicine*, translated by Dr. Bazire. Vol. i. p. 513. London, 1868.

and there being neither fever nor sickness.   A discharge from the left ear had persisted since an attack of scarlatina some two years previously.

The appearances presented by the membranes after death from meningitis are necessarily of a fluctuating nature, much depending upon the severity and duration of the disease. Thus, if the case have run a very rapid course, the membranes are particularly vascular and dry ; when the disease has continued for some days, there will be an effusion of purulent serum or of pure pus in the sac of the arachnoid and in the connective tissue of the pia mater ; while supposing the morbid action to have had a still longer spell, layers of lymph may be found, together with concrete pus in the meshes of the pia mater upon and between the convolutions.   Moreover, as the vascular pia mater not only invests the brain but is prolonged into its interior, forming the velum interpositum and choroid plexuses of the fourth ventricle, so the traces of inflammatory action can perhaps be traced into the nervous matter itself.   Sometimes, even the lateral ventricles contain false membranes.   Or the mass of the brain may be œdematous ; a condition more frequently found in children, than in adults.

2. CEREBRITIS AND ABSCESS.—Partial inflammation of the brain, without meningitis, is of the rarest occurrence.   Indeed, the membranes may be said to be always affected ; though the energy of the mischief is found to be expended on the brain tissue. The inflammation is either spontaneous, or traumatic ; the latter being the most common.   Concussion, fracture of the bones of the skull, disease of the ethmoid, and mischief about the petrous portion of the temporal bone, are frequent antecedents.   Sunstroke is also said to be an occasional cause.   The most remarkable symptoms appear to consist of persistent, deep-seated pain in the head ; general malaise and vomiting ; impairment of vision and hearing ; confusion of ideas, with failure of memory ; rigors ; rapidly progressive emaciation ; increasing weakness ; and convulsive paroxysms, ending in paralysis or coma.   The mental disturbance varies considerably according to the seat of the disease.   At the end of three or four days there may be a copious effusion of serum, followed by all the symptoms of compression.   Sometimes the inflammation ends in abscess, the latter perhaps forming without exciting any suspicion in the minds of the attendants.*   No active

* The two following remarkable instances serve well to exemplify the obscurity which surrounds some of these cases :—
i. A youth, aged eighteen, applied as an out-patient at the Hôpital St. Louis, on account of a purulent discharge from the ear. So little inconvenience did he feel, that it was with difficulty he could be persuaded to enter the hospital.   Though appearing in excellent health, death took place suddenly the next day, immediately after the occurrence of a convulsive paroxysm. At the autopsy, the petrous bone was found diseased, but the dura mater covering it had not undergone any change. The cavity of the tympanum

treatment is of any avail in warding off a fatal conclusion. If by a fortunate chance recovery should occur, it may be partly due to good management,—decidedly not to the use of drugs.

An *abscess of the brain* has been found in all parts of the cerebral hemispheres, in the corpus striatum, the optic thalamus, the pons Varolii, the cerebellum, and the medulla oblongata. There has been one abscess, or several collections of pus have been discovered. The abscess has been surrounded by cyst-walls of some thickness; or there has been no enclosing capsule, but merely disorganized

was filled with pus, which obtained an exit both by the external auditory meatus and the Eustachian tube. All the convolutions of the left cerebral hemisphere had become effaced, while a collection of pus occupied the whole of the middle and posterior lobes of the brain. Very small abscesses were scattered throughout the anterior lobe. This patient had never manifested the slightest intellectual disturbance; and no symptom indicated the existence of cerebral lesion, until the pus, bursting into the lateral ventricle, caused instant death.—*Gazette Hebdomadaire de Médecine et de Chirurgie*, p. 743. Paris, 15 Novembre 1861.

2. A soldier of the French line, being on parade, was suddenly seized with vertigo. He passed his musket to a comrade, staggered a moment, and dropped senseless. Carried to the hospital, he remained for some time comatose; with his limbs relaxed, his pupils dilated and immoveable, and his pulse full and slow. He then fell into a series of epileptiform convulsions, and died. The following history was obtained:—Two years previously this man had stolen out one night from barracks, and in order to re-enter unperceived, had to climb a rampart. He tumbled into the ditch, pitching on his head; but on recovering consciousness, returned to his quarters without saying a word about the accident. He continued to perform actively the duties of sergeant, and was never suspected of ill-health; nevertheless, it was remembered that from time to time he had complained of violent headaches attended with great prostration, and the sufferer himself seems to have attributed them to the fall. These headaches, after lasting from six to twenty-four hours, would pass off in a very heavy sleep. Not the slightest disturbance of intellect or locomotive power made its appearance. A few months before death, the surgeon of the regiment had noticed that the sergeant was much changed in appearance; the face was pale and of a *leaden hue*, and there was considerable loss of flesh. A careful physical examination produced no elucidation of the mystery.—On *post-mortem* inspection, no external trace of wound was found upon the head, nor was there any evidence of fracture, old or recent. The veins of the dura mater were gorged, but there was no bloody effusion. The left hemisphere was much enlarged, and on palpation of its convex surface extensive fluctuation could easily be perceived. On slicing the brain, the left lateral ventricle was found distended with liquid blood, which seemed recently effused; the third ventricle was similarly filled, and a rent communicated between the two. The cerebral substance in front of the left lateral ventricle was the seat of a spherical cavity the size of a walnut, full of blood, and communicating with the ventricle by an opening which would admit a common quill. Along with the blood in this cavity there was also found a considerable layer of concrete pus, lining its walls, from which, however, it was separated by a whitish grey pyogenic membrane. The series of events, then, in this case were:—(1) Formation of an abscess in the anterior lobe, in consequence of the blow on the head; which abscess was the cause of the intermittent headache, and latterly of the failure in general nutrition. (2) Rapidly fatal hæmorrhage into the ventricles, produced by the sudden rupture of the wall of the abscess.— *Gazette des Hôpitaux.* Quoted from the *London Medical Review*, p. 333. December 1862.

brain structure. According to Rokitansky, the recent abscess consists of an irregular cavity in the parenchyma of the brain ; the walls being composed of suppurating cerebral tissue, sloughing shreds of which hang into the collection of pus, while the brain all around is in a state of inflammation. The pus in such cases is thick and greenish, and has a fetid phosphorescent odour.

Although a cerebral abscess is usually soon fatal, yet when encysted it may not destroy life for some time. In a very few cases it is even possible that restoration to health has taken place ; the pus cells having undergone fatty degeneration, the fluid contents having become absorbed, and the capsule having contracted. If in any given case we sought to effect a cure our only chance would lie in enforcing mental and bodily rest ; in allowing a plain nourishing diet, with plenty of milk and no stimulants ; and in keeping the patient in pure air. For many months after the cessation of all symptoms care would still be needed to prevent any mischief from being again started in the brain tissue around the cyst.

There are records of the skull having been trephined in a few cases, for the purpose of giving exit to pus ; but recovery did not follow in a single instance, so far as I have been able to learn.

3. ACUTE ENCEPHALITIS.—This disease may be roughly described as a morbid process which gives rise to more or less complicated phenomena during life, according to its degree and the extent to which the brain and its membranes are involved. After death, traces of its power are found in the form of meningeal congestion, with effused lymph or serum or pus ; an appearance of vascularity, varying from bloody points, or a scarlet tinge, to a dusky redness about the affected part of the brain ; with occasionally softening, or suppuration, of the cerebral substance.

Causes.—They are often difficult to detect. Inflammatory affections of the brain sometimes arise without any appreciable reason. Plethoric persons, and such as have short necks, are said to be more liable to them than others. Occasionally these attacks come on in the course of continued fever, or of measles, or of scarlatina ; or they may follow upon wounds, blows, or other injuries ; or they will be due to disease of the bones of the ear or of the nose, or to poisoned blood, or to intemperance ; or they may be owing to suppressed evacuations. Dr. Abercrombie in speaking of the causes of encephalitis states that—" One of the most common examples of this is suppression of the menses, which in young women of unsound constitution is very often followed by dangerous affections of the brain. Headache, or any symptom in the head occurring under such circumstances, is always to be considered as requiring most minute attention."[*] According to my own experience, the symptoms which occur under these circum-

* *On Diseases of the Brain and Spinal Cord.* Fourth Edition, p. 148. Edinburgh, 1845.

stances, are much more frequently the result of anæmia than of inflammation.   It need scarcely be said the distinction is of just as great importance, as is that between hydrocephalus and hydrocephaloid disease.

Symptoms.—The chief and earliest indications of encephalitis, or phrenitis [from Φρὴν = the mind, with the terminal *-itis*], or meningo-cerebritis, as it is more appropriately termed, are—fever, nausea and vomiting, acute headache, sharp and hard and irregular pulse, constipation, impatience of light and sound, watchfulness, a look of oppression or sullenness, suffusion of the eyes, and confusion of thought or even delirium.   These symptoms are most marked where the meningitis predominates.

At the end of from twelve hours to two days, the second stage of the complaint sets in—the period of collapse.   The patient falls into a state of stupor; his articulation is rendered difficult or indistinct; his vision and hearing get dull; the pupil (from having been contracted to a pin's point) becomes dilated; there may be squinting, and paralysis of the muscles of the eyelids; and there are frequent twitchings of the muscles.   Then the countenance gets ghastly; sordes form on the gums and teeth; and the body is covered with cold sweats.   Finally the sphincters relax; and there are a few convulsive paroxysms, paralysis and profound coma, which usually soon terminate in death.

Occasionally the first symptom that attracts attention is a sudden attack of convulsion; in some cases occurring without any previous illness, at other times preceded for a few days by headache and slight complaints which have passed on unnoticed.   The convulsion is generally long and severe; it may be followed immediately by coma, which in a few days is fatal; or it will perhaps recur frequently at short intervals, and pass into coma at the end of twenty-four hours.   Sir Thomas Watson thinks that when nausea and vomiting are the earliest symptoms, the inflammation has had its origin in the cerebral pulp—in the substance of the brain; and that when the attack commences with a convulsion, the inflammation has started from the pia mater or the arachnoid.

In all the forms of this dangerous complaint there is a great uncertainty about the symptoms; while much observation will be necessary to put us on our guard against the insidious characters which many of the cases assume, and the deceitful appearances of amendment that often take place.   Fortunately the disease is not of frequent occurrence.   It either ends fatally in a few days; or the patient may struggle on for two or three weeks.

Diagnosis.—To distinguish encephalitis from the delirium of fever and from delirium tremens is sometimes difficult.   The history will often throw light on the matter.   In phrenitis the delirium is an early symptom, and it is usually violent; the pulse is sharp, hard, and often irregular; and there is generally sickness. In fever, the delirium is an after symptom.   In delirium tremens, the soft and frequent and compressible pulse, the busy delirium or wandering, the loquacity of the patient, the trembling of his hands, and generally the ease with which he is temporarily roused to answer questions rationally, are important diagnostic signs.   Moreover, as Dr. Bence Jones has shown, in acute inflammations of the brain there is an increase in the earthy and alkaline phosphates of the urine ; while in delirium tremens there is a marked diminution of them.   And again, in inflammation the chlorides in the urine are greatly diminished, if not entirely absent ; while in the delirium from drink or exhaustion these salts are unaffected.

Morbid Anatomy.—The post-mortem appearance most commonly found is more or less vascularity of the substance of the brain ; a condition indicated by the existence of numerous bloody points in the medullary portion, giving an appearance as if it had been sprinkled with red dots.   In other instances the vascularity is much greater, sometimes being so excessive that the part is of a dusky red hue.   There may be an exudation of pus, either upon and between the convolutions, or collected in one or more abscesses in one of the hemispheres.   Softening of a part of the cerebral substance is not uncommon ; the softened portions sometimes resembling thick cream, so that they are readily washed away by a gentle stream of water.   Moreover, we may have copious serous effusions beneath the pia mater and into the ventricles.

The dura mater is seldom involved in the morbid action, unless the inflammation be the result of violence.   In such cases there may be a deposition of false membranes between the bone and dura mater, or between the dura mater and arachnoid ; or we shall find thickening of all the membranes.

Treatment.—The principal measure usually recommended is a strict observance of the antiphlogistic regimen.   In other words, the practitioner has been advised to put his trust in a diet of the lowest kind, general and local bleeding, antimonials in some stages of the disease, digitalis, active purgatives, mercury, blisters to the back of the head and neck, mustard pediluvia, and the constant application of cold to the scalp after the hair has all been shaved off. With regard to venesection it has been suggested that the blood ought to be allowed to flow until a decided impression is made upon the pulse, or until the patient faints ; which will perhaps happen when some twenty-four ounces have come away.   Afterwards, it is said that leeches or cupping may be resorted to.

When it is remembered that encephalitis is one of the most quickly depressing and fatal diseases which can affect the human body, it may readily be imagined—from what has been already stated —that its dangers are not lessened by the foregoing treatment. And such seems really to be the case ; for one of the strongest advocates of this practice, Dr. Abercrombie, in speaking of the results of a course of these so-called remedies, says :—" The cases which thus terminate favourably, form, it must be confessed, but a small proportion of those which come under the view of a physician of considerable practice ; but they hold out every encouragement to persevere in the treatment of a class of diseases, which, after a certain period of their progress, we are too apt to consider as hopeless." With the greatest respect for this clever physician's opinions, it rather seems to me that the extensive failure of one plan of treatment should decidedly lead us either to test another, or to hold our hands. We talk of the vis medicatrix naturæ, but it is seldom allowed fair play. Here at least is a good opportunity for trying whether this force, perhaps gently guided, may not carry a patient through a disease where the efforts of our art are notoriously so futile. If it fail, we must strive again and again after a better course. But in such a contingency, drugs are not to be used at haphazard—on the mere chance of their doing good. And until we have more light, let us at least determine not to thwart the natural efforts at reparation, as we may easily do by acting upon the fallacious notion that the free loss of blood is well borne ; neither let us credit those who assert that antimony or mercury is capable of effecting a cure in these distressing diseases. It may be said that in these observations I am combating shadows. That the treatment condemned, is that of past days. This is not so, however. A writer of great ability, in one of the most important medical works published during 1868, says that the treatment of acute meningitis can only be successful when employed very early ; and that it consists of bloodletting, hard purging, and cold to the head. The patient is to be bled in a sitting posture, from a large opening in a vein in the arm ; the blood being allowed to flow till syncope is induced. The bleeding is to be repeated as often as the symptoms require it, or to be followed by leeches behind the ears and to the temples. Moreover, mercury is to be so administered by the mouth and by inunction as to bring the system quickly under its influence. In alluding to these recommendations, I hope it will not be thought that I am improperly criticising them. They are mentioned in justification of my own remarks. Less could hardly be said, inasmuch as my distrust of violent attempts to cure these meningeal and cerebral inflammations is so great ; and seeing also my belief that we may do good if we can but be contented with prescribing for the urgent symptoms as they arise,—endeavouring to calm excitement by sedatives, to lessen increased heat of body by diluents and tepid sponging, to prevent accumulations in the intestines by purgatives, and to diminish maniacal delirium by the application of cold to the head.

Active cathartics of calomel and jalap, followed in three or four hours by an aperient draught, are often deemed indispensable (F. 140, 159). The compound decoction of aloes (from one to two ounces), repeated once or twice, forms a favourite remedy with me ; or simply such a saline aperient as F. 152 may be recommended. Croton oil (F. 168) is a most valuable purgative in some of these cases where there is obstinate constipation. Dr. Abercrombie rather illogically says (*Opus jam citat.* p. 153) :—" Although blood-letting is never to be neglected in the earlier stages of the disease, my own experience is, that more recoveries from head affections of the most alarming aspect take place under the use of very strong purging than under any other mode of treatment."

The application of cold to the head, after it has been shaved, is a remedy of importance. Pounded ice in a bladder, or a cold evaporating lotion (F. 273), or especially the pouring of cold water in a stream upon the vertex of the head, will best effect our object of reducing the temperature and calming excitement. By the cold douche, used with discretion, a strong man in the highest state of maniacal delirium may often be subdued in almost a few minutes ; but it must be particularly remembered that this practice, if long continued or too often repeated, has a very depressing influence. I feel bound to add this caution having seen the imprudent use of both the ice bag and the cold douche productive of mischief.

With regard to medicines for directly modifying the morbid action, I know only of one on which the least reliance can be placed, and that is the iodide of potassium. Of course, the use of this drug is imperative where the diseased action is in any way connected with the poison of syphilis. But I have also seen this salt of iodine, in doses of three to eight grains repeated every four or six hours, do so much good in a few apparently hopeless cases where no evidence of venereal infection could be obtained, that I think it ought to be tried. I have, of course, often found it fail ; but in my hands it has never done mischief. The iodide of potash may often be advantageously given at the same time that stimulants are being cautiously employed.

When, from exhaustion of the nervous force, an extreme degree of collapse sets in, the only chance of rescuing the patient will consist in the administration of stimulants and nutriment; such as ammonia, spirit of ether, milk, raw eggs, strong beef tea, wine, or brandy. In all stages of this disease the practitioner ought to watch his patient almost hour by hour, must ascertain that he is kept dry and clean, and will have to be careful that the bladder does not become over-distended.

Should the disorder happily yield to these measures, great attention will be requisite for some time (especially with regard to diet and the avoidance of all excitement) to prevent a relapse.

4. CHRONIC ENCEPHALITIS.—This is a disease which may follow an attack of acute meningo-cerebritis, or it can come on independently as the primary disorder. The term *chronic* is used not merely in the sense of prolonged duration, but also as implying a series of symptoms of a subacute character.

The phenomena presented by chronic encephalitis are singularly diversified ; but they may be briefly said to be commonly allied to those which mark the commencement of insanity. Hence, we find either great mental excitement or depression. Some absurd whim exists, to gratify which everything must be sacrificed; and the patient believes that he is either about to make a fortune, or to become a parish pauper. Amongst the general symptoms, hesitation in speaking or a slight stammering, a stiffness of some of the muscles, noises in the ears, troublesome headache, vertigo on walking, loss of appetite, constipation, and irregularity of the pulse, are perhaps the most prominent. As the disease slowly progresses, however, the evidences of cerebral disorder become fully developed: the memory fails, the external senses get impaired, there is a constant tendency to somnolence, paralysis shows itself, and the general health completely breaks up.

The symptoms of chronic inflammation of the meninges in aged persons are obscure. The mental faculties are dulled, there is a loss of all vivacity and energy, the speech is somewhat indistinct, and the gait is tottering. Constipation, giddiness, noises in the ears, headache, and fits of irritability are common. But there is nothing in all this which can lead to a positive diagnosis. The indications are those of some cerebral mischief; but whether it be inflammation, softening, œdema, &c. can scarcely be determined. The patient gradually passes more and more of his time in bed; sores are very apt to form upon the sacrum; and death at length occurs from exhaustion. A subsequent examination reveals opacity and thickening of parts of the arachnoid; with probably a similar condition of the pia mater. The serum in the ventricles may likewise be much increased in quantity.

Chronic encephalitis sometimes runs its course in a few months, or it may last for years. In our treatment we can only attempt to combat the symptoms as they show themselves, while trying by judicious hygienic measures to support the general health. Stimulants usually do harm, and so does tea or coffee. For all of these, milk proves an admirable substitute; and particularly is this the case with the aged. Repeated small blisters behind the ears, the use of a seton in the nucha, and perhaps the free inunction of the shaved scalp with the iodide of potassium or red iodide of mercury ointment, may be of some utility. The state of the bowels, as well as of the uterine functions in women, ought to be looked to. In the advanced stages, the patient ought to lie on a water-bed; exhausting and troublesome sores being easily produced by any unequal pressure upon the nates and sacrum. The catheter will also have to be used in many instances.

5. ŒDEMA OF THE BRAIN.—Congestion of the brain and its membranes may give rise to different conditions, which either prove transitory or become developed into serious maladies. The feverish attack sometimes spoken of as "brain fever" is one of the simplest effects of congestion: an apoplectic fit, or a so-called paralytic stroke, must be regarded as among the most grave. In the latter class we have also to place œdema of the brain ; a condition which will be either acute or chronic.   The cerebral substance becomes infiltrated with serum ; and this freely exudes on a section being made.   A higher degree is marked by the brain substance being converted into a soft diffluent pap.   Examples of *acute œdema* are observed in cases of tubercular meningitis, when the cerebral matter around the lateral ventricles (which are full of serum) is found in a pulpy condition ; as also in the tissue surrounding cancerous or fibrous tumours, or patches of inflammation.   The effusion when rapidly developed, proves fatal by its pressure : in other instances it soddens the affected parts, causing these portions of the brain to soften and break down.

Chronic œdema of the brain is oft-times met with, especially in advanced life.   It occurs, like the acute variety, as the result of persistent venous congestion.   This congestion has its origin in some impediment to the circulation, such as may be produced by a dilatation of the right side of the heart, with diminution of power and valvular competency ; or by pulmonary emphysema, chronic asthma, infiltration of part of the lungs with fibroid material or with tubercle, chronic renal disease with albuminuria, &c.   The symptoms are those of cerebral compression.   They come on in a tardy and very gradual manner, especially where the brain has lost some of its volume by previous atrophy.   The intellectual faculties are blunted, and at length get more or less abolished ; there is muscular weakness, which increases until the patient is bedridden ; while the general sensibility becomes more and more torpid.   Frequently there is drowsiness during the day ; often followed at night by a continued babbling of sentences without meaning, carried on in a low tone of voice.

Cases of chronic cerebral œdema are to be seen in the infirmaries of most workhouses.   The sufferers are helpless, quiet, and uncomplaining : they give some little trouble as it is necessary to keep them dry and clean, and generally to feed them.   They require nourishing food, of a kind which can be easily digested ; while a brisk aperient draught ought to be given every three or four days to relieve their constipated bowels.   The effect of a few loose stools on the mental faculties is often remarkable.   The pressure on the brain gets lessened by absorption of some of the serum ; so that the individual seems to wake up, and in some measure to become himself again.   His old feelings and failings partly return, and he may get angry and almost violent if thwarted.   This change is of brief duration.   The effusion continuing, the symptoms produced by the pressure gradually reappear.   Every now and then, death seems to happen rather suddenly ; when it is usually registered as due to serous apoplexy. In other instances, there is progressive enfeeblement of the functions of the nervous system. Attacks of quiet delirium supervene ;

leaving the patient imbecile, and almost deprived of voluntary muscular power. Then follows an interval of mere animal life. Perhaps for two or three days, a feeble circulation and respiration alone continue; with occasional involuntary twitchings of the muscles of the face and limbs. And then life ceases; the fragile connecting link being so gently severed, that those around the bed are doubtful if all is over.

6. **SOFTENING: INDURATION: TUMOURS.**—The results of these different morbid states are of great importance. With regard to *softening of the brain* there are three varieties; which are respectively known as white or atrophic softening, red softening, and yellow softening.

White or atrophic softening (ramollissement non-inflammatoire) is that form in which the cohesion of the cerebral texture becomes loosened and lacerated by an interstitial exudation of serum. It occurs in the white substance of the hemispheres. The affected part may only have its consistence slightly lessened, or it will perhaps be rendered as diffluent as cream. The softening is the consequence of imperfect nutrition, or of the strength of the brain tissue being exhausted. Either because sufficient healthy blood does not reach the affected parts, or because the latter are no longer capable of repair, degeneration sets in. Hence the subjects of this condition are in general weakly individuals advancing towards old age; while they sometimes are suffering from renal or cardiac disease, or from disease of the coats of the cerebral and other arteries. It has been already pointed out that the detachment of small fibrinous deposits from the valves, or interior of the left side of the heart, and their circulation with the systemic blood until they become arrested in one of the cerebral arteries, may (by impeding the transit of a due quantity of blood) lead to imperfect nutrition, and hence to softening.

Red softening or acute ramollissement has long been regarded as one of the terminations of the inflammatory process; although recent researches have cast much doubt upon this view. Indeed, it seems much more probable that the cause of this form is the sudden withdrawal of blood from the affected part, by the abrupt obstruction of an artery. This variety of softening is met with in either the grey or white substance of the brain; it may be slight and partial, or diffused and extensive; it may render the affected tissue pulpy, or so thin that it can be poured away merely leaving an irregular cavity; while the colour of the softened structure is found to vary from a brown or purple to a rosy hue.

The third form or *yellow* softening occurs as an idiopathic disease in circumscribed patches. According to Rokitansky,* at the affected part (which varies from the size of a bean to that of a hen's egg) the cerebral substance looks as if converted into a moist tremulous pulp, of the colour of sulphur. When cut across it rises above

* *A Manual of Pathological Anatomy.* Vol. iii. p. 419. London, 1850.

the level of the section ; while a nearly clear yellow fluid oozes out. To the naked eye no trace of natural structure is presented. The transition from healthy to diseased tissue is somewhat abrupt ; there being no reddening or vascularity around the morbid part. The most frequent seat of yellow softening is the cerebrum ; the fibrous structure and the central masses of grey matter being both attacked. It is very rare in the periphery of the brain. This species of softening may be found surrounding a patch of inflammation, an apoplectic clot, or any adventitious product. It is most common in middle and advanced age ; and it runs a rapidly fatal course. Rokitansky looks upon the theory which ascribes the origin of yellow softening to inflammation as quite untenable.

The general symptoms of cerebral softening are,—more or less severe and persistent pain in the head; with attacks of vertigo coming on suddenly, and soon passing off. There is a diminution of intellectual power, an embarrassment in answering questions, depression of spirits, and a susceptibility to shed tears on the slightest excitement or emotion. Prickings and twitchings of the limbs are common : sometimes there is pain and oft-times numbness. A tendency to stupor, especially after food, is not uncommon ; and there is often more or less impairment of vision and hearing. In the red variety the symptoms are of a more acute character. The headache is very severe, at times preventing sleep during the night : the limbs are frequently the seat of painful cramps, stiffness, or contractions ; and the general sensibility is heightened.

The second stage of either of the forms of cerebral softening may end suddenly in a fatal apoplectic seizure, in convulsions, or in delirium. But in more chronic cases there will often come on paralysis of a limb, or of one half of the body ; with all the usual phenomena attendant on such a state. Thus, there is a loss of power in the affected limbs ; questions are answered slowly, and the patient has a difficulty in making himself understood ; there is great general feebleness, with a weak and intermitting pulse ; there will usually be attacks of sickness and constipation ; and there is a difficulty in emptying the bladder, while the stools are passed involuntarily. Then the respiration gets laboured, towards the last becoming stertorous ; and a state of coma comes on, which may perhaps pass off in a day or two, but only to return and become more profound, until it ends in death. Although softening can occur at any period of life, it is most common after the fiftieth year.

In one of his clinical lectures Dr. Brown-Séquard related some interesting examples of *softening of the cerebellum*. He alluded to the great variety of symptoms present in these affections, and pointed out the chief differences between cerebral and cerebellar inflammatory ramollissement. In all except two of his cases there was a fixed pain at the back of the head, and generally on the side corresponding to the diseased hemisphere of the cerebellum. Amaurosis occurred complete in both eyes in two of eleven in-

stances, though the disease only existed in one half of the cerebellum : in one case there was loss of sight only in the right eye,
with disease of the left half of the cerebellum. Hemiplegia was
complete in two cases, incomplete in one. Paraplegia existed in
only two. The other symptoms were a tendency to walk backwards,
tottering gait, vertigo, an emotional and semi-convulsive agitation
of the limbs, obtuse hearing, and aphonia. Vomiting existed in
none ; though it is frequent in other diseases of the cerebellum.
No two of the cases recorded were alike, but all showed great
differences from cerebral softening. There were none of the referred or local sensations or pains in the paralysed limbs which
are so characteristic of the red cerebral softening. The various
kinds of involuntary movements were absent ; while there was no
muscular rigidity. No irregularity of pulse was noticed, either as
regards rapidity or strength.

Induration of the brain (sclerosis) is found in its most marked
degree in counexion with cerebral atrophy. The whole brain may
be affected, or only portions. This increase of consistence has
been detected in epilepsy, rickets, and after death during some of
the continued or eruptive fevers. The whole cerebral mass may become as tough as leather. In other instances, the indurated portion
is of small extent ; presenting the appearance of wax, or of white
of egg boiled hard. The change is probably due to a great increase
of the albumen.

Tumours—both simple and malignant, *deposits of tubercle, blood-
clots, cysts, abscesses, chalky concretions, syphilitic gummatous growths,*
as well as *cysticerci* and *hydatids* have also been found in the brain.
Primary *cancer* of this organ is a very rare disease : it is perhaps
more common in males than females, and occurs more frequently
between the thirtieth and fortieth years than at any other age.
Gliomata are growths formed by a localized hyperplasia of the
neuroglia—as the interstitial connective tissue of the brain and
spinal cord has been named by Virchow. A microscopical examination of neuroglia shows that it consists of a fibrillated substance,
in the meshes of which are cells of different shapes ; many of these
cells resembling colourless blood corpuscles. The glioma is an
overgrowth of this tissue. The tumour is vascular, and generally
solitary ; it will be either soft or hard ; and it may be of the size
of a walnut, or even larger.

The indications of either of the foregoing occurrences are
usually very obscure ; varying with the situation of the morbid
product, its size, and the condition of the nervous tissue around it.
Probably the most common symptoms are headache, sickness,
giddiness, an unsymmetrical state of the pupils, mental depression
with confusion, partial paralysis, and epileptiform convulsions.

The coats of the cerebral arteries occasionally become affected
with fatty degeneration (*atheroma*) ; with calcareous infiltration
(*ossification*) ; or with uniform dilatation of all their coats causing

aneurism. One or more of these vessels may also get obstructed from local coagulation of fibrin (*thrombosis*); or in consequence of a coagulum being carried from a distant part, and getting impacted there (*embolism*).

7. **TUBERCULAR MENINGITIS.**—Acute inflammation of the brain is a very common disease of early life—of children under five years of age. It rarely occurs, however, in such as are previously healthy : where it does so, it may be regarded as simple encephalitis. When it is the result (as it most frequently is) of tubercular deposit in the brain or its membranes, when it occurs, in fact, in scrofulous children, it is then known as tubercular meningitis. Formerly the name of acute hydrocephalus was given to this disorder; but this term was evidently badly chosen, since it referred only to one of the possible results of the disease, not to the disease itself.

Symptoms.—The symptoms of tubercular meningitis are various and uncertain. For convenience, they may be arbitrarily considered as exhibiting three stages. The *first* or *premonitory stage* is attended with indications of mal-nutrition ; and there are more or less perfect signs of the strumous diathesis in the child or its parents. There is often a short and dry cough; with much peevishness, intolerance of light and sound, headache, giddiness, and other warnings of cerebral congestion. In addition we notice general fever, presenting exacerbations and remissions at irregular periods. The skin is hot ; the appetite capricious—sometimes bad, sometimes voracious ; the tongue is furred, and the breath offensive ; there is often nausea and vomiting ; and the bowels are disordered—generally constipated. The child is drowsy, yet restless ; he sleeps badly, moans or grinds his teeth, screams and awakes suddenly in alarm without any apparent cause ; while often there is delirium.

At the end of four or five days, the disease, if unchecked, passes into the *second stage ;* when its nature becomes very apparent, and a cure almost hopeless. The child only wishes to remain quiet in bed ; his countenance is expressive of anxiety and suffering, and is alternately flushed and pale ; the eyes are closed, and eyebrows knit ; and he is annoyed by light or the least noise. If old enough to reply to questions, the little one complains of headache, weariness, and sleepiness ; crying out frequently, " Oh, my head !" As this stage advances, the pulse—which has hitherto been rapid—becomes irregular and diminished in frequency, often falling in a few hours from 120 to 80 ; the slightest exertion, however, at once accelerates it. Moreover, a remarkable remission of all the symptoms may now take place ; so that pain ceases, while the general condition improves. But the amendment is not of long duration. Stupor and heaviness gradually come on ; there is often squinting ; the helpless patient lies on his back almost in a state of insensibility, perhaps picking, with tremulous fingers, his nose and lips; convulsions frequently occur, with now and then paralysis; while, at the same time, the fæces and urine are passed unconsciously. The latter is now and then albuminous.

The transition to the *third stage*, at the end of a week or two, is not unfrequently effected very gradually by the drowsiness passing into profound coma, from which it is impossible to rouse the child; while the pulse gets feeble, the extremities lose their warmth, and a cold clammy sweat breaks out over the body. In other instances the child becomes comatose quite suddenly; immediately afterwards being attacked with paralysis and convulsions, which often put an end to the painful scene. Occasionally, however, death does not occur until the lapse of several more days.

M. Bouchut was the first to make use of the ophthalmoscope in the diagnosis of tubercular meningitis; and he asserts that in some cases, but not in all, characteristic appearances may be observed before the convulsive period sets in. These are,—(1) Peripheral congestion of the papilla, with spots of congestion in the retina and choroid. (2) Dilatation of the retinal veins around the papilla. (3) Varicosity and flexuosity of these veins. (4) Thrombosis of the same. And (5) in some instances, retinal hæmorrhages from rupture of the veins.*

When tubercular meningitis occurs in the adult, there will generally be found a history of previous lung affection; which affection seems to become ameliorated as the cerebral disorder sets in. The symptoms may early assume an apoplectic or a convulsive form. More frequently they come on gradually with vomiting, slight fever, and most acute pain in the head; the patient seems unable to collect his thoughts, and is peevish and irritable, desiring only to be left quiet; there may be mutism and somnolence; and the pulse is irregular and feeble. In the second stage the depression increases, there is greater mental dulness or delirium, and there are clonic or tonic spasms. Then in the third stage the sphincters relax; while there is increasing stupor and paralysis, followed by death.

Post-mortem Appearances.—Those usually discovered consist of traces of inflammation of the membranes of the brain; especially effusion of serous fluid beneath the arachnoid and in the meshes of the pia mater. False membranes are usually observed between the arachnoid and pia mater at the base of the hemispheres. The cerebral substance often contains scrofulous tubercles; while granular tubercular deposits may be seen scattered upon and between the membranes, and especially in the pia mater lining the fissure of Sylvius. But the characteristic morbid appearance consists of softening of the central parts of the brain, with effusion of thin watery serum into the ventricles. In the majority of cases tubercular matter is found in the lungs, or in the glands of the mesentery.

* *Gazette des Hôpitaux*, pp. 225. 469. Paris, 15 May and 9 October 1862.

Treatment.—The treatment of tubercular meningitis has always been said to be beset with difficulties; inasmuch as, being an inflammatory affection, it was thought to demand remedies which the patients (strumous subjects) could not bear.   Fortunately the difficulty is abolished, if the observations made in the preceding pages are at all sound.   For my own part, having long acted upon rules deduced from these doctrines, I can express my firm belief, that the more we act up to their spirit, and the less we deplete in this disease, the greater the chance of the ultimate recovery of our patient. * It is only fair to mention, however, that several authors agree that lowering measures are not to be had recourse to under the present circumstances without great consideration; that if there is much doubt, the practitioner should first try the effect of a strong purgative; and that if it be necessary to take blood, local bleeding (by leeches) will generally answer every purpose.   At the same time, these gentlemen forget that it is impossible to effect local bleeding, in the sense intended.

In almost all instances two or three doses of some purgative are very useful; and I think perhaps that most good is derived especially at an early stage, from such as contain or consist of mercury.   After the bowels have freely acted, I am in the habit of trusting to the iodide of potassium; which is administered in doses varying from half a grain to three or four grains, every four or six hours.   The employment of cold to the scalp is likewise an important remedy.   A piece of muslin or thin rag wetted with cold water, or with an evaporating lotion (F. 273), laid on the child's head and frequently renewed, will prove soothing.

When the infant is teething, many practitioners resort, as a matter of course, to scarification of the gums; unmindful of the fact that the irritation often arises from the passage of the tooth through the bony canal of the jaw, rather than from pressure on the gum.   Such practice is a piece of barbarous empiricism.   On the other hand when the gum is really tender and hard and swollen, then the use of the lancet gives great relief.—Supposing that the vital powers become much depressed, either from the course of the disease or from the action of the remedies, stimulants must be freely had recourse to.   I have frequently given a child of from six to twelve months old a teaspoonful of equal parts of port wine and water, or of port wine and beef-tea in the same proportions, every hour, or every second hour, with the greatest advantage. Cream is also useful; and so is the essence of beef, or simply raw meat (F. 2).   If physic be preferred, some ammonia or a mineral acid, with spirit of ether may be ordered.

8. HYPERTROPHY AND ATROPHY.—*Hypertrophy* of the cerebral hemispheres has once in a way occurred during childhood, but in the majority of recorded cases the individuals have been between 20 and 30 years of age. In some instances, the skull increases in size as the brain itself becomes over-developed; and then there may be an absence of all symptoms, until perhaps death takes place in a sudden attack of convulsions. But if the bony case does not become enlarged, indications of compression necessarily ensue; and hence there will be mental disturbance varying from slight dulness of intellect to complete idiotcy. The other prominent symptoms consist of paroxysms of headache, attacks of vertigo, impairment of the power of motion ending sometimes in general paralysis, an unaltered or very slow pulse, and more or less severe epileptic convulsions. Death will perhaps occur during one of the latter attacks, or in a state of coma coming on subsequently.

The opposite condition, that of *atrophy*, may vary from a complete absence of the cerebral hemispheres incompatible with extra-uterine life, to a simple incomplete development of certain convolutions above the ventricles. When the atrophy exists only on one side, life may not be interfered with for a long time. Andral states that he has seen cases of the following kind:—Above the lateral ventricle of one side there has been no nervous substance, the arachnoid usually covering the convexity of the hemispheres, being found in apposition to that which should line the parietes of the ventricles; while these two folds of one and the same membrane have been separated from each other by an areolar tissue, provided with a great many vessels. He mentions one remarkable instance where this alteration seems to have commenced twenty-five years before death; the latter being produced by an attack of peritonitis. Up to the last moment there was a perfect preservation of intelligence; although the autopsy revealed no trace of nervous substance between the meninges and the ventricles on the right side.

II. CHRONIC HYDROCEPHALUS.

Hydrocephalus [from "Ὕδωρ = water + κεφαλή = the head], or dropsy of the brain, is met with in children at various ages, as the result of a great variety of circumstances. When congenital, as it often is, we generally find it associated with some cerebral malformation. It is sometimes the result, never the precursor, of tubercular meningitis; so that this latter affection used to be spoken of as *acute hydrocephalus*. When the dropsy is congenital, or when it arises slowly from constitutional causes, it is termed *chronic hydrocephalus*.

The head attains a very great size in this disease, the unossified sutures readily yielding to the pressure of the liquid. One side of the cranium is now and then larger than the other, the bones are mostly thin and transparent, while the membranes of the brain are thickened. The serum is usually contained in the lateral ventricles, which are often expanded into one large cavity; but occasionally it is collected in the sac of the arachnoid, when it may compress the brain to a remarkable extent. The quantity of the fluid varies from two or three ounces to as many pints. In the well-known history of a man named Cardinal, it is reported that the head measured in circumference thirty-three inches; while after death nine pints of water were found in the cavity of the arachnoid, together with one pint within the ventricles.

The bodily functions are frequently but slightly impaired, occasionally not at all, till a short time before death; while it is remarkable also how little the mental powers are affected in some subjects. Heberden has related an instance where there were no signs of dropsy of the brain during life, and yet eight ounces of fluid were found in the ventricles after death. Although essentially an affection of childhood, yet cases are recorded in which it has affected adults. Thus amongst others, the celebrated Dean Swift suffered from it. According to Dr. West, almost every example is fatal. Professor Gölis, of Vienna, affirms, on the contrary, that of the cases which commenced after birth, and which were seen and treated early by him, he saved the majority.

The *causes* of this affection are obscure. The children of drunken, scrofulous, or syphilitic parents seem most likely to be sufferers from it. Exposure to cold, insufficient nourishment, breathing impure air, blows upon the head, the sudden retrocession of cutaneous disease, dentition, intestinal worms, tubercular deposit on the membranes of the brain, or the extension of inflammation from the petrous portion of the temporal bone, may all be regarded as likely to excite it. In some instances it has followed the eruptive fevers—especially scarlatina and measles.

The *symptoms* generally begin to show themselves before the infant is six months old, in cases where they do not exist from birth. Although the child takes its food eagerly, it does not thrive; and consequently, after a few weeks, the marasmus becomes extreme. The wasted appearance of the body makes the increased size of the head the more remarkable; so that he who has once noticed the small face with the prominent heavy forehead, the protrusion and downward direction of the eyes, and the extended globular cranium with its open sutures and fontanelles, needs no pen-and-ink sketch of the hydrocephalic infant to fix the features upon his memory. The intelligence may (as before mentioned) be unaffected, although often it is much enfeebled: there is great irritability and peevishness, a morbid susceptibility to noise and light, oft-times a liability to epilepsy, while the muscular weakness is occasionally very great. A peculiar rolling movement of the eye-ball can often be noticed; and there may be strabismus, with occasionally amaurosis. Recurring attacks of headache and nausea seem particularly troublesome; there is constipation, with dark-coloured offensive stools, and pains about the belly; and there is grinding of the teeth during sleep, with frantic screams on awaking. Moreover, the position of the head, often drooping helplessly on one side, is remarkable; this being due to the muscles and vertebræ being too weak to maintain it in the erect position.

During the second stage there is generally more stupor, great pallor, a slow pulse, and dilatation or contraction of the pupils; while the little fingers are constantly picking the nose and lips. When the disease is about to terminate favourably, the lethargy, pallid hue of skin, and irritability gradually subside; and then a desire for food is evinced, the muscular power increases, and the emaciation gets less marked. But in other instances excessive prostration sets in, the pulse becomes rapid, there may be paralysis, and coma or convulsions follow, which end in death.

With regard to the *diagnosis*, care must be taken to distinguish dropsy of the brain from *spurious hydrocephalus* or *hydrocephaloid disease*. Weakly children are especially the subjects of this latter morbid condition; which produces heaviness of the head, drowsiness, great languor, unhealthy stools, alarm at slight noises and at strangers, freaks of temper, irregular breathing, and coolness of the skin. Above all, the surface of the fontanelle is found depressed; whereas it is prominent in dropsy. If these symptoms are insufficient to teach the practitioner the difference between the two disorders, the treatment will show him how little they are allied to each other. Purgatives, diuretics, and all the salts of iodine will rapidly increase the severity of the symptoms in spurious hydrocephalus; which disease imperatively demands the administration of pure milk, beef tea, perhaps raw meat, steel or bark, and port wine or brandy in arrowroot.

Many plans of *treatment* have been practised in hydrocephalus with a small amount of success. The favourite remedies appear to have been purgatives, bloodletting, blisters, and mercury to salivation. The cases which have come under my own care have occurred chiefly in hospital practice; and I have trusted to gentle aperients, plain but nourishing food, cod liver oil or glycerine, with sometimes iodide of potassium or iodide of iron. As regards the iodide of potassium I can only say that my faith in its efficacy yearly increases; but to do any good it ought to be freely given (one grain every six hours to a child one year old), while it must also be persevered with for a few weeks, or perhaps even for two or three months.

The course advocated by Professor Gölis, after great experience, consists in the administration of calomel in quarter or half-grain doses, twice daily; together with the inunction of one-eighth or one-fourth of an ounce of the mild mercurial ointment (Phar. Lond. 1836) into the shaven scalp once in every twenty-four hours. At the same time the head is to be kept constantly covered with a flannel cap, to prevent all risk of the perspiration being checked. If no improvement be perceptible after a lapse of six or eight weeks, diuretics (the acetate of potash, or tincture of squills, or both) are to be combined with the treatment; and an issue may be made in the neck or on each shoulder, to be kept open for months. When convalescence is once established, he thinks benefit is derived from small doses of quinine—a quarter of a grain three or four times daily.

Two remedies—*compression* of the head, and *puncturing* it—have been strongly advocated by several writers. Compression is well effected by bandaging; or, better still, by the methodical application of strips of adhesive plaster over the whole of the cranium, so as to make equal pressure on every part. In cases where there are no symptoms of active cerebral disease, pressure will probably do good; and from my own experience I am inclined to think favourably of it. Puncture is performed with a small trocar and cannula at the coronal suture, about an inch and a half from the anterior fontanelle, so as to avoid the longitudinal sinus. The fluid ought to be evacuated slowly, as much as will flow being allowed to come away; while gentle pressure must be kept up both during its escape, and afterwards for some weeks. This operation is only to be had recourse to when other means have failed. It has occasionally proved successful in very young children.

Sir Thomas Watson mentions two hopeless cases successfully treated on a plan suggested by Dr. Gower.* Ten grains of crude mercury were rubbed down with twenty grains of manna and five grains of fresh squills. This formed a dose which was taken every eight hours, for three or four weeks. It caused a profuse flow of urine, great debility, and emaciation; but there was no ptyalism. When the symptoms of hydrocephalus had disappeared, the health was restored by the exhibition of steel.

The foregoing remarks show the necessity of attending to *prophylactic* measures. A child with any tendency to hydrocephalus should be reared so as to strengthen its system as much as possible. Accordingly, care is to be taken that it has sound sleep at night; it ought to have a nourishing diet, with animal food and as much milk as can be fairly digested; a salt water tepid bath had better be used every morning, followed by friction of the skin; the nursery and bedroom are to be properly ventilated; and plenty of exercise is to be taken in pure air. In some instances residence at the sea-side, with the administration of cod liver oil, may be needed. Stimulants had better always be avoided. And then only the most gentle attempts at education are to be permitted; the lessons being made short, of a varied character, and as interesting and little fatiguing as possible. The child is almost certain to be precocious; and often will be only too happy to over-work its brain, if permitted to do so.

III. APOPLEXY.

By the term Apoplexy ['Aπὸ – from, or by means of, + πλήσσω = to strike,—because those attacked fall down as if from a blow] is

---

* *Principles and Practice of Physic.* Third Edition, vol. i. p 458. London, 1848.

meant a fit of sudden insensibility.   There is a complete loss, for
the time, of consciousness and sensation and power of voluntary
motion; together with a more or less severe disturbance of the
functions of respiration and circulation.   It is a state of coma
occurring suddenly from pressure upon the brain; the compressing
power having its seat within the cranium.

There is a popular belief that patients suffer from three different
attacks of apoplexy; the first being mild, the second followed by
paralysis, and the third ending in death.   Without subscribing to
the literal truth of this conceit, it can at all events be allowed
that the danger greatly increases with each attack.

Causes.—Whatever tends to induce cerebral congestion may
produce apoplexy; and therefore amongst the causes we must set
down the immoderate use of intoxicating drinks, tobacco, and
opium.   These agents can act as direct provocatives of a fit, or
indirectly by inducing disease of the nervous or vascular structures.
Great heat or cold, sudden excitement, mechanical violence, plethora from the sudden suppression of an accustomed hæmorrhage,
and in short anything which tends to produce congestion and to
lower the tone of the capillaries, will possibly give rise to an attack.

In the greater number of instances some disease of the cerebral
bloodvessels is found.   Fatty degeneration of the arterial tunics is
perhaps the most common; but there may be ossification or calcification, or some intra-cranial aneurism.   The cerebral bloodvessels are more apt to be the seat of aneurism than is generally
believed; but to detect such, after rupture, will often require a
cautious dissection.   Cases of renal disease not unfrequently end
in apoplexy, the same degeneration of the coats of the vessels
occurring in the brain as in the kidney.   Hypertrophy of the left
ventricle of the heart, independently of valvular affection, may
cause a fit; owing to the blood being propelled with greater force
than the vessels can bear.   This hypertrophy often exists in combination with granular degeneration of the kidneys.   So also
valvular disease of the heart, ossification of the aorta, the pressure
of an overloaded stomach, &c., can all be the source of a seizure
by offering an impediment to the natural circulation of the blood.

Diagnosis.—It is often a matter of difficulty to discriminate between apoplectic coma, and that due to a narcotic poison or to
drunkenness.   The distinction is most important as regards the
treatment.   The coma is profound in each instance, though arising
from so different a cause : the history of the case, the general appearance and age, and the presence or absence of the odour of
spirits in the breath, are the points which chiefly help to solve the
embarrassment.

Speaking generally, it may be said that in intoxication the
person may often be momentarily roused, so as to give an intelligible answer to a distinct question; though of course if he be
dead drunk, he is as senseless as a mass of inanimate matter.   The

pulse is frequent; but in deep alcoholic coma it will be found infrequent and small and laboured. The respirations are perhaps slow : stertorous breathing is either absent or not loud. The pupils may be contracted or dilated, though the latter appearance is most common. The face is either flushed or pale. The power of motion is impaired or entirely abolished ; as is sensation. Reflex action is often absent. The characteristic odour of alcohol is appreciable; though implicit reliance must not be placed on this point, because a man who has been drinking may have cerebral hæmorrhage. In drunkenness the urine is frequently limpid and abundant : where a large quantity of spirit has been taken, the specific gravity of this secretion may even be found to be below that of water. According to Dr. Anstie the presence of a poisonous dose of alcohol in the system can be determined, if the addition of one drop of the urine to fifteen minims of the chromic acid solution turns the latter immediately and decidedly to a bright emerald green colour. This chromic acid solution is made by dissolving one part of bichromate of potash in three hundred parts (by weight) of strong sulphuric acid. As regards poisoning from opium, contraction of the pupils is not always present in the advanced stage. Nitro-benzole has caused several deaths, in four or five hours, after giving rise to symptoms resembling those of drunkenness, followed by sudden coma. The peculiar smell of the poison causes it to be easily recognised. In apoplexy the patient cannot be roused ; the pulse is infrequent and slow, rather than frequent and quick ; the pupils are perhaps unequal ; and the stertor is often well-marked.

So many cases of apoplexy occurring in the streets have been mistaken for intoxication, that no person found insensible by the police (whatever the *supposed* cause may be) ought to be placed in a cell until a cautious examination has been made by a medical man. Even if the individual be " dead drunk," remedies are urgently demanded, to prevent fatal poisoning or apoplexy. Especially ought the stomach-pump to be employed : first, for the removal of any alcoholic fluid not already absorbed ; and secondly, for the injection of strong coffee. Moreover, cold affusion over the drunkard's head and chest is very often valuable ; taking care to follow up its employment by warmth to the surface of the body where the temperature is depressed. But in the case of apoplexy, putting aside the question of treatment, the feelings of the relatives surely deserve some consideration ; for it must be no small aggravation of their grief to find, that one they have respected and cherished has been locked up on a charge of drunkenness.

Varieties.—The state of coma in apoplexy may cease in three different ways. Either it will gradually pass off, leaving the patient well ; or it terminates in incomplete recovery, the mind being impaired, and some parts of the body paralysed ; or it ends in death. In the latter case, on examining the brain we find either no appearance whatever of disease ; or extravasated blood is discovered ; or there is effusion of serum into the ventricles or beneath the arachnoid. Dr. Abercrombie calls the first, or that which is fatal without leaving any traces, *simple* or *nervous* apoplexy (uræmia ?) ; the second is *sanguineous* apoplexy, or *cerebral hæmorrhage ;* the third, *serous* apoplexy (cerebral œdema ?). During life we are unable positively to distinguish, by the symptoms presented at the time of the fit, between these three varieties.

Warnings.—This dreadful visitation is seldom experienced without some previous threatenings ; which properly interpreted, should put the patient on his guard. There are fugitive attacks of cerebral congestion ; these being indicated by mental confusion and dulness, distension of the veins of the neck and temple and forehead, a duskiness of the lips and conjunctivæ, a feeling of heat about the head with coldness of the extremities, and a diminished secretion of urine with constipation.

The following individuals may be said to be predisposed to apoplexy :—Those whose ancestors suffered from it. Men and women of a peculiar habit of body, of sedentary habits, accustomed to high living, with protuberant bellies, large heads, florid features, and short thick necks. Individuals advanced in life, beyond fifty. A strong predisposition will also be engendered by disease of the kidneys, of the heart, or of the cerebral bloodvessels ; by intemperance ; and by the cessation of habitual discharges.

Among the prodromata, such as these are the most important :—
(1) Headache and giddiness, experienced particularly on stooping.
(2) A feeling of weight and fulness in the head ; with roaring noises in the ears, and temporary deafness. (3) Transient attacks of blindness, or sometimes double vision ; and especially the formation of minute clots in the retinæ, as seen by the ophthalmoscope. (4) Repeated˙ epistaxis ; fits of nausea ; and a sluggish state of the bowels. (5) A loss of elasticity in walking ; a tendency to lean forward ; a sense of pins and needles in the feet, or a feeling as if marbles or some foreign body were in the boot ; perhaps with numbness in the limbs. (6) Loss of memory, great mental depression, and peevishness ; the use of wrong words in talking ; occasional incoherent conversation ; indistinctness of articulation ; and transient delusions. (7) Drowsiness with heavy sleep, and a tendency to dreaming or nightmare. And (8) partial paralysis ; sometimes affecting a limb, sometimes the eyelids, and sometimes only causing a slight drawing of the face to one side without any palsy of the orbicularis palpebrarum.

Modes of Seizure.—Dr. Abercrombie has shown that the apoplectic seizure commences in three different ways :—" In the *first* form of the attack, the patient falls down suddenly, deprived of sense and motion, and lies like a person in a deep sleep ; his face generally flushed, his breathing stertorous, his pulse full and not frequent, sometimes below the natural standard. In some of these cases convulsions occur ; in others rigidity and contraction of the muscles of the limbs, sometimes on one side only." This kind of seizure is not uncommon in renal disease.

In the *second* form, the coma is not the first symptom, but complaint is made of a sudden attack of pain in the head. Then the patient becomes pale, sick, and faint; sometimes he vomits; while frequently he drops down in a state resembling syncope. Occasionally he does not fall, the sudden attack of pain being merely accompanied by slight and transient loss of consciousness. After a few hours, however, the headache continuing, he becomes heavy and oppressed and forgetful; and gradually sinks into perfect coma, from which recovery is rare. A large clot is usually found in the brain. The coats of the cerebral vessels are often diseased.

The *third* form of apoplectic seizure begins by an abrupt attack of paralysis of one side of the body, sometimes with deprivation of power of speech, but no diminution of consciousness. The paralysis may pass gradually into apoplexy; or the hemiplegia will remain without further urgent symptoms; or, in certain favourable cases, the palsy slowly goes off and the patient recovers.

Phenomena during the Fit.—The duration of the apoplectic fit varies from two or three hours to as many days; throughout which time there is total unconsciousness. The pulse, at first infrequent and small, becomes more frequent and larger and harder according as the system recovers from the prostrating shock : it usually remains less frequent than natural, and is sometimes intermittent. Respiration is slow, embarrassed, and often accompanied by stertor : perhaps the cheeks puff out with each expiration. There is frothy saliva about the mouth. In bad cases, the body gets covered with a cold clammy sweat; the face becomes pale; the eyes appear dull and glassy, with one or both of the pupils dilated and immoveable; the teeth are firmly clenched; and all power of deglutition is lost, or much impeded. The bowels are torpid; or, if they act, the motions are passed involuntarily. There is either involuntary micturition, or (as most frequently happens) retention of urine, until the bladder becomes distended and overflows, as it were, causing the urine to be constantly dribbling away. When the patient recovers incompletely, more or less paralysis of the limbs usually remains.

Prognosis.—A guarded opinion must always be given. The danger at the time is great; being somewhat in proportion to the depth of the coma, the amount of stertorous breathing and puffing out of the cheeks, the degree of prostration, and the difficulty of swallowing. Where the coma has been preceded by one or more attacks of convulsions, the hope of restoration is small. Supposing the loss of consciousness to continue beyond twenty-four hours, and that there are thoracic râles with a frequent pulse, the prognosis is most unfavourable. The longer the insensibility lasts, the greater is the fear that the clot is large and the ploughing up of the nervous tissue considerable. Partial recovery having taken place, there is still a fear, especially during the first fortnight, that the hæmorrhage may recur ; or that the clot will act as an irritant, and set up inflammation in the nervous tissue. The more decided the hemiplegia, the greater the fear that the mischief is extensive.

Where the symptoms gradually diminish, there is first a recovery of the mental power. This may be imperfect, so that the patient becomes childish ; or his memory will be impaired, so that he cannot express his wants in proper language, or he cannot read, &c. Then, sensibility is restored to the affected limbs ; and at a still later stage there may be a gradual improvement in the power of motion. In the latter case, the capability of movement is first experienced in the paralysed lower extremity, then in the arm, and subsequently in the hand.

According to Dr. Duchesne, contraction of the muscles is evidence of spinal action, increased by the persistent central mischief removing cerebral control. Flaccidity of the muscles, on the other hand, is the secondary result of long-continued inaction ; this inaction having been produced by the cerebral disease. The same author has also noticed, that active tonic contraction of the muscles is indicative of inflammation in the walls of the cyst.

In fatal cases of apoplexy death does not usually happen immediately, as it occurs from heart disease, rupture of an aneurism, a broken neck, or poisoning by prussic acid or nicotine. There is almost always an interval between the fit and the cessation of life, —an interval of at least some hours. The distinction between death occurring *rapidly* and *instantaneously* is not to be overlooked. Even when blood is effused into the pons Varolii life may continue for two or three hours.

The deaths registered in England, as due to apoplexy, during the year 1866, were $\frac{\text{Males 5121}}{\text{Females 5176}} = 10,297$. This is the average for the last ten years, making allowance for increase of population. Of the above total, 670 were children under five years of age. More fatal cases, in both sexes, occur between sixty-five and seventy-five than during any other decade.

Post-mortem Appearances.—It is only necessary to notice those which are discovered in cases of sanguineous apoplexy. The blood may be effused upon or between the membranes of the brain ; as on the outside of the dura mater, into the sac of the arachnoid, or into the meshes of the pia mater. It will perhaps be poured into one of the ventricles, or into the cerebral substance itself. In the latter case, the blood is usually found in the most vascular parts ; that is to say in the corpora striata, the optic thalami, or in that portion of the hemispheres of the brain which is on a level with these bodies. Dr. Craigie arranges the parts which may be the seat of the hæmorrhage in their order of frequency, thus :—The corpora striata, optic thalami, hemispheres, pons Varolii, crura of the brain, medulla oblongata, and cerebellum.

Where death occurs within a few hours of the effusion upon or between the membranes of the brain, the cerebral substance will usually be seen simply flattened from the pressure which the extravasated blood has exerted; this blood being either liquid or coagulated. But if some days have elapsed, there will probably be evidence of meningitis as well as of softening of the convolutions. Moreover, in the latter case, the blood may be found fixed to the arachnoid by a delicate transparent membrane. Supposing the vital fluid to have been poured into the substance of the brain, a cavity (varying from the size of a barleycorn to that of a hen's egg) will be seen, containing semi-coagulated blood and softened cerebral matter. At a rather later period the clot will probably be much firmer; while the walls of the cavity may have undergone some amount of inflammatory softening. And lastly, when life has been prolonged for about twenty-five days, the coagulum may be discovered small and isolated, a membrane can be detected around it, and the cerebral walls of the cyst will be found to be perceptibly getting indurated. At this time, moreover, the walls of the blood corpuscles will have ruptured through endosmosis ; and the contents of these cells having escaped and crystallized, blood- or hæmatoid-crystals may be discovered on a microscopic examination.

The point of rupture in the vessel cannot always be made out. Where the walls of the carotid, basilar, or meningeal arteries have given way through ossification, or aneurismal dilatation, there is no difficulty in showing the source of the hæmorrhage; but it is not so easy if only one or more of the minute vessels have broken down, probably owing to fatty degeneration of the coats.

Treatment.—This may be divided into that which is prophylactic, and that required when an attack has occurred.

The remarks that are needed on the *prophylactic* management are few and plain. When a predisposition to apoplexy is suspected, the individual should avoid strong bodily exertion, venereal excitement, the stimulus and irritation of anything approaching to drunkenness, violent mental emotion, exposure to extremes of temperature, straining at stool, long-continued stooping, tight neck-cloths, and warm baths. He (or she) ought to observe a moderately spare diet, almost free from alcoholic drinks ; heavy meals at long intervals being bad, partly because an overloaded stomach will obstruct the circulation by its pressure, and also for the reason that any sudden increase in the quantity of the blood may cause a diseased vessel to give way. Sleep should be sought with the head high, on a mattress rather than on a feather bed, in a cool well-ventilated room, and for not more than eight hours out of the twenty-four. Daily exercise ought to be taken in the open air, but without over-fatigue ; while attention is also to be paid to the bowels. Washing the head in the morning with cold water is often useful ; or establishing a drain near the occiput, by means of an issue or seton in the neck, will perhaps do good. When giddiness, headache, throbbing of the arteries of the head, and epistaxis are present, much benefit will result from active purging for a day or two ; as well as from blistering the nape of the neck. On the contrary.

where there is anæmia, small doses of steel, good easily digested food, and plenty of milk will be needed.

But supposing that *an attack has occurred*, what are we to do? Formerly the treatment of every case of apoplexy was commenced by bleeding; and statistics prove that the more freely the blood was taken away the greater was the mortality.* This is what might be expected, for we only see the patient when the mischief is done : rupture with extravasation of blood has taken place, and bleeding will not remove it. Moreover, we are seldom able to learn the cause of the fit,—the nature of the antecedent disease of the cerebral vessels, or of the brain itself. When such disease is in existence, or where there is a morbid state of the heart or kidneys, will such conditions be improved by loss of blood? How are the reparative powers, the action of which is so indispensable, to be encouraged by bleeding? But, it is said, depletion will prevent further extravasation. I believe, with Mr. Copeman, that so far from doing so, it promotes it; partly by inducing greater thinness of the blood, and partly by diminishing the power of coagulation. In proof of this it is only necessary to read the reports of not a few cases, where it is distinctly stated that the abstraction of blood was immediately followed by an aggravation of the symptoms and by paralysis. As regards my own practice, it may be mentioned that among the several cases which formerly came under my care in dispensary and hospital practice I never saw one in which I considered bleeding necessary; and certainly the majority of the cases, at least, recovered. The lessons then learnt have since guided me in treating this disease; for I cannot recollect having met with an instance where venesection or leeching has been called for. And, moreover, the most unfavourable cases which I have seen in consultation have been those where one or the other practice has been employed.

The best rule to adopt is that laid down by Cullen—*to obviate the tendency to death*. If the tendency be towards death by coma; if the pulse be full, or hard, or thrilling; if the vessels of the neck are congested; and if the face be flushed and turgid, then a small bloodletting may perhaps be called for. But, on the contrary, when

---

* " The universal *remedy*, as it is called, for apoplexy is bloodletting; at least so generally has it been employed, that of 155 cases in which the treatment is specified, 129 were bled, and only 26 were not : of the 129 who were bled, 51 recovered and 78 died—the cures being 1 in 2⅓, the deaths 1 in 1⅔; of the 26 who were not bled, 18 were cured and 8 died, the proportion of cures being 1 in 1½, and of deaths 1 in 3¼. But the mortality varies a good deal according to the particular method in which bloodletting was performed. In 2 cases the temporal artery was opened; both died. In 11 cases cupping only was employed; 6 were cured and 5 died. 14 were treated by leeching; 4 cured, 10 died. 17 were bled in the foot, a plan strongly recommended by M. Portal, of which 13 were cured and 4 died. 85 were bled generally and copiously, of which number 28 recovered and 57 died; that is to say, 2 in every 3 cases terminated fatally."—*A Collection of Cases of Apoplexy*, p. 6. By Edward Copeman. London, 1845.

the patient is dying from syncope,—where there is a feeble or almost imperceptible pulse, with a cold clammy skin, then bleeding will only ensure a speedily fatal termination. In either case, the patient ought to be removed into a cool room; he may be placed in a reclining chair, but any way the head should be raised; all the tight parts of the dress must be loosened, especially the cravat and shirt collar; and cold is to be applied to the head by means of pounded ice in a bladder. Supposing the practitioner thinks it proper to bleed, let him do so by opening a vein in the foot, as recommended by Portal: or let him take only a very small quantity of blood from the nape of the neck with the cupping glasses.

Active purgatives are at times serviceable. If the patient can swallow, a full dose of calomel and jalap followed by the common black draught may be given (F. 140). Where the power of deglutition is lost, two or three drops of croton oil should be put on the back part of the tongue. Stimulating enemata (F. 189, 190, or 191) ought also to be thrown up the rectum. Pediluvia containing mustard, or sinapisms to the legs, can seldom do any harm; while their employment gratifies such friends of the patient as expect that "something" should be done. Blisters, applied over the scalp or to the neck, are to be avoided. The catheter is to be used if there be retention of urine. Some practitioners recommend emetics; but unless the attack were clearly due to an overloaded stomach, I should avoid them. Even then it must be remembered that these agents cause a determination of blood to the head; and hence their effects must be narrowly watched.

Supposing the patient to recover from the fit, great care will afterwards be required to prevent a second attack. Strong medicines, great excitement, or much mental occupation are to be avoided. The diet ought to be light but nutritious; milk is useful taken to the extent of a pint and a half or two pints, in the day; while, as a rule, only small quantities of light French, Hungarian, Austrian, or Greek wines should be allowed.

IV. CONCUSSION OF THE BRAIN.

Concussion of the brain is signalized by fainting, sickness, stupor, more or less insensibility, and loss of all muscular power; these symptoms succeeding immediately to a heavy blow or to some act of external violence. The patient may rally quickly, or not for many hours; or he will perhaps die suddenly, or at the end of some days. After death, either no lesion of the brain can be detected; or a laceration of some portion of it will be found; or there may be discovered a general softening of its substance.

Symptoms.—These will vary according to the degree of concussion. When the shock has only been slight, the person soon recovers from the state of unconsciousness; complaining merely of confusion of ideas, faintness, sickness, chilliness, a desire for sleep, and ringing noises in his ears.   In a more severe case, the insensibility continues longer : the patient lies as if in a deep slumber, his pupils are insensible to the stimulus of light, he is pale and cold, the muscles are flaccid, the pulse is fluttering or feeble, the sphincters are relaxed, and the breathing is often scarcely perceptible.   After a variable interval, when partial recovery ensues, there is great confusion of thought, often an inability to articulate distinctly, frequently severe vomiting, and sometimes paralysis of one or other of the extremities.   Even though more complete restoration take place, still the individual will never be the man he was prior to the accident.   In the worst forms of concussion, the individual is felled to the ground by the shock—whatever it may be, and dies upon the spot.

The whole nervous system seems now and then to receive a bruise or jar by a *railway accident*, without any immediate indications of mischief being developed.   There may be no external manifestations of injury,—no wound or abrasion, no contusion or ecchymosis.   But in the course of a few days, pains in the head with nervous depression are complained of; or some slight diminution of the power of motion will probably be noticed.   There may even be an attack of epilepsy, or of epileptoid convulsions.   Sometimes the sense of sight becomes impaired, or squinting may take place ; or there will be deafness and troublesome noises in the ears. These symptoms perhaps persist for a longer or shorter time, and then pass off; while occasionally they prove to be the precursors of serious cerebral or spinal disease.   More than once, a general shake of the nervous system, combined with constitutional shock and fright, has caused death some time after the accident; and though a careful necroscopy has been made, yet the pathologist has been unable to detect any trace of mischief.   These points ought all to be recollected in the examination of sufferers from railway accidents ; especially when we are called upon to give evidence upon this subject in the courts of law.   As Dr. Buzzard* remarks, the symptoms are for the most part " subjective."   There is little or nothing which we can discern for ourselves, with absolute precision.   Dependence must be placed on the statements of the patients themselves.   We should endeavour to test the assertions by looking at the consistency of the complaints, and by regarding the statements of trustworthy friends.

Diagnosis.—The following circumstances (according to Chelius) distinguish concussion from pressure upon the brain caused by extravasation of blood.   In concussion which immediately follows external violence, the patient usually recovers himself to a certain degree.   In extravasation he lies in an apoplectic state, with snoring and difficult breathing; he has a hard, irregular, inter-

* See an excellent series of papers by this gentleman,—" On Cases of Injury from Railway Accidents ; their Influence upon the Nervous System, and Results."   *The Lancet*, vol. i. pp. 389, 453, 509, and 623.   London, 1867.

mitting pulse; his pupils are widely dilated; but there is no vomiting. In concussion, the body is cold; the breathing easy; the pulse regular and small; the countenance little changed. Extravasation and concussion may, it must be remembered, occur together; but then there will be other evidence of a severe accident.

There will occasionally be a difficulty in distinguishing between concussion and drunkenness. The history of the man, his general appearance, and the smell of his breath (see p. 366), are the chief points to attend to. But where there is any doubt, the practitioner had best refrain from giving an opinion, while he also keeps the patient under close observation so long as the insensibility continues.

Prognosis.—The prognosis must in all cases be made with wariness and deliberation. In every severe form of brain bruise or concussion, there is peril at first from the prostration, and afterwards from excessive reaction. Moreover, it is difficult to say at once that there is no rupture of any fibres of the brain, and no compression. These events being wanting, and the dangers of great enervation and undue reaction being passed, the convalescence is always tedious; while the shock frequently leaves behind it permanent impairment of the memory, irritability of temper, loss of smell or taste, squinting, and weakness of sight or even amaurosis.

Treatment.—It is essential that the patient be kept very quiet. Not unfrequently, this will form all the treatment a judicious practitioner can resort to. If, a few hours after recovery from the shock, the reaction seem to be intense, the head should be elevated, and cold applied : two or three drops of croton oil may also be placed on the tongue. Generally speaking, however, the depressing effect on the system is so great, that mild stimulants are necessary ; and a little wine, or brandy and water, had better be cautiously administered. At the same time, while the surface remains cold, warmth must be applied by means of blankets, bottles of hot water, hot bricks, &c. In the after-management of these cases, a mild unstimulating diet, absolute rest from all mental occupation, bodily repose and quiet, perhaps with an occasional gentle bitter aperient, will alone be necessary.

V. SUNSTROKE.

Sunstroke (*Coup de soleil, Insolation, Heat apoplexy, Heat stroke,* or *Erethismus tropicus*) is a disease allied to simple apoplexy. It usually follows exposure to the direct rays of the sun, especially if the injurious effects of great heat be encouraged by unfit clothing, or exhaustion. The mortality is variously estimated at from 40 to 50 per cent. of those attacked. During the summer of 1868, the great heat which prevailed in this country for several weeks was the cause of many fatal cases of sunstroke. The persons affected were, for the most part, those engaged in field labour.

Causes.—In its perfect form it is seldom met with except in the tropics ; in which region it is often fatal to the European soldier, especially at seasons when the heat is very oppressive.   The more severe the regimental duty, the more the men are harassed or depressed, the more defective the commissariat arrangements, the worse the supply of drinking-water, and the more close and contaminated the atmosphere,—the more liable will the soldier be to this affection. It has been noticed that those attacked have often been affected for a few days previously with suppression of perspiration. The urine, at the same time, has been abundant and limpid ; while there has been either an inability to retain it, or the desire to pass it has recurred very frequently.   The nights have been sleepless ; and attacks of vertigo, with a sense of weariness, have been complained of. Such men, too, may have been irregular in their habits ; while perhaps they have also been indulging freely in alcoholic drinks, and prowling about under exposure to an almost vertical sun for two or three days previous to the seizure.

Symptoms.—There is generally faintness, thirst, great heat and dryness of the skin, with prostration.   In many cases, vertigo and a sense of tightness across the chest are complained of.   Frequently the pulse is quick and full, but sometimes it is thin and so feeble that it can scarcely be felt.   As the disease advances the heart's action becomes violent, the man can scarcely be roused, the face gets pallid, and probably an attack of vomiting ushers in the stage of coma.   When the patient is comatose the skin is found very hot, the breathing is performed with difficulty, the pupils are contracted, the conjunctivæ are congested, and the action of the heart is intermittent. Just before death the pupils dilate, the respiration gets gasping, and the patient perhaps vomits.

This affection sometimes comes on very insidiously.   A man will be seen to be listless and stupid ; but he makes no complaint beyond saying that his head feels a little queer.   Yet in twelve hours he may be dead.   In several instances, after exposure to the sun, the individual has fallen down insensible, made one or two gasps, and at once died from syncope.   This form of insolation is that described by Dr. Morehead as the " cardiac" variety.   Mr. Cotton, surgeon of a regiment of infantry, met with twelve cases of sunstroke when at Meerut.   The seizure usually happened towards evening, with symptoms of stupor and insensibility.   Then followed loss of speech ; burning of the skin ; at first contraction, and afterwards dilatation, of the pupils ; with great rapidity, hardness, and fulness of the pulse.   In some of these soldiers tetanic convulsions occurred.   They almost all sank very rapidly ; death ensuing in the greater number within two or three hours from the commencement of the attack.

The occurrence of prolonged insensibility, convulsions, and a rapid tumultuous action of the heart, are very unfavourable indications.   It is usually allowed that the patient cannot be considered free from danger until the skin gets cool and moist. In the event of recovery taking place, the convalescence will often be retarded either by deranged secretions, continued fever, persistent headache, obstinate dyspepsia, constipation, pulmonary congestion, epilepsy, or simply by great prostration of strength. Moreover, many months after an apparent cure symptoms of some obscure derangement of the nervous system or even of insanity, may set in; while if these miseries be escaped, the individual will hardly ever be as strong and healthy as he was prior to the attack.

Post-mortem Appearances.—It is seldom that any cause for the symptoms can be detected. Sometimes there is found an effusion of serum at the base of the brain; or the vessels of the membranes are turgid with dark blood. The brain itself is usually healthy. The kidneys are very often much congested; the lungs are sometimes engorged; but the other viscera present no changes of any importance. Dr. Morehead agrees with those observers who refer the phenomena of sunstroke to depressed function of the cerebrospinal and sympathetic nervous systems.

Treatment.—The course which has often been pursued consists of venesection, cold to the head, and blisters to the back of the neck. The fatality attending bleeding has been such, that the practice is only mentioned in order that it may be unreservedly condemned. Even leeching, after the subsidence of acute symptoms, ought certainly to be avoided for the future.

The remedies upon which it is probable that most reliance may be placed are cold douches to the head and neck and chest, with the frequent administration of iced water or cold tea. Rubbing the head and body with pieces of ice, for an hour or longer, has been successfully practised by Dr. B. Darrach of New York. After the assiduous use of the douche, evaporating lotions to the scalp, or a bladder containing ice, may be advantageously employed. The nape of the neck can also be painted with blistering liquid— liquor epispasticus. The occasional application of ammonia to the nostrils, while the patient is being fanned, helps to restore sensibility. If stimulants are absolutely needed owing to the failure of the heart's action, the best are ammonia and brandy; given in doses proportioned to the depression, and persevered with to the last. Sinapisms or turpentine stupes to the extremities may do good. Attempts have been made to induce sweating by wrapping the patients in the wet sheet; but the proceeding has not been successful. Where the heat of the skin is great, a bath at a temperature varying between 75° and 90° according to the state of the pulse, might prove valuable. Certainly it is most important to reduce the temperature of the body to its normal standard if possible. Dr. Edward Smith has proved that all animal foods, alcoholic drinks, and coffee lessen the activity of the skin, in the first stages of their digestion; but that tea and sugar have the opposite effect. He therefore urges that an infusion of good tea should be very freely given in this disorder; since beyond its effects on the skin it tends to directly stimulate the nervous system, and has also a powerful effect in increasing the respiratory functions. Consequently it may be found to meet three of the most urgent wants in sunstroke, viz., cooling of the body, removal of the listlessness and oppression, and increase of the respiratory action. The same writer also suggests that, as the act of vomiting tends to induce perspiration, so it might be useful to give ipecacuanha as an emetic early in the attack.

Assistant-Surgeon Chapple, of the Royal Artillery, says that he has saved a few cases which had advanced to the stage of coma; and he attributes his success chiefly to the employment of stimulant enemata. He remarks that there is a failure of nervous energy from the commencement, and that therefore our chief endeavours ought to be directed towards supplying this defect. The patients, in fact, generally die quite worn out.

Amongst the means of *preventing* sunstroke and other serious effects of excessive heat, the most important are the following :— The body is to be bathed every morning in cold water, so as to insure a free and clean skin. All intoxicating fluids are to be avoided. Water, tea, lemonade, and other simple diluents are to be freely partaken of. The meals should be at regular hours, with good properly cooked food. Natural perspiration is not to be checked. Light and loose flannel clothes are better than most other kinds. The head should be covered, when exposed to the sun, with thin folds of white linen or serge : this covering may be kept wet with cold water, if the heat be very great. A light-coloured umbrella affords great protection. Directly there is experienced any sense of pain or tightness about the forehead, or dizziness, or weakness, the sufferer ought to retire into the shade, lie down, and have cold water poured gently over the head. Until medical assistance can be obtained, he may also take plenty of iced water, or cold tea.

With regard to the management of soldiers travelling in tropical climates Dr. Aitken gives some excellent directions, which I have ventured to abbreviate thus :—When a march is to be undertaken in India during hot weather, the weak and sickly had better be left behind. The costume should be suitable for the early morning hours before sunrise, as well as for the scorching heat which follows. A flannel shirt is a safeguard against sudden chills : a flannel belt is an advantage, except in the hottest weather. The shirt collar ought to be open. A light knapsack should be allowed, which does not require the use of crossbelts over the chest. The troops should march "easy" and loosely clad ; at a pace not exceeding three and a half miles an hour : with halts when the men are exhausted ; and with a longer halt half way, so that each man may have a biscuit and cup of coffee. The men ought to arrive on the *new* ground about an hour after sunrise. The camp should be formed on as high and open ground as possible.   The men ought to be provided with an ample supply of water.   And lastly, all rations of spirits should be discontinued.

VI. APHASIA.

Aphasia [from 'Α = priv. + φάσις = speech] is a term first adopted by Trousseau to denote that form of speechlessness which is of cerebral origin.   There may be a loss only of the faculty of articulate language; or, as is much more frequently the case, there is likewise an inability to express the thoughts by writing or by gestures.   In other words there is a failure, in a greater or lesser degree, of the memory of words, and of the memory of those acts by means of which words are articulated; there being at the same time a diminution of intelligence.   Dr. Hughlings Jackson puts the matter very clearly when he says, that talking implies three distinct things—voice, articulation, speech.   The first produced by the larynx, is for sound; the second formed by the lips and tongue and palate, is for utterance of words; the third, having its source in the brain, is for expression of ideas.   It is this third condition which is affected in aphasia,—the loss of language is the result of the mental defect.

Aphasia is sometimes transitory; lasting only for a few minutes, or for hours, or for a week or two.   During convalescence from severe attacks of fever there may be this variety of aphasia, perhaps due to passive congestion of some portion of the brain.   But cerebral speechlessness is also often permanent; being the consequence of apoplexy, or of cerebral softening from embolism, or of the pressure of some syphilitic deposit or any other kind of tumour. So again, aphasia may either be complete, so that no syllable can be uttered; or it will be partial, one or two words being articulated more or less distinctly, though they are used in a wrong sense and to express every variety of want.   And then also, this form of speechlessness is found to occur alone, or to be accompanied by hemiplegia; while if the latter be present, the paralysis is almost invariably found to affect the right side of the body.

Examples of "loss of speech," or of a "loss of the memory of words," have been met with by most practitioners, and have been noticed as "curious cases" almost since medicine possessed a literature.   They have been carefully distinguished from instances of deprivation of voice (aphonia) the consequence of disease about the larynx, or of some affection of the organs of articulation; as well as from the silence of the deaf-mute, and of the lunatic who can speak but perhaps will not utter a syllable for several months. But it is only within a comparatively recent date that any attempt, founded on clinical observation with dissection after death, has been made to connect aphasia with a lesion of a particular and limited portion of the brain.   The question is now being investigated on all sides; the animated discussions on this subject at the French Academy of Medicine, in 1865, having more particularly excited the attention of numerous scientific men.

Many years have elapsed since Gall conjectured that the faculty of language was seated in those parts of the anterior cerebral lobes which lie upon the supra-orbital plates, without any restriction as to side; while he professed that pre-eminence as an orator was indicated by prominence of the eyeballs.* The localization of the faculty of speech in the anterior lobes of the brain, was regarded with great favour by Bouillaud as early as 1825; who believed, from cases observed by himself, that whenever the faculty of speech had been abolished during life, disease of these lobes was always to be found after death. This opinion he repeatedly advocated; and he seems to have maintained it as lately as 1865. During the year 1836, however, a more definite step was made by Dr. Marc Dax; who taught that disturbances in the faculty of speech were invariably connected with lesions of the left hemisphere—never with those of the right. He had observed that aphasic patients when paralysed had hemiplegia of the right side, so that the lesion was of course situated in the left hemisphere. Then, some five and twenty years later (in 1861), M. Broca announced his conviction that the seat of the faculty of articulate language is in the posterior part of the third frontal convolution of the left lobe of the brain. This is therefore called "the convolution of articulate language." The term *aphemia*, proposed by M. Broca for this affection, has generally been rejected in favour of *aphasia*. During 1863, Dr. G. Dax attempted to prove that the lesion in aphasia is not only invariably seated in the left hemisphere, as his father had insisted; but that it is to be found in the anterior and outer portion of the middle lobe of that hemisphere,—that portion which borders on the fissure of Sylvius. Again, according to views published in 1864, Dr. Hughlings Jackson concludes that the most frequent cause of hemiplegia with loss of speech is obstruction of the middle cerebral artery, or of some of its branches. Now and then it is due to syphilis, sometimes to injury. But any disease, whether softening from embolism, apoplexy, tumours &c., will affect speech if situated in a certain region of the hemisphere; which region, whatever its precise limits may be, is at all events near to the (left?) corpus striatum. Dr. Jackson does not accept the old view that the brain is a double organ, nor the new one that the faculty of language resides only in the left hemisphere. All that he wishes emphatically to teach at present

* The earliest notice of Gall's intention to publish his elaborate work on the Exercise of the Brain, and the possibility of recognising the Faculties and Propensities from the Form of the Head and Skull, appears in the *London Medical and Physical Journal*, vol. iv. p. 50. London, 1800. The desire was that the volume should be got out in England and Germany at the same time. It was subsequent to this publication, that Spurzheim, having been the pupil of Gall, became his associate.

is, that when hemiplegia attends loss of speech the palsy is almost invariably on the right side of the body. And now lastly, in 1869, Dr. Bastian has suggested, that as speaking and writing are processes which so far differ that one power may be lost while the other remains intact, so it will facilitate the future consideration of this subject to classify the various cases of loss of power of expression under three heads. The divisions he proposes, and which it seems to me might well be adopted, are these :— (1) *Aphasia*, including persons who can *think*, but cannot *speak* or *write*. This class will contain the largest number of cases. There is mental impairment, from a degree well nigh inappreciable to almost complete abolition of mind. There is usually hemiplegia. (2) *Aphemia*, including those who can *think* and *write*, but cannot *speak*. The intellect may be unaltered : there is no hemiplegia. (3) *Agraphia*, including persons who can *think* and *speak*, but cannot *write*. Such individuals on being told to write (their names for example), produce a meaningless assemblage of letters. There are usually also, defects in the power of speaking, such as using wrong words.

A fair consideration of the views which have been put forward as to the seat of the faculty of articulate language serves to show, that hesitation and doubt are the fittest attitudes to assume at this crisis. So much evidence confirmatory of M. Broca's views has been put on record, that to pretend to be perfectly free from any bias is surely unnecessary. But it is one thing to wish a particular view to be true, and another matter to believe that it is so. The two points which may be held to at this juncture are,—that in the greater proportion of recorded examples of decided aphasia there has been left-sided cerebral lesion ; while in a large number of these again, the lesion has involved the third frontal convolution. Then, on the other hand, a few cases have been observed by Trousseau and others which presented appearances incompatible with those that should have obtained had we successfully localized the faculty of speech. The argument, also, of this physician and of Vulpian, that an organ so symmetrical as the brain cannot have one function assigned to one half, and another power to the other half, is clearly not unreasonable if the premise be sound. But the question is, does this symmetry exist ? Todd and Bowman, in their work on Physiological Anatomy, state distinctly that the convolutions of the right and left hemispheres do not present a perfect symmetry ; while they notice as not a little remarkable, that in general, the lower the development of the brain, the more exact will be the symmetry of its convolutions. Thus, the imperfectly developed brain of the child exhibits this symmetry ; as does that of the inferior races of mankind. Whether the researches of Gratiolet will decide, as he believes, that the convolutions of the anterior lobe of the left hemisphere are developed at an earlier date than those of the right side, I do not know. At present this opinion is not to be received as a fact.

Although, however, objections derived from mere anatomical considerations seem undeserving of much attention, still it must be granted that decisive evidence cannot at present be brought forward from the domain of pathology. Even M. Broca, when advocating his views before the members of the British Association for the Advancement of Science in 1868, did not shed new light on the subject. He again, fully explained his theory of the localization of articulate language in the third frontal convolution of the left side, and argued for the corpus striatum as merely the medium of connexion. Amongst other cases he cited one, in which a pistol-ball lodged in this third convolution, without further damage ; and in this instance articulate speech alone was lost, no other faculty being affected. At the same time, he admitted there were apparent exceptions to his rule ; and he especially drew attention to cases of aphasia (or, as he still prefers to say, " aphemia") from disease of the island of Reil, with integrity of the convolution of articulate language. In these instances, however, this convolution is cut off from the corpus striatum ; being thus practically destroyed, by its isolation, so far as utterance of words goes.

With regard to the general symptoms it may be noticed that usually the deprivation of speech occurs suddenly. Perhaps, in a short time, two or three words can be uttered, which are then used in reply to all kinds of questions. The face is intelligent. The movements of the lips and tongue and palate and larynx are healthy. As so often mentioned, if there be hemiplegia it will almost constantly be found that the right is the side paralysed. There may be consciousness of what is wished to be expressed, and yet complete inability to express the thoughts by speech, gestures, or even (frequently) by writing. Aphasic patients know the use of objects (such as spoons, night-caps, pipes, &c.) though they cannot name them.*   Moreover, they can often play correctly at cards, back-

---

* The case related by Trousseau, of a Russian gentleman, resident in Paris, furnishes a good example of aphasia.   Mr. T. spoke French like a Parisian, yet after his attack was unable to speak a word of French.   When questioned he smiled and said " *da*," a Russian word meaning *yes*.   He was unable to construct even part of a sentence in his own language.   When shown a spoon he could make gestures showing its use : and yet had forgotten its name in Russian and French.   Nevertheless, he could play at whist correctly, and noticed any errors of his adversaries by making a gesture.—In another example, a young man 25 years old, was attacked with hemiplegia of the right side and aphasia.   Some power of moving the right leg, and then of the arm, returned ; but he could only articulate two words,—*No* and *Mamma*. " What's your name ?"—" Mamma."   " What's your age ?"—" Mamma no." Yet he knew that his reply was incorrect.   He had taught himself to write with his left hand, as far as signing his name.   He wrote this legibly.   But on being told to say " Guénier" as he had written it, he made an effort and said " Mamma."   " Say Henri," and he replied " No, mamma."   On being told to write " mamma," he wrote " Guénier."   " Write no :" and he again wrote " Guénier."—A third instance, was that of the mother-in-law of a medical man.   Whenever a visitor entered her room, she rose from her chair

gammon, dominoes, &c.; but too much importance must not be attached to this fact as an indication of intelligence, since many confirmed lunatics are able to do the same. The aphasics can perhaps read; but if they understand what they peruse they forget it directly, as they will pore over the same page again and again.

In cases of aphasia without hemiplegia recovery may occur spontaneously. Probably every kind of treatment (by drugs, bleeding, or blistering) is injurious. In aphasia with hemiplegia medicine is powerless to effect a cure; save in cases dependent on syphilis, when iodide of potassium or some preparation of mercury will be the remedy. Possibly, cod liver oil, with the hypophosphite of soda and bark (F. 419), might do some good where there is softening of the brain of very limited extent.

VII. ALCOHOLISM.

Alcohol is an agent which, through the medium of the blood, seems especially to affect the nervous system, and more particularly the brain. When taken in a large dose it may immediately destroy life, like any other active poison. In smaller quantities, frequently repeated, its effects are very prejudicial; for it has a tendency to accumulate in certain structures (the nervous centres and the liver), in spite either of its destruction within the economy, or of its elimination by all the excretory organs—especially the lungs. The consequences of alcoholism must be considered under the two divisions of delirium tremens, and dipsomania.

1. DELIRIUM TREMENS.—Delirium tremens (*Delirium è potu*, or *Delirium ebriositatis*) is still, unfortunately, a common disease in this country. It may be described as an acute attack of poisoning by alcoholic drinks. The delirium is characterized by hallucinations, fear, trembling of the muscles of the extremities, weakness, and watchfulness. The natural tendency of this disorder is to terminate in a critical sleep, at the end of from forty-eight to seventy-two hours from the commencement of the delirium.

The number of deaths which occur annually, in England and Wales, from excessive drinking can only be very imperfectly ascertained. According to the returns of the Registrar-General, it seems that during the ten years 1857-66 the deaths reported from delirium tremens amounted to 4958, while there were also 3447 from intemperance. In 1866, the mortality from delirium tremens was $\frac{Males\ 430}{Females\ 57} = 487$; that from intemperance being $\frac{Males\ 308}{Females\ 138} = 446$. Of course, these figures teach us nothing of the much larger indirectly fatal consequences of alcoholism.

with an amiable look, and pointing to a seat exclaimed—" Pig, animal, stupid fool." She did not in the least understand the meaning of these insulting expressions. Her son-in-law had to explain her wishes.

Symptoms.—These are chiefly—sleeplessness, a busy but not a violent delirium, constant talking or muttering, tremors in confirmed dram-drinkers, hallucinations of sight and hearing, a dread or suspicion of every one, mental with bodily prostration, and a generally excited and eager manner. The skin is commonly moist or clammy, from copious perspiration; the face is sometimes pale, but often flushed and wild-looking; the tongue is moist, and covered with a white fur; and the pulse is frequent and soft. In severe cases there is an increase in the sulphates and in the urea, with a diminution in the quantity of phosphates contained in the urine; while in phrenitis, on the contrary, the phosphates are in excess. There is a complete loss of appetite, attacks of sickness are common, the bowels are confined, and pain may be complained of in the epigastric or right hypochondriac regions. The symptoms generally become aggravated towards night, while early in the morning there appears to be greater weakness.

The delirium is always peculiar. Often the patient will not allow that there is anything the matter with him; but he answers questions rationally, puts out his tongue in a tremulous manner, and does whatever he is bid at the moment. Then he begins to wander again, gives orders about his business to absent servants, refers to some imaginary appointment he must keep, or speaks of all he has been doing through the night. A publican will have been drawing beer for hosts of customers, a lawyer has been making an effective appeal to a jury. A medical man who was under my care three or four times, was engaged during each attack in delivering "no end of women." The patient is also distressed or perplexed, and suspicious of all around him. Rats, mice, beetles, or other animals, are about or under his clothes; strangers are in his room, or they will insist upon getting into his bed; listeners are at the door or behind the curtain. With all this there is incessant restlessness; his hands are in tremulous motion, while his features are constantly twitching; and he talks rapidly and continuously. He is perpetually wanting to get out of bed, though easily persuaded to lie down again; but if not watched, will soon be downstairs, and perhaps out in the street. There is but little fear of his harming himself or others; yet it is a wise precaution to remove his razors, fasten the windows, and so forth.

In favourable examples the critical sleep comes on about the beginning of the third or fourth day, when the patient falls into a sound slumber, which lasts for twelve or more hours. From this he awakes very feeble, but cured of his disease. On the other hand, in the examples of cases about to end fatally the watchfulness continues; the temperature of the body rises—perhaps as high as 107° or 108°; there is muttering delirium, subsultus tendinum, and exhaustion; followed by great prostration, coma, or convulsions. Death most commonly takes place between the third and seventh days. Occasionally this result occurs rather suddenly, the patient being active in his delirium until the moment of his ceasing to breathe.

Causes.—Men are much more subject to this disorder than women. It arises from the excessive use of ardent spirits, wine, beer, or some fermented liquor. The habitual use of opium, excessive mental excitement, and venereal excesses, will occasionally produce an affection resembling, but not identical with, it. Individuals with an irritable nervous system, who are subjected to any prolonged mental strain, may induce this disease by smaller quantities of alcoholic drinks than would be required to excite it under other circumstances. But in all instances it is almost certain that the poison, in some form or other, has been taken; for there seems to me every reason to believe that delirium tremens is a specific toxæmia, due to alcoholic excess.

According to some authors the symptoms of delirium tremens may set in either after a protracted debauch of six or eight days, or upon the sudden withdrawal of the accustomed potations. The latter observation has been repeated so frequently that at last it has become a sort of recognised law; and yet for all that it is, in my opinion, a mistake. Evidence derived from hospital practice, from houses of correction and convict-prisons, and from asylums for inebriates in the United States, seems directly to negative it; and it may now be said to be at least highly probable, that a person accustomed to the very free use of stimulants can at once give them up without any danger whatever. In fact, as with other poisons, the only risk to be feared is from continuing their employment.

Treatment.—The great point, it has always been thought, is to check the incessant restlessness—to procure sleep. For this purpose opium has been given in full doses; either morphia, or solid opium, or Battley's liquor opii sedativus, or the common tincture. At the same time stimulants have been deemed necessary; and as a rule, that stimulant has been considered the best to which the patient has been accustomed. Thus, supposing he has generally besotted himself with beer, good ale or porter has been freely administered; while if brandy or gin has been the favourite liquor, he has been supplied according to his depraved taste.

Now it is not pretended that this plan of adding fuel to the fire is always prejudicial; but it seems certain that when indiscriminately practised, as it has been, great mischief must often result. The cases to which it is applicable are, indeed, the exceptional ones; while in the majority of instances, it is as absurd as it is injurious to treat a case of alcoholic toxæmia by continued doses of the very poison that has caused all the mischief. The practice to adopt is to bring about the critical sleep as soon as possible by removing the cause of the disease; to give ice, and perhaps salines, to cool the irritable, if not inflamed stomach; and to support the strength by milk, raw eggs, beef tea, &c. The wet-sheet packing (F. 136) has frequently a most soothing influence. Sometimes a cold shower-bath affords so much relief, that the patient will ask to have it repeated. Where the depression is very great, stimulants must undoubtedly be administered, as in other cases of prostration ; and in such, a well-timed dose of opium with ipecacuanha and a little belladonna will often prove useful. In three or four instances, where the delirium and constant talking seemed to be rapidly exhausting the patient, I have resorted to the use of chloroform with manifest advantage ; but I have also seen this anæsthetic act prejudicially, the excitement returning in an aggravated form so soon as the influence of the vapour has subsided.

The late Mr. Jones of Jersey stated that for twelve years he treated all his cases of delirium tremens by large doses of digitalis, with a remarkable degree of success. He was accustomed to give half an ounce of the tincture (Phar. Lond. 1851) with a little water, for a dose. In some few instances, one dose was sufficient ; but generally a second seemed to be required four hours after the first. Very seldom a third dose of two drachms was called for, owing to the absence of sleep. The effect was to produce a warm skin, a fuller and more regular pulse, and six or eight hours' good sleep.* My own experience with this drug is not very large, but as far as it has gone it confirms Mr. Jones' statements. At the same time I should never think of administering digitalis to all cases without distinction—a practice as injudicious as that of giving large quantities of brandy and opium simply because the individual is delirious. Foxglove has appeared to me to answer best when the symptoms have assumed a resemblance to those of acute mania, and where there has been decidedly increasing exhaustion.

Occasionally it is thought necessary to restrain the patient's movements by strapping him down to his bed, or by fastening a folded sheet across the chest and abdomen, or by putting on a strait-waistcoat. This should never be done, however, if it can possibly be avoided ; as it always increases the excitement and prevents sleep. It will invariably be much better to have a good attendant at the bedside to calmly control him. The apartment occupied by the patient should be darkened, kept quiet, and well ventilated ; while nothing is to be done in any way calculated to produce that violent irascibility, which is so easily provoked in these cases by a want of tact on the part of the friends.

2. DIPSOMANIA.—Within the last few years the word Dipsomania [from Δίψα = thirst + μανία = madness] has been revived, to express that craving for intoxicating liquors which, according to some physicians, partakes of the character of insanity. Now, although a fit of intoxication is undoubtedly an attack of temporary mania, yet it appears a highly unphilosophical view (and one, too, which is fraught with the greatest danger to society) to regard a dipsomaniac as an irresponsible being ; to look upon him, in fact, as an individual affected by some recognised form of lunacy. Hard-

* *The Medical Times and Gazette*, p. 301. London, 29 September 1860.

drinking is a degrading vice ; and, like many other vices, the more freely it is indulged in the more difficult becomes its discontinuance. It is a cause of insanity, and a cause of crime, though I believe its influence in these respects has been much overrated.* The drunkard is artful and especially untruthful ; he breaks every promise he makes ; and he is perfectly regardless of the feelings and happiness of others. His good resolutions are few and written in sand ; his temptations and failings appear innumerable and insurmountable. Nevertheless it is absurd to say that the desire for alcoholic stimulants is a disease—that it is symptomatic of some abnormal cerebral condition, unless indeed we allow the same of every act of wickedness or folly. Not only is the experience of the dead-house against such a view ; but if this evidence be set aside, as of little value, we yet know that there is no difficulty in curing the most inveterate sot, provided we are but able to deprive him of his poison. The fact is indisputable, that many who drink to excess can be persuaded to abstain temporarily, if only a limit to their abstinence be fixed, so that they may enjoy the anticipation of a debauch ; while a few can be so influenced that they renounce this habit entirely.

The drunkard is a nuisance to himself and to all who are brought into contact with him ; and it is to be regretted that there are no legal means of controlling him until he is cured of his folly. The man who attempts suicide by some summary process is liable to imprisonment ; while he who slowly poisons himself can proceed to certain destruction with impunity. He may ruin himself and his family, but so that he breaks only moral laws and obligations he cannot be stopped in his downward career. The welfare of society demands some place of detention for such men ; and even if an Act of Parliament could not be obtained to sanction the necessary interference with the liberty of these misguided people, yet I believe that there are many who would voluntarily enter and submit to the rules of an institution for the cure of drunkenness.

* Lord Shaftesbury says—" From my own experience as a Commissioner of Lunacy for the last twenty years, and as Chairman of the Commission during sixteen years, fortified by inquiries in America, I find that fully sixtenths of all the cases of insanity to be found in these realms, and in America, arise from no other cause than habits of intemperance."—Quoted from Dr. Belcher's pamphlet on *Reformatories for Drunkards*, p. 9. Dublin, 1862. Also from *How to Stop Drunkenness*. By Charles Buxton, M.P. London, 1864. Reprinted from the *North British Review*, 1855.
This statement is just one of those which tell with great force at temperance meetings. But after all is it correct ? I can only say that none of the Asylum reports with which I am acquainted afford any evidence in confirmation of it ; and surely the physicians to these institutions ought to be able to arrive at the truth on this point as readily as Lord Shaftesbury. If we take Dr. Hood's *Statistics of Insanity*, we shall find " the apparent or assigned causes" given as regards 3668 cases (male and female), admitted into Bethlem Hospital from 1846 to 1860 inclusive. Out of this total the disease is said to have been produced by intemperance in 177 ; but according to Lord Shaftesbury the number ought to have been 2200. May not his " experience" be like that of so many other men—fallacious ?

c c 2

Mr. Dickens in his "American Notes" mentions the case of a man who got himself locked up in the Philadelphia prison, so that he might rid himself of his propensity to drink ; where he remained, in solitary confinement, for two years, though he had the power of obtaining his liberty at any moment that he chose to ask for it. Patients have more than once told me that they would gladly submit to any treatment or surveillance ; but they have also said that without restraint all else would be useless, for they could not trust themselves.*

Our knowledge of the precise effect of alcohol upon the living body is becoming more and more perfect, though many points still remain for elucidation. A series of experiments ·led MM. Ludger Lallemand, Maurice Perrin, and J. L. P. Duroy,† to teach that alcohol is not only separated from the blood by the tissues of the body—especially the substance of the brain and of the liver, but that the excretory organs freely help to eliminate it ; the length of time required for its entire removal from the circulating current depending of course upon the quantity introduced into the system. The experimenters believed themselves justified in deducing the conclusion, that alcohol is neither transformed nor destroyed in the living body, but that the whole of what is ingested is excreted unchanged ; so that this substance has no claim to be regarded as a producer of heat—as a true food, but must be placed in the same category with the medicinal or toxic agents whose presence in the living body exerts a most important influence on its functions, though they do not themselves enter into combination with any of its components. These opinions are directly contradictory to those which have been accepted from Liebig ; who ranked alcohol among the heat-forming aliments, capable of replacing the

* Institutions for this purpose have been formed in the Isle of Skye. Dr. Christison, in relating an account of a visit to one of these establishments, where whisky could only be obtained by a walk of twelve miles, remarks,— " Here we found ten gentlemen—cases originally of the worst forms of ungovernable drink-craving—who lived in a state of sobriety, happiness, and real freedom. One, who is now well, had not yet recovered from a prostrate condition of both mind and body. The others wandered over the island, scene-hunting, angling, fowling, botanizing, and geologizing; and one of these accompanied my companion and myself on a long day's walk to Loch Corruisk and the Cuchullin Mountains. No untoward accident had ever happened among them. I may add, that it was impossible not to feel that, with one or two exceptions, we were among a set of men of originally a low order of intellect. Radical cures are rare among them ; for such men, under the present order of things, are generally too far gone in the habit of intemperance before they can be persuaded to submit to treatment. Nevertheless, one of those I met there, a very bad case indeed, has since stood the world's temptations bravely for twelve months subsequently to his discharge."—*A Lecture delivered before the Royal College of Surgeons of Edinburgh*, 19 March 1858. Since the delivery of this lecture this establishment has been given up. But there are others in various parts of Scotland; and among them an excellent one, on a limited scale, at Ostaig in Skye, under the care of Dr. Macleod. There are also four " Inebriate Asylums" in the United States.

† *Du Rôle de l' Alcool et des Anesthésiques dans l'Organisme ; Recherches expérimentales.* Paris, 1860.

fatty, starchy, and saccharine elements of food. Hence they have not been allowed to pass unchallenged ; and M. Edmond Baudot, Dr. Hugo Schulinus, and Dr. Francis E. Anstie have, by their independent researches, shown the incorrectness of the total elimination theory.

Briefly stated, the opinions of these three gentlemen seem to be as follows :—Thus, according to M. Baudot's[*] conclusions it is allowable to believe that alcohol is destroyed in the organism, and that it fills the office of respiratory food, as asserted by Liebig. To this M. Perrin[†] has replied, reiterating his assertion that alcohol is neither transformed nor destroyed in the organism ; that it is eliminated by the various excretory organs ; and that it offers none of the characters of food. Then the researches of Dr. Schulinus[‡] have led him to make these deductions :—(1) The effects of alcohol on men and animals are uniform. (2) The largest portion of any ingested dose of alcohol is always in the blood, and not in the nervous centres or liver. (3) The greatest portion of any dose of alcohol which may be taken is always decomposed in the organism. And (4) the proportion of alcohol which escapes unchanged in the breath, sweat, and urine, is trifling relatively to the amount which is utilized in the body. Finally, Dr. Anstie,[§] whose views on stimulation in febrile diseases are so well known, has stated positively that it is impossible any longer to deny that alcohol is a food. The quantities in which it can be taken without causing visible toxic effects would alone establish this, unless we were at liberty to suppose that it was rapidly eliminated in bulk. Such elimination, however, is now finally disproved.

The pernicious effects of the excessive use of alcoholic stimuli, as revealed after death, are found to be induration of portions of the nervous centres, congestion of the respiratory organs, amyloid and fatty degeneration of the liver, chronic inflammation and thickening of the walls of the stomach, with disease of the substance of the heart and kidneys. Cirrhosis, or gin-drinker's liver, with all its painful train of symptoms, is a common result. Dipsomania may also lead to tuberculosis, though it probably does so indirectly, by taking away all desire for food and so lowering the powers of life. But it must be remembered that these morbid changes are the consequences (not the cause) of the abuse of stimulants ; for in no instance is it pretended that the condition of brain has been demonstrated, which according to some writers gives rise to the propensity to drink.

The evils which afflict the drunkard are so great that it is unnecessary to resort to fables to point any moral. For example, spontaneous combustion from the excessive use of alcoholic stimuli, is only a silly fiction ; its gross absurdity, however, being a power-

* L'Union Médicale, pp. 272, 357, 374, 390. Paris, November 10, 21, 24, 26, 1863. † Idem, p. 582. 23 December 1863.
‡ Archiv der Heilkunde, pp. 97-128. Leipzig, 1866.
§ The Lancet, p. 120. London, 25 January 1868.

ful recommendation to the lovers of the marvellous. It would not be difficult to collect fifty recorded examples of it ; just as fifty sane people might easily be brought together to testify to the truth of spirit-rapping, table-turning, clairvoyance, and so forth. But the physician credits none of these idle tales. His character, like that of the true philosopher as described by Herschel, " is to hope all things not impossible, and to believe all things not unreasonable."

A few words must suffice on the medical treatment of *chronic alcoholism ;* which differs from delirium tremens inasmuch as it is not an acute disturbance of the functions of the nervous system, but a protracted state of general depression with restlessness. The chief points that demand attention are these :—To enforce total abstinence at once ; since I believe it to be more easy for the habitual drinker to renounce all stimulants, than to practise moderation. Then, to guard against sleepless nights by the exhibition, when needful, of the extract of henbane or hop, or even of opium ; to afford mental occupation and amusement, and especially out-door recreation in cheerful society ; to administer tonics and such remedies as will give nervous and gastric tone ; and to regulate the diet. In almost hopeless cases an attempt may be made to substitute opium for alcohol. The opium-eater is at all events not an annoyance to others ; he is much less likely to commit criminal acts than the drunkard ; while he injures his health in a smaller degree than the sot. Of two evils we may well choose the least. Dr. Marcet states that the nervous symptoms present in these cases may be best relieved by the oxide of zinc ; which is to be given in two-grain doses, twice a day, gradually increasing the quantity until twelve or sixteen grains are taken in the twenty-four hours (F. 415). The reputed effects of this powder are to induce sleep, to remove the tremor of the limbs, to relieve the headache and giddiness, and to destroy all hallucination. In my hands, however, it has not answered these expectations. More reliable remedies are, I believe, to be found in the hypophosphite of soda, or in ammonia and bark, the mineral acids and gentian, quinine and citrate of iron, pepsine and reduced iron, and phosphate of zinc with nux vomica. It is often a question as to what shall be substituted for beer or wine at meal times, and I generally recommend milk or some agreeable fruit-syrup in soda water.

In conclusion, I would venture to give a word or two of warning to practitioners as regards their manner of prescribing stimulants, and to urge the necessity for ordering these remedies with great care and discretion. In acute diseases more prudence is usually exercised than in chronic affections. It is in these latter, that so much mischief is apt to arise from recommending " a little brandy and water occasionally ;" or from sanctioning " a glass or two of wine" for faintness or low spirits. Having seen again and again the mental misery and physical destruction produced by a craving for strong drink, when once the desire has been started, I feel it impossible to be silent on this head. It is also the more necessary to speak, seeing that a tendency exists on the part of the public to trace the origin of not a few cases of confirmed drunkenness to the careless advice of medical men. This is not the place, however, to enquire if the charge be just, or to assert that it has been over-strained : suffice it to remark our practice should be such, that even suspicion cannot attach to us. And consequently, when it is neces-sary to recommend the use of some alcoholic stimulant not only is the kind to be specified, but also the exact quantity ; while the times at which the doses are to be taken ought to be mentioned. I would even go further and say, that in many cases (and perhaps always in the instance of a reclaimed hard-drinker) it will be better to order a medicine like the carbonate of ammonia or the spirit of ether, where a stimulant is required, than to recommend brandy, or gin, or wine, &c. Without a doubt, the examples of chronic disease where beer and wine are needed except at meals are exceptional ; while a number of persons who consume these fluids then, would in all probability be much better without them.

VIII. INSANITY.

1. GENERAL OBSERVATIONS.—Few subjects more deserve the careful study of the medical practitioner than the diseases which affect the intellectual functions, and few have been more neglected until a comparatively recent date. " The care of the human mind," says Gaubius, " belongs to the physician,—it is the most noble branch of our office."

Several *definitions* have been attempted of insanity ; but though unsoundness . of mind is for the most part easily recognised, it cannot be satisfactorily defined. As a rough description which is sufficiently definite to embrace all forms it may be said,—In-sanity consists of a functional or organic disease of the grey matter of the cerebral hemispheres ; this disease giving rise to illogical or erroneous ideas, to disordered actions, and to that general mental condition which hinders a man from discharging his duties to his God, his neighbour, and himself. This definition is open to many objections ; and let doctors and lawyers vex themselves as they may, every endeavour to form one will be so. For, as nothing can be more slightly defined than the line of demarcation between sanity and insanity ; so if we make the definition too narrow it becomes meaningless, and if too wide the whole human race may be involved in it.*

* The *Report from the Select Committee on Lunatics*, ordered by the House of Commons to be printed, 27 July 1860, shows that the number of lunatics in England and Wales in 1844, 1858, and 1859, was as follows :—

	1st January 1844.	1858.	1859.
In Private Establishments	3,790 ...	4,612 ...	4,762
In Pauper Asylums, Workhouses, &c.	16,821 ...	30,735 ...	31,230
Total	20,611 ...	35,347 ...	35,992

Thus, it seems, that the increase of lunatics is much in excess of the exten-

The *indications* of impending cerebral mischief may generally be detected by the careful physician some months before they attract the serious attention of the patient or his friends. The chief premonitory symptoms or prodromata have been especially pointed out by Dr. Forbes Winslow; who forcibly insists upon the fact that cerebral affections are not suddenly developed, while they are often rendered incurable by a neglect of treatment in the early stages. The threatenings of incipient insanity which should excite alarm, are—headache, attacks of giddiness and mental confusion, paroxysms of irritability and loss of temper, inaptitude for usual occupations, a weariness of life, a state of sleeplessness or of lethargy, loss of memory, some marked deviation from the usual line of conduct, defective articulation, dimness of sight, and flightiness of manner. The patient feels too that he is not quite right, yet he does not like to consult a physician. He also shuns his old friends; is tortured with nonsensical, blasphemous, or obscene thoughts; has restless nights, or disturbed sleep with frightful dreams; while generally he suffers from dyspepsia.

Mental diseases are not only dependent on temporary or permanent faulty nervous structure, but are likewise frequently accompanied with symptoms of a variety of bodily disorders. Even the Greek and Roman physicians were aware of this fact; yet in the present day it is often forgotten, and the physical disorder (other than the cerebral) is allowed to pass on unnoticed, simply because it is not at first apparent. Diseases of the lungs are frequent; especially the low forms of pneumonia, pulmonary gangrene, and tubercular consumption. In their early stages, these diseases are apt to escape notice. Thus many insane patients have died of pneumonia without manifesting any symptoms of pulmonary inflammation; so that the existence of this affection has not been suspected until its discovery in the post mortem room. It is always a safe precaution to examine the chest, when a lunatic seems even slightly ill. Probably one-fourth of the deaths which occur in asylums are due to pulmonary consumption. Many observers have remarked upon the supposed predominance of heart affections in the insane; but if the statistical reports of a

sion of the population between the above periods; but allowance must be made for improved registration, as well as for the diminished mortality among the insane. The figures, however, show that at least one person out of every 600 in England and Wales was incapable of managing himself and his affairs. Doubtless a vast proportion of these were cases of idiocy, or of mental imbecility from age, fits, &c. These are always incurable; but of the rest, some 50, 60, or perhaps 70 per cent., may be deemed to have been curable if they were taken in time and carefully treated.

The total number of Private and Pauper Lunatics and Idiots in England and Wales, as known to the Commissioners of Lunacy on the 1 January 1868, was $\frac{\text{Males } 15,734}{\text{Females } 17,479} = 33,213$. Of these only 3384 were deemed curable; 435 had been found lunatic by inquisition; and 675 were criminals. The foregoing total of 33,213 does not include 274 private patients under single care.

large number of asylums be examined, no evidence can be obtained to show that cardiac diseases are more rife among the inmates than in the sane. The occurrence of insanity with paralysis, and with epilepsy, will be noticed presently. Diseases of the stomach and intestines and liver are far from rare. The sexual organs, especially in women, may be the seat of morbid action or of growths. Lallemand has described the case of a patient who believed himself to be a woman, and who wrote letters to an imaginary lover. The necroscopy revealed enlargement and induration of the prostate gland, abscesses, obliteration of the ejaculatory ducts, and enlargement of the vas deferens with dilatation of the vesiculæ seminales.

2. **VARIETIES OF INSANITY.**—Much diversity of opinion exists as to the best classification of mental diseases. As an intelligible and serviceable one for clinical instruction, I shall adopt that proposed by Pinel and Esquirol; who arranged the various forms of insanity under the heads of *mania, monomania, dementia,* and *idiocy.* To these classes a fifth must be added—the *paralysis of the insane.* With regard to the first four divisions it ought to be remembered, that the differences between these varieties are almost always imperfectly marked; that the descriptions laid down in books are extraordinarily distinct compared with the medley of symptoms presented by real cases; and that the various forms frequently run into each other.

(1) *Mania.*—Mania [Μαίνομαι = to rage], or raving madness, may be said to be characterized by *general* delirium. The reasoning faculty, if not completely lost, is disturbed and confused; the ideas are abundant, erroneous, absurd, wandering—not under control. The manners are violent, excited, and exceedingly mischievous.

Although mania rarely makes its incursion suddenly, still it is that form of insanity which most frequently does so. Repeatedly there are premonitory symptoms, such as,—neglect of family and business, change of moral character, distrust of relatives, fits of passion, despondency, insomnia, &c. When the disease sets in the delirium becomes general, and the fury extreme. Then it is that maniacs often destroy themselves, either from not knowing what they do, or from despair—being conscious of their condition, or from accidentally injuring themselves. The difficulty of describing the symptoms of mania is extreme. "Where is the man," says Esquirol, "who would dare to flatter himself that he had observed and could describe all the symptoms of mania, even in a single case? The maniac is a Proteus, who, assuming all forms, escapes the observation of the most practised and watchful eye." Mania may become complicated with epilepsy: it oft-times ends in dementia and paralysis.

In general, maniacs soon become weak and emaciated. The mere physical exertion which they go through, very commonly talking, shouting, howling, laughing, reciting, &c., for hours together ; often furious, destructive, and rapidly moving about :—the fatigue of all this would quickly exhaust a strong man. In addition there is a want of refreshing sleep, night after night, and not unfrequently an aversion to all food. Oft-times the patient has incontinence of urine ; while this secretion perhaps contains an excess of phosphates. The temperature of the body is above that of health : it is especially raised during the evening. Where recovery takes place, it is invariably preceded by sleep and a desire for food. There is then a gradual cessation of the agitation and delirium.

Puerperal Mania is a peculiar affection occurring to women almost immediately, or about the fourth or fifth day, after delivery. A similar disease sometimes attacks pregnant women long before labour ; or it sets in months afterwards, as a consequence of undue lactation. Puerperal mania commences usually with symptoms of agitation and excitement ; though now and then there is only great moroseness and obstinacy, this last feature being often most evinced in a persistent refusal to take food. Under any circumstances, a great dislike is apt to be early shown towards the husband and infant. There is also considerable restlessness, insomnia, severe pain in the head, and a diminution of the secretion of milk. Sometimes there is no fever, on other occasions the skin is hot and dry ; while the pulse is full and frequent, and the tongue thickly furred. Constipation is the rule ; with a diminution of the secretion of urine. The lochia may cease abruptly. Formerly it was believed that inflammation of the brain and its membranes was the cause of this disease. No one holds such an opinion now, so far as I know. In the cases which I have seen there has been great debility ; the patients having been prostrated, either by floodings during their labours, or by the presence of a morbid poison (as that of erysipelas) in the system, or by some other cause which has lowered their vital powers. The delirium is often violent ; there may be a strong tendency to suicide or child-murder ; and there is either great general irritability, or an appearance of deep melancholy. The prognosis is generally favourable with respect to the ultimate restoration to mental health. The fact of one pregnancy being followed by mania, should make us very watchful on subsequent occasions. Contrary to many authorities, I think the recurrence of the disease is much to be feared. As regards their treatment these cases of puerperal mania require particular care. The indications are to rouse and support the powers of the patient ; and to allay the irritability of the brain and the nervous system. The first is to be accomplished by a cordial, stimulant, and nutritious diet. One of the brandy and egg mixtures (F. 17) will often be very useful, in oft-repeated doses. Ammonia and bark (F. 371), quinine and phosphoric acid (F. 379), and cod liver oil (F. 389), are all efficacious remedies. Good beef tea and wine also prove beneficial. The cerebral excitement is to be calmed, and sleep procured, by sedatives; especially by full doses of the extract of stramonium (F. 323), or of the extract of opium (F. 343), or of camphor with henbane (F. 325), or of morphia and Indian hemp (F. 317). The subcutaneous injection of morphia (F. 314) often procures sleep when other remedies fail. The constipation is to be overcome by small doses of castor oil, given in hot and salt beef tea; or by mild aperient pills, or the confection of senna. The patient must be controlled effectually, but mildly, by a humane nurse accustomed to the management of these cases. Moreover, she had better never be left alone, lest a sudden impulse to commit some act of violence overcome her. It is almost always desirable to remove the infant from the sick room; for suckling by the mother is not to be thought of. When the disease threatens to be of considerable duration, the sufferer should certainly be separated from her family and friends.

(2) *Monomania.*—Monomania [Μόνος = alone + μαίνομαι = to be furious,—irrationality on one subject only], or partial insanity, is that form in which the understanding is deranged to a certain degree, or is under the influence of some one particular delusion. The mind is vigorous : the ideas are few, erroneous, fixed, not under control. The manners are in accordance with the predominant idea or train of ideas. At one time the intellectual disorder is confined to a single object, or to a limited number of objects. The patients seize upon a false principle, which they pursue logically; and from which they deduce legitimate consequences that modify their acts and affections. Thus, a monomaniac will insist that his body is made of glass, and being thoroughly impressed with this idea, will reason correctly that slight causes may injure it; he consequently walks with care, and avoids any rough handling. Aside from this partial delirium, he often thinks, reasons, and acts like other men. Another, in the belief that he is a bad half-crown, will go round to the neighbours warning them not to take him in payment or to give change for him when his wife offers him at the counter. Again, a third will fancy himself suspected of some horrid crime, or may think he is possessed of a demon or evil spirit, or will believe himself to be a god—imagining that he is in communication with Heaven. Occasionally, under the idea that he is a divine instrument of vengeance, the monomaniac commits murder. He will often be happy, full of joy, and communicative; unless rough attempts are made to control him, when he becomes wild and furious. Such individuals ask the most extraordinary favours, and make the most absurd demands. The following copy of a letter, presented by a monomaniac to Dr. Conolly, is a good example :—
" In the name of the Most High, Eternal, Almighty God of Heaven, Earth, and Space, I command you to procure me the following articles immediately :—A Holy Bible, with engravings, &c.; a Concordance; a Martyrology, with plates; some other religious books; a late Geographical Grammar, a modern Gazetteer, news-

papers, magazines, almanacks, &c., of any kind or date ; musical instruments and music ; large plans, guides, maps, directories,"— and many other works, concluding with—" wines, fruit, lozenges, tobacco, snuff, oysters, money—everything fitting to Almighty God.   Answer this in three days, or you go to hell.   P.S.—A portable desk and stationery, and a dressing-case."

A remarkable and not uncommon effect produced in the mind by insanity, is the hypochondriacal supposition of the existence of venereal disease (see the section on Syphiliphobia, p. 337).   In one instance related by Sir W. C. Ellis, although there was no possibility of the disease having existed, the patient fancied she had been infected ; while she could not rest satisfied until put under a course of what were believed to be mercurial medicines.   After having taken pills made of bread-crumbs for several days, the patient, from the expectation that they were to produce salivation, spat such a quantity of saliva as to require a vessel constantly by her side for that purpose.   When this had persisted for some time, she imagined that the medicine had produced its effect ; the bread pills were discontinued, and the excessive action of the salivary glands ceased.

Almost every insane patient labours under hallucinations of one or more of the senses,—he sees or converses with imaginary beings.   When he is satisfied by the evidence of his other senses that what he sees or hears is only an *illusion*, he is said to labour under a *hallucination ;* whereas when he believes in his false perceptions, the hallucination becomes a *delusion*.   Some authors use the terms hallucination and illusion in a somewhat different sense. Thus if a man hears voices speaking to him which no one else can hear, or sees objects no one else can discover, they say he labours under a hallucination ; but to lay the foundation for an illusion there must be present some material object,—thus the clouds are formed into angels sounding trumpets, the windmill is regarded as a giant, and so on.   Hallucinations may exist where the senses of sight and hearing are absent, but illusions of course cannot do so. Illusions are frequently observed in a state of mental health, being then corrected by the reason.

The actions of lunatics are at times most contradictory and undecided.   Frequently, the sufferer is puzzled ; being tormented by the commands of different spirits.   For example, a gentleman, after recovery, recollected that various spirits would assail him at breakfast.   One said, eat a piece of bread for my sake, &c. ; another at the same time would urge, refuse it for my sake, or refuse this piece for my sake and take that ; others would direct the tea to be taken or declined.   He saw that he could not comply with one, without disobeying the other; so that there was hesitation at every morsel put in the mouth.   Again, it is occasionally sufficient for the good or bad or indifferent spirits to order a thing to be done, for the lunatic to refuse to do it.   Mr. Perceval, who has detailed in full the treatment he was subjected to in different asylums,* states,—"I disobeyed the voices in doing so, but it was usually a reason for me now to do anything, if I heard a spirit forbid it." The love of contradiction, however, is not always shown thus. The same author says in his narrative, that it was always a great delight to get his hand loosened from the strait-waistcoat,—"and the first use I usually made of it was to strike the keeper who untied me; directed by my spirits to do so, as the return he desired above all things else; because he knew I was proving my gratitude to the Lord Jehovah, at the risk of being struck myself." And again, when being shaved he used frequently to ask the barber to cut his throat,—"in obedience to voices I heard; but I did not want it."

Sometimes the symptoms are so far obscure, that although the conduct of the patient, the expression of his countenance, and his demeanour suggest mental delusions, yet he manifests nothing of the sort in his conversation. The insanity may then frequently be detected by the written letters. Such a case occurred in my own practice :—I was sent for one morning to see a young gentleman whose manners were peculiar, but who spoke rationally. A few hours afterwards he wrote to me—"I find that after a physician has received his fee he must do whatsoever the patient wishes, unless he (the physician) can and does certificate that to be peculiarly hurtful and detrimental. I require you to come prepared to lave my bowels completely, and apply the anti-costive oil; prepare the perineum for a blister; and put three ounces of castor oil in the bladder. I have got a preparation made to keep the blister open."—In another example a well-conducted youth, who had only evinced a few vague symptoms of depressed mental and bodily health, left his home in town to spend a few days at the seaside. His respectable, but poor and hard-working relatives were startled at the end of a week by getting a short note asking for twenty pounds, as he had purchased a horse. Unable to gratify this request, the next day they received the following letter, written in an almost undecipherable hand on several smudged and blotted sheets of paper :—"I think your conduct is disgraceful. I have not only bought a horse but a basket chaise. You have put me to great inconvenience. I think it will be a long time before we are again friends. You are damned fools, do you think when a fellow buys a horse he is obliged to keep him. A horse a horse my kingdom for a horse. At length I have got one and moreover a beauty a highflyer. I took him out this morning—I put him in a gallop away the beggar went still I stuck like wax—The

* A Narrative of the Treatment Experienced by a Gentleman, during a state of Mental Derangement; designed to explain the causes and the nature of Insanity, and to expose the injudicious conduct pursued towards many unfortunate sufferers under that calamity. London, 1838. In a second work with the same title, published in 1840, the writer gives his name—"John Perceval, Esq.," and acknowledges the authorship of the first volume.

cabmen of course chaff'd me hold on I needed not their advice. I thought I was riding a race.   Fortunately I pulled up and a gentleman helped me off.   He said he never in his life saw a horse so seated and I was worthy of being Cavalry officer in the Artillery.   I think without exception you are all the most disagreeable family exhisting. I shall not remain at——thats certain. The horse is mine, a carriage bought by my own money.   You have inconvenienced me exceeding in not sending me a £5.   All this disarrangement of the family—arises entirely from your unsisterly and disgraceful conduct towards me I despise *you*, Your Brother."   Again, Dr. Noble mentions the instance of a youth, twenty-one years old, the son of a publican, who had become reserved, disdainful, and totally changed in disposition shortly before being seen.   No perversion of ideas was apparent, excepting from his demeanour.   Attempts to gain an explanation were quite vain ; still the intuitive good sense of those about him suggested that he was not in his right mind.   An accident at length revealed the fact.   The draft of a letter to the Queen Dowager was found, showing that he believed himself to be her son, and was indignant at being temporarily deprived of his birthright.*

That form of monomania which is characterized by fear, moroseness, and prolonged sadness, has been separately described by some authors as *lypemania* [Λύπη = sadness + μανία] or *melancholia* [Μέλας = black + χολὴ = bile].   Such cases are most painful to have charge of, the despondency is often so great.   Everything that is done to relieve them becomes a new source of suffering : they are incapable of experiencing pleasure from any acts of kindness or attention : no pursuit has the slightest charm for them.   A lypemaniac is unwilling to move, or talk, or to take food ; he is morose, capricious, contradictory, quarrelsome, and discontented ; while he will often remain a whole day without change of posture, or without uttering a word.   He now and then wishes to be alone, and yet dreads solitude ; sleeps but little ; sometimes tortures himself by the anticipation of never-ending punishment hereafter ; while at other times he is bent on severely maiming or destroying himself, or on murdering others.

The attempt to commit suicide [*autophomania*, Αὐτοφόνος = a self-murderer] is not, as a general rule, made from any sudden impulse, but rather from a long premeditated determination ; and often when patients find that they are so watched that it is impossible for them to carry out their designs, they will assume a cheerful manner for days or weeks so as to lull suspicion, and then avail themselves of the first opportunity which offers.   Hanging seems to be a favourite mode of self-destruction among the insane of this country.   When a would-be suicide has determined (usually after much consideration) upon the manner in which he shall destroy

* *Elements of Psychological Medicine*, p. 125.   Second Edition.   London, 1855.

himself, it may be practically useful to remember, that he will very often wait and neglect all other means which may present themselves until he can accomplish his death after his own fashion. Sir W. C. Ellis mentions the case of an old gardener who one day consulted him as to the best mode of destroying himself, since he said that he had made up his mind not to live any longer. The heinousness of the crime contemplated, and the fact that hanging was a most painful death, were pointed out; his wife was directed never to leave him alone; and he got better by the use of medicines which restored the healthy character of the secretions. Some time afterwards, however, he was discovered dead in a little shed in his garden, where he used to keep his tools. It appeared that so determined had he been to die by hanging, that though the place was so low he could not stand upright in it, and he had not a rope or even a string with which he could suspend himself, yet he contrived to carry out his wishes by getting a willow twig and making it into a noose, which he fastened to one of the rafters. He must have stooped to put his head through it; and then pushing his feet from under him, suspended himself until he died. Had he not made up his mind to destroy life in this particular manner, he might have done so much more easily by drowning himself in the pond which was in his garden, or by cutting his throat with the knife which he always had about him.—In many instances, melancholics having a tendency to suicide will resort to modes of destruction such as baffle all ordinary precautions. For example, they will set fire to their clothing, and while parts of the body are burning appear neither to suffer pain nor fear, but rather to triumph in their martyrdom. A lady, the subject of religious mania, as her clothes were burning on her, said—"Let me die; the pain of my body is nothing compared to the pain of my mind." And even during the few hours that she lived after setting herself on fire, with the right side of her body all charred, she showed signs of suicidal tendency as great as ever. So a man who recovered after cutting away the whole of his genital organs, still evinced so strong a desire to operate further upon himself, that he had to be most carefully watched. Such is their singular tenacity of purpose, that suicidal patients will tear their night dresses, and by stuffing the shreds into their mouths endeavour to produce suffocation. Again, cunning lunatics, while taking pills containing narcotics, have been known to hoard successive doses, until they have accumulated a poisonous quantity.

Another variety of monomania has also been described as *moral insanity*; in which there is perversion of the natural feelings, affections, temper, habits, and moral dispositions, without at first any remarkable disorder of the intellect. Eccentricity of conduct, an impulse to commit crime, a propensity to every species of mischief, are often the leading features. These cases sometimes assume an uncontrollable destructive tendency [*androphomania,*

'Ανὴρ = a man + φονεύω = to kill], and the lunatic commits murder ; or there may be a propensity to set houses or other property on fire [*pyromania*, Πῦρ = fire] ; or the disease will possibly give rise to an irresistible desire to steal [*kleptomania*, Κλέπτω = to steal], things being often pilfered for which the madman has no use, or which he could easily purchase if needed.

In *erotomania* ["Ερως = love + μανία], according to Esquirol, amatory delusions rule, just as religious delusions predominate in *theomania* [Θεὸς = God] or religious melancholy. Erotomania may be only an excessive degree of a chaste and honourable affection ; or it will be combined with *nymphomania* [Νύμφη = the nympha] in women, or with *satyriasis* [Σάτυρος = a satyr] in men. In all these forms there is usually great mental and bodily depression ; women suffer the most frequently, especially those who are single; and the phenomena are often connected with some malformation or organic disease of the sexual organs.

The occurrence of *insanity with epilepsy* is said by Esquirol to be incurable, and the experience of most physicians will confirm this remark. The conduct of insane epileptics is often characterized by the most ferocious, murderous, or suicidal aberrations ; it is frequently also most filthy and disgusting. Notwithstanding these unfavourable symptoms, however, residence in a well-ordered asylum can do much to induce a certain amount of mental tranquillity ; whilst a good diet and daily exercise will contribute to the physical improvement. By some practitioners bromide of potassium is said to reduce the frequency of the fits, as well as to soothe nervous irritability. If early death do not result, the disease usually subsides into incurable dementia.   .

Dr. Bucknill states that in epileptic cases where no considerable amount of dementia has resulted, the brain is not found atrophied or presenting any appearances of disease. Not unfrequently indeed, the weight of this organ is much increased. The heaviest brain weighed by Dr. Thurnam was that of an uneducated butcher who could only just read, and who died of epilepsy combined with mania, after about a year's illness. This man's brain weighed 62 oz. avoir.* Dr. Thurnam remarks that epilepsy is often connected with an unusually large brain. In the case of a male epileptic, 37 years of age, seen by Dr. Bucknill, this structure weighed 64·5 oz. In the examination of thirty-three brains of epileptics, this gentleman only once found a spicula of bone projecting from the cranium, and once only a tumour.

The connexion of homicidal and suicidal impulses with epilepsy is very remarkable. An epileptic may commit the greatest violence directly after a fit, without any subsequent recollection of what he has done. Sometimes, instead of the epileptic seizure occurring in the usual form, it seems to burst into an attack of

* *On the Weight of the Human Brain, and on the Circumstances affecting it*, p. 32. London, 1866.

acute mania. In a few days, or perhaps hours, the symptoms pass away; the individual remaining sensible and well behaved until the recurrence of the epilepsy. Possibly, however, in the first fit he may destroy himself. The medico-legal bearings of such cases are highly important.

(3) *Dementia.*—Dementia [*De* = priv. + *mens* = the mind] or incoherence, is that condition in which a general weakness of the intellect, induced by disease or age, is the prominent feature. The mind is altogether feeble; the ideas are confused, vague, and wandering; and the memory daily becomes more and more impaired. There are paroxysms of restlessness and excitement. The patients are ignorant of time, place, quantity, property, &c. They forget in a moment what they have just seen or heard. Their manners are undecided, childish, and silly: their conversation is incoherent, and they repeat words and entire sentences without attaching any precise meaning to them. They have neither partialities nor aversions; neither hatred nor tenderness. They see their best friends and relatives without pleasure, and they leave them without regret. Now and then they are constantly but slowly moving about, as if seeking for something; on other occasions, they will pass days in the same place and almost in the same attitude. They have little or no control over the bladder or rectum. The phosphates of the urine are diminished: there may be albuminuria. Their temperature is below the normal standard. The ultimate tendency of mania and monomania is to pass into dementia. It is a condition which is very rarely, if ever, cured; and in its last stage there is complete paralysis. Cerebral atrophy is a constant concomitant of dementia, its extent varying with the loss of mental power.

(4) *Paralysis of the Insane.**—This important variety of mental disease has received considerable attention from physicians of late years. It is an affection sui generis: a combination of insanity with a gradually increasing loss of motor power. Not very uncommonly it is ushered in merely by symptoms indicative of a gradual waning of the intellect. More frequently, however, there are prominent delirious conceptions. These may, or may not, take the form of very exalted notions with regard to self-importance; or of extravagant delusions respecting the possession of wealth and power and wonderful abilities. There are also frequent attacks of frontal headache, perhaps so severe as to make the patient strike the part with his fist, or knock it against the wall; while neuralgic pains in different parts of the body may perhaps increase the suffering. With all this there are the symptoms of progressive paralysis of the muscular system. The disease has been thought to be caused by sexual excesses, intemperance, and

* The synonyms of this disease are numerous. The principal are,—General paresis [Πάρεσις = want of strength, from παρίημι = to relax]; Insanity with general paralysis; Progressive paralysis of the Insane; Paresifying mental disease; Dementia paralytica; Paralysie générale incomplète; and Geisteskrankheit mit Paralyse.

those evils which result from leading " a fast life." A history of hereditary tendency to insanity is often to be procured. Excessive or prolonged emotional agitation exerts an influence in producing it. The disorder rarely occurs before the age of forty; while it is the general opinion that men are much more liable to it than women. According to Foville, 31 general paralytics (22 males and 9 females) were found in 334 insane.

Esquirol first drew attention to the incurable nature of this malady; and we now know that paralytic lunatics seldom live more than from one to three years. Perhaps the progress of the disease has now and then been arrested, but only for a time. At whatever period the paralysis supervenes its commencement is generally unmarked by any striking symptoms, beyond the marked weakness of the intellectual powers, or the delirious conceptions already mentioned; while it may come on in any variety of mental disease, increasing as the power of the mind diminishes. The first direct indication is commonly an impediment in the movement of the lips and tongue; the articulation becoming muffled and imperfect. This impediment increases, so that there is confirmed stuttering or mumbling. It is followed by tottering, uncertain, and vacillating movements in walking; or the impairment of locomotion may even be the earliest symptom. The same difficulty exists in co-ordinating the movements that is seen in locomotor ataxy. The handwriting is changed. The affected muscles always contract under the influence of galvanism. Then also, there is want of expression in the countenance—a heavy vacant look; the intelligence and judgment are greatly lessened; while fits of irritability, hallucinations, and illusions are common. There is loss of memory; a marked falling off in disposition, especially as regards energy and decision; with great debasement of the moral character. The pulse gets feeble and frequent; the tongue on being protruded moves tremulously from side to side; usually the mobility of the pupils is lessened and often they are of unequal size, or one pupil may be dilated and sluggish while the other is permanently contracted; the excretions escape involuntarily either from want of attention, or from paralysis of the sphincters; and there is exaltation of the mind, with the formation of childish hopes and schemes. Epileptiform convulsions are apt to occur. Hemiplegic seizures, attended with convulsions or coma, are not uncommon; but they generally pass off after the use of stimulating enemata, and the removal of any collection of hardened fæces. According to Dr. Allbutt, an ophthalmoscopic examination of the eyes shows an atrophic condition of the optic nerves, through the whole course of the disease, in nearly every case. As the disorder progresses, the patients become unable to articulate a single word; they continually grind their teeth, often producing a most discordant noise during the stillness of the night; their weakness is such that they cannot walk or even stand; bed sores form upon the back; all traces of intelligence become abolished; they get motionless and insensible; and their torpid existence is reduced to a kind of slow death, unless they happen to be more quickly carried off by diarrhœa, bronchitis, pneumonia, or some other complication.

Concerning the exact nature of this disease much has yet to be learnt. Dr. Conolly says :—" It appears to originate in a general affection of the brain, scarcely indicated after death by more than greater softness or greater firmness, general or partial, of the cerebral substance, and by ventricles full of serum, combined merely with other appearances common to all chronic cases of mental malady : and it leaves the practitioner, after the longest reflection, ignorant of its primary nature, and helpless as to its cure."* Since this was written Wedl has demonstrated that in every instance there is hypertrophy of the connective tissue of the small arteries and veins in the pia mater and cortical portion of the brain. In consequence, there follows degeneration of the vascular walls; and hence derangement of the circulation, with disturbed nutrition. The increasing and destructive formation of connective tissue in the cortical substance, leads to the destruction of nerve-cells and nerve-tubes.† Dr. W. H. O. Sankey, who shows by the by that the credit thus given to Wedl is in reality due to Rokitansky, states than an examination of the capillaries in about twenty cases of insanity, of which seven were from patients who died of general paresis, has led him to the conclusion that these vessels in the cortical substance are more or less diseased in every case of this form of paralysis.‡ The morbid state consists of some degree of tortuosity; amounting to a curve or twist, a kinking of the vessel, or the formation of little varicose knots. And lastly, in protracted cases of general paralysis Mr. Lockhart Clarke has also found the spinal cord more or less affected. Sometimes, parts have been softened to the consistence of cream : in other instances numerous areas of granular and fluid disintegration within and around the grey substance, have been discovered.§

With regard to treatment, all that can be done is to relieve any painful symptoms, to give sleep by large doses of henbane, and to support the strength by a nourishing diet and warmth and cleanliness. Mr. Austin states‖ that when the patient is not very feeble, twenty grains of the extract of henbane is not too large a dose to begin with ; and that this quantity may be gradually increased to thirty grains, twice or thrice a day.

(5) *Idiocy.*—This condition is characterized by partial or com-

* *On the Treatment of the Insane without Mechanical Restraint*, p. 72. London, 1856.
† *Beitrage zur Pathologie der Blutgefässe.* Wien, 1859. Quoted from Dr. Ernst Salomon's essay on *The Pathological Elements of General Paresis.* Translated from the Swedish by Dr. W. D. Moore. London, 1862.
‡ *The Pathology of General Paresis.* (Reprinted from the Journal of Mental Science, No. 48), p. 21. London, 1864.
§ *The Lancet*, p. 230. London, 1 September 1866.
‖ *General Paralysis: its Symptoms, Causes, Seat, &c.*, p. 208. London, 1859.
D D 2

plete absence of the intellect, owing to imperfect organization of the brain. It is congenital. The mind is not developed : there are no ideas, or they are few. The manners are childish, with occasional transient gusts of passion. The countenance is vacant, and void of aught approaching to intelligence. The articulation and the gait are often imperfect. And occasionally the idiot ['Ιδιώτης = a private individual,—one unfit for society] is a blind deaf-mute.

Curious examples are recorded of the recovery of idiots after some injury to the head, which though inexplicable are not therefore to be discredited. Dr. Prichard says,—" I have been informed on good authority that there was, some time since, a family consisting of three boys, who were all considered as idiots. One of them received a severe injury of the head : from that time his faculties began to brighten, and he is now a man of good talents, and practises as a barrister. His brothers are still idiotic or imbecile. Van Swieten mentions the case of a girl who was imbecile till she received an injury of the head, and underwent the application of a trephine for the removal of a depressed portion of skull : she recovered and became intelligent. Haller has reported the case of an idiot whom a wound in the head restored to understanding."* Dr. Forbes Winslow notices the history of Father Mabillon, who was said to have been in his younger days an idiot, and to have continued in this condition until the age of 26.   He then fell with his head against a stone staircase, and fractured his skull. He was trepanned. After recovering from the effects of the operation and injury, his intellect fully developed itself. He is said subsequently to have exhibited, " a mind endowed with a lively imagination, an amazing memory, and a zeal for study rarely equalled."†

The weight of the brain of an adult man may be estimated at about 48 ounces, or 3 lbs. avoirdupois (see pp. 340, 400). Dr. John Thurnam weighed, or caused to be weighed, the brain of nearly every insane patient who died under his care. Thus he accumulated notes of 470 cases. Before taking the weight, the cephalo-spinal fluid, effused serum, and blood were allowed to drain away ; the dura mater was removed ; but the arachnoid and pia mater were retained. The weights are given in ounces (avoirdupois) and tenths. The average weight of the brain, for all ages, in the insane (including idiots and congenital imbeciles,) as deduced from the tables, is as follows :—

	Brains of Men. oz.	Brains of Women. oz.	Excess per cent. in Men.
Cerebrum	40·2	35·6	12·
Cerebellum	6·	5·4	10·
Encephalon	46·2	41·	12·

* *A Treatise on Insanity, and other disorders affecting the Mind*, p. 203. London, 1835.

† *On Obscure Diseases of the Brain, and Disorders of the Mind.*   Second Edition, p. 433. London, 1861.

The maximum weight of the encephalon in man, out of 257 cases, was 62 oz. The minimum was 32 oz. The maximum weight of the encephalon in women, out of 213 cases, was 53·2 oz. The minimum, 30·7 oz.

With regard to idiocy and brain-weight the following cases may be noticed :—Dr. Peacock found the brain of an idiot boy, who died of scarlet fever when nearly eleven years old, to balance only 21 oz. 3½ dr. avoirdupois ; its proportion to the whole body being . as one to 16·2. Dr. Todd also dissected the brain of an adult idiot, which was 20¼ oz. avoirdupois : Dr. Tuke mentions the case of an idiotic female, who died at the Retreat at York, at the age of 70, in whom the brain weighed 23¾ oz : Dr. Down found the brain of an idiot boy, 18 years old, who died at Earlswood, to be only 15 oz. : in the Museum of St. Bartholomew's Hospital there is the brain of a male idiot, aged 22, which weighed 13 oz. 2 dr. avoirdupois. Lastly, Professor Marshall has given an account of the brains of two idiots of European descent,—one, that of a woman, who died of phthisis at the age of 42, and whose recent brain without the membranes weighed 10 oz. 5 grs. ; the other, that of a boy, who died when 12 years old of spinal and pulmonary abscess, and whose fresh brain with the membranes weighed only 8½ oz.*

3. PRINCIPAL CAUSES.—These are often very difficult to detect. Insanity is no doubt frequently hereditary ; or it can sometimes be traced to marriages among near relatives, " breeding in and in," as the farmers say ; or it may perhaps be due to syphilis in the system of the parents, or to drunkenness on their part, or to scrofula and tubercle. Defective mental education—imperfect training of character, parental mismanagement, the encouragement of too eager a desire for learning or riches or worldly position, as well as the fostering of extreme religious feelings, are all so many predisposing causes of mental alienation. Among the more immediate causes are injuries of the head ; the abuse of alcohol, or of narcotics—as tobacco and opium ; sexual excesses, and particularly masturbation ; somewhat rarely, perhaps, continence ; fevers ; and the retrocession of erysipelas or gout in persons predisposed to insanity. Then there are certain moral causes, as blighted ambition, disappointment in love, distorted views on the subject of future rewards and punishments, immoderate grief, long-continued anxiety and distress, prolonged intellectual exertion, and pecuniary reverses. I think it is Dr. Noble who remarks, that the more advanced the civilization of any community, the more abundant are the diseases of the mind. Humboldt states that he looked in vain for cases of insanity among the native Indians of America. But in this remark he probably referred to acute mental disease ;

* *Philosophical Transactions of the Royal Society of London,* vol. cliv. p. 527. London, 1865.

since savages, like children, may surely suffer from congenital imbecility or idiocy.

A disregard of everything but self—a forgetfulness of his due relation to all other creatures, is a characteristic of the lowest order of man. " All the diseases of the mind leading to the fatalest ruin consist primarily in this isolation. They are the concentration of man upon himself, whether his heavenly interests or his worldly interests, matters not; it is the being *his own* interests which makes the regard of them so mortal. Every form of asceticism on one side, of sensualism on the other, is an isolation of his soul or of his body; the fixing his thoughts upon them alone : while every healthy state of nations and of individual minds consists in the unselfish presence of the human spirit everywhere, energizing over all things; speaking and living through all things."* If we seek for an illustration of mental disease thus set up, we shall find it in the insanity of women. Man having selfishly and uncharitably appropriated the right of entering and working in the various labour markets, the so-called weaker sex has become practically debarred from all honourable occupation. Women being educated with but one purpose—that of marriage, what is to befall them if they fail in their aim of life; or if their wedded portion prove only a misery and debasement. Having no healthy life-giving career, driven to a morbid egoism, perhaps carried away by ungratified sexual passions, is it to be wondered at that so many of the sex suffer from all forms of nervous disorder,—passing through the various grades of restlessness and irritability and hysteria, until their wretchedness finally culminates in madness.

One undoubted cause of insanity, though only recognised of late years, is defective nutrition of the brain. The ultimate effect will be the same whether there exist a morbid condition of the blood, or some obstruction to the capillary circulation. The nervous centres require a rapid renewal of healthy arterial blood : if the blood be impure (as from use of alcohol, opium, chloroform &c.), or if congestion take place, mental activity ceases. Want of refreshing sleep interrupts the restoration of nervous force most seriously ; and many patients after recovery, have attributed their disease either to complete insomnia, or to their repose having been long disturbed by frightful dreams. Those slumbers which are " but a continuation of enduring thought " must necessarily be quite opposed to the nutritive regeneration of that part of the cerebral organism on the action of which the emotions depend.

In individuals predisposed to insanity, local irritation may give rise to an attack. In a case which I saw a few years ago, a large abscess in the loins had this effect. I have also observed severe hysterical mania result from acute ovaritis, the mental disease ceasing as the ovarian pain was relieved.

Men and women suffer in nearly equal proportions from in-

* *Modern Painters.* By John Ruskin, M.A. &c., vol. v. part ix. chap. ii. p. 206. London, 1860.

sanity. In this country the females under control are somewhat in excess of the males. It must be recollected, however, that in England and Wales, the women are in excess of the men. Thus, in the middle of 1866, the estimated population was $\frac{\text{Males } 10,771,700}{\text{Females } 10,976,320} =$ 21,210,020. The age at which mental disease appears to be most common is between twenty-five and fifty : in women, perhaps between thirty-five and forty-eight, and in men between twenty-five and fifty when the nervous system is often most severely taxed.

4. DIAGNOSIS AND PROGNOSIS.—The *diagnosis* of insanity is on many occasions attended with great difficulty. In examining a lunatic we may perhaps find that several of his actions are not more extravagant than those of many peculiar though sane men ; but we shall probably learn from those about him that his conduct is totally at variance with that which he manifested prior to his attack. In short, the individual is not what he was. There has been a gradual change of demeanour, perceptible to all acquainted with him ; while no satisfactory reason can be given for the alteration. Thus the temperate man has more or less gradually become a drunkard : the good husband has given himself up to every kind of licentiousness : the individual with kind friends has become imbued with the belief that everyone's hand is against him. I have known a gentleman, remarkable for his morality and tenderness of disposition prior to the setting in of mental disease, boast of " keeping several women ;" and while informing his wife of the fact, reproach her harshly for her tears, remarking that he could not see what she had to complain of. Frequently, there is some difficulty in finding out the patient's delusions, and on this point we have to make close inquiries of the friends. But with regard to all hearsay evidence, both as to the antecedents and the existing state, the physician must be cautious ; inasmuch as, without any wish to deceive, it often happens that the friends have a bias towards which they may unconsciously lean.

When insanity is feigned, the trickster may usually be detected. Give him time, and he is certain. to betray himself. He overacts his part ; performing antics which he thinks are characteristic of lunacy, but which are never seen in an asylum. It becomes tolerably clear that he, being a sane man, wishes to be thought mad : he is violent, incoherent, talks absurdly on many topics, and makes exertions which quickly tire him. The lunatic, on the contrary, shows no evidence of fatigue for a long time : he talks rationally on several subjects, and takes all the pains he can to be regarded as sane. The difficulty is greater if the impostor maintain a sullen silence ; but even then he will surely be found out by carefully observing him when he believes himself unseen.

It has long been known that the insane are prone to suffer from changes in the form of the external ear, and particularly from sanguineous tumours (*Hæmatoma auris*) about the outer surface of the auricle. By some these have been attributed to mechanical violence, but this opinion seems untenable. The peculiar condition is often symmetrical. Dr. Laycock, after a careful study of the symptomatology of the ear, has come to these conclusions :—" 1. That the states of the circulation, nutrition, and development of the tissues which make up the ear-lobule, and cover the helix, very commonly coincide with similar conditions of the encephalic tissues. And 2. that the development of the cartilages of the external ear, and of their several parts, is in relation with the encephalic and cranial development of the individual."*

This is hardly the place perhaps to enter upon the consideration of the treatment of lunatics in our courts of law. But it is impossible not to see that in this matter there is a decided leaning to undue severity. A scientific witness may entertain no doubt as to the insanity of a particular criminal; and yet if he cannot assert that the prisoner at the time of his committing the act was ignorant of the wrong he was doing, the law will not heed the evidence. In many instances the life or death of a man rests upon the answer given by the physician to this question,—Did the prisoner know the difference between right and wrong when he committed the crime? If the principle here involved were acted up to generally, half of the asylums might be closed for want of inmates. Why the whole management of lunatics in the present day depends upon moral control,—upon teaching them that they must behave properly. But daily experience proves that a man may be quiet and harmless in an asylum, who would be very dangerous if he were his own master. A madman bent on committing suicide knows that it is a wrong act, and will regret his tendency to it, and beg to be restrained. Yet the next hour he may attempt self-destruction. A wise and benevolent dispenser of justice should endeavour to learn if the general tenour of the man's life has been that of a sane or insane man; whether there has been any gradual alteration of character; and if any cause has been in action likely to induce imperfect nutrition or actual disease of the brain. In short, he should be bent upon simply discovering the truth, in a possibly obscure case, rather than of confounding "the mad doctor," and exposing him as an enemy to society. No lawyer, however great his general abilities and legal knowledge may be, should expect to be able to form a sound opinion as to whether a given individual is, or is not, of unsound mind, without having studied the subject of lunacy. Hence, science and humanity alike demand that if the judges are to define in set terms what is meant by insanity, they ought first to visit the asylums and watch the behaviour of their inmates. They might then see how variable in kind and degree are the symptoms of brain diseases; while they would likewise learn that it is no more absurd to believe that some of these disorders lead to "uncontrollable impulses," than that certain other affections of the nervous system interfere with the power to govern choreic and sundry irregular muscular movements.

* *Medical Times and Gazette*, p. 289. London, 22 March 1862.

With regard to the *prognosis*, it may be said that it is more favourable when an acute disorder of the whole system, or some cerebral malady attended with fever, has constituted the beginning of the mental aberration, than it is in those cases where the alienation of mind has slowly exhibited itself (perhaps almost imperceptibly at the onset) and advanced progressively to confirmed insanity. At the same time it must be remembered that one attack predisposes to another. The recovery may appear complete; but often the malady is only dormant, and slight causes will serve to rekindle it perhaps in an aggravated form. Of the cases discharged as cured from the public asylums, probably at least one-fourth relapse.

Where physical violence sustained by the head is the cause, the prognosis is uncertain, inasmuch as very severe lesions of the encephalon may thus arise. Moreover, where the mind has been overthrown by sudden and severe calamity, the prospects of recovery are great. Again, if the mind breaks down after protracted cares, the case is bad; especially if the physical energies also become depressed. When insanity is complicated with general paralysis or with epilepsy, it is generally quite hopeless. Probably more cases of mania are cured than of any other form of insanity; the likelihood of restoration being very much greater in the earlier than in the advanced periods. Melancholia, however, if the patient be properly and promptly treated often proves curable. According to Esquirol the most favourable age for recovery is between twenty and thirty, few being cured after fifty: most authors assert that insanity in women is more curable than in men. And lastly, when the mental disease is connected with some bodily disorder which admits of removal by the progress of age, or by medical treatment, the grounds for hope are much increased. To form a correct prognosis, no link in the chain of circumstances must be overlooked. Dr. Noble well observes:—"The causes, moral and physical, predisposing and exciting; the history of the invasion and progress; the actual state, and the reactions taking place under influences of every kind,—must all be known and rightly appreciated if an opinion is to be formed of the slightest value."

In advanced insanity, when the patient is happy in his delusions, he often gets robust; for he sleeps nine or ten hours out of the twenty-four, his appetite is good, he takes no heed of the future, and his morbid ideas give him no trouble. It is an unfavourable symptom for the bodily health to improve, without the mental disease becoming at all alleviated.

A common cause of death in the insane is some disease of the thoracic viscera, especially of the organs of respiration. The slightest symptom of bronchitis or pneumonia ought to claim attention. To prevent any insidious development of phthisis from being overlooked, it is well to weigh each patient (especially in large asylums) every month.

Supposing recovery to take place from acute insanity, the time which has intervened between the onset of the disease and its ter-

mination now and then appears like a sleep; or it is perhaps regarded as a frightful dream.   When George the Third, in November 1810, had so far recovered from an attack of mania as to be
able to receive a visit from the Lord Chancellor, he enquired of his
physicians how long he had been ill.   On being told that it was
some eighteen days, he replied that he had no recollection of the
time.   This, he said, had been the fourth blank in his life; at the
same time enumerating his three former illnesses and the length
of time they had lasted.[*]

5. **PATHOLOGY AND MORBID ANATOMY.**—The two
chief postulates as to the nature of insanity which are entertained
in the present day are,—the *metaphysical* or *spiritual* theory, and
the *cerebral* hypothesis.   The first conjecture, that insanity is a
disorder of the immaterial principle, and not of the material instrument by which the mind manifests itself, seems untenable;
although it has been adopted by many psychologists.   The second
theory is the only plausible one—viz., that the brain, or nervous
structure on which all mental action is dependent, is the part affected.
According to the observations of many physiologists a general
agreement seems to be now arrived at, that complexity and richness
of the convolutions, depth of the sulci, and thickness of the grey
matter are the conditions found where there has been high intelligence.   In the drawings and descriptions given by Professor Wagner
of the brains of five men eminent in different branches of science, the
complex arrangement of the convolutions is certainly remarkable.
Consequently, it is to these parts we direct our attention in cases
where there has been morbid mental action.   The cerebral disease
may be such as is visible on examination after death, or it will
consist of some change which we cannot discover.   If the brain be
imperfectly nourished, through any morbid condition of the blood,
we may have diseased action without any structural change being
left which can be detected by an ordinary examination.   Schroeder
van der Kolk says, however, that he does not remember to have
performed the dissection of a lunatic during the last twenty-five
years, without finding a satisfactory explanation of the phenomena
observed during life.   And indeed, it seems far from impossible,
that in the course of time as chemical analysis in conjunction with
microscopical investigation gets perfected, we may become acquainted with the changes which occur in the nerve cells; so that
the brain of a lunatic being given, the pathologist shall be able to
say exactly what the main features of the disease have been,—
whether there has been intellectual disorder, or melancholia, or
idiocy, or failure of memory &c.
The retrograde changes of tissue which have been most frequently found in the brain after insanity consist of softenings of
the grey substance, perhaps reducing parts of the convolutions to

* *Memoirs of the Life and Reign of King George the Third.*   By J. Heneage
Jesse.   Vol. iii. p. 557.   London, 1867.

a mere pulp; of an increase in the amount of connective tissue, and consequent atrophy of nerve cells; together with fatty, amyloid, pigmentary, and calcareous degenerations, occurring in the walls of the smaller vessels, in the nucleated cells of connective tissue, and in the nerve cells. There may be an increase in the volume and consistence of the whole cerebrum; or a state of atrophy, affecting one or more convolutions, or the entire cerebral mass; or an œdematous condition, with cerebral anæmia. The ventricles too are frequently found somewhat dilated, and containing more fluid than in health; this being especially the case in acute insanity from drunkenness. An indurated condition of the nervous substance, making the texture as firm as cheese, is generally the result of hypertrophy of the connective tissue.

With regard to the alterations in the brain case, it need only be noticed that the bones of the skull have sometimes been found abnormally thick; the hypertrophy of osseous tissue being important or not, according as it has affected the intracranial space. Syphilitic exostosis, as well as osseous tumours, may be present. The dura mater is occasionally appreciably increased in density; and at the same time unduly adherent to the inner table of the frontal, parietal, and occipital bones. The arachnoid will frequently be opaque in parts, thickened, and congested: extravasations of blood into the sac of the arachnoid, or hæmatomata, are said not to be uncommon in cases of general paralysis. After violent mania intense congestion of the pia mater has been seen, in conjunction with a red coloration of the subjacent cortical substance. Under other circumstances, this vascular membrane has been found in a pallid anæmic state: it may also present an œdematous condition.

The observations of Drs. Bucknill and Sankey on the brains of the insane and the sane give us the following results:—(1) The absolute weight of the brain is increased in insanity, though the absolute size relatively to the capacity of the cranium is diminished. (2) The greater heaviness depends upon increased weight of the cerebellum, compared with the cerebrum, pons, and medulla oblongata; so that the cerebellum is heavier in relation to the cerebrum in the insane than in the sane. (3) The increased weight of the cerebellum is found to be the greatest in general paralysis, and least in acute mania; the first being a disease of very much longer duration than the second. (4) The specific gravity of both the grey and white portions of the brain is increased in the insane. (5) Dr. Bucknill seems to think that the most essential change consists in the existence of two kinds of cerebral atrophy,—namely, that which is positive, and that which is interstitial or relative. By positive atrophy he indicates an actual shrinking of the brain; while by relative atrophy, which may or may not be coexistent, he means an interstitial change, wherein the active cerebral molecules suffer diminution, inert materials being deposited.

It must not be thought because structural disease of the brain exists, even to a considerable extent, that amelioration of symptoms may not take place for a time. As a fact, amendment does now and then occur, especially shortly before death. Sir Henry Holland* alludes to a case of mental derangement (and says that he has met with similar instances) where the post-mortem examination showed great organic changes in the brain; many of them, obviously of long standing, and upon which it was next to certain that the symptoms depended. Yet in this instance there occurred not long before death a lucid interval, so far complete and prolonged as to afford hopes of recovery where none had existed; and where the event proved that none could be reasonably entertained.

6. GENERAL TREATMENT.—Assuming that the physician is fortunately consulted when the symptoms are merely threatening, he may often effect a cure. This is to be attempted by quieting the nervous system; by insisting on rest from all professional and mercantile pursuits; by taking care that there is a due amount of sound sleep in every twenty-four hours; and by attending to the functions of the skin, liver, kidneys, and alimentary canal. Where there is no symptom of active disease in the head, morphia or extract of opium often proves invaluable; or Indian hemp, henbane, stramonium, or chloroform, may be useful. Some forms of excitement are best treated by thirty-minim doses of tincture of digitalis, repeated every eight or twelve hours. If the vital powers be depressed, tonics—such as quinine and iron, phosphate of zinc and nux vomica, hypophosphite of soda and bark, cod liver oil, &c., must be given. The diet is to be nourishing, and the amount of stimulants to be regulated. Gentle travelling amidst beautiful scenery may be recommended; especially if the patient can be accompanied by an affectionate and judicious relative.

On examining a person supposed to be insane, the duty of a medical man, as Dr. Conolly has pointed out, is twofold, viz.—1st, to determine whether the individual in question be of sound mind; and, 2nd, to give an opinion regarding the treatment required, and especially concerning the necessity of restraint and its degree and nature.—The practitioner will have learned from the preceding observations how to answer the first question. With respect to the second (the medical treatment) it must of course depend upon the state of the patient; but it may be positively asserted that under no circumstances can an antiphlogistic course of remedies be borne.† Even when exacerbations occur at the menstrual

* *Chapters on Mental Physiology.* Second Edition, p. 68. London, 1858.
† This opinion is in its main features acquiesced in by all physicians. One of the most careful recent writers on this subject draws the following conclusions from his experience :—Insanity, in any form, is not of itself an indication for bloodletting; on the contrary, its existence is of itself a contra-indication; hence the person who is insane should, other things being equal, be bled less than one not insane; insanity may coexist with plethora, a tendency to apoplexy or paralysis, and sometimes sthenic congestion or

periods, and the flow is scanty, we must not do more than apply a few leeches to the neck of the uterus; while nourishing food ought to be freely allowed to prevent the loss of blood from causing general depression. Indeed, our general object clearly must be to restore and maintain the bodily functions; while we also remove any disorders in other parts of the system, such as skin diseases, uterine disturbances, gastric and intestinal irritations, &c. which may be connected (or coexistent) with the cerebral affection. We shall perhaps persevere the more, when we remember that many lunatics have been cured by improving their general health, even after suffering for some years. In an ordinary case of insanity, I should especially take care that the patient had a nutritious diet, warm clothing, out-door occupations and amusements, healthy evacuations from the bowels, and sound sleep at night. Attention would quietly be paid so as to prevent all bad habits, as onanism, &c.; persevering attempts would be made to give repose to the nervous system; I would endeavour to impart power to the body, if necessary, by tonics; and then at length would gently try to revive the affections, to send a glimmer of hope into the dark spirit, as well as to strengthen the bewildered intellect. While following such a plan as this no mechanical restraint ought on any account to be resorted to; and as much cheerful occupation and recreation should be afforded as the lunatic could beneficially enjoy.

From this it will seem that stimulants, tonics, mild warm purgatives, and narcotics (especially opiates, in combination or not with belladonna, or Indian hemp, or henbane) must usually prove invaluable remedies. The subcutaneous injection of morphia (F. 314), with or without a small dose of atropine, can be practised without fear or trouble. The douche, shower, or simple warm bath may perhaps be used, but only according to the ordinary principles of medicine. The regular employment of the Turkish bath is often of service; partly by improving the function of nutrition, as is evidenced by a gradual increase of weight. In acute mania especially, the wet-sheet packing (F. 136) with a full dose of henbane will often prove most useful. The diet of the insane should undoubtedly, as a rule, be generous and of the most nourishing kind. It not unfrequently happens that all food is refused, especially perhaps by those who have morbid ideas on religious subjects. Such patients will fancy that they are commanded to fast, and will perish from inanition rather than disobey the imaginary precept. In other cases the functions of the stomach and bowels are deranged, and the refusal is merely due to com-

inflammation, which call for the abstraction of blood; therefore venesection in mental disorders should not be absolutely abandoned, although the cases requiring it are very rare. As a general rule *topical* is preferable to *general* bleeding. Insanity following parturition, other things being equal, is to be treated by bleeding less frequently than that which has its origin in other causes.—*An Examination of the Practice of Bloodletting in Mental Disorders.* By Pliny Earle, M.D. New York, 1854.

plete loss of appetite; the food being eagerly taken when the intestinal evacuations have become free and healthy. If we can, therefore, find any physical cause for the abstinence, it must of course be removed; but otherwise we may try and persuade the patient to eat by tempting him with dainties, or by putting food where he can help himself when unseen, or by feeding him with a spoon like a child. These plans failing, we must resort to *forced alimentation* to sustain life. This may be effected by injecting nutritious fluids through the nasal passages or by the mouth. If we adopt the first mode, it is only necessary to have a funnel with a long flexible tube attached to it; which tube, on being passed through the posterior nares and œsophagus, will convey any liquid by simple gravitation. In the second case, while the patient is firmly held by two or three attendants, we employ the gag and stomach-pump; by means of which I have often injected mixtures of strong beef tea, milk, bark, cod liver oil, brandy, and flour. The use of nutrient enemata in these cases is not advisable.

As regards the moral treatment of insanity, no rules can be of universal application. I will only say, therefore, that it ought to be regulated by kindness and a feeling of sympathy with misfortune; and that no harshness or means which induce fear should be tolerated. Any practice, moreover, which is meant to supersede constant personal surveillance on the part of the nurses is bad. The faulty habits of the insane are to be met by careful management, by unwearying attention. Attendants who are impatient, who will not take trouble, who cannot sacrifice their own comfort to duty, have mistaken their calling. There is too much reason to fear that many of the patients in public and private asylums are even now sometimes cruelly ill-used. Uneducated and coarse keepers seem incapable of understanding that kind words and encouraging smiles are more efficacious than blows and curses. A convalescent who was an eye-witness of the misery caused by rough hands; and who had to look on while one attendant flung a lunatic on the floor and knelt upon him, while a second wrenched open the mouths of helpless patients and crammed the food down their throats, while a third threw the potatoes and hunches of bread and butter upon the table as if they were bricks &c., and while a fourth irritated and knocked about a poor nervous fellow who rebelled against being undressed,—this witness says,—" The doctor never saw these things—how could he? He was never there, but when, like the hands of a clock, the appointed hour was come, or when sent for; and *then* all things were straight, the rooms were still, and the speech as soft as any silk. His rule was regularity; his guide, punctuality. To see everything clean and beautiful and trim was his hobby—to make them *appear* so, the attendants' aim."*

* *Life in a Lunatic Asylum: an Autobiographical Sketch*, p. 68. London, 1867.

Concerning the physician's bearing, few I hope will deem it in bad taste if I venture to urge that he should endeavour to obtain the confidence of his unfortunate patients. In this he will be successful by showing an interest in their well-doing, by listening to the recital of their ailments, by never making a promise without keeping it, by visiting them at unexpected times so as to see that they are properly cared for, and by allowing as much indulgence as is compatible with the proper treatment of their disease. He ought to remember that although lunatics are frequently shy and nervous, yet they are often prompt and acute to see through any mystification; that they appreciate truth and fair dealing; and that any attempt to deceive them is sure to weaken his power over them. Then, if he have a pleasing and friendly address, with kind but firm manners, he may feel confident of maintaining a greater degree of influence than can ever be acquired by severity. It can rarely, if ever, be advantageous to reason with a lunatic presenting acute symptoms. But when recovery has commenced, when the patient may be said to be convalescent, then his questions should be kindly considered; the semblance of treating his observations and complaints with contempt must be guarded against; while his natural longing for home ought to be combated by urging the disadvantage of returning there too soon. Dr. Noble mentions the histories of three inmates of an asylum, each of whom fancied himself the Holy Ghost. On their being brought together, one was cured of his delusion: he saw there could not be three Holy Ghosts. But I cannot suppose that Dr. Noble regards the discussion as the agent that effected the cure; if indeed a cure was effected, for it is not stated whether there were other delusions, or what was the ultimate result of the case.

The existence of any degree of insanity is sufficient to render an individual incapable of executing a will. According to the law, as explicitly laid down by Sir James Wilde in the case of Mrs. Tebbitt against the legatees of Mrs. Thwaytes, August 1867, —"A person who is the subject of monomania, however apparently sensible or prudent on all subjects and occasions other than those which are the special subject of his apparent infirmity, is not in law capable of making a will."

In order to render restraint imperative, I believe a lunatic should either be dangerous to himself or to others; or else seclusion must be deemed necessary as part of the curative treatment. Although the quiet and regular mode of life led by patients in well-ordered asylums is often most efficacious as a remedial agent, yet I am thoroughly convinced that many institutions contain harmless though incurable lunatics, who would be much happier and in no degree injured by residence elsewhere; but who, unfortunately, have relations and friends that will not be troubled with them. At the same time I am not an advocate for either qualified or unqualified medical practitioners receiving single cases of mental disease into their homes. The experience of the Commissioners of Lunacy has shown conclusively, that in many instances where this plan has been adopted, the treatment has proved positively injurious.* What might in all probability answer well, if placed in healthy rural districts, would be colonies for the insane, like that of Gheel, in Belgium ; where patients could be allowed to enjoy a certain amount of liberty, and to mix with the families in the farmhouses where they boarded. At all events, modifications of the present system are needed. For although very much has been done within the last few years to improve the appearance and character of our asylums, nevertheless much remains to be accomplished. They are not yet properly converted into *Hospitals for the Cure of Insanity*. The sites of several are bad. The buildings, in too many instances still retain to an injurious degree the look and nature of prisons ; while the parsimonious way in which some are furnished, and the especially wretched appearance of many of the night-cells, are circumstances positively disgraceful. The days of rotatory chairs, manacles, stripes, head-shaving, baths of surprise, prolonged and violent shower baths, chambers without bed or bedding, dark rooms,—in short, of punishments of all kinds—have, it is to be hoped, gone for ever. Nevertheless, if any one doubts that we have yet much to do, let him read the suggestive and valuable Reports of the Commissioners in Lunacy.

IX. HEADACHE.—VERTIGO.

1. **HEADACHE.**—Headache, or technically cephalalgia [Κεφαλὴ = the head + ἄλγος = pain] is of common occurrence ; since it is present as a prominent symptom during some part of the progress of most acute, and of many chronic diseases. The pain or uneasiness is usually in the head ; although it is often hard to be distinguished from the suffering connected with rheumatism, or neuralgia, or inflammation of the scalp, or with syphilitic affections of the pericranium and bone.

Four principal varieties of headache may be noticed. Arranged in the order of their importance, they may be thus treated of :—

---

* When a medical man receives a patient of unsound mind into his house, he must take care to obey the law of the land. The Commissioners of Lunacy have very properly shown their determination to insist on the salutary provisions of the Lunacy Acts being carried out ; and it is certainly quite time that all violations of the statute should be punished. Over and over again it has been stated by the public press that, although the friends of a lunatic have a right to take care of him themselves, if there is no other person in the house similarly affected, and if no profit is made out of the charge ; still, if any person takes a lunatic into his house and derives profit from so doing, he must comply with all the provisions of the Act of Parliament. He is bound to have an order, and two medical certificates ; while it is also imperative that he should send a statement of the particulars of the case to the Commissioners in London.

The first, or *organic headache*, is due to disease of the brain or its membranes, and especially of such iu an early stage.   It is generally accompanied by attacks of vertigo, occasionally by fits of vomiting, sometimes by confusion of the mind, and frequently by rumbling noises or murmurs in the ears.   The pain may be sharp or dull, lancinating or throbbing.   Diseases of the meninges are attended with more severe headache than those of the nervous substance itself.   In abscess, as well as in cancerous tumours of the brain, paroxysmal attacks are common.   Dr. Forbes Winslow appears to confirm the opinion of Hasse, that pain in the head always exists in central softening of the cerebrum involving the corpus callosum, septum lucidum, fornix, and the ventricular parietes.   When due to inflammation, the pain is often most intense; while it is confined to one portion of the cranium, is increased by warmth or movement or noise, and is lessened by elevating the head.   At times it remits in severity.   There are no symptoms of gastric disturbance, or of sluggish action of the liver.

The second, or *plethoric headache*, is dependent upon fulness of blood : the cerebral vessels become congested.   There is a sense of pulsation in the ears; together with giddiness on stooping   Persons who live too freely, who take but little exercise, who rise late in the morning, &c., are liable to it.   This variety afflicts robust middle-aged men who " make blood too fast ;" as well as plethoric women with irregularity of the catamenia.   Certain forms of cardiac disease, by retarding or hindering the return of blood from the brain, may set up venous congestion and headache.

The third, or *bilious headache*, will either be temporary or constant.   When temporary, it generally arises from some unusual excitement, or an error of diet—any excess either in food or wine ; while it is most severe in the morning on awaking from an unrefreshing sleep.   The suffering for the time is often great.   There is perhaps an inability to keep the head on the pillow, and yet every attempt to sit up brings on violent retching.   The throbbing is so violent, that each beat seems to lift the head from the pillow.   One patient compared this pulsation to the force of steam raising the lid of a kettle up and down as the water boils.   Fortunately, in the course of twelve or twenty-four hours all uneasiness passes off as the cause ceases.—The constant sick headache occurs in persons of weak stomach, who are almost always suffering from indigestion, or who have a tendency to gout.   Such individuals take too little exercise, and often too much unwholesome food.   The stomach and duodenum get out of order ; as is evinced by the coated tongue, the offensive breath, the flatulence, the low spirits, and the nausea which exist.   The hepatic functions are also ill-performed, and the stools are clay-coloured ; while the urine is scanty and of a brown tint.   There is seldom any disposition to vomiting.

The fourth, or *nervous headache*, is often due to debility and exhaustion.   Poverty of blood from renal disease, hæmorrhage, &c.,

may induce it. The irritation of diseased stumps and decayed teeth is I believe a frequent cause; though most sufferers are either incredulous or angry when told that they ought to go to the dentist. Headache is a common symptom in valvular disease of the heart ; being due to the interference with the regular and perfect supply of blood to the brain which is induced. In one variety of this disorder— known as *hemicrania,* or *brow-ague*—the symptoms assume an intermittent character; the pain recurring, every day or each second day, with the same degree of regularity as a regular fit of ague. Although this form prevails in damp and marshy districts, yet it may arise in healthy parts of the country from other causes than malaria, and especially from constitutional debility. Weakly women, who exhaust themselves by over-lactation, &c., are frequently the victims of a variety of nervous headache known as *megrims;* which may assume an intermittent character like hemicrania. And, lastly, hysterical girls are very liable to a kind of nervous headache; which, when confined to a single spot, is known as *clavus hystericus,* because the pain is said to resemble that which it is supposed would arise from driving a nail into the head.

Pain in the nerves of the scalp can scarcely be mistaken for headache the result of organic disease. In the former there may be considerable sharp suffering, but it is not of the sickening and confusing and depressing nature of an inflammatory headache. Frontal neuralgia, the most common variety, has its seat in the supra-orbital branches of the frontal nerve; or the suffering may extend along the whole of this nerve (virtually the continuation of the ophthalmic division of the fifth), causing severe orbital and frontal pains. Suffering of this kind can frequently be relieved by a dose of ammonia and quinine ; while a strip of muslin well moistened with tincture of belladonna mixed with a little tincture of aconite and a few drops of chloroform, and laid along the forehead, will often give immediate ease. To put off the recurrence of the attack for as long as possible, few drugs are more to be relied upon than phosphate of zinc and nux vomica (F. 414). These not succeeding, trial should be made of the chloride of ammonium (F. 60). Where this fails, steel will now and then succeed.

Headaches, of whatever kind, occur more frequently in persons of adult life than in extreme youth or advanced age; and in the brain-workers rather than among the mechanics. Their occurrence is favoured by hereditary predisposition. Habitual dwellers in towns suffer more than residents in the country; females more than males; the nervous and delicate more than the robust; and the middle and higher classes of society more than the lower. And then lastly, Dr. Wright says that all pains in the head " especially affect persons who neglect the many little attentions and cares that our civilized, and therefore in some measure artificial mode of life requires. I may especially instance regularity in diet, carefulness in adapting the clothing to the requirements of our variable climate, attention to the action of the bowels, and a sufficient amount of exercise, as essential objects of our care."*

The indications for *treatment* are to relieve the congestion of the head and the dyspeptic symptoms, while at the same time attempts should be made to give tone and strength to the system. The diet ought to be regulated, only such food being allowed as can be usefully assimilated. Many individuals afflicted with headaches, tremors, and restless nights would derive great benefit from leaving off tea. Coffee is seldom as mischievous ; while in some forms of sick headache it positively gives relief at the time, and also tends to keep off the attacks. I look upon tobacco in every shape as injurious where there is a tendency to headache of any kind ; though I am occasionally told that a cigar eases, or even dispels the pain. Mild purgatives, such as rhubarb and senna (F. 146), nitric acid and taraxacum (F. 147), rhubarb and blue pill (F. 171), podophyllin and henbane (F. 160), or alkalies with compound decoction of aloes (F. 148, 149) will frequently be useful. When the pain is connected with the gouty diathesis, colchicum is the proper remedy (F. 46). We may also often effect a cure in bilious headaches by pepsine (F. 420) ; or by quinine with ipecacuanha, or rhubarb (F. 384, 385), to aid digestion. In these cases also the patients must take daily exercise in the open air, and avoid too much sleep. All alcoholic stimulants, but particularly beer and port and sherry, can frequently be given up with great advantage by those subject to this kind of headache. On the other hand, in many nervous headaches, stimulants and tonics—particularly the nitro-hydrochloric acid (F. 378), are to be tried ; in hemicrania, quinine or arsenic (F. 52, 379), will be needed ; while in hysterical women we must resort to shower or douche baths, with nux vomica or zinc or steel (F. 394, 410, &c.)

Holding the arms high above the head produces a marked effect upon the cerebral circulation. Hence this proceeding will once in a way check troublesome bleeding from the nose ; while I have frequently seen it relieve the severity of that peculiar morning headache, with which some persons constantly awake. Again, compression of the temporal arteries with a couple of pads and a bandage, may sometimes be of service. Without pretending that there is anything curative in this proceeding, I am sure it will often be the means of affording much relief at the time of greatest suffering.†

* *Headaches, their Causes and their Cure*, p. 12. London, 1856.

† This effect of pressure did not escape the observation of Shakespeare. When Othello, after listening to the insinuations of Iago (act iii. scene 3), tries to conceal his feelings from Desdemona by the plea that he has a pain upon his forehead, she replies,—" Faith, that's with watching ; 'twill away again : Let me but bind it hard, within this hour, it will be well." And so again, in the scene between Hubert de Burgh and young Arthur (*King John*, act iv. scene 1), the latter attempts to excite Hubert's compassion by reminding him,—"When your head did but ache, I knit my handkercher about your brows, The best I had, a princess wrought it me, And I did never ask it you again ; And with my hand at midnight held your head."

In addition to the foregoing we shall occasionally have to try the effect of iced water, cold lotions, eau de Cologne, &c., to the head; the application across the forehead of a thin piece of muslin soaked in tincture of belladonna; sinapisms, dry cupping, or blisters, or setons to the nape of the neck; the removal of decayed teeth or stumps from the mouth; and change of air. It need hardly be added that in *organic* headaches arising from some cerebral mischief, the disease and not the symptom must claim the greatest share of the practitioner's attention.

2. **VERTIGO.**—Giddiness, or vertigo [from *Verto* = to turn round] consists of a transitory sense of whirling round, or of falling. Surrounding objects appear to be in motion. The sufferer loses his balance for a second or two, but often recovers himself without dropping, provided he can grasp some firm support; and then he asks to sit down immediately. The attack is followed by headache.

Vertigo is most prevalent in advanced life. It is perhaps a more important symptom of incipient disease of the brain, than headache. When frequent seizures are complained of, they assume a really serious bearing; being generally the precursors of impairment of the mental powers, as well as of actual lesions of nervous tissue. The difficulty of relieving these seizures is painfully great.

The practitioner should always endeavour to trace the attack to its origin. In several instances it betokens general weakness; as is seen in the vertigo which arises on assuming the erect posture, during the early stages of convalescence from acute disease. It may be due to some poison in the blood; examples of which are common from the abuse of alcoholic drinks, a dose of opium, and the use of tobacco by one unaccustomed to it. Now and again it is merely symptomatic of some gastric or intestinal irritation: of some disturbance of the liver: of chronic kidney affection, particularly of such as is accompanied with albuminuria: or of disease, functional or organic, of the heart. Disease or weakness of the walls of the right auricle will give rise to vertigo, by its influence in retarding the return of blood from the brain: in the same way headache is produced. Venereal excesses cause giddiness. With women, attacks of menorrhagia often induce it; and so does prolonged lactation, more especially if the catamenia are regular.

Vertigo very frequently arises from some evident disturbance of the cerebral circulation. Indeed, any circumstance which suddenly modifies the circulation of the blood through the brain will produce it; whether the occurrence act so as to accelerate the flow or to retard it,—to cause plethora or anæmia. In the mild form of epilepsy (epileptic vertigo), the two chief, or indeed only symptoms, are giddiness and faintness. "Swimming in the head" is also often a forerunner of apoplexy and paralysis: it is an accompaniment of cerebral tumours. Paroxysmal attacks are not uncommon in the aged, unattended by other symptoms. A diseased condition of the coats of the arteries of the brain, in advanced life, is a frequent cause of very troublesome giddiness. Less com-monly it is connected with a gouty state of the system.

In the majority of cases there are indications of depressed vital power. And it must be recollected that this is the case, even when the vertigo is connected with a fulness of the cerebral vessels; the congestion consisting of passive venous hyperæmia much more frequently than of active arterial determination of blood. Hence, as a rule, tonic and antispasmodic remedies are more frequently called for, than those which have a tendency to lower the system. The latter, however, will be needed in persons of a full habit of body; in those whose heads are hot and throbbing, whose arteries are pulsating with undue force, and who complain of buzzing noises in the ears. In such, a plain nourishing diet without any alcoholic stimulants, mild doses of alterative and purgative drugs (F. 171), small blisters behind the ears, or setons in the nape of the neck, may prove useful. On the contrary, where there is evidence of anæmia, where the nervous system has been over-worked or insuf-ficiently nourished, there the chloride of ammonium, cod liver oil, chalybeates, plenty of animal food with wine or malt liquor, and change of air must be prescribed. For those attacks of temporary dizziness to which the aged are liable, small doses of corrosive sub-limate (F. 27) and bark are often valuable.

X. DISEASES OF THE SPINAL CORD.

Experiment and clinical observation have taught us that the spinal cord in connexion with the brain is the instrument of sensa-tion and voluntary motion to the trunk and extremities. The continuity of the cord with the encephalon is absolutely essential; for let it be destroyed, and then sensation and voluntary motion must necessarily be abolished in all those parts of the body sup-plied by spinal nerves below the seat of injury. The nearer the seat of interruption to the encephalon, the greater will be the paralysis and the more rapidly will life be extinguished; so that if the cord be severed at its junction with the medulla oblongata (as when an animal is " pithed"), death will result immediately. To Dr. Marshall Hall, however, we are mainly indebted for proving that the spinal cord may be the instrument for the excitation of movements, *independently* of volition or sensation; either by the direct irritation of its substance, or through the influence of some stimulus carried to it from a portion of the trunk or extremities by nerves there distributed.

The spinal cord, surrounded by the dura mater and arachnoid and pia mater, occupies the superior two-thirds of the vertebral canal; its weight, when freed from the membranes and nerves, being about one ounce and a half. Above, opposite the upper border of the atlas, the cord ends in the medulla oblongata; while below, on a level with the intervertebral substance separating the first and second lumbar vertebræ, it terminates among the leash of nerves known as the cauda equina. Of a flattened cylindrical form, the cord is divided by an anterior and a posterior median fissure into two symmetrical portions; each of these divisions being so fissured that it consists of four columns,—an anterior, a lateral, a posterior, and a posterior median. On making a transverse section of the cord we find it to consist of grey or vesicular, and white or tubular matter. The grey matter, made up of nerve filaments and countless corpuscular or multipolar cells, is placed in the interior of the cord, in the shape of two crescentic masses; each mass being in a lateral half of the cord, each having an anterior and posterior horn, and each being joined to the other by a band of matter called the grey commissure. The thirty-one pairs of nerves which issue from the cord have each two roots,—an anterior purely motor, and a posterior purely sensitive; these roots by their union forming a compound nerve. From the labours of Schroeder Van der Kolk it seems certain, that the anterior roots of the spinal nerves have their origin from the grey ganglionic cluster of cells of the anterior horn; the anterior medullary fibres of the cord being the channels through which the influence of the will is conveyed from the brain to these ganglionic clusters or plexuses. The posterior roots have two rootlets, one of which seems to ascend in the white substance to the brain, thus forming the channel of sensation; while the other penetrates the white substance, and appears to be lost in the ganglionic cells of the posterior horn and centre of the grey matter. These latter rootlets of the great posterior or sensitive roots are thought to consist of the filaments for reflex action. Thus it is said that the two horns of grey matter stand in the closest relation to motion; the anterior being the direct sources of motion, while the posterior serve for reflex action and co-ordination. (The cause of the co-ordination of movements is therefore situated in the spinal cord, and not in the cerebellum). The medulla oblongata is believed to be the common central point, where reflex action crosses to either side; and on the irritated state of which, general spasms—as convulsions and epilepsy—are thought by Van der Kolk to depend. The white or medullary matter consists of gelatinous nerve-substance and extremely minute nerve-filaments.

The structure of the medulla oblongata extends upwards through the pons Varolii to the crura cerebri; while below it is continuous with the spinal cord, of which indeed it may be said to be the superior enlarged portion. This pyramidal-shaped body is divided into two equal portions by an anterior and a posterior groove. Each lateral half thus produced is subdivided by minor grooves into four columns or eminences,—the anterior pyramids, the lateral tract and olivary body, the restiform body, and the posterior pyramid. About one inch below the pons Varolii (the bond of

union between the cerebrum, medulla oblongata, and cerebellum),
if the anterior pyramids be separated from each other, it will be
seen that the innermost fibres of these pyramids decussate with
one another. Consequently, disease on one side of the brain
manifests its effects on the opposite half of the body. With regard
to the functions of the medulla oblongata, besides exhibiting the
property of reflex action, and besides being the tract of communication between the brain and cord, it is a nervous centre of the
greatest importance ; since on the integrity of its structure depend
both respiration and deglutition.

In the hope that these remarks will facilitate the comprehension of much that follows, I proceed to a consideration of the
diseases of the cord.

1. SPINAL MENINGITIS.—Acute inflammation of the membranes of the cord (sometimes termed *acute paralysis from inflammation of the membranes of the spinal cord*) is seldom met with. The
disease terminates either in resolution, or in the effusion of serum,
or in softening or suppuration. The morbid action when acute,
may be associated with disease of the cerebellum or of the cerebral membranes ; while when chronic, it is mostly found associated
with caries of the bodies of the vertebræ.

The *symptoms* which have been described as indicating inflammation of the meninges of the cord, are very severe. Thus there
is always high fever with sleeplessness. There are acute pains,
often of a burning character, extending along the spine and
stretching into the limbs, aggravated by motion and pressure,
and often simulating rheumatism. In one case which was under
my care, the patient remained coiled up in the middle of the
bed in a characteristic manner ; dreading to move, and in fact
declining to do so for some sixty hours : she would not even
allow her position to be altered when the catheter was required,
so severe had been the paroxysms of pain along the spine and
limbs on any movement being attempted. As the disease continues we find rigidity or tetanic contraction of the muscles of
the neck and back, varying in degree, but amounting sometimes
to opisthotonos ; with feebleness of the limbs. This feebleness
does not prevent motion, if the patient will make an attempt to
move. Where there is much effusion, we may detect paralysis of
the lower extremities, the loss of power gradually extending upwards as the effused serum increases in quantity. When the disease
gets fully developed there will be more or less difficulty of breathing,
sometimes so severe during the paroxysms as to give rise to suffocating sensations ; a feeling of constriction in the neck, back, and
abdomen ; retention of urine ; occasionally priapism ; and obstinate constipation, oft-times succeeded by diarrhœa with pale offensive stools. Great prostration sets in towards the close ; while
there may be feverish delirium and coma.

Males appear to suffer more often from spinal meningitis than females.   The disease is most common between the second and seventh year, and then between the twentieth and twenty-fifth year ; while exposure to wet and cold in rheumatic subjects seems to be its most frequent cause, mechanical injuries taking the second rank.   The changes found after death are great congestion, chiefly confined to the pia mater ; effusions between the arachnoid and pia mater of serum or pus ; with perhaps softening of the cord.   Lastly, the treatment of this for the most part fatal disease must be that recommended when speaking of inflammation generally.   It has indeed been allowed by some who have resorted to bleeding and mercury, that success has not followed the use of these remedies, though they account for the failure on the ground of the practice not having been adopted with sufficient energy.*

2. MYELITIS.—Myelitis [Μυελὸς = marrow + terminal -*itis*], or inflammation of the substance of the spinal cord, is not marked by any very uniform set of symptoms.   The features of the disease will be found to vary with the severity of the attack, its duration, and the portion of the cord affected.

Tracking the inflammation from above downwards, the following are the chief *symptoms*.   When the *cranial* portion is affected, we find deep-seated headache, convulsive movements of the head and face, inarticulate speech, trismus, difficult deglutition, impeded spasmodic breathing, irregularity in the heart's action and in the pulse, with hemiplegia or other form of paralysis.   As the fatal stage approaches, there is great prostration, feeble circulation, increased dyspnœa, and involuntary escape of the excretions.   Where the inflammation affects the whole thickness of the cord above the origin of the phrenic nerves, life is at once extinguished by the cessation of the action of respiration.—Supposing the inflammation is in the *cervical* portion, the prominent signs will consist of difficulty of deglutition, impossibility of raising or supporting the head, acute pain in the back of neck, great dyspnœa, a sense of pricking and formication in the arms and hands, together with paralysis of the upper extremities.—In inflammation of the *dorsal* region, there is pain in this district, numbness or pricking sensations in the fingers and toes, convulsive movements of the trunk, paralysis of the arms and lower extremities, short and laborious respiration, great palpitation, &c.—When, as is most commonly the case, the *lumbar* portion is attacked, the paralysis of the lower extremities becomes more marked ; there is great pain in the abdomen, with a sensation as of a cord tied tightly round it ; there are convulsions or paralysis ; while paralysis of the bladder and sphincter ani ensues, leading to retention which is followed by incontinence of urine, and involuntary stools.

The pain in the affected part of the cord is less severe than in

* *Diseases of the Spinal Cord and its Membranes.*   By Charles Evans Reeves, M.D., &c., p. 45.   London, 1858.

meningitis : it is increased by the application of heat (as of a sponge dipped in hot water), or by firm pressure. Care must be taken not to attribute the pain to lumbago. The loss of sensation in the palsied limbs is complete. Probably myelitis often coexists with pneumonia and gastro-enteritis.

The disease seems usually to be *excited* by cold and damp, or by wounds and contusions ; while sometimes it occurs during the progress of fever. The *prognosis* is always grave ; but there is no reason to doubt that many cases recover, where the inflammation has only been of short duration, and especially where only the lower half of the cord has been affected. It may, however, terminate fatally in the acute stage, or afterwards from the occurrence of ramollissement or of suppuration. Ramollissement is the most frequent result; which cannot be distinguished from non-inflammatory softening by the naked eye. Sometimes one part of the cord is found softened, and another portion indurated. Occasionally an abscess has been discovered in the substance of the cord.

The *treatment* proper in inflammation of the cord and membranes is the same as that previously recommended for inflammation of the brain and its membranes. Better results may be hoped for from iodide of potassium than from any other drug. Where there is any suspicion that a syphilitic taint is at the root of the mischief, mercury ought to be given. Great care must be taken to keep the patient dry and clean, as well as to empty the bladder frequently with the catheter; remembering that incontinence of urine generally arises from the bladder being over-distended,—literally from the urine overflowing. Bed sores will most likely be prevented by placing the patient on a water-bed ; or in the absence of this, by the use of the soft amadou plaster.

3. **SPINAL HÆMORRHAGE.**—Apoplexy of the spinal cord is more infrequent than cerebral hæmorrhage. The paralytic and other effects are due to the effusion of blood into the spinal canal, or into the sac of the arachnoid, or into the substance of the cord.

The *causes* are chiefly blows and falls, over-exertion, acute inflammation of the cord or membranes producing softening of the cord, fatty degeneration of the coats of the bloodvessels, and caries or other disease of the vertebræ. Remains of old apoplectic clots have been found external to the dura mater, or between the membranes, or in the substance of the cord—even in the medulla oblongata. Such signs of bygone hæmorrhage and recovery are very uncommon. Where the effusion is abundant, death may ensue at once ; but when this does not happen, a fatal result will perhaps take place after the lapse of some time owing to chronic softening of the cord.

The *symptoms* will depend upon the seat of the ruptured vessel. When the blood is effused between the membranes, it will necessarily gravitate to the lowest part of the spinal canal ; and hence will arise abrupt paraplegia, which gradually ascends. There will also be acute and sudden pain in the back, and sometimes in the head ; severe convulsions often set in ; the breathing will be difficult when there is pressure on the upper part of the cord ; the heart's action is usually much depressed ; the skin is pale and cold ; but there is no loss of consciousness.—Effusion into the substance of the cord produces sudden paralysis in all parts supplied with nerves below its seat ; unless the hæmorrhage be very slight, when the loss of power may occur slowly after the lapse of several hours.

The object of our *treatment* must be to check the effusion of blood by absolute quiet, and the application of ice along the spine.

4. TUMOURS.—Paralysis may arise from the long-continued pressure of tumours upon the cord, producing partial atrophy. The morbid growth will consist either of tubercle, or cancer, or bone, or hydatid cysts, or aneurisms, or small syphilitic gummata. Exostosis of the odontoid process of the second cervical vertebra has occasionally been found. Sometimes the pseudo-tumour has had its origin in syphilitic caries of the vertebræ.

The *symptoms* come on very slowly, paralysis occasionally not being manifested until great pressure is exerted. The paralysis of motion always precedes that of sensation. There is usually a severe neuralgic kind of pain over the seat of the growth ; while cramps, with convulsive movements of the extremities, are not uncommon. Malignant fungoid growths have been found on the dura mater. Where any kind of tumour is associated with scrofula or syphilis or cancer, there will be other manifestations of the particular affection.

The *treatment* must be chiefly constitutional ; though occasionally counter-irritants to the painful part of the spine do good. Iodide of potassium, cod liver oil, and a nourishing diet, are the remedies from which most good may be expected.

5. HYDRORACHIS AND SPINA BIFIDA.—Hydrorachis is a term applied to abnormal collections of fluid within the spinal column. When the fluid has been present for some time it produces, by its pressure, atrophy of the cord.

Hydrorachis is generally congenital, and associated with *spina bifida*. Where the latter is unaccompanied by hydrorachis, the deformity consists in absence of the spinous processes of the vertebræ ; the vertebral arches being bent towards each other so as to leave only a very slight space between them. In the greater number of cases, however, the spinous processes and laminæ of some of the vertebræ are widely cleft, or deficient. Consequently, the cord and its coverings being deprived of support, protrude and form a fluctuating tumour, varying in size from an orange to an adult head ; the serous fluid which naturally lubricates the medulla and its membranes being secreted in excess. The tumour is generally covered with skin ; under which is areolar tissue, and then dura mater. If the child live, the dura mater becomes thicker and harder as age advances. "The connexion," says Mr. Prescott Hewett, " which generally exists between the cord or the nerves and the walls of the sac, is a point of the utmost importance.   Some cases are related, by various authors, in which neither the cord nor the nerves had any connexion with the sac; these parts followed their usual course down the spinal canal, but in by far the greater number of cases that have been placed upon record, the nerves presented some kind of connexion with the sac.   Of *twenty* preparations of spina bifida occupying the lumbo-sacral region, which I have examined in various collections, I have found but *one* in which the nerves were not connected with the sac.   If the tumour corresponds to the two or three upper lumbar vertebræ only, the cord itself rarely deviates from its course, and the posterior spinal nerves are generally the only branches which have any connexion with the sac.   But if the tumour occupies partly the lumbar and partly the sacral region, then generally the cord itself and its nerves will be found intimately connected with the sac.   M. Cruveilhier believes, from his dissections, that this connexion is constant."*

Before birth, spina bifida does not seem to affect the fœtal health; while afterwards, the noxious effects vary with the seat of the tumour, and its contents.   When the cleft is in the cervical portion, it is generally fatal a few days after birth : it is the least dangerous when seated in the lumbar and sacral regions, some few individuals having lived with it for twenty or thirty years, or even for the natural term of life.   If complicated with hydrocephalus, the prognosis is very unfavourable ; and such is also the case when there is paralysis of the lower extremities, or when the tumour continues to enlarge, or when its walls enlarge and burst.   There is frequently, moreover, great irritation and discomfort from excoriations about the perineum and thighs, produced by an inability to retain the urine.   The sphincter ani is generally weak.   This malformation is said by Chaussier (whose opportunities for observation at the Paris Maternité have been large) to be met with about once in every thousand births.

As a general rule, the less the tumour is interfered with the better ; all operations being attended with danger.   In those cases, however, where the fluid contents are rapidly increasing in quantity, it is certainly justifiable to try the effects of puncture, followed by compression.   Two rules laid down by Mr. Hewett must be observed :— 1. The tumour should never be punctured along the mesial line, especially in the sacral region, for it is generally at this point that the cord and its nerves are connected with the sac. The puncture is to be made at one side of the sac, and at its lowest part, so as to diminish the risk of wounding any of the nervous branches.   2. The instrument ought to be a needle or a small trocar ; for if a lancet is used there will be a greater risk of

* *Remarks on Cases of Spina Bifida,* by Prescott Hewett.   *Medical Gazette,* vol. xxxiv.   London, 1845.

wounding some important structure contained in the tumour. Compression by air-pads and bandages ought to be resorted to after evacuating the fluid.   The most remarkable example of this practice I have seen, is the following :—On the 21 March 1860, I tapped the tumour of a little girl four years of age, removing eight ounces of a clear limpid fluid.   A cleft was distinctly felt in the sacral vertebræ.   In spite of pressure, the cyst refilled and appeared to be as large as ever two days after the operation.   Nevertheless, the child is still living (1869), and in the enjoyment of tolerable health.

Iodine injections have been proposed and practised by M. Chassaignac, and in one case at least with apparent success. More evidence, however, is required of the safety and utility of this mode of treatment before its adoption can be recommended. Cases are also said to have been cured by pressure alone,—even by such an amount as can be produced with collodion !

In all instances attention should be paid to the general health. The diet ought to be nutritious ; while in the case of an infant at the breast, great care must be taken that the nurse is strong and healthy. If residence at the sea-side can be obtained, so much the better.

6. CONCUSSION.—It is rather remarkable, that while considerable attention has been paid to the subject of concussion of the brain, very little notice has been bestowed upon the same condition as it affects the spinal marrow.   The little knowledge which I possess on this matter will perhaps be best conveyed to the reader, by a concise reference to two well-marked cases of concussion of the cord which came under my notice during the year 1860.   In one case the lady fell while walking upon some rocks on the Devonshire coast ; in the other a jump from a high phaeton was the cause of the accident.   Neither lost consciousness in the slightest degree, both felt the peculiar tingling in the hands and feet called pins and needles, and both were able to walk some little distance after the shock.   The first patient did not apply to me till six weeks after the fall ; when she complained of nervousness and general weakness, some difficulty in passing urine, a sense of cold and deadness in the legs, startings at night, with a steadily increasing difficulty in walking.   Perfect rest in bed for one month, with the daily application of the extract of belladonna down the course of the spine, effected a cure.

The second patient consulted me on the day following the mischief, inasmuch as she was frightened because she felt so sore and bruised that she could scarcely move.   There was, however, no real paralysis.   The bladder was unaffected.   The pain was correctly attributed to the jump, though surprise was expressed at the severe result, inasmuch as she alighted safely upon her feet.   She was kept in bed for many days until every symptom had vanished ; and no ill consequence ensued on her afterwards walking about.

Where cases like the foregoing are neglected, and when the

sufferers continue to take exercise, there is a fear of degeneration and softening of the marrow setting in; which conditions are very likely to end in more or less extensive incurable paralysis, or even in general muscular atrophy and death.   Mr. Hilton, in his lectures at the Royal College of Surgeons during 1860, mentioned the case of a gentleman who had had a fall upon his back, a few years previously, owing to the giving way of some scaffolding.   Directly he fell he experienced the sensation of pins and needles in his legs. Having been told, when a boy, that in the event of an accident of this description the best plan was to "run it off," he immediately started away and quickly walked six miles.   Within a very short time he began to experience spinal-marrow symptoms, which have resulted in complete and irremediable paraplegia.   Mr Hilton stated his belief, that if the man had gone home directly after receiving the injury, and had kept himself quiet for a considerable period, he would have been quite well in a few weeks.

One more example will complete all that need be said on this subject.   The particulars of the case are as follows :—A stout but feeble man, between sixty and seventy years of age, trod on a piece of orange-peel, and fell; the lower part of his sacrum striking the pavement with great force.   He was taken in an insensible condition to Charing Cross Hospital, where he soon recovered his mental faculties, but both his upper and lower extremities were motionless.   On the fourth day he was conveyed home, and was seen by Dr. C. E. Reeves; when it was noted that his voice was weak and interrupted, his breathing slow, the heart's action weak, the urine scanty, and the extremities motionless and insensible.   Galvanism and stimulating embrocations were tried, but the patient was found dead in his bed on the twelfth morning. At the necropsy, the cord was discovered of a bluish tinge and pulpy to the touch; while the brain presented a similar but less marked appearance.   The heart and large bloodvessels, moreover, contained fibrinous clots.

7. **SPINAL IRRITATION.**—The existence of spinal irritation as a distinct and idiopathic disease has been denied by some writers; and it is my duty to confess that the greater the attention which I have bestowed upon this subject, the more inclined I am to believe that there is no affection deserving the name.

In the second and third editions of this volume the symptoms of spinal irritation were said to consist of pain about the thorax, mammæ, abdomen, or uterus; this pain having some remarkable connexion with the spine, since, wherever the suffering might be, it was increased on pressing certain of the spinous processes of the vertebræ, which were also themselves exceedingly tender. Moreover this tenderness was sometimes confined to one spot, sometimes diffused over a large portion of the spinal column; while it was most common in the lumbar and sacral regions.   The disease would seem to depend (it was observed) upon congestion of the spinal venous plexus ; this hyperæmic condition causing pressure upon, and consequent irritation of, the origins of the nerves.

Owing to doubts which I have for some time entertained, I have scrupulously availed myself of every opportunity, during the last nine years, to carefully examine examples of so-called " Spinal Irritation," or " Spinal Disorder ;" and the result has been this— that in every instance the suffering has appeared to be due to a combination of myalgia and hysteria with constitutional debility. The history has always shown that the patients, almost without exception, were delicate women ; and that prior to the illness for which relief was sought, they had undergone great fatigue, or had been living badly, or had indulged in excessive sexual excitement, or had long suffered from a copious leucorrhœal or menstrual discharge.   Frequently, they have retroflexion of the uterus.   Moreover, the seat of the pains has usually corresponded with the insertions of important muscles ; there has been a marked freedom from suffering so long as the recumbent posture has been maintained ; and more or less well-marked symptoms of hysteria have coexisted.

The *treatment* of these cases has served to confirm the statements just made ; for under the influence of rest, belladonna plasters, nourishing food, cod liver oil, bark or steel, and attention to the position and functions of the uterus, many cures have been effected with comparative ease.   To prevent any misunderstanding, it must be mentioned that, with regard to rest, I merely mean that for a few weeks the patient shall retire to bed at nine or ten o'clock at night, and remain there until about the same hour the following morning ; and not that she shall be confined to the recumbent posture for several months together.   A short time since, I saw a delicate young lady, who, under the advice of an irregular practitioner, had actually kept her bed for five years ; but who, I believe, might have been cured of her pseudo-spinal disorder in as many weeks by confidence in a physician who knew his business, sea air, moderate exercise, and a nourishing diet.

XI. PARALYSIS.

By paralysis [Παραλύω = to relax—to affect with paralysis], or palsy, is meant a total or partial loss of sensibility or motion, or of both, in one or more parts of the body.   All paralytic affections may be divided into two classes.   The first division includes those in which both motion and sensibility are affected ; the second, those in which the one or the other only is lost or diminished.   The former is called *perfect*, the latter *imperfect* paralysis.   Imperfect paralysis is divided into *acinesia* ['A = priv. + κίνησις = motion], paralysis of motion ; and *anæsthesia* ['A = priv. + αἰσθάνομαι = to perceive by the senses, to feel], paralysis of sensibility. Again, the paralysis may be *general* or *partial*, as it affects the whole body or only a portion of it. Partial paralysis is arranged into *hemiplegia* [Ημισυς = half + πλήσσω = to strike], when it is limited to one side; and *paraplegia* [Παραπληξία = partial paralysis; from Παραπλήσσω = to strike badly], when it is confined to the inferior half of the body. The term *local paralysis* is used when only a small portion of the body is affected; as the face, a limb, a foot, &c. In *reflex paralysis* [*Reflecto* = to turn back] the irritation extends from the periphery to the centre. Diseases of the urinary organs, uterus, and intestines are the most common causes of this form. And then there is that peculiar disease known as *progressive muscular atrophy* or *wasting palsy*, the prominent symptom of which is a remarkable degeneration and wasting of the disabled muscles.

Paralysis of the eye, or loss of sensibility of the retina to the rays of light, is called *amaurosis* ['Αμαυρόω = to obscure] ; paralysis of the levator palpebræ superioris muscle, allowing the upper eye-lid to fall over the eye, *ptosis palpebræ* [Πτόω = to fall] ; insensibility to the impression of sounds, or deafness, *cophosis* [Κωφὸς = deaf] ; insensibility to odours, or loss of smell, *anosmia* ['A = priv. + ὄζω = to smell] ; while loss of taste is technically known as *ageustia* ['A = priv. + γεῦσις = the act of tasting].

Locomotor ataxy can scarcely be correctly classed with paralytic diseases strictly so called. It is more properly a disease of the posterior columns of the spinal cord, producing a loss of the power of co-ordinating movements. Still there are advantages in treating of this affection in the present section. The disease was formerly described under the name of *Tabes dorsalis*, and was erroneously believed to be always the result of exhaustion from masturbation. In extreme cases, this pernicious habit leads to a wasting of the spinal cord ; but this wasting can also be produced by other causes. With regard to masturbation it may be remembered that a frequent cause of self-abuse in boys is the irritation produced by sebaceous matter lodging between the glans penis and prepuce ; under which circumstance the operation of circumcision proves very valuable. Women suffer less frequently from the evil consequences of bad habits than young men. Many instances of so-called " spinal irritation" are, however, due to them ; while they probably have a considerable influence in the causation of hysteria and other nervous affections.

In *hysterical paralysis* there is probably neither organic disease of the nervous centres nor of the motor nerves. It occurs in hysterical women ; and is produced by fright, over-excitement, ovarian irritation, &c. The paralysis may affect the muscles of both lower extremities (hysterical paraplegia) ; or the muscles of the arm and leg on the same side (hysterical hemiplegia) ; or only one or two particular muscles will be attacked. There are generally, but not always, other symptoms of hysteria. Many cases get well by recourse to remedies which improve the general health ; but frequently electricity will effect a more speedy cure.

In *rheumatic paralysis* the lower extremities are often affected, or the extensor muscles of the fore-arm, or the deltoid and trapezius causing a difficulty in raising the arm. It comes on suddenly or gradually, with pain or numbness, and it is curable. Sometimes, at least, the palsy is connected with rheumatic spinal meningitis.

The peculiar feature of *diphtheritic paralysis* is the manner in which it comes on just as the physician is congratulating himself that the patient is convalescent. The greater number of cases recover. All this, however, will be mentioned by and by.

Then there are, likewise, certain forms of paralysis induced by the use of metallic poisons, as *mercurial palsy* or *tremors*, and *saturnine* or *lead palsy* ; there is the rare affection termed *scrivener's palsy* ; and, lastly, there is that very peculiar affection known as *paralysis agitans*, readily recognised by the incessant trembling, &c.

To conclude this summary, before proceeding to the consideration of each form of paralysis in detail, it must be added that the palsy in the foregoing instances may be due either to disease of the brain arising from apoplexy, abscess, softening, induration, tubercular or cancerous or syphilitic or aneurismal tumours, epilepsy, or chorea ; to disease of the spinal cord, such as inflammation, atrophy, solution of continuity, &c. ; to diseases of the investing parts of the brain or cord, acting by the pressure they produce ; to simple lesion or compression of a nerve, by which its conducting power is impaired ; to the effects of diphtheria, hysteria, or rheumatism ; or to the influence of such poisons as lead, mercury, &c.

1. GENERAL PARALYSIS.—General paralysis, or complete loss of sensation and motion of the whole system, cannot take place without death immediately resulting. This term therefore is only applied to palsy affecting the four extremities, whether any of the other parts of the body are implicated or not. In most cases the loss of motion is more marked than that of sensibility ; the intelligence also soon becomes affected. It must not be confounded with the general paralysis of the insane.

Dr. Defermon[*] has related a remarkable case in which the power of motion in every part of the body was lost, with the exception of the muscular apparatus of the tongue, and that of the organs of deglutition and respiration. The sensibility was also wholly destroyed, barring that of a small patch on the right cheek, by tracing letters on which the patient's friends were enabled to communicate with him ; while the intellect was perfect.

2. HEMIPLEGIA.—This term is used to denote paralysis of one side, extending almost invariably to both the upper and lower extremities. It is most times the result of a fit of apoplexy.

* *Bulletin des Sciences Médicales*, tome xiii. p. 6. Paris, 1828.

Hemiplegia is the most common form of palsy. It is usually spoken of as "a paralytic stroke;" and the left is affected more frequently than the right side. When only one extremity suffers, it is generally the arm. Very rarely, the upper limb of one side and the lower of the opposite are paralysed, forming what is termed *transverse* or *crossed palsy*. Generally, the facial nerve or portio dura of the seventh pair is not involved in the paralysing lesion; but the fifth nerve is affected, so that the palsied cheek drops loosely, while the angle of the mouth is drawn slightly upwards and to the sound side,—clearly because the muscles on that side are no longer counteracted and balanced by the corresponding muscles of the paralysed side. The tongue also is often implicated; so that when protruded, its point is turned towards the palsied side. This is owing to the muscles which protrude this organ being powerless on the diseased side, while they are in full vigour on the other; so that the sound half of the tongue is pushed out further than the other half, and consequently it bends towards the affected side. The articulation is imperfect, in consequence of the palsy of the ninth and fifth nerves. And then if the third nerve be involved, the upper eyelid will drop, there will be a dilated pupil, and a divergent squint.

The paralysis in hemiplegia is always limited to one half of the body, the median line being the boundary. In most cases there is anæsthesia. The mental faculties are sometimes uninjured, but more frequently they are irreparably damaged. The memory especially becomes weakened; while at the same time there is a peculiar tendency to shed tears, and to be much distressed by slight causes.

The effect of paralytic disorders upon the memory is often very remarkable. In hemiplegia of the right side there is sometimes a curious forgetfulness and misplacement of language, so that the sufferer cannot find words to express his ideas, or he substitutes expressions having no relation with the sense intended. Sir Henry Holland refers to a case of slight paralytic affection, in which the perceptions from the senses were unimpaired, the memory of persons and events seemingly correct, the intelligence only slightly affected, the bodily functions feeble but not disordered, and yet the memory of words for speech so nearly gone that the single monosyllable "yes" alone remained as the sole utterance of all the patient desired to express. Even when a simple negative was intended, no other word was used. These cases of cerebral speechlessness have already been treated of under the head of *aphasia* (see p. 379).

In paralysis from red softening of the brain, the muscles of one of the affected limbs are sometimes rigid and contracted; owing to irritation of that part of the cord from which the nerves of the paralysed member arise, by the propagation to it of excitement from the diseased portion of the brain.

Supposing recovery to take place, the symptoms of amendment

are first noticed in the leg.   In hopeless cases, the limbs waste ; their nutrition and temperature get diminished ; and they become atrophied.   It is of practical importance to recollect that they are unable to resist the influence of cold or heat equally with the sound parts.

Hemiplegia is generally the result of organic lesions of the brain ; while most frequently perhaps the lesion is in the corpus striatum and the optic thalamus.   An apoplectic seizure is the cause of sudden and perfect hemiplegia in the great majority of cases. Where the palsy comes on gradually and slowly, then the cerebral lesion is of the nature of softening (possibly the result of obstruction of the middle cerebral artery by a clot), or of a tumour, or of a syphilitic gummatous growth, or of an abscess, or a hydatid cyst, &c.   When the intelligence and memory are affected, we may be sure that the convolutions of the cerebral hemispheres are involved, either directly in the lesion, or indirectly by pressure upon them. It must be remembered that the disease is not, as a rule, found on the side of the brain corresponding to the affected half of the body, but on the opposite ; the cerebral portion of the centre of volition for the left side of the body being situated on the right side, and *rice versâ*.   The decussation of the fibres of the anterior pyramids at the junction of the medulla oblongata and medulla spinalis, accounts for this phenomenon.   This form of paralysis may also be due to some lesion of one-half of the spinal cord, just below the decussation of the pyramids ; and then the palsy will be on the same side as the disease.   Hence the term hemi-plegia may signify *cerebral* paralysis, or *spinal* paralysis (very uncommon).   So also the hemiplegia may be transient and caused by a fit of epilepsy ; or it can happen in connexion with preg-nancy ; or it may follow chorea, and pass away ; or it may be due to some distant irritation (reflex hemiplegia) such as a colon loaded with unhealthy fæces, or persistent dyspepsia, in which the disease creeps from the periphery to the centre ; or, lastly, an imper-fect form will temporarily occur in some nervous women—hysterical hemiplegia, which may be diagnosed by the way in which they drag the limb while walking without attempting to lift it, whereas in true hemiplegia the patient drags the leg at the same time that he lifts it from the ground.   In all forms the paralysis of motion is the prominent symptom ; but sensation is sometimes more or less impaired.

In hemiplegia from disease of the brain, although the sufferer cannot by his own will move the palsied limb, yet irritation of the sole of the foot (as with a feather) will excite active movements ; these reflex actions often causing no little astonishment to the patient.   To distinguish between cerebral and spinal paralysis is not easy.   According to Marshall Hall the condition of the irrita-bility or contractility of the muscular fibre in the paralytic limbs must be our guide in diagnosis : since,—(1) In pure cerebral paralysis—or that in which the influence of the cerebrum alone is removed, there is augmented irritability and reflex action. (2) In spinal paralysis—or that in which the influence of the spinal marrow is also removed, there is diminished irritability and reflex action. The galvanic current is the test of the amount of irritability.* Dr. Todd, however, denied the correctness of these views, and asserted that the contractility or irritability of the muscles of paralysed limbs bears a direct relation to their nutrition; that the excitability of the paralysed muscles to galvanism varies with the condition of their nerves, more than with that of the muscles themselves; that, in the majority of cases of cerebral palsy, the contractility or irritability of the paralysed muscles is less than those of the sound side, simply because their nutrition is impaired by want of exercise; and lastly, that no diagnostic mark to distinguish between cerebral and spinal palsy can be based on any difference in the irritability of the paralysed muscles, for the muscles in spinal paralysis exhibit the same states as those in cerebral paralysis.†

Dr. Althaus has tested the muscular irritability in nineteen cases of cerebral paralysis, and has arrived at the same conclusions as Dr. Todd. The former gentleman found that in a certain number of cases the contractility was diminished, the muscles were flaccid, and the polarity of the nerves depressed. In another class the contractility was increased, there was early rigidity of the muscles, and an irritative lesion of the brain. While in a third set of cases there was no difference between the contractility of the healthy and the paralytic limb. Dr. Althaus employed both modes of experimentation, viz., sending the current through the limb, and localizing the current in the tissue of the muscles. The two methods yielded nearly the same results; but by localizing the electric current in the muscles, the difference of muscular contractility appeared more striking. This gentleman's conclusions, which seem to have been carefully deduced and therefore to be trustworthy, are these:— The muscles of paralysed limbs may present three different conditions when subjected to the action of the electric current, and this may enable us in certain cases to diagnose the paralysing lesion. " 1. If the excitability of the muscles—or rather the polarity of the motor nerves—be *increased* in the paralysed limbs, the case is one of *cerebral paralysis*, connected with an irritative lesion within the cranium. 2. If the excitability of the muscles be nearly or totally *lost*, we have in all probability either *lead palsy* or *traumatic paralysis;* but it must be kept in mind that certain hysterical and rheumatic palsies of long standing present the same peculiarity; and that it also may be found in cases of disease of the brain and the cord. 3. If *paralysed muscles respond readily to the electric current*, there is no lead in the system, nor is the connexion between the

* *Medico-Chirurgical Transactions*, vol. xxii. p. 191.   London, 1839.
† *Idem*, vol. xxx. p. 227.   London, 1847.

motor nerves of the paralysed muscles and the cord interrupted ; but if such cases are of *long standing*, they are due to *brain disease:* and if they are of *recent standing*, they are generally instances of *hysterical, rheumatic*, or *spontaneous* paralysis."*

In the *treatment* of hemiplegia, even when seen early, it must not be forgotten that the mischief is done; and we cannot remedy the evil by taking away blood. Indeed, the patient will require all the power which he possesses to enable him to recover from the shock which his system has received; and hence depletion can only do harm. Benefit may, however, be very frequently and reasonably expected from cathartics ; particularly such as jalap and scammony, or calomel, or croton oil, or stimulating purgative enemata. Some authors recommend blisters to the scalp, or to the nape of the neck, or the use of a seton. In all cases the practitioner should flex the fore-arm upon the arm, and the leg upon the thigh ; taking care to observe if any of the muscles offer resistance to these movements. Where the muscles of the palsied limb are perfectly flaccid, we may feel satisfied that the cerebral lesion is of an atrophic nature— probably white softening due to defective supply of blood ; and consequently that wine and nourishment, cod liver oil, ammonia and bark, are needed. On the contrary when there is resistance, the brain lesion is of an irritative kind—such as may be produced by an apoplectic clot which has lacerated or ploughed up the nervous substance in its vicinity ; and then purgatives, blisters, and iodide of potassium will be called for. With respect to reflex hemiplegia, the cause must be ascertained ; and then, if possible, removed.

When the paralysis becomes chronic, stimulants—especially such as act on the paralysed parts, are to be had recourse to. Strychnia in small doses (the twentieth or thirtieth part of a grain thrice daily) should be cautiously tried ; always provided we can reasonably hope that there is no disease of the brain, nor the remains of any blood-clot which may be easily excited into an irritating foreign body. And again, local stimulants had better be employed. Thus frictions with the hand or flesh-brush, as well as stimulating liniments of turpentine, ammonia, tincture of cantharides, croton oil, &c., have been used with occasional benefit.

Electricity and galvanism have long been extensively employed ; but when there is any structural disorganization they do harm. Thus, they aggravate the mischief in cases of cerebral hæmorrhage, in softening and atrophy of the cerebral substance, in pressure from tumours, and in paralysis due to disease of the spinal cord. But after reparation of the mischief (as by complete absorption of the clot, the nervous substance being left uninjured), when paralysis remains without any muscular rigidity, galvanism will do good. It is also useful in hysterical, rheumatic, and lead palsy ; as well as in reflex paralysis from disease of the urinary organs, in diphtheria, fever, &c. Moreover, in cases of mal-nutrition and atrophy of muscular tissue it acts well, by augmenting chemical changes in

* *A Treatise on Medical Electricity*, pp. 230 and 246. London, 1859.

the muscles and increasing therefore the supply of blood to them. Induction currents are to be used, so as to excite the vitality of the motor nerves; the continuous current proving useless in the cases under consideration. Opinions differ widely as to the *direction* in which the induced current should be sent through the paralysed limb. Naturally the course of nervous influence is from the trunk towards the extremities, and hence it has been argued that the induced electric current should be made to travel through the nerves in the same direction,—in other words the *direct* current is to be used, and not the *inverse*. But this view is not born out in practice; and the inverse current is generally employed, because it excites stronger contractions in the muscles than the direct. At first a gentle current is to be applied, the intensity being gradually increased; while as a rule the administration should not last for more than fifteen minutes at a time, even if for so long a time.

3. **PARAPLEGIA.**—Paraplegia, or paralysis of the inferior half of the body, arises from organic or functional disease of the spinal cord or its membranes. It most frequently commences slowly and insidiously, with weakness and numbness of the feet and legs, or with tingling and formication of these parts, unattended by pain. By degrees the weakness increases, until there is complete loss of sensibility and motion of the lower extremities, with paralysis of the coats of the bladder and the sphincter ani. The patient is obliged to remain in the horizontal posture; while from imperfect nutrition and pressure sloughs form on the hips and sacrum, which by their irritation and exhausting discharges accelerate death. If the urine be allowed to collect in the bladder in any quantity, it will soon get ropy, fetid, and alkaline; owing probably to the coats of the bladder becoming diseased and pouring forth unhealthy mucus, in consequence of the paralysis. Dr. Bence Jones has remarked, that the urine when secreted is healthy; but admixture with the diseased mucus contaminates it, decomposes its urea, and gives rise to the formation of carbonate of ammonia thus rendering it alkaline.

Although voluntary motion is completely abolished in the lower limbs, involuntary movements and spasms of the muscles are not uncommon. Patients are thus often tormented and rendered sleepless at night by involuntary startings of the lower extremities. The cause of this is to be found in some exacerbation of the primary disease in the spinal marrow; the excitement being propagated upwards to that portion of the cord in contact with the brain, as well as downwards below the lesion. Reflex movements can be excited much more frequently in paraplegia than in hemiplegia.

Paraplegia may happen from various injuries of the spinal cord or its membranes; from inflammation, congestion, or hæmorrhage; from non-inflammatory softening; from the pressure of tumours;

and also from affections of the bones and cartilages of the vertebral column. Most authorities now clearly distinguish two classes or kinds of paraplegia ; viz., that which is due to disease of the spinal cord or its membranes, and *reflex* paraplegia—*i.e.*, that produced by an excitation which has reached the spinal cord from a sensitive nerve. In these latter cases Dr. Brown-Séquard believes that the palsy is accompanied, and perhaps produced, by an insufficient amount of blood in the spinal cord. With such the irritation may have its starting-point either in the viscera, the skin, the mucous membranes, or the trunks of nerves ; while no direct treatment of the paralysis is of use, so long as the cause of irritation remains. Moreover, in reflex paraplegia there is an absence of the special symptoms of organic disease of the spinal column or its contents ; while the paralysis of the lower limbs is incomplete, and comes on gradually after the existence of disease in the urinary or genital organs, or in the thoracic or abdominal viscera, &c.

As regards the *treatment* of paraplegia we have first to decide whether there is any congestion or inflammation of the spinal cord or its membranes, or simply the very opposite condition. Dr. Brown-Séquard shows that when the amount of blood is increased (*e.g.* in chronic local myelitis), we find symptoms of irritation of motor nerve-fibres, such as convulsions, cramps, twitchings, erection of penis; indications of irritation of sensitive nerve-fibres as itching, pricking pains, abnormal sensations of cold or heat, &c. ; together with signals of irritation of vaso-motor or nutritive nerve-fibres, such as wasting of muscles, bedsores, alkaline urine, and so on. There is pain corresponding with the upper limit of the inflammation ; with tenderness on pressure at the same part. The application of a sponge, dipped in warm water, along the spine, causes a natural sense of heat in all parts above the seat of inflammation, but a burning sensation at its upper limit ; while the passage of a piece of ice over the vertebral column produces a sense of cold everywhere except at the level of the inflammation, at which part a feeling of heat is experienced. In attempting to cure these cases our object must be to diminish the quantity of blood sent to the spinal cord ; and for this purpose it seems no agents are so efficacious as the ergot of rye and belladonna, since they both produce contraction of the vessels of the cord and its membranes. The ergot should therefore be given in five- or six-grain doses twice a day, while a large belladonna plaster is to be applied over the spine. If no benefit ensue in the course of a few weeks, the iodide of potassium must be given in conjunction with the other medicines. Cod liver oil can also be often beneficially added to the treatment. If there be much restlessness, henbane or conium or Indian hemp had better be exhibited; but opium is to be avoided, since it produces congestion of the cord. The diet should be generous ; beer or wine often being needed. The nutrition of the limbs is to be maintained by the use of stimulating liniments, or by shampooing ; and subsequently by having recourse to a gentle galvanic current.

For paraplegia due to diminished nutrition of the cord (as that caused by white or non-inflammatory softening, and reflex para-plegia) a directly opposite course is to be pursued. Consequently where we find no signs of irritation or congestion, or of increase in the vital properties of the cord, we endeavour to give such food and remedies as will improve the quality of the blood, will cause an increased quantity of it to be sent to the cord, and will augment the vital properties of this nervous centre. Strychnine is here the remedy ; one-twentieth of a grain being given daily, or one-thirtieth of a grain if combined with opium. Sulphur baths may also be used ; quinine and iron will occasionally do good ; and the patient when in bed should lie on his back, with his head and shoulders and lower extremities elevated, so that the blood may gravitate to the vessels of the cord.

Dr. John Chapman claims to have discovered that a controlling power over the circulation of the blood in the brain, in the spinal cord, in the ganglia of the sympathetic, and through the agency of these nervous centres in every other organ of the body, can be exercised by means of cold and heat applied to different parts of the back. In this manner the reflex excitability, or excito-motor power of the spinal cord, and the contractile force of the arteries in all parts of the body can be immediately modified. In order to lessen the excito-motor power of the cord only, he applies ice, in an indian rubber bag about two inches wide, along that part of the spinal column on which he wishes to act. On the same principle, the vitality of the cord may be increased by em-ploying hot water and ice alternately, each in a proper bag, where very energetic action is required ; but if less vigorous effects are alone necessary, he uses ice or iced water only, resorting to it several times a day, for a short time on each occasion, with a long inter-val between each application. Thus for example, intending to direct a fuller and more equable flow of blood to the brain, he ap-plies ice to the back of the neck and between the scapulæ ; in-creased circulation in, and warmth of, the upper extremities will be induced in the same way ; the thoracic and abdominal viscera can be influenced in like manner by applications to the dorsal and lumbar regions ; while the legs and coldest feet may have their circulation so increased that they become thoroughly warm by the icebag applied over the lower part of the back.*

It need only be further added, that while in reflex paralysis we endeavour by the foregoing plans to relieve the palsy, we must also try to remove its exciting cause ; as by the expulsion of intestinal worms, relieving irritability of the urinary or sexual system, and curing all skin diseases, &c. In reflex paraplegia from onanism, the penis should be painted every night with the tincture of iodine, so as to make it too sore to allow its being handled. If this prove insufficient, blistering fluid may be used so as to produce a raw surface. Where there is irritation from the retention of sebaceous

* *The Medical Times and Gazette*, p. 60. London, 18 July 1863.

matter between the glans penis and the prepuce, the latter should be cut off. The cold douche will also be useful in these cases.

4. **LOCOMOTOR ATAXY.**—The symptoms and pathology of this remarkable disease have been worked out by different authorities. In the first place, Romberg, the eminent Professor of Medicine at the University of Berlin, described the prominent features of the disorder under the very old name of *tabes dorsalis*. Then Dr. R. B. Todd, after teaching in his hospital wards the features distinguishing this affection from ordinary paraplegia, published some remarks upon it about the year 1847 ;* these observations though brief, really containing the pith of the matter. Subsequently, in 1858, Dr. Duchenne's first memoir on this subject appeared ; and to him we are indebted for an excellent clinical study of it. He also selected the name of progressive locomotor ataxy (*ataxie loco-motrice progressive*), by which it has been subsequently recognised. And finally, Mr. Lockhart Clarke has shown the nature of the peculiar change which takes place in the posterior columns of the spinal cord, as well as in the posterior nerve-roots.

Locomotor ataxy [from 'A = priv. + τάσσω = to place or order,] is characterized by such a diminution of the power of co-ordinating the action of the muscles required for the performance of certain movements, that those movements cannot be made steadily in response to the will. As a rule, the abolition of this faculty of co-ordination commences in the lower extremities; so that loco-motion is accomplished in a disorderly manner, with an uncertain or staggering gait. There is no true paralysis, but the sensibility of different textures becomes more or less impaired. Neuralgic pains in the legs and feet are among the most constant phenomena presented. Moreover, the loss of power is progressive; a fact however, which can be recollected without prefixing this hopeless word to the disease as it stands in our nomenclature.

* "Two kinds of paralysis of Motion," says Dr. Todd, "may be noticed in the lower extremities, the one consisting simply in the impairment or loss of the voluntary motion, the other distinguished by a diminution or total loss of the power of co-ordinating movements. In the latter form, while considerable voluntary power remains, the patient finds great difficulty in walking, and his gait is so tottering and uncertain that his centre of gravity is easily displaced. These cases are generally of the most chronic kind, and many of them go on from day to day without any increase of the disease or improvement of their condition. In two examples of this variety of paralysis, I ventured to predict disease of the posterior columns, the diagnosis being founded upon the views of their functions which I now advocate; and this was found to exist on a post-mortem inspection ; and in looking through the accounts of recorded cases in which the posterior columns were the seat of lesion, all seem to have commenced by evincing more or less disturbance of the locomotive powers, sensation being affected only when the morbid change of structure extended to and more or less involved the posterior roots of the spinal nerves."—*The Cyclopædia of Anatomy and Physiology*, vol. iii. p. 721 B. London, 1839-1847.

Very little information can be given with regard to the *etiology* of this disease. Summarily it may be said, that males suffer much more than females ; while the former are most liable to it between the ages of thirty and fifty. Hereditary predisposition to diseases of the nervous system has an undoubted influence. The causes mostly assigned, however, are prolonged exposure to cold and damp, insufficient food, drunkenness, over-fatigue, sexual excesses —especially masturbation, and possibly mental anxiety acting on a weak frame for a long period. Some patients have attributed it to operations for the cure of hæmorrhoids ; but seeing that whatever depresses nervous force will have some influence in producing ataxy, it is not unlikely that the loss of blood which accompanied the piles before the surgeon was consulted had much more to do with the subsequent mischief than the operation. Rheumatism, gout, syphilis, and gonorrhœa have severally been blamed ; but in all probability without sufficient reason.

The *symptoms* of this chronic disease have been usually divided into three stages. If the arrangement is arbitrary, it is convenient. In the first stage, there is usually a temporary loss of power in one of the motor nerves of the eye, disordered vision, paroxysms of neuralgic pain, and spermatorrhœa or impotence. After an interval varying from a few months to some years, the second stage sets in ; being characterized by a difficulty in standing or walking with steadiness, diminution of sensibility, constipation, and probably some trouble in retaining the urine—especially at night. Then follows the third stage, which is marked by the symptoms of the two preceding divisions becoming more marked and painful. The loss of power often becomes more general, though it continues most apparent in the legs and feet ; and death happens from exhaustion, or from the occurrence of some complication.

The difficulty of co-ordinating the movements usually begins in the lower extremities, and makes the greatest progress in them. After a time, the hands and arms may get affected ; while one case has been reported where these limbs were alone attacked during the whole course of the disease. The unsteadiness of gait is peculiar. The patient starts off nervously and hurriedly, and then walks like a drunken man ; but as soon as a little confidence has been acquired he shows less fear of losing his balance, and his gait gets less tottering. A stick, or the arm of a friend, proves a grateful support to him. He fixes his eyes on surrounding objects at first ; but in a later stage watches his feet, and tries to assure himself by his sight that they are firmly planted on the ground. If the upper extremities are unsteady, there is a similar difficulty in carrying out the mandates of the will. To pick up anything, for example, the patient is obliged to use both hands—one being employed to steady the other. As the disorder progresses, the movements of the limbs become more and more uncertain. The legs are jerked forward, or they are thrown to the right and left ;

while the knees and ankles seem about to give way, the effort to be steady or to produce any desired movement causing much exhaustion.   At length, all attempts at walking fail; and without the support of two persons, there is an inability to stand.   Nevertheless, the muscular power is still so considerable, that when the patient is lying down it is very difficult to flex or extend his legs against his will.

These ataxic symptoms are accompanied by other nervous affections.   The most common appear to be strabismus, ptosis, double vision, and diminished acuteness of the retinal perception.   The strabismus and ptosis are often temporary; but the indistinctness of sight frequently merges into complete amaurosis, the result of atrophy of the retina.   Deafness is very rare: difficulty of mastication, and dysphagia are more common.   The intellect and memory usually remain unaffected; though the general sensitiveness gets blunted, so that the grave nature of the condition is fortunately not appreciated.   The pains are for the most part distressing; being sometimes sharp and sudden like shocks of electricity, on other occasions wearying and gnawing or boring and deep seated. Every now and then days of respite are obtained; to be succeeded suddenly by two or three bad days, the suffering passing from the legs to the arms, from the latter to the head and face.   The severity of the pain is aggravated by cold and damp, constipation, fatigue, or any kind of debauchery.   Amongst other important symptoms, there is a loss of sexual power; an inability to retain the urine; constipation, paralysis of the sphincter ani permitting of involuntary stools being very uncommon; numbness of the feet and legs, hands and arms; and a sensation as of a cord tied round the chest or abdomen.   The power of distinguishing between heat and cold is only exceptionally impaired.

The *diagnosis* may be facilitated in many ways, during the early stage.   Thus, an ataxic patient finds his difficulty in walking greatly increased by shutting his eyes.   If he stand up with the inner edges of his feet applied to each other, he can only maintain this position, so long as his eyes are open: directly he closes them, he seeks some support to prevent his tottering limbs from failing to support him.   Ataxy is at first most likely to be confounded with disease of the cerebellum; from which, however, it can be distinguished by the absence of that frequent vomiting and pain at the back of the head so characteristic of cerebellar affections.

The ultimate unfavourable *termination* of locomotor ataxy may be almost positively predicated.   The only hope indeed is, that its progress will possibly be retarded.   Cases which have remained stationary for several years are known.   In many instances, although the tendency has been steadily from bad to worse, yet a fatal result has been deferred for six or eight or more years. On the contrary, the unfavourable symptoms have sometimes run on so rapidly, that within six months from the commencement all power of standing without support has become abolished.   Death from some intercurrent affection—such as bronchitis, pneumonia, erysipelas, &c.—is not a rare event.

From *pathological anatomy* we learn that the spinal cord is always structurally affected in locomotor ataxy; the changes being most marked in the lumbar and lower part of the dorsal regions. The vertebræ, spinal canal, and membranes, are generally found healthy; though sometimes the posterior surfaces of the latter have been seen to be congested, or to be thickened by some exudation, or to be adherent to each other.   These conditions, however, are not essential.   The pathognomonic appearances are to be detected in the posterior columns of the cord, including the posterior nerve-roots.   There is a destruction of nervous matter.   According to Mr. Lockhart Clarke,—" the alteration is peculiar, and consists of atrophy and disintegration of the nerve-fibres, to a greater or less extent, with hypertrophy of the connective tissue, which gives to the columns a grayish and more transparent aspect, and in this tissue are embedded a multitude of corpora amylacea.   Many of the bloodvessels that traverse the columns are loaded or surrounded, to a variable depth, by oil-globules of different sizes. For the production of ataxy it seems to be necessary that the changes extend along a certain length—from one to two inches— of the cord.   The posterior nerve roots, both within and without the cord, are frequently affected by the same kind of degeneration, which sometimes extends to the surface of even the lateral columns, and occasionally along the edges of the anterior.   Not unfrequently the extremities of the posterior cornua, and even deeper parts of the gray substance, are more or less damaged by areas of disintegration."*   If it be asked whether the change in the cord precedes that in the nerve-roots, the answer must be in the affirmative.   With regard to other parts of the cerebro-spinal axis it is only necessary to say that the cerebellum has always been found healthy; while the cerebral nerves, excepting the fifth and seventh and eighth pairs, have been more or less diseased in different cases.   The optic nerves especially have been seen to be almost destroyed; the mischief having extended from them as far as the corpora geniculata on the sides of the optic tracts.   Mr. Lockhart Clarke has pointed out, that when the cerebral nerves are affected the morbid action travels from the periphery towards the centre; instead of from the centre to the periphery, as obtains with the cord and posterior roots.

I do not recollect having seen a case of locomotor ataxy where the patient has not previously learnt from experience the inutility of medical *treatment*.   In former times, I doubt not but that he was even more unfortunate; for if he were capable of analysing the results which followed from the employment of setons and

* *St. George's Hospital Reports*, vol. i. p. 103.   London, 1866.   A more complete account is also given in *The Lancet*, p. 618.   London, 10 June 1865.

issues and blisters, cupping and leeches, shocks of electricity, and the ingestion of a heap of drugs, he could only have concluded that his miseries had been greatly aggravated by the doctor.   But it is to be hoped, that in the present day we are more careful to do no harm where we cannot effect real good.   There is certainly a much more happy desire to treat incurable diseases by attention to the diet and hygienic surroundings of the patient, than by physic.

With regard to medicines, in the present instance there is not one that deserves any confidence so far as curing the disease goes. The utmost that can be said in favour of the oxide of silver, nitrate of silver, hypophosphite of soda or lime, quinine, iron, and so on, is that they have no injurious influence.   Yet this negative merit ought not to induce us to prescribe them.   And I cannot help feeling that we are better discharging our duty when consulted in these cases by recommending warm clothing, a nutritious diet table, together with rest of those limbs which are gradually becoming incapacitated for all movement; than by leading the sufferer to believe that medicines, mineral waters and baths, methodical flagellation, blisters and galvanism, have virtues which they in reality do not possess.

At the same time that I profess this creed, it is not to be thought a patient must be told his sufferings cannot be relieved. A fair quantity of animal food, with stimulants and milk and cod liver oil, will do much to lessen or postpone the neuralgic pains; though it may also be necessary to afford that comfort which can be given by properly regulated doses of opium, belladonna, or Indian hemp. So, likewise, the appetite will perhaps flag; and yet it can often be restored by quinine, or salicin, or small doses of the mineral acids with bitter tinctures.   Again, sulphur baths occasionally seem to mitigate the numbness and general uneasiness during the earlier stages of the complaint.   Hence they may be tried; though the patient need not be sent abroad to use them.   And lastly, attention will be needed to prevent constipation, which is apt to occur and to aggravate the pains.   There is no objection therefore, to the occasional exhibition of a mild purgative; though as a general rule, simple enemata will answer every purpose.

5. INFANTILE PARALYSIS. — Speaking generally, this disease is by no means the same alarming affection as paralysis in the adult; for though infantile paralysis is often obstinate and occasionally incurable, yet it is not perilous to life.   Moreover, it is very rarely the result of the same serious disease of the brain or spinal cord.   The terms *myogenic paralysis*, and *essential paralysis of infants*, have been applied to these cases of partial muscular paralysis, arising independently of any appreciable lesion of the nervous system.   The palsy often attacks only a single limb as one leg, or very seldom one arm, or one side of the face, or even a single muscle like the sterno-mastoid, or a group of muscles; or

one whole side of the body may be affected—hemiplegia; or the
lower half of the body—paraplegia.   The disease often dates from
such an early period, that it appears most probably to be due to
some defect of conformation.   Such cases can of course only be
remedied by well-adapted mechanical means to lessen the inconvenience of the deformity.

The evils which result from a persistence of the paralysis are
very great; for if it is seldom followed by death, still it produces
an altered condition in the nutritive functions of the affected muscles,
and often leads to incurable deformity.   Not only do the affected
parts cease to grow in the same proportion as the healthy, but the
limbs waste, owing to their being imperfectly nourished; while
although they do not seem to want sensation, yet their power of motion is lost or diminished. Consequently if the child begins to walk,
the leg drags; and as it fails to support the body, the little sufferer
tumbles down.   Supposing one arm to be paralysed, it will soon
be noticed that it is not used equally with its fellow; and that
when raised it falls, as if dead, by its own weight.   In many
instances, partial or complete loss of power over certain limbs or
particular muscles of a limb, is noticed after slight and brief cerebral disturbance; while in other cases, the paralysis comes on
during that irritable state of nervous system which coexists with
teething.   Sometimes, again, the palsy appears after either of the
eruptive fevers; and frequently it supervenes suddenly, without
any apparent constitutional derangement.

These paralytic affections have been mistaken for the stiffness
of rheumatism, and occasionally for hip joint disease.   The absence
of pain in palsy ought to be sufficient to prevent such errors.   For
although there is sometimes, especially in the early stages of
paralysis, an exalted sensibility of the affected muscles or limb,
still this is very different to the suffering caused by an examination of a diseased joint.   Now and then a more cruel blunder is
committed, and the child is thought to be malingering.   On this
principle he may be harshly treated ; just as children have been
whipped for wetting the bed, when the involuntary micturition has
been due to an irritable condition of bladder, or a long prepuce, or
a morbidly acid state of the urine.   One other caution is necessary,
and that is not to express too sanguine a hope of cure.   The practitioner loses caste when it is found that his promises are not
brought to pass; and when it is seen that a loss of power which
it was said would be temporary, shows every probability of becoming
permanent.   Recovery occurs often,—not always.

The paralysis which at times attends dentition happens more frequently during the eruption of the permanent than of the temporary
teeth.   Where there is nervous disturbance with the first dentition,
it occurs for the most part in the form of convulsions: in the
second dentition, especially as the molars are being cut, there is a
fear that paralytic affections may supervene.   The following suc-

cession of events is now and then observed. A child goes to bed quite well, but passes a miserable and restless night. The next morning, when about to be dressed, the nurse finds that one arm, or an arm and leg, cannot be moved. There is probably no fever, neither are there any head symptoms. While there is loss of power, there is very slight, if any, diminution of sensibility. The parents hope that the numbness is temporary, and of no consequence. Only as it becomes evident that there is paralysis, and that it is not passing off, is alarm felt. In such cases, the palsy either subsides in some ten or fourteen days, or in a month or two, or it proves to be incurable. In the latter case, indications of disease about the nervous centres sometimes set in at the end of a few years or even earlier. But more frequently the patient grows up, having a paralytic and withered limb for the remainder of life.

The pathology of these cases is at present obscure. That there is some disease of the spinal cord can scarcely be doubted; though it seems certain that the alteration is often only temporary. Possibly, as I think Dr. C. B. Radcliffe believes, the palsy may arise from spinal congestion.

The treatment of infantile palsy must vary according to the cause. In all cases the general health is to be attended to, and the functions kept as nearly normal as possible. Mild purgatives will often be needed, perhaps followed by tonics and nervous stimulants. Small doses of mercury, given as an alterative for a long time, have occasionally produced a remarkable amount of amendment; and so has the iodide of potassium with bark, or iodide of iron. The little patient, if under two years of age with palsy of one lower extremity, is to be taught to walk while being supported in a go-cart, or in a baby-jumper; or if old enough, by means of a pair of crutches. It is of the greatest importance that the muscles of the arm or leg be daily exercised : hence friction and shampooing should be systematically and perseveringly used, together perhaps with very gentle shocks of electricity. The limb is also to be kept warm by wrapping it in flannel or chamois leather. With regard to special drugs, in addition to those already mentioned, it is to be remembered that cod liver oil often does great good by nourishing the system. Small doses of steel, especially the chemical food (F. 405), ought to be given where there is anæmia. Sometimes too, I have seen good in chronic cases from minute doses of strychnia. For a child four years of age, half a minim of the officinal solution (equivalent to about the two hundred and fortieth part of a grain of the salt) may be administered thrice daily ; the strength of the mixture being cautiously and slowly increased to two minims. At the same time the food is to be good, with plenty of milk. A residence at the sea-side, with tepid salt water bathing, will greatly increase the chances of cure.

Facial hemiplegia is not unfrequently seen in infants soon after birth. It is probably caused by some injury to the branches of the seventh pair of nerves either by the use of the forceps, or from pressure during the passage of the head through the pelvis. The distortion usually diminishes in a few hours, and quite disappears by the end of a week or two without any treatment.

6. SCRIVENER'S PALSY.—This disease may be defined as a spasm or cramp of certain muscles, which is only manifested when the sufferer attempts to execute some long-practised and very familiar movement requiring the co-ordination of these muscles. There is, in fact, a partial loss of controlling power; so that the will can no longer compel a set of muscles to perform a series of acts to which they have so long been habituated that the necessary motions had become almost mechanical. The affection is named *scrivener's palsy*, or *writer's paralysis*, or *writer's cramp;* designations, however, which are not very appropriate inasmuch as the artist, musician, compositor, shoemaker, saddler, sempstress, and even the milkmaid, are all liable to become incapacitated for their special work in exactly the same way. The penman does not really suffer more frequently than the members of any other class. He seems to do so, simply because the art of writing is universally acquired and practised.

The *cause* of the disease is obscure. Of course, the suggestion naturally arises that it is due to overwork; but an examination of recorded cases seems almost to negative this view. If, however, undue exertion cannot be set down as the starting point, it is certain that exercise of the affected muscles materially serves to increase the disorder.

The *symptoms* make their appearance insidiously. At first, there is only a stiffness of the muscles of the arm, or forearm, or fingers of the right limb; and this comes on at the end of the day's labours, disappearing after a night's repose. Soon there is an unsteadiness of movement; so that the writer or artist every now and then produces an irregular scrawl or daub that was not intended, or the musician plays one or more false notes. Then an uncomfortable burning sensation is often experienced in the muscles of the hand or forearm, together with more or less aching; both of these symptoms, however, passing off after a few hours rest. As the disorder progresses, so the inconvenience increases. Directly pen or pencil is taken in hand the spasm comes on. The thumb gets drawn into the palm, while the index and middle fingers become rigidly contracted. It is as if there were a limited chorea. And just as a child with St. Vitus' Dance cannot put out its tongue, or walk, or sit still, as it could when well; so a man with scrivener's palsy cannot quietly hold his pen, or sign his name legibly, though he may previously have been remarkable for his handwriting. At the same time, curiously enough, he can employ his hand for other purposes. I have seen a law-stationer's clerk cut up his food, comb his hair, fasten his clothes, use a buttonhook,—in short, do anything but that by which he had been getting his living for nearly twenty years.

With regard to the *pathology* of the disease nothing is known. The disturbed force may commence in the spinal cord ; but this is only a guess, and is not unlikely to be wrong. As scrivener's palsy does not destroy life the opportunities for examining the cord are very rare.

The *treatment* consists in giving complete rest to the affected hand. The clerk must forego writing, the artist should put away his pencil, the sempstress will have to use the sewing machine. Without rest, all remedies are useless : with it, a cure may be hoped for at the end of a few months provided the means have not been rejected until too late. Where our plans are not fettered by the straitened circumstances of the patient the prescription should run thus,—Perfect rest of the affected hand. Mountain or sea air : a long voyage will be of great service. Nourishing food, with plenty of milk. Cod liver oil.

Where drugs are demanded, the hypophosphite of soda, with bark or steel, will not do harm. Neither will quinine, or phosphate of zinc, or phosphate of iron. They may prove useless; but they cannot cause mischief, as is certain to ensue from strychnia, arsenic, mercury, iodine, nitrate of silver, electricity, cold douches to the head and neck, Turkish baths, &c.

Oft-times the patient is driven to confess that rest and starvation are with him convertible expressions. Can he be helped for a time ? Well, he may learn to write with his left hand, without much difficulty ; but then, after an interval, this hand will probably suffer like the right. He is not unlikely to derive partial relief from using Perry's orthodactylic penholder ; on the handle of which there are fixed three oval plates for resting the thumb and first two fingers. I have seen an invention of M. Velpeau's, consisting of a pear-shaped knob, with a tube at its apex for carrying a pen, and rests on the handle for the index and middle fingers. The knob is held in the palm of the hand ; the relief, I suppose, arising from the spasm being kept off while the hand has something which it can firmly grasp. And lastly, instrument makers contrive simple leather or gutta percha pads, by which the affected parts are supported. These pads are inexpensive ; and can be made to fix the flexors of the thumb and index and middle fingers, so as to prevent their otherwise uncontrollable spasm.

7. HYSTERICAL, RHEUMATIC, AND DIPHTHERITIC PARALYSIS.—In *hysterical* palsy there is neither organic disease of the nervous centres, nor of the motor nerves. The affection is manifested in hysterical women ; and is sometimes directly traceable to fright, over-excitement, ovarian irritation, loss of blood, insufficient nourishment, &c. The muscles of the lower extremities may be affected—hysterical paraplegia ; or the muscles of the arm and leg on one side—hysterical hemiplegia; or the loss of power will be limited to one particular muscle, or to a group of muscles. There are almost invariably other symptoms of hysteria present; while the uterine functions are scarcely ever performed in a regular and painless manner. Constipation and indigestion with flatulence, backache and tenderness all over the sacrum, bearing-down pains, irritability of the bladder, neuralgic pains about the inside of the thighs, with a more or less copious leucorrhœal discharge, all betoken derangement in the functions of the pelvic viscera. The pathology of all forms of hysterical paralysis seems to be, that there is a state of imperfect nutrition, which especially lowers the tone of the nerves of the palsied muscles, and very probably affects the nervous centres also. How far this state of mal-nutrition is brought about by moral causes, and to what extent the latter are influential in keeping up the palsy, we need not now enquire. The pivot on which our treatment must turn is the existence of this depraved state of general nutrition. Hence, the remedies are steel, quinine, cod liver oil, cold or tepid bathing, mental occupation, and good food; together with friction and galvanism of the affected limb. By these agents, always in co-operation with tact and unwearied patience on the part of the practitioner, a cure can be achieved; so that, as Carlyle says, the patient shall remain " no longer the victim of nerves, but the vanquisher."

Rheumatic paralysis may attack the muscles of one or both lower extremities; or the extensor muscles of the forearm; or only the deltoid or trapezius, rendering it impossible to raise the arm. The symptoms of loss of power, the increased sensibility of the parts affected, and the general depression, will come on suddenly or gradually. It is not improbable that the affection has its origin in rheumatic irritation or inflammation of a limited portion of the membranes of the spinal cord. At all events, the remedies which mostly succeed are iodide of potassium and cod liver oil; with the warm douche, hot air or vapour baths, shampooing, and electricity.

Among the other secondary nerve affections which follow *diphtheria*, paralysis claims a prominent position. Generally it comes on a few days after convalescence has set in. According to most authorities, there is a primary peripheral change in the nerves of the part which has been affected; this alteration being propagated to the spinal centre. The muscles of the soft palate, fauces, and pharynx suffer the first and most severely, causing the act of deglutition to be performed with difficulty. The loss of power, and especially that of swallowing of fluids, will now and then persist for months. The muscles of the neck are occasionally palsied, so that the head cannot be properly supported; or one or more of the limbs are attacked; or there is paralysis of the ciliary muscle (?) causing defective vision. Together with the loss of motor power in the constrictors of the pharynx, there may be more or less anæsthesia; and consequently, without considerable caution, food will lodge in the gullet and produce fatal choking.   The length of time that the paralysis lasts, is liable to great variety. The important point is, that ultimately the power becomes restored; recovery being the rule, and not the exception.   The chief remedies are rest, animal food with milk, cod liver oil, steel, and strychnia.

8. **LOCAL PARALYSIS.**—Of the different varieties of local palsy, I shall only mention *paralysis of the face*, the effect of pressure on, or injury to, the portio dura or facial portion of the seventh pair of nerves; a nerve which is very rarely affected by disease of the brain. As one-half only of the face is usually palsied, the appearance is remarkably striking.   All symmetry between the two sides of the countenance is destroyed; the profile on the paralysed half being blank, unmeaning, and void of expression.   The features get drawn up on the healthy side.   The orbicularis palpebrarum muscle is powerless, and therefore the patient is unable to close the eyelid sufficiently to cover the eyeball.   Moreover, he cannot frown on the affected side, the nostril does not dilate, the cheek hangs loose, he cannot blow, and the angle of the mouth droops. The fifth pair of nerves is usually unaffected; for the muscles of mastication act properly, while there is no loss of sensibility.   The food, however, gives trouble by lodging between the cheek and teeth on the palsied side; while the saliva also dribbles from the same angle of the mouth.   Where the motor branch of the third division of the fifth nerve is involved, there will be palsy of the movements of the jaw on the affected side.   In any case the paralysis is generally free from danger, being but rarely connected with intracranial disease.   There is no loss of hearing, sight, or speech : if the latter be at all affected it will be in the pronunciation of labial consonants and vowels, and then perfect power can be restored by supporting the drooping angle of the lower lip with the finger.   The more complete the palsy, the more favourable may our diagnosis be; inasmuch as partial palsy (e.g. ptosis, or an inability to lift the upper eyelid from loss of power in the superior branch of the third nerve) is more frequently the result of cerebral disease, than of temporary external mischief.

Paralysis of the portio dura on both sides is a rare affection. Owing to the symmetrical nature of the disease in such cases there is no distortion of the features, as happens when one nerve only is affected.   But, on close examination, the lineaments will be found fixed.   The nostrils are motionless; the cheeks flat and relaxed; there is inability to close the eyes completely; and there is defective articulation with regard to the sounds formed by the lips, while the lingual articulation is unimpaired.

Exposure to cold is a frequent source of paralysis of the portio dura; and so is debility from any exhausting influence.   In cases where no appreciable cause can be detected, the mouth should be examined; so that if there be any decayed teeth or stumps they may be extracted.   In children, otitis leading to caries of the petrous portion of the temporal bone not unfrequently produces the loss of power.

Pure facial palsy may have a duration of from ten days to many weeks. Where it does not get quite well, there is no fear of its shortening life, unless there be disease of the temporal bone. The patient's mind must be made easy with respect to this absence of danger; while aperients, tonics, iodide of potassium, warm douches, shampooing, and galvanism, are the remedies to be resorted to.

9. PROGRESSIVE MUSCULAR ATROPHY.—This curious disease has only been recognised as a distinct affection since the year 1853. It has been described under various names,—such as *Creeping palsy*, or *Peripheric paralysis*, or *Lead palsy without lead*, or *Paralysie musculaire atrophique* (Cruveilhier), or *Atrophie musculaire avec transformation graisseuse* (Duchenne). Dr. W. Roberts, in an excellent essay on the subject, states that he was inclined to call it *Idiopathic degeneration of the voluntary muscles;* but as this name was too cumbrous, and might not prove correct in the end, he preferred the more homely one of *Wasting palsy.* This title, however, will have to give way to that of *Progressive muscular atrophy,* according to the Nomenclature proposed by the Royal College of Physicians.

Symptoms.—The pathognomonic feature of this disease is a degeneration, and consequent loss of volume and power, of the voluntary muscles; there being no diminution of the intelligence, or of the sensibility of any part of the body. The first symptom has sometimes been pain in the ball of the thumb; followed by weakness of the upper extremity. The atrophy will occasionally be confined to this arm, or it affects both upper limbs, or the lower limbs, or more rarely the voluntary muscles of the entire body—of both the trunk and the extremities. Fibrillary tremors or convulsive quiverings of some of the fasciculi which form the muscle, can often be noticed by the attendant, though the patient may be quite unconscious of their occurrence. Anything which irritates the skin will produce these muscular vibrations. There is weakness that increases daily, though slowly; and which patients at first describe as an unwonted lassitude of the limbs. The wasting of the muscles gives rise to a peculiar withered look in the parts affected; while as the muscular atrophy is often unequal on the two sides of the body, distortions arise—the muscles least diseased overcoming the resistance of those most affected. Tactile and common sensibility are usually unimpaired; there is no tremulous agitation, as in paralysis agitans; occasionally neuralgic or rheumatic pains are complained of; and there is great sensitiveness to cold. The intellectual powers are undisturbed, and the judgment remains sound; while the general health long continues moderately good, unless there be difficulty in taking food owing to the muscles of both mastication and deglutition being involved. In one distressing

G G 2

example which I have seen, there was no diminution of sensibility, but simply a complete inability to move either the upper or lower extremities ; so that the patient was obliged to be fed and carried about like a child. Death, I believe, occurred from an attack of bronchitis. Fatal asphyxia is a very common termination of these cases. For when the diaphragm and intercostals become involved, the thoracic movements get reduced to a slight motion of the lower ribs ; and consequently if any mucus be poured out, it must accumulate and produce suffocation, since no sufficient efforts can be made to dislodge it.*

* Few of the reported examples of wasting palsy are more interesting than the one published by Cruveilhier (*Archives Générales de Médicine*, cinquième série, tome i. p. 571. Paris, 1853), and I shall therefore give a condensed account of it. This case is the more deserving of attention since from it Cruveilhier first determined the existence of a new form of paralysis, unconnected (as he believed) with either cerebro-spinal disease, or metallic poisoning. The chief points are these :—A mountebank, thirty-two years of age, came under observation in July 1850, suffering from atrophic muscular paralysis, which had already become almost general. According to his account, in September 1848 he passed the night in the open air, on the muddy pavement; and awaking, found his right side, on which he had slept, quite benumbed. The warmth of a tavern soon restored both sensation and motion ; but three weeks afterwards he noticed a weakness of the right hand, he could not take hold of objects, and was henceforth unable to play the cornet-à-piston. For a year the weakness was confined to the muscles of the hand ; but he then passed another cold wet night in the open air, and afterwards felt a great weakness in the lower limbs. From this time the muscular paralysis progressed rapidly ; so that when he entered Cruveilhier's wards, in July 1850, not only were the extremities affected, but also the facial muscles and those concerned in articulation and deglutition and respiration. Still the patient could dress himself and walk, though with trouble; while he was able to feed himself and to articulate intelligibly. The muscles were agitated with a fibrillary quivering or tremor—a kind of twitch, such as would be produced by an uninterrupted succession of mild electric shocks. The tactile sensibility was developed to its highest degree ; the organs of special sense were remarkably delicate, the intelligence was perfect, and he used thus to describe his condition :—" I am not ill, but my strength is gone, and my weakness increases daily. There is a feeling of great lassitude in my limbs, which torments me every hour, but especially at the time of awaking from sleep." At the end of 1851, this man could not walk at all, neither had he the power to change his position without help. His food was given to him, and he was put to bed like a little child. The saliva could not be swallowed, but ran from his mouth. The buccal portion of the act of deglutition could not be effected, owing to almost complete paralysis of the tongue : twice he was nearly choked by pieces of vegetable lodging in the pharynx : and his appetite was voracious. To feed him, the nurse was in the habit of thrusting the spoon filled with food down low into the pharynx : considerable efforts at swallowing on the spoon and its contents were then made, and the former being withdrawn, repeated attempts at deglutition followed. In trying to swallow liquids, the greater part was always returned. The power of articulation being lost, the wants were made known by nods, by the eyes, and by a guttural nasal sound. The respiration was very incomplete ; so that it seemed certain that the unhappy man, whose intelligence was unimpaired, was menaced every moment with asphyxia. On the 15 January 1853, he was seized with the prevailing influenza, and being unable to expectorate the mucus, was one morning found quite dead.
At the autopsy it was shown that the *brain* was perfectly healthy, and

Prognosis.—The duration of wasting palsy may be said to vary from nine months to five or six years ; although in one instance death did not occur till after the lapse of more than twenty years from the commencement of the symptoms. In some few instances complete recovery seems to have taken place ; whilst in a larger number the progress of the disorder has been permanently suspended. When the disease has invaded the trunk, the prognosis is most unfavourable ; but as long as it is confined to the extremities, there is hope of arresting it. Most frequently, however, death results from it sooner or later.

Etiology.—General muscular atrophy—that of the trunk and extremities, spares neither children nor adults nor aged people ; whereas the partial form would appear to be most common between thirty and fifty years of age. Males are much more liable to the disease than females, perhaps owing to their occupations. It is certainly hereditary. Exposure to wet and cold, or very hard work, are often the assigned causes ; blows upon the spine, and shocks to the cord, seem to have had an influence in producing it in some of the reported cases ; while Dr. Roberts shows that when it arises from cold the atrophy is much more likely to extend to the muscles of the trunk, than when it has its origin in overwork.

Pathology and Morbid Anatomy.—We are perhaps scarcely yet in a position to decide upon the nature of this disease. According to some authorities it has its starting-point in the nervous system, the affection of the muscles being secondary. Three or four years since, most observers were inclined to agree that this position was untenable ; and it was generally believed that the disorder consisted of a granular and fatty degeneration of the muscular fibre, similar to that which is observed in fatty heart. It was said, that although there is no general depression of the nutritive functions, yet there is an error of nutrition affecting the muscular fibre, owing to some unknown constitutional peculiarity.

The post-mortem appearances seemed to confirm these remarks.

weighed 36 ounces 163 grains avoirdupois. The *spinal cord* was sound, and of the usual bulk, consistence, and colour. The *anterior roots of the spinal nerves* were remarkably small compared with the posterior : for whereas in health the posterior or sensitive roots are to the anterior or motor as 3 to 1 in the cervical region, 1½ to 1 in the dorsal, and 2 to 1 in the lumbar ; here the proportion was as 10 to 1 in the cervical, and 5 to 1 in the dorsal and lumbar regions. Moreover, many of the anterior cervical roots were reduced to mere neurilemma, and presented no trace of nervous tissue when examined with a lens. The *muscles* of the pelvis and thigh had escaped the atrophy ; while the elevators of the lower jaw, the muscles of the pharynx, those of the supra- and infra-hyoidean regions, the platysma on both sides, and the zygomatics had undergone simple atrophy or emaciation. Other muscles were wasted and pale ; while most had undergone atrophy with fatty degeneration. Several seemed at first sight to have disappeared, so thin and slender were their remains. There was not a single muscle of the upper extremities unaffected ; those of the hand being the most atrophied, then those of the shoulder, forearm, and upper arm. The tongue was changed into a fatty mass, in the midst of which appeared a number of vertical muscular bundles.

The heart, liver, kidneys, and spleen have been always found healthy; as have also the brain and medulla oblongata. In two thirds of the reported cases the spinal cord was said to be in a normal condition ; while in three instances there was inflammatory softening, and in one amyloid degeneration of the posterior columns. The anterior roots of the spinal nerves were diminished in size in some instances, but by no means in all ; although such a change has been carefully looked for, since Cruveilhier imagined that he had discovered the essential nature of the disease in this alteration.

There is a great probability, however, that in some of those instances where the cord is said to have been found healthy it has not been properly examined (see p. 342). In one instance widespread degeneration of the spinal marrow was detected. Then in another example, where Mr. Lockhart Clarke minutely examined the spinal cord a few days after its immersion in a weak solution of chromic acid (gr. 3 to each ounce of water), this gentleman found a peculiar degeneration and softening of particular points of the grey substance of the cord ; from which he concluded that the disorder began in the cord, and not in the muscles as a consequence of defective nutrition.

The muscles which had lost all power during life have always been found after death to be wasted, and sometimes to be really annihilated. At most examinations it is reported that the muscular fibres were of a pale red or buff colour ; while often to the naked eye they presented evidence of fatty degeneration. From the results of the microscopic examinations it may be said, that the muscular fibrillae had degenerated into a granular amorphous substance, or into fat globules ; the empty sarcolemma or tunic of the elementary fibre having been broken up, so that only a little connective tissue was left. The degeneration sometimes appeared to be entirely granular and not fatty ; while in other instances the fat was abundant.

Treatment.—It may be instructive to mention that amongst the remedies which have certainly failed to do good, we must place strychnia and nux vomica ; setons, issues, or blisters, over the vertebræ ; and cold baths during the active stage. With one exception, mercury and iodide of potassium have proved useless ; and it is very doubtful if there has been any greater success with tonics and cod liver oil.

Wunderlich and Vulpian have obtained good results from the administration of nitrate of silver ; the first physician employing this salt in doses of gr. $\frac{1}{10}$ thrice daily, while the second gives gr. $\frac{1}{4}$ twice or thrice in the day. Under its use the sense of touch has been rendered more acute, the neuralgic pains have ceased, the sensibility to cold has diminished, the appetite has increased, and the general nutrition has improved. It is much to be feared, however, that no such favourable consequences as these will be obtained in this country, from this or any other silver salt.

Galvanism applied locally to the wasting muscles is said by Dr. Roberts to be the most effective remedy. Duchenne seems to have been particularly successful in the treatment by localized Faradisation (the electricity of the induced or secondary current in the helix round the magnet, discovered by Faraday); but he advises the careful use of this agent, not giving more than one minute to each affected muscle lest it become fatigued and exhausted, and not prolonging each sitting for more than ten or fifteen minutes. With galvanism there may be combined gentle frictions, occasional warm sulphur baths, the use of such remedies as will improve the quality of the blood, and methodical exercise.— When the disease has become stationary, galvanism may be more freely resorted to, together with cold bathing.

10. **MERCURIAL PALSY.**—Mercurial palsy, or mercurial tremor as it is sometimes termed, consists of a kind of convulsive agitation of the voluntary muscles, which is increased when volition is brought to bear upon them. In advanced stages of the disease, articulation and mastication and locomotion are performed with difficulty; while the use of the hands is almost entirely lost. The tremor prevents the performance of most combined movements. The skin acquires a brown hue, and the teeth turn black. Workmen exposed to the fumes of mercury,—such as gilders of buttons, glass-platers, barometer-makers, &c., are very liable to it.

In the *treatment* of mercurial palsy the patient must be withdrawn from the injurious atmosphere. If the case be taken in time, sulphur baths, good diet, sea-air, and iodide of potassium (for reasons to be presently mentioned) will generally effect a cure.

11. **LEAD PALSY.**—This is an affection which usually follows or accompanies *colica pictonum*, though it may exist independently. The poison of lead appears to exert some peculiar noxious influence over the nerves of the forearm and hand. In consequence of this the extensor muscles of the hands and fingers become paralysed, so that when the arms are stretched out the hands hang down by their own weight; or, as the patients say, the *wrists drop*. The inferior extremities are very rarely affected. The sufferers frequently experience attacks of lead colic. The odour of the breath is peculiar (saturnine), and there is a similar kind of taste. A characteristic symptom of the presence of lead in the system is the existence of a blue or purplish line—the sulphuret of lead—round the edges of the gums, just where they join the teeth; a very important aid to diagnosis, for the notice of which we are indebted to Dr. Burton.* Plumbers, painters, colour-grinders, typefounders, &c., are the usual sufferers from this affection. Occasionally it is met with on board ship, during long voyages, owing to the use of minium in the apparatus employed for distilling sea water. Zinc pipes containing lead are also now and then impro-

* The formation of the blue sulphuret of lead is probably due, as was suggested by Dr. Pereira, to the action of sulphuretted hydrogen (evolved by the decomposing particles of food lodged between the teeth) on lead contained in the saliva and buccal mucus.

perly employed. The use of snuff which has been packed in lead has caused symptoms of incipient palsy.   But cases of lead poisoning are sometimes met with among the public generally; the source of the mischief being in most instances traceable to the employment of water which has either been kept in, or transmitted through, leaden vessels.

The question naturally suggests itself,—What is the particular organ affected in the cases where the mischief arises from the handling of lead compounds ? Dr. Todd answered this moot-point by stating his belief that the muscles and nerves are early affected, and that subsequently the nervous centres become implicated.   The muscles being contaminated by the lead, their nerves participate in this contamination.   The nervous system is therefore first vitiated at the periphery, in the nerves ; and the poisonous influence continuing, the deterioration gradually advances to the centres.   This is thought to be proved by the occurrence first of local paralysis in these cases, and subsequently of epileptic convulsions or other symptoms of centric disease.

The operatives in lead-works and in mines suffer much from the saturnine emanations.   The work-rooms where the manufacture of white lead is completed, have the atmosphere loaded with minute particles of lead-compounds, so that the men and women employed in them get their systems contaminated chiefly through the respiratory organs.   They become " leaded ;" and hence are rendered the victims of paralysis, colic, gout, spasms of the respiratory muscles, and sleeplessness.   They get wan, pallid, feeble, and suffer much from neuralgia.

Death may occur when the system has been long exposed to the influence of lead ; this termination being most common in those addicted to intemperance.

The *treatment* of lead palsy has been very much facilitated by the hypothesis promulgated by M. Melsens, that the baneful effects of lead and mercury are caused by the chemical combination of these metals with the tissues of the body, or by their being present in intimate union with these tissues in some analogous manner. The therapeutical application of this theory necessarily was, as pointed out by Dr. J. R. Nicholson, that the action of the curative agent must be directed to the conversion of the poisonous metal into a compound having less affinity for those tissues, and which therefore can be readily eliminated from the body.   Now it has been shown that iodide of potassium possesses the requisite conditions for becoming a curative agent in lead diseases, according to this theory ; and consequently this drug has superseded all others.

Dr. Nicholson has published a very interesting case in which the lead, after the administration of the iodide of potassium, could be distinctly detected in the urine, notwithstanding it was not to be found before the commencement of the treatment.   In this instance the colic entirely ceased, but the palsy persisted.   Galvanism was then used in conjunction with the iodide of potassium, and the patient went to his work, about fifty days after the commencement of the treatment, without any trace of paralysis. From this result it is concluded :—First, that the iodide of potassium acts as a curative agent in lead-poisoning, by converting the lead into a form which can again be readily taken up by the blood, and evacuated by one of the natural outlets. Secondly, that the iodide acts most speedily in conjunction with galvanism, when employed for the relief of lead paralysis.*

Finally, in addition to the iodide of potassium (gr. 5—10 thrice daily) the patient may use warm or sulphur baths (F. 125) ; while galvanism and friction to the paralysed limb, a nourishing diet, and exercise in the fresh air ought generally to be had recourse to. To prevent any injurious influence, Liebig recommends all workers in lead to drink sulphuric acid lemonade daily. This acts probably by converting the salt of lead, as it enters the system, into an insoluble sulphate. Cleanliness is also an excellent prophylactic.

12. PARALYSIS AGITANS.—This disease is characterized by a tremulous agitation—a continued shaking—usually commencing in the hands and arms, or in the head, and gradually extending over the whole body. Mr. Parkinson has well defined the disorder thus :—" Involuntary tremulous motion, with lessened muscular power, in parts not in action, and even when supported, with a propensity to bend the trunk forward, and to pass from a walking to a running pace ; the senses and intellects being uninjured." The disease progresses slowly. When it is far advanced the agitation is often so violent as to prevent sleep. The patient cannot carry food to his mouth ; while deglutition and mastication are performed with difficulty. He is liable to trip, owing to his hurried and shuffling gait. The intellect is unimpaired. Mental excitement always aggravates the tremor. As the disease extends, the body becomes inclined forwards, and the chin bent on the sternum. The wearisome movements cause exhaustion ; the agitation gets extreme ; and the violent tremors do not even cease at night. It soon becomes evident that the constitutional powers are daily getting lessened ; food can hardly be swallowed ; the urine and fæces pass involuntarily ; and coma with slight delirium closes the scene.

As regards the remedies for paralysis agitans I can say but little, since I know of no measures likely to do much good. I should, however, try the effects of pure air, nourishing diet, simple warm or sulphur baths, ferruginous tonics, cod liver oil, and occasional opiates. A cure is said to have been effected by the employment of the continuous galvanic current, such as may be derived from a Pulvermacher's chain-battery of 120 links.

XII. CONVULSIONS.

The subject of convulsions is a very complicated one. To endeavour to simplify it, an arbitrary arrangement of the matter

* *The Lancet.* London, 14 October 1854.

will be made ; so that this symptom of disease as it occurs in adults, in children, and in pregnant or parturient women, will be considered separately. It is distinctly to be understood, however, that this plan has little or nothing to recommend it beyond expediency.

1. **CONVULSIONS IN ADULTS.**—Amongst the many prominent symptoms which accompany disturbances of the nervous system few occasion greater alarm to the friends of the patient than an attack of convulsions or " fits." This is partly due to the suddenness with which the paroxysm comes on, the general struggles and the distortion of countenance which it produces, and the complete loss of consciousness that attends it.

By way of definition, convulsions [from *Convello* = to overthrow, to annihilate &c.,] may be said to consist of violent and involuntary contractions of the muscles of the body ; occurring in paroxysms, and often associated with insensibility. Sometimes the contractions are partial, of considerable duration, attended with hardness of the affected muscles, and not accompanied by unconsciousness ; such being known as *tonic* spasms [from Τείνω = to strain or tighten], or as *spastic* contractions [from Σπα'ω = to draw + the terminal -ικος]. Examples of these are seen in tetanus and common cramp. In another variety there are rapidly alternating contractions and relaxations—*clonic* spasms [from Κλονέω = to put in commotion] ; subsultus tendinum, or that catching of the tendons of the hands and feet which occurs in the last stages of low fever, being an instance of this kind. And again there are *epileptiform*, or *epileptoid* attacks [from *Epilepsia* + the terminal *-ides* = resembling epilepsy], in which we find sudden loss of consciousness and voluntary motor power, with clonic spasms ; the fit lasting from one or two to twenty minutes, and ending in more or less exhaustion with a tendency to sleep.

The *causes* of an attack of general convulsions are to be found in all those conditions which suddenly arrest the nutrition of the brain. Hence a seizure may be due to cerebral hæmorrhage, to thrombosis and embolism of the cerebral arteries, to the rupture of an intra-cranial aneurism, to concussion of the brain, and possibly to some sudden congestion of a syphilitic or cancerous tumour within the skull. Attacks are readily produced by quickly cutting off the supply of healthy blood to the nervous centres ; so that we generally find convulsions preceding death from rapid hæmorrhage. Animals killed in the slaughter house by dividing the large vessels in the neck are violently convulsed before death. So also convulsions were frequently seen in the sick room some thirty years back, when patients were bled to " incipient syncope" for the purpose of diagnosis ; and when, for extinguishing inflammation, Wardrop and Marshall Hall were in the habit of taking away from one hundred to one hundred and twenty ounces of blood in a short space of time. Strange to say, venesection was lauded as the most valuable of remedies; though the last-named physician allowed that in his own practice, as well as in that of others, excessive bleedings often occasioned convulsions which endangered the patients' lives. Convulsions from a morbid state of the blood are far from uncommon. They are witnessed when the due oxygenation of the circulating fluid is suddenly impeded; as from mechanical obstruction and spasm of the glottis, or the inhalation of poisonous gases. In acute atrophy of the liver death is usually preceded by convulsions. When, in renal disease, urea and other ingredients of the urine are not properly eliminated, the nervous system gets poisoned and convulsions may ensue. The uræmic convulsions of pregnant and parturient women are examples of this condition. And lastly it seems certain, that the abnormal excitement of organs distant from the brain can provoke convulsions; probably by irritation of the vaso-motor nerves causing spasm of the muscular coats of the cerebral arteries. In this way, fits take place in young children from teething, the presence of indigestible food in the stomach, the irritation of thread worms in the rectum &c.

Speaking very generally of the *symptoms* of convulsions it is to be noticed, that with or without premonitory indications, there is a sudden loss of consciousness, accompanied by irregular and powerful contractions of the muscles. The limbs are affected with clonic spasms, and at the end are spasmodically extended. All the voluntary muscles may be attacked; or there will be only spasms of the features, or of one half of the body, or of a single limb. During a general paroxysm the countenance is much distorted; the face being commonly pallid or livid. The eyeballs seem staring and motionless; there is generally insensibility to light; and the pupils are usually widely dilated, though not as much so as in poisoning by belladonna in which the irides are sometimes scarcely to be seen. Grinding and gnashing of the teeth, protrusion of the tongue and injury of this organ from its being bitten, laborious respiration, stertorous breathing, involuntary evacuations, &c., are commonly observed. As the attack subsides, it leaves a disposition to sleep. In adults a fatal result is rare unless the convulsion have its origin in severe cerebral or renal disease.

The *treatment* of convulsion as an entity, so to say, calls for little comment. The difficult point, though one always to be attempted, is to trace this symptom to its cause. Of course, if this be impossible, we must place the patient in such a condition as to help his recovery; even if this is only to be temporary owing to some incurable primary malady. His dress is to be loosened and all clothing about the neck removed. He is to be placed so that pure and cool air may be breathed, while care is taken to prevent his falling off the bed. Subsequently, cold can be applied to the head if there be much heat or flushing; with warmth and sinapisms to the extremities. The practitioner who, knowing nothing of the source of the disturbance, feels that he must still do something more, can select what he likes from such remedies as purgative and antispasmodic enemata, ammonia to the nostrils, spirit lotions for the scalp, chloroform inhalation, dry cupping, &c.   It is, however, rather confusing to find a gentleman with a self-applauding air applying cold affusion to the head of his patient, a blister to the nape of the neck, mustard to the feet, and croton oil to the tongue; then hesitating as to whether he shall select leeches or venesection or galvanism, the inclination being towards the first; and all for what?   Because the unfortunate sufferer has had a fit of convulsion owing to the rupture of a cerebral aneurism, and is lying in a state of deep coma. So again I have seen a young child with its upper and lower gums deeply gashed, the diagnosis being— "convulsions from teething;" the real sequence of events having been mild scarlet fever, acute renal disease with albuminuria, and uræmic poisoning. As before remarked, there is often very great difficulty in finding out of what disease the convulsion is a symptom; while sometimes it is impossible to form any conclusion as to whether the nerve tissue is simply irritated, or badly nourished, or poisoned, or irreparably injured.   Unhappily, there is an equal difficulty in persuading the practitioner to hold his hand under such circumstances. He is impatient to do battle with his enemy— disease, though he cannot distinguish him; forgetful that in the mêlée he is just as likely to favour as to oppose the progress of his foe.

2. INFANTILE CONVULSIONS.—From the time of birth until the end of the seventh or eighth year, convulsions are of rather frequent occurrence, inasmuch as they are produced by a variety of circumstances; but they are most common during infancy, since this is not only an excitable period of life, but the immature nervous centres are exposed to peculiar sources of irritation.   The attacks very commonly (supposing they are not symptomatic of severe cerebral disease) pass off without any bad result. When, however, they recur frequently they are very likely to weaken the intellect, and to impair the general health; while in some instances they prove the immediate cause of death.

A few days after birth, the young child is apt to suffer from slight convulsive movements, to which nurses give the name of "inward fits."   The baby lies as though asleep, rolls its eyes about or has the corneæ drawn up under the upper lids, moans gently, breathes with a little difficulty, and has twitchings of the muscles of the face: sometimes there is a livid ring round the mouth. This condition arises from flatulence and indigestion; and is a warning that the quality of the food should be looked to. It is relieved by gentle friction over the abdomen; together with the administration of two or three drops of aromatic spirits of ammonia, the same quantity of spirit of ether, and a teaspoonful of dill water.

Causes.—Anything which rapidly depresses the nervous system, or which interferes with the due performance of the functions of the nervous centres, is likely to induce a fit of convulsions. Hence the fits may arise from structural disease such as tubercular meningitis, phrenitis, apoplexy, &c. ; from an insufficient supply of blood to the brain, as may be noticed in weak and badly nourished children, or in those debilitated by profuse diarrhœa ; or from a supply of impure blood, examples of which occur at times during the course of the eruptive fevers, or the progress of renal disease. Again, these seizures are now and then due to distant irritation reflected to the brain, such as arises from the pressure of a tooth upon the inflamed gum during dentition, or from intestinal worms, or the passage of a renal calculus, or simple indigestion, or a pin or needle sticking in the body ; to general irritation produced by exposure to a cold and damp atmosphere ; and lastly they may be produced by fright, and by causes which we cannot discover. Moreover it may be noticed that all such circumstances as would give rise to delirium in the adult, will probably induce convulsions in the infant.

Mr. North observes, that the children of parents who marry at too early or at too advanced an age are more susceptible of convulsions, than the progeny of those persons who marry in the prime of life. Hereditary predisposition has been also observed. Thus Boerhaave states that all the children of an epileptic man died of some convulsive affection. A remarkable instance of this derivative proclivity has been narrated by Dr. Duclos.* The case is that of a woman, aged 34, one of eleven children, six of whom had died of convulsions. She had herself had frequent attacks of eclampsia until her eighth year; which attacks had left slight deviation of the mouth, with ptosis of the left upper eyelid. This woman had ten children, who all had convulsions; five having died in the first two years of life, and one when three years old.

The frequency and the fatality of convulsions diminish in a marked degree as the organization of the nervous system becomes more perfect. This is clearly shown by a reference to the reports of the Registrar-General. Taking the last of these, we find the deaths in England from "convulsions" during the year 1866 were registered as 27,431 ; of which number 26,847 occurred in children under five years of age, 24,577 of these being infants under one year. These figures do not include the deaths from epilepsy, which disease was fatal in 1866 to 2468 persons ; only 145 being children under five years.

Symptoms.—In slight cases the symptoms are merely such as I have just described as inward fits : generally they are much more severe. The attack comes on suddenly, like a fit of epilepsy, and without warning. Sometimes the child utters a sharp cry, sometimes there is no sound. It perhaps looks unusually bright for a a few seconds, stares vacantly, loses consciousness, has the respiration momentarily suspended, and has its body rendered stiff and immoveable. Then the seizure may end. Most times,

* *Etudes Cliniques pour servir à l'histoire des Convulsions de l'Enfance,* p. 75. Paris, 1847.

however, clonic spasms set in.   The muscles contract and relax involuntarily ; the limbs are quickly flexed and extended ; the hands are generally firmly clenched, while the thumbs are turned inwards on the palms ; and the head is jerked backwards and forwards, or laterally.   The countenance is rendered frightful, for the muscles of the face twitch violently and rapidly, and the lips are drawn in all directions ; while the integuments of the head and face become red and then livid.   There is often convergent strabismus : the eyes roll and start, and the pupils are dilated and usually insensible to light.   The respiration is irregular and laborious.   The pulse is very frequent and small.   The spasmodic action of the abdominal muscles causes the contents of the bladder and rectum to be voided involuntarily.   At the end of some eighty to one hundred and sixty seconds (the time seeming much longer) a deep inspiration announces that the fit is over.   The limbs and features relax, and the natural appearance returns : the blood becomes properly oxygenated, and the lips and face assume their healthy hue. The child perhaps looks frightened and cries ; but more frequently it falls into a sound sleep directly.   During this, its body gets bathed in perspiration.   In unfavourable cases the child sinks into a state of complete coma, and perhaps dies.   It is rare for the fit to be single : usually it returns after a longer or shorter interval.   Occasionally only one side of the body is convulsed ; or only one limb ; or merely the muscles of the face are affected.   In all cases the muscular actions are rarely equal on the two sides of the mesial plane ; and therefore the eyes, countenance, and general frame appear greatly distorted and make the aspect of the little patient perfectly distressing.   The more feeble the attack, the longer its duration. Sometimes the convulsive phenomena appear to be almost continuous for several hours ; so short are the intervals between the fits. Not uncommonly they cease for three or four hours and then return ; so that there may be half a dozen paroxysms during the day.   The sequelæ most to be feared are infantile palsy ; hemiplegia ; permanent squinting ; some defect of sight or hearing or power of speech ; and disorder of the mind, varying from the slightest form of disturbance as shown by an uncontrollable temper, to complete idiocy.

Treatment.—This will of course vary according to the circumstances of each case, and the exciting cause of the attack.   Nevertheless, the broad principles of treatment are as follows :—During the fit it will be advisable to avoid all unnecessary interference ; it being generally sufficient to rapidly loosen the clothing about the neck and chest and waist, and to admit plenty of fresh air.   The head can be raised and the face sprinkled with cold water, if the practitioner have any faith in such proceedings.   Subsequently, if a recurrence of the fit be feared the warm bath may be of signal service, cold being at the same time applied to the head ; or a gentle douche of cold water over the occiput will possibly be beneficial.   Wet cloths, as well as bladders containing pounded ice laid upon the top and back part of the head, only do harm. When the bowels are confined, gentle antacid purgatives will be needed; when there is much flatulence, carminatives; when the stomach contains undigested food, emetics. Supposing the irritation is due to dentition, and the tense gum appears to offer an obstacle to the passage of the tooth, lancing this fibrous texture is to be had recourse to. Then, as a medicine from which more may be hoped for than from any other, I would advise the exhibition of the bromide of potassium; giving it even in enemata of beef tea, when there is an inability to swallow. Subsequently, where there is restlessness, sedatives—especially the hydrocyanic acid with a few drops of tincture of hyoscyamus, had better be prescribed. If there are intestinal worms they must be got rid of by suitable anthelmintic drugs. When the blood is watery and deficient in red globules, ferruginous tonics are the suitable remedies. In all instances, leeches and blisters, calomel and grey powder and antimony, merely serve to lessen the chances of recovery.

One important agent remains to be noticed, namely the inhalation of the vapour of ether or chloroform; or, as I greatly prefer, of a mixture of the two. There are probably few practitioners who have seen much of the diseases of children that have not become impressed with the value of producing anæsthesia in those cases where the convulsive attacks follow each other in rapid succession. At the same time, I would not trust to anæsthesia alone; it being advisable, in the greater number of cases, to administer the bromide of potassium simultaneously.

3. **ECLAMPSIA NUTANS.** — Eclampsia nutans [from Ἐκλάμπω = to emit brilliant light; Nuto = to nod], or the "Salaam" convulsions of infancy, is an important but very rare malady—so rare that the majority of practitioners never see an example of it. The disease probably bears some relation to both convulsions and paralysis agitans. Like epilepsy, from which it is distinguished by the absence of loss of consciousness, it may lead to impairment of the intellect. Thus, of four cases (the histories of which have been collected by Mr. Newnham*) two terminated in complete idiocy, and two in impairment of the intellect. The ages of the sufferers were 16 months, 4½ months, 12 months (?), and 6 months respectively. Of two cases recorded by Dr. Faber of Wartenberg, one became epileptic with an imbecile appearance. Other instances are likewise known where either hemiplegia or paraplegia has been the unfortunate termination.

Symptoms.—The pathognomonic symptom by which this affection is distinguished—and which induced Sir Charles Clarke to denominate it "the Salaam" convulsion, is a peculiar and involuntary bowing backwards and forwards of the head, and occasionally of the

* Clay's *British Record of Obstetric Medicine and Surgery*, vol. ii. Manchester, 1849.

body; the bowings being repeated in rapid succession, and the attacks coming on in paroxysms several times daily.   The severe seizures appear usually to commence in the morning on awaking from the night's sleep.   There is frequently headache, perhaps with a tendency to drowsiness; and the tongue may be coated. Squinting, with one or both eyes, is not uncommon.   The bowels are usually sluggish, or even obstinately confined.   Then, by and by cerebral symptoms with general convulsions arise, or pure epilepsy; there may be hemiplegia or paraplegia; and the little patients pine and waste away.   In more favourable cases, after the lapse of several months, the symptoms remit; and then at the end of two or three years the bodily health will be partially restored.   The causes of this affection are involved in obscurity.

Pathology.—Mr. Newnham believed that the essential character of this malady is inflammatory action of a weak or strumous character.   This probably commences in the membranes investing the medulla oblongata, and extends to those at the base of the brain. Hence exudations of coagulable lymph or serum occur, which cause pressure, and consequently paralysis.   The regular nutrition of the brain is also interrupted, and its manifestations blunted; while in the more aggravated cases, the organ becomes so deteriorated, as to lose all power of carrying on the intellectual functions, it having in all probability, partaken of the same kind of inflammatory action as first appeared in its investing membranes.

Treatment.—The chief points to attend to are these:—To see that the child is placed under the most favourable hygienic conditions; to keep the secretions in order by rhubarb and magnesia, or by mild doses of aloes; and at the same time to support the powers of life by bark, or by quinine combined with some preparation of steel. Cod liver oil does good service.   It may be well given with the so-called chemical food (F. 405).   One case has been reported as cured by the use of blisters behind the ears, keeping the bowels regular with castor oil, and the prolonged administration of iodide of potassium with quinine.   In some of the other instances above referred to, hydrocyanic acid palliated the symptoms, while opium aggravated them.   I do not know whether chloroform has been fairly tried.   Bromide of potassium would probably be serviceable.

Tepid or cold bathing will be useful, especially at the sea-side. Shower baths and cold affusions do harm.   The diet must be nourishing, and should contain a free amount of fatty matters—especially milk.   The body ought to be warmly clad, while the head is kept cool.   All quick movements, and all harshness or anything which produces mental excitement should be carefully avoided.

4. ECLAMPSIA OF PREGNANCY AND PARTURITION.— Considering that this subject has been treated of somewhat fully in the section on Uræmia (p. 31), it will not be necessary to do more than supplement the remarks already made by a few notes.   I

shall offer these in the form of aphorisms, thus :—(1) The eclampsia of pregnant and parturient women is characterized by the sudden occurrence of violent tonic and clonic spasms, with complete loss of consciousness ; the convulsive seizure ending in more or less profound stupor. Usually, the convulsions are general—they affect the whole body. Exceptionally, they are partial ; perhaps involving only one-half of the body, consciousness remaining unimpaired.—(2) The attack commonly comes on for the first time during the last three months of pregnancy, and especially just as labour is commencing. It is from this latter circumstance that the disease is usually spoken of as " puerperal convulsions."—(3) Primiparæ are more liable to convulsions than multiparæ.—(4) The eclampsia is a symptom of blood poisoning from functional or organic disease of the kidneys ; in either case, the renal affection being attended with albuminuria.—(5) According to my own experience the occurrence of convulsions is more to be feared where the albuminuria is due to some unknown condition set up by pregnancy, and when it is therefore temporary, than where this state of urine is the consequence of old-standing structural disease of the kidney.—(6) The urine has generally been albuminous for some weeks previous to the convulsions ; although a few cases are recorded where the albumen has only been found shortly after the first fit. The albumen being abundant in the urine, it may be taken for granted that the urea is proportionately scanty ; so that as the blood becomes deficient in albumen its impurity gets greater. In addition to the albuminous state of the urine, the face and hands and arms will generally be found œdematous ; or this condition may perhaps chiefly affect the feet and ankles, or the labia majora.—(7) When the fits once come on, they usually follow each other in rapid succession, being often repeated several times in the day ; the patient being not only insensible during the paroxysm, but most frequently also in the interval. The duration of each fit, inclusive of the stage of convulsion and that of coma, varies from half an hour to two or three hours, or even longer. As the symptoms remit, consciousness returns very gradually ; a confused dull headache being complained of, though there is no recollection of what has happened.—(8) Spontaneous premature labour is common in eclampsia ; but it is quite exceptional for the child to be born alive particularly after numerous paroxysms.—(9) The prognosis must always be guarded. From the statistics which I have collected it is inferred, that the mortality is at least thirty per cent. The termination is in recovery or death ; protracted illness, as a result, being very rare, except where there has been renal disease prior to the pregnancy. When mischief is set up, it is mostly some form of paralysis or of mania.—(10) The principal remedies consist of the following :—Inhalation of chloroform, or of chloroform and pure ether mixed in equal proportions. Antispasmodic and purgative enemata. Large doses of bromide of potassium ? The induction of labour, so as to empty the uterus speedily : the convulsions often cease, however, as soon as the liquor amnii is evacuated. When the attack occurs during the act of parturition, the labour is to be expedited by turning or by the application of the forceps. On all grounds I maintain, that the employment of venesection, leeches, blisters, or mercury, is to be deprecated.

XIII. EPILEPSY.

Epilepsy [Ἐπιλαμβάνω = to attack unexpectedly] is a complicated disease of the nervous system, which has attracted attention from the earliest times. The leading symptoms are usually,— sudden loss of consciousness and sensibility, with clonic spasms of the voluntary muscles, followed by exhaustion and coma ; the attack varying in intensity and duration, and having a tendency to recur at intervals. The paroxysmal loss of consciousness is, however, the prominent or important element present in every instance ; while not unfrequently it is the only one, there being no evident spasmodic movements of any kind.

Warnings.—There are sometimes, though not in the majority of cases, premonitory symptoms sufficient to warn the patient of an approaching seizure. These warnings differ both in character and the length of time they last. In some cases they are too short to allow the sufferer to dismount from horseback, or to get away from the fire, or even to lie down ; while in other instances, many minutes, or even hours, elapse between their occurrence and the attack. Dr. Gregory of Edinburgh, was assured by an epileptic that when a fit was approaching, he fancied he saw a little old woman in a red cloak advance towards him, and strike him a blow on the head ; on which he at once lost all recollection and fell down. In a patient of my own, the fit is always preceded by rushing noises in the ears ; which noises rapidly increase in intensity and velocity until they seem to come into collision. Directly this happens consciousness is lost. On one occasion there was an opportunity of testing the duration of these noises before evidence of the fit was given ; and it was found to last two minutes and twenty seconds. Spectral illusions, headache, sickness, giddiness, dimness of vision, tremor or twitching, confusion of thought, a vague sense of fear and terror, and especially that peculiar blowing sensation known as the *aura epileptica*, constitute the most frequent premonitory symptoms. The epileptic aura is differently compared by patients to a stream of cold water, or a current of cold or warm air, or the creeping of an insect ; the sensation commencing at the extremity of a limb, and more or less rapidly ascending along the skin towards the head. Directly the aura stops the paroxysm takes place.

Symptoms.—The commencement of a typical seizure is generally characterized by a cadaverous pallor of the countenance, and the utterance of either a loud piercing shriek or a kind of suppressed groan ; immediately after which the individual falls to the ground senseless and violently convulsed.　Hence the disease has been called by the vulgar the *falling sickness*, or more vaguely *fits*. During the attack, the convulsive movements continue violent. There is gnashing of the teeth, foaming at the mouth, and the tongue is thrust forward and often severely bitten ; the eyes are partly open and suffused, the eyeballs rolling, and the pupils dilated and insensible to light ; the pulse becomes feeble, or it may remain natural ; and the skin is generally cold and clammy. There may be involuntary defecation and micturition, with or without vomiting ; the breathing is laborious or almost suspended ; while the face gets flushed, and then livid and turgid.　In fact, death seems about to take place from suffocation ; when gradually these alarming phenomena subside, the extremities of one side are jerked about, and shortly afterwards all convulsive movements cease.　The paroxysm leaves the epileptic insensible, and apparently in a sound sleep ; from which he recovers exhausted and with slight mental confusion or headache, but without any knowledge of what he has just gone through.　An attack of vomiting will sometimes follow the attack ; while generally there is a copious secretion of almost colourless urine, of low specific gravity, for many hours after the fit.

The average duration of the fit is three or five or eight minutes ; it may, however, last for half an hour or more.　The periods at which the seizures recur are variable.　At first there is often a respite for three or four months ; this time of freedom being perhaps followed by a bad day, on which as many as half a dozen fits may quickly succeed each other.　Then as the disease progresses the intervals become shorter, lasting a week or two ; until at length hardly a day passes without one or more paroxysms.　In recent cases especially, the fits often take place in the night, either on just going to sleep or on awaking.　The repetition of the seizures has a tendency to impair the memory, to weaken the understanding, and to produce a sense of mental depression or melancholy.　Beyond these, no other consequences have been seen sufficiently often to enable any conclusion to be drawn as to the influence of epilepsy on the health.　As will readily be imagined, various accidents are likely to occur from the epileptic falling into the fire, or into the water, or upon the sharp angles of furniture, &c.

The epileptic fit may be either severe or very slight, constituting the *grand mal* and the *petit mal* of the French.　Instead of the severe well-marked phenomena just described there will perhaps be only a momentary loss of consciousness, so that the sufferer does not even stagger or fall (epileptic vertigo).　For example, a child may be seized in the middle of its play, which it will resume immediately after the paroxysm, though probably slightly scared ; there having been neither convulsion nor staggering,—

simply a sudden but complete blank lasting a few seconds. Such a seizure in an adult might be preceded by vertigo; so that he would be glad to hold some object, to which he would be fixed, as it were, during the attack. So again, with the scarcely more than momentary loss of consciousness, there may be twitchings of the muscles of the face and neck, dilatation of the pupils, and pallor of the countenance; succeeded by a dazed feeling, which the individual shakes off with one or two deep inspirations, and an exclamation of being "all right again." A lady under my care, whose fits at times recur twice a day, loses consciousness without falling, and often endeavours to strike any one near her; but she always tries, wherever she may be, to undress herself. In about five minutes there is recovery, as if from a dream.

The face of the epileptic frequently wears a peculiar expression which it is difficult to describe. In many cases there can be observed an immobility of the countenance—a sort of fixed state of the muscles, with a strange staring appearance about the eyes. The patient looks as if he were going to have a fit, though nothing of the kind happens. There is frequently also a dilated and sluggish condition of the pupil, with a want of brightness in the eye. In another class there appears to be a general torpid state of the system, with a disposition to suffer from frequent attacks of headache.

Epilepsy is now and then *feigned*; but the imposition may be detected by observing that the eyes are closed, the pupils contract to the stimulus of light, the skin is hot from the necessary exertion, the tongue is not bitten, and neither the urine nor fæces are voided. The foaming about the mouth is abundant; either because there is naturally plenty of saliva, or in consequence of a pellet of soap having been worked into a froth. The impostor also selects a time and situation for his manœuvres, when attention will be attracted to them. Proposing to apply the actual cautery, or to cut off the hair, will often effect a speedy cure; or an ingenious passer-by may blow some dry snuff up the nostril with a quill, and change the fit into one of sneezing. One cunning rascal is reported to have worn over his chest, so that it attracted attention directly his coat was unbuttoned, a large card with this memorandum,—"I must not be bled. A glass of hot brandy and water revives me."

Causes.—The tendency to epilepsy is often hereditary: probably in one-fourth of the cases that come under observation there can be traced a history of epilepsy, or of insanity, or of some marked disease of the nervous system in the parents or grandparents. The two sexes are equally liable to this disease. Malformations of the head are frequent predisposing causes. Perhaps infants whose heads have been greatly compressed during birth are more subject to epilepsy than others who have been brought into the world without the aid of forceps or extra violence. It is more common for the first attack to occur between the ages of twelve and twenty than at any other period; while in women at this time it is often

accompanied by some derangement of the catamenia,—menorrhagia or dysmenorrhœa, more frequently than amenorrhœa.   Debauchery of all kinds, indulgence in alcoholic drinks, the practice
of masturbation, &c., may give rise to it.   Amongst other causes
must be also mentioned fright, grief, blows upon the head, pregnancy, intestinal worms, and the irritation of teething. Poisoning
of the blood in acute rheumatism or scarlet fever or diphtheria, and
its impoverishment in renal disease, &c., may induce it.

Associated with epilepsy we often find dyspepsia, constipation,
sleeplessness, great nervousness and depression, leucorrhœa in
women, involuntary seminal discharges in men, &c. &c.

Morbid Anatomy and Pathology.—Uncomplicated epilepsy is so
rarely fatal, that it is difficult to give precise information as to the
appearances most commonly found, or to determine the value of the
variety of lesions which have been discovered.   When an epileptic
dies who has only laboured under the disease for a short time, no
appreciable alteration of any part of the nervous system can, as a
rule, be detected.   If death occur during a paroxysm, the pia mater
is often found more or less congested.   In cases of long standing,
disease of the cerebral bloodvessels, with softening or induration
of the brain, may be present; while in such the weight of the
brain is usually above the average.   Occasionally the bones of the
skull are thickened or otherwise diseased.

Dr. Todd held that the peculiar features of an epileptic seizure
were due to the gradual collection of some morbid material in
the blood; the accumulation going on until it reached such an
amount as to act upon the brain in, so to speak, an explosive manner. Schroeder Van der Kolk concludes from his researches that the
first cause of epilepsy consists in an exalted sensibility and excitability of the medulla oblongata, rendering this part liable to discharge its force in involuntary reflex movements, on the application of irritants which excite it.   This irritation may be external
(of the fifth pair of nerves), or it may be in the brain, or in the
intestines.   In children, intestinal worms and torpidity of the bowels
are common causes; in adults, it may be due to irritation of the
intestines, but especially to onanism.   Amenorrhœa, chlorosis,
congestion of the uterus, hysteria, &c., must also be remembered
as causes.   In the commencement there is only exalted sensibility,
which may be removed and a cure effected; but when the disease
becomes of long continuance, organic vascular dilatation takes
place in the medulla, too much blood is supplied, and the ganglionic
groups are too strongly irritated.   Every attack increases the
mischief by promoting the vascular dilatation.   Moreover, increased
exudation of albumen ensues from the constantly distended vessels;
and the coats of these organs get thickened, the medulla becomes
hardened, and we have fatty degeneration, softening, &c.

The deaths registered as due to epilepsy, in England, for the
year 1866, are $\frac{\text{Males 1277}}{\text{Females 1191}} = 2468$, which is about the average
number for each of the last ten years.

Treatment—This must have reference to the measures to be adopted during a fit, and those to be employed in the interval.

During the fit—the patient ought to be laid on a large bed, or on the floor, air is to be freely admitted around him, his head is to be raised, and his neckcloth (together with any tight parts of the dress) loosened. A piece of cork or soft wood should, if possible, be introduced between the teeth, to prevent injury to the tongue. Cold affusion to the head will sometimes be useful; especially where the countenance is turgid and congested; but generally speaking it is better to do nothing. With regard to those cases where the fit is preceded by the epileptic aura, the application of a ligature between the region from which the sensation starts and the trunk, has been said to prevent the attack. I know a lady who says she has a warning in the shape of a blowing sensation commencing at the fingers of the right hand. By getting somebody to grasp her arm very tightly just above the wrist, she escapes the fit for the time. On this principle the testicles have been removed or a limb amputated, when the aura has appeared to proceed from these parts; and although success seems once in a way to have followed, yet this practice would hardly be adopted in the present day.

In the interval—we must endeavour to improve the patient's general health, and especially to give tone and firmness to the nervous system. Amongst those physicians who have recently paid attention to this disease, there are very few who do not agree in believing that everything tending to depress the vital powers does harm. Mineral tonics, especially quinine (F. 379, 386); or the salts of iron (F. 380, 390, 394, 405), or of zinc (F. 410, 413, 414), are consequently to be employed. Phosphorus is beneficial in some cases; the best preparation being the hypophosphite of soda (F. 419). There can be no doubt but that the bromide of potassium, in doses varying from ten to fifty or sixty grains thrice daily, is of remarkable efficacy in a large number of cases. Where it acts favourably, however, it seldom produces a radical cure; and I am inclined to think that most of the exceptions to this rule will be found in children. The bromide of potassium may certainly be continued for many months without injury, and perhaps for years. To gain any real amendment the remedy has generally to be given in full doses, while it must be steadily persevered with. Another drug which likewise acts as a valuable sedative in epilepsy is henbane. The good effect, however, has only persisted in my hands so long as the remedy has been regularly taken. A lady who has long been under my care, and who has suffered from severe epilepsy for many years, now passes from twelve to fourteen weeks without an attack, so long as she takes twelve fluid drachms of the tincture of henbane every night. This dose has, of course, only been gradually reached. She is not conscious of its producing any effect upon her system, beyond keeping off the fits.

The general health ought always to be attended to. The cold shower bath may be recommended, if it can be well borne; otherwise the tepid sponging bath should be substituted. Care is to be taken that refreshing sleep is obtained : it will be advantageous for a mattress to be used, with a large firm pillow, so that the head may be high. The diet must be simple but nutritious; including animal food, milk, raw eggs, and a moderate quantity of wine or bitter ale. Cod liver oil (F. 389) is often useful. The patient's habits must also be regulated by such rules as common sense will dictate—daily exercise, early hours, quiet occupation at home, and attention to the alvine and urinary secretions being necessary; while excessive mental excitement or exertion is, on the other hand, especially contra-indicated.

In some cases, those more particularly which are dependent upon a thickening of the cranial bones or membranes, iodide of potassium, or a gentle long-continued course of mercury, does good. Foville had great faith in the oil of turpentine in half-drachm doses, repeated every six hours; and Sir Thomas Watson seemed at one time to think it more useful than any other single drug. Camphor, valerian, assafœtida, naphtha, cajuput oil, and the various preparations of ether, are often very valuable adjuvants. The nitrate of silver long enjoyed great but undeserved reputation; while its tendency to blacken the skin ought to be sufficient to interdict its further employment. Again, the juice of the cotyledon umbilicus has been much vaunted; but my own experience coincides with that of many practitioners who have tried it and found it valueless. The expressed juice of the galium album or "ladies' bedstraw," has been said to act "with almost uniform success;" an assertion which all physicians who have had much to do with epileptic patients can rightly interpret. Dr. Marshall Hall recommended strychnia in *tonic* not *stimulant* doses (F. 407, 408); while, following a suggestion of Dr. Todd's, I have used the vapour of chloroform, and believe that the fits have diminished both in severity and number from its employment. The truth probably is, however, as Esquirol shrewdly remarked, that epileptics improve for a time under every new plan of treatment. Undoubtedly, hope and confidence are important elements in the treatment of this disease, and the physician should therefore never appear to despond nor allow his patient to do so.

Dr. John Chapman, whose views have been already referred to (p. 439), gives the following directions for the cure of epilepsy. The object to be kept in view is to lessen the excito-motor power of the cord, by diminishing the amount of blood circulating in it, and to prevent those spasmodic contractions of the cerebral arteries which induce the sudden loss of consciousness constituting the first phase of an epileptic fit. The rules are,—(1) Apply ice, in an india-rubber bag, to some one part, or to the whole length of the back, for from two to eighteen hours a day, according to the special character of the case under treatment. (2) If the extremities be cold, their wonted warmth is to be restored by frequently immersing them in hot water and by friction, during the first day or two of treatment. Also, in winter, by clothing the arms and legs in flannel. (3) As auxiliaries, abundant physical exercise, use of dumb bells when practicable; to arrange the dress and hair so as not to impart warmth to upper and back part of neck; promote mental activity by healthy study, or some interesting employment; and to have the dress along the centre of the back light and cool. I am only personally acquainted with one patient who I believe was thoroughly treated on these principles; and in this case, no benefit was derived. The experience of some other physicians is also very unfavourable to the practice. Dr. Chapman, however, has recorded instances in which he has been successful.

Mr. Tomes has published an instructive case that occurred in the Middlesex Hospital, where the derangement of the nervous system was due to diseased and exostosed teeth.—" A lad, a farmlabourer from Windsor, was admitted into the hospital for epilepsy. The usual remedies were tried for six weeks without effect. His mouth was then examined, and the molar teeth of the lower jaw were found to be much decayed, and of some of these the fangs only remained. He did not complain of pain in the diseased teeth or in the jaw. The decayed teeth were, however, removed, and the fangs of each were found to be enlarged and bulbous from exostosis. During the eighteen months that succeeded the removal of the diseased teeth, he had not suffered from a single fit, though for many weeks previous to the operation he had two or three per day. This is a case of singular interest, inasmuch as there was no complication of maladies, and hence there could be no doubt as to the cause of the disease, seeing that it immediately subsided when the teeth were removed."*

These remarks will hardly be complete without a brief notice of one or two other points. For example, Mr. Baker Brown has proposed the operation of clitoridectomy, as one calculated to effect a cure in a considerable proportion of epileptic women. The general voice of the profession has, however, been so strong in condemning this proceeding, that probably many years will elapse before it is again revived.—Where these fits have been supposed to be due to masturbation in boys and young men, circumcision has been had recourse to. Supposing that the opening of the prepuce is so small that it cannot be drawn back for purposes of cleanliness, removal of the foreskin will be an unobjectionable measure; but whether any case can be shown where this proceeding has proved successful in curing epilepsy may be doubted.—Dr. Marshall Hall entertained strong opinions as to the efficacy of tracheotomy in some forms of epilepsy, not so much as a curative proceeding, but to avert the dangers of the paroxysm, to convert

* *A System of Dental Surgery*, p. 443. London, 1859.

the disease into a milder variety, and to give time for a trial of remedies.* Two or three cases have been recorded where this practice has been adopted; but probably no practitioner would now resort to it.—Again, caustics to the larynx have been applied; though, as might be expected, without benefit.—Compression of the carotids just before the fit may prevent it (see p. 491).—Brown-Séquard cauterizes the nape of the neck, or the part where the aura originates, using the moxa or the red-hot iron; but I know not what amount of success has justified this treatment.—And lastly, on the principle of attempting to relieve the congestion of the medulla oblongata, Schroeder Van der Kolk employs setons or issues placed high up in the neck. That counter-irritants over the upper cervical vertebræ, perhaps, with the administration of bromide of potassium or henbane, and the removal of all external sources of irritation, will often prove most useful, admits of no question.†

XIV. HYSTERIA.

Dr. Copland defines hysteria thus :—" Nervous disorder often assuming the most varied forms, but commonly presenting a paroxysmal character; the attacks usually commencing with a flow of limpid urine, with uneasiness or irregular motions and

* Dr. Marshall Hall says—" There are two cases of epilepsy in its direst forms, in which the propriety and efficacy of tracheotomy admit of no doubt: these are—first, Epilepsia laryngea, with spasmodic laryngismus, threatening the extinction of Mind; second, Epilepsia laryngea, with paralytic laryngismus, threatening the extinction of Life. . . . . . The diagnosis must be established by observing the state of the larynx, of the neck, of the face, and of the cerebrum. In the absence of laryngismus, the deep purple lividity and tumefaction, and the subsequent deep coma, &c., are equally absent, and tracheotomy of course *hors de propos.*"—*Lancet,* pp. 308, 309, 14 October 1854.

† In proof of this statement I may mention the case of a gentleman upwards of fifty years of age, who has been subject to epileptic fits for many years. To obtain relief he has consulted several physicians, and has taken large doses of bromide of potassium without any benefit. Under my advice he has half an ounce of tincture of henbane every night; and is provided with the blistering fluid of the British Pharmacopœia, to be used when necessary. His wife always knows when an attack is coming on, inasmuch as for a few hours before it occurs he speaks incoherently. Generally he rouses from his first sleep at about midnight. He wakes his wife, talks rubbish (knowing all the time that what he says is unintelligible, though he cannot help saying it and cannot give any explanation), goes to sleep again, and then in the course of the night has a severe fit. But since he has been under my care, his wife applies the blistering fluid freely to the back of his neck, directly he wakes in the semi-delirious state; and now, on almost every occasion, the seizure is prevented. From frequent observation this lady feels certain that the counter-irritant has a most decidedly valuable effect. She thinks the tincture of henbane alone has diminished the number of the attacks; but with this and the blister she feels almost sure of warding them off. The sore neck tells the patient in the morning what has happened during the night. He has no recollection, however, of having been awake.

rumbling noises in the left iliac region, or the sensation of a ball (*globus hystericus*) rising upwards to the throat, frequently attended by a feeling of suffocation, and sometimes with convulsions; chiefly affecting females from the period of puberty to the decline of life, and principally those possessing great susceptibility of the nervous system, and of mental emotion."*

I shall consider this disease as it occurs in paroxysms, as it affects sensibility, and as it mimics other affections. The name hysteria ['Υστέρα = the womb] has been applied to it, owing to its supposed origin in the uterus. The term is inappropriate, on several grounds; but particularly so since the disease is not necessarily connected with any derangement of the female sexual system, while it is occasionally seen in the male sex.

Causes.—There is no one prominent circumstance which can be brought forward as a cause of hysteria. Disturbed cerebral nutrition may be said to be its foundation; using the word "nutrition" in its broadest sense, and considering the proper performance of this function to involve the healthy action of every organ in the body. Sex, celibacy, and age influence the origin of this disease.

Females are greatly more predisposed to all forms of hysteria than males. This is said to be due to *the greater susceptibility of the nervous system* in women; a vague phrase, however, having more sound than meaning. With a much greater show of reason I think it may be suggested that the explanation lies in the different way in which the two sexes are trained and educated. The disease usually begins about the time of puberty: in about 70 per cent. the first manifestation of it will be found to happen during the decade of 16 to 25 years. Single women suffer more frequently than married: among the latter, those who do not become pregnant are most susceptible to it. Hysteria is almost unknown among prostitutes; and hence it must be inferred that excessive sexual intercourse has no influence as an exciting cause. There can be little question but that want of occupation has a very injurious effect upon both mind and body, and that one of these effects is the production of the hysteric condition. Disappointment and vexation, especially if these emotions are called into play by "love affairs," are active causes of this disorder. Examining my numerous notes of cases of hysteria which have accumulated during twenty years, I cannot learn that there is any relationship between the development of this disease and the occurrence of amenorrhœa, dysmenorrhœa, or menorrhagia. There is often some disturbance of the uterine functions, but not of one kind more frequently than another.

With regard to males the disease has seemed due in the instances which have come under my own observation to mental overwork, to an unwise curtailment of the hours for sleep, to all

* *Dictionary of Practical Medicine;* article "Hysteria," vol. ii. p. 272. London, 1858.

kinds of dissipation, or to the influence of long-continued anxiety or grief. Hereditary tendency to nervous disorders may have existed.

Symptoms.—The symptoms which characterize the *hysteric paroxysm* or fit are,—convulsive movements of the trunk and limbs; violent beating of the breasts with the hands clenched, and tearing of the hair or of the garments; together with shrieks and screams, violent agitation, and the globus hystericus. The attack ends with tears, convulsive outbreaks of crying or laughter, and sometimes with obstinate hiccup. Occasionally, the patient sinks to the ground insensible and exhausted: she remains so for a short time; and then recovers, tired and crying. The fit is often followed by the expulsion of a quantity of limpid urine; while occasionally this secretion is passed involuntarily during the tumult.

The paroxysm differs from epilepsy, inasmuch as the hysteric fit is almost peculiar to women, it continues longer, the pupils are not affected, and there is seldom loss of consciousness — the patient being aware of all that is passing around her. The convulsive movements are also of a different character, much noisier though in reality less severe, and not more marked on one side of the body than the other. Moreover, the respirations are never suspended; the tongue is not bitten; and the attack is not followed by coma, as epilepsy is.

It has been well pointed out by M. Briquet that hysterical patients frequently suffer from *hyperæsthesia,* or increased sensibility of various tissues. The fleshy portions of the muscles are very liable to become so affected. This is particularly the case with the muscles of the frontal and temporal regions of the cranium; with those of the epigastric region, often in association with dyspepsia; with those of the back, especially on the lower part and left side of the vertebral column, sometimes leading to the erroneous opinion that there is spinal disease; with those of the side of the thorax, especially the left, giving rise to symptoms likely to be confounded with the suffering produced by pleurisy or intercostal neuralgia; also with those of the walls of the abdomen, the pain of which can hardly be mistaken for that of metritis or ovaritis if its superficial character be observed; and, lastly, with the superficial and perhaps the deep-seated muscles of the upper and lower extremities. The pain is generally aggravated by pressure, by movement, by moral emotion, and by even a mild electric current; while it is relieved by resting the affected muscles. Moreover, it varies in intensity from mere uneasiness causing slight inconveniences, to the most acute suffering destroying all repose and inducing fever with general disturbance; and it is generally accompanied by weakness and mental depression. There is none of the heat, redness, tension, or pulsation of inflammation; and the pain may disappear for a time, soon to return in an aggravated form, and to prove very rebellious to all kinds of treatment.

The opposite condition of *anæsthesia*, or loss of sensibility, is a prominent phenomenon in some instances; and it is probable that nervous women and magnetic somnambulists, whose insensibility is supposed to be a trick, are often merely hysterical women thus affected. The anæsthesia may be only temporary, or it may last for years; the skin being most commonly affected. The left side of the body also suffers more often than the right; while the conjunctiva is frequently insensible, especially that of the left eye. The muscles of the extremities may be rendered so devoid of sensibility, that pins and needles can be thrust into their substance without causing the least manifestation of pain.

In some chlorotic and hysterical subjects the appetite for food becomes diseased, and the most improper and indigestible substances will be eaten. Occasionally, the appetite is preternaturally diminished; and weak girls, wishing to make themselves objects of pity and wonder, will pretend to subsist without any nourishment at all. Allied to these cases are those where young women thrust needles into various parts of their bodies, or produce ulcers by pressure, or pass various substances into the vagina, or resort to other means to excite the compassion of their relatives.

Although *hysteria may simulate almost every disease* in our nosology, yet there are certain favourite maladies for imitation. The most common seem to be,—suppression of urine, calculus of the bladder, inflammation of the peritoneum, pleurisy, consumption, laryngitis, stricture of the œsophagus, aphonia or loss of voice, paralysis, and disease of the spine or of one or more of the joints. Hysterical cough, dyspnœa, sneezing, yawning, panting, sighing, sobbing, or wearying hiccup may be continuous for hours, or even days; until, indeed, considerable exhaustion sets in. In all forms, the individual deceives herself and tries by strong expressions of suffering to mislead others. A practised eye is seldom, however, long imposed upon by such patients; although undoubtedly cases are met with, and especially among the upper classes of society, where the diagnosis is surrounded with difficulty. There is a peculiar expression about hysterical women impossible almost to define, yet readily recognised when once it has been studied. Moreover, there is a fulness of the upper lip, and a tendency to drooping of the upper eyelids; the self-tormentors answer questions in an unpleasant manner, often only in whispers and monosyllables; and their pains are always said to be most acute, and to be increased by pressure, or almost even by pretended pressure. The catamenia are generally irregular, and there is frequently profuse leucorrhœa.

And here the important question may be asked,—Are these pains and sufferings, described as being so acute, simply feigned? Is the patient merely playing at disease or shamming? There can be no hesitation in replying,—Undoubtedly not. Of course, exceptions to this rule are to be met with; but, speaking generally, the hysterical woman believes herself to be grievously afflicted. Her sensibility is undoubtedly altered,—perhaps exalted, perhaps depressed. Her will for good ends seems almost powerless, and only to be roused by some strong emotion. The intelligence is much more commonly above than below that of average women, while often there is great ability and acuteness. Yet with all this, many valuable years may be wasted, owing to a long series of morbid feelings. Sir Henry Holland has well observed that the hypochondriac, by fixing his consciousness with morbid intentness on different organs, not merely creates disordered sensations in them, but even disordered actions. Examples of such can easily be called to mind. Thus there may be palpitation of the heart, hurried or choked respiration, flatulence and other diseases of the stomach, irritation of the bladder, and vague neuralgic pains, all arising from this morbid direction of attention to the organs in question. It is also certain that many of the secretions are immediately affected by mental emotions; and the same results ensue from simple sustained attention to the parts concerned in these functions.

Under the name of "The Bed Case," Dr. Walter Channing has described a peculiar affection which I cannot but regard as a not uncommon form of hysteria.* The subjects of it live in bed; they are tranquil, cheerful, have good digestions, and like the kind attentions showered upon them by sympathizing friends. They are often firmly impressed with the belief that there is serious disease in the spine, or in the womb; and there are generally certain movements which they think cannot be made without "horrible" pain. Menstruation is frequently attended with suffering, and there is vaginal or uterine leucorrhœa. Amongst the seven or eight examples of this pseudo-disease which have come under my observation, the most marked was that of a single lady, thirty four-years of age, who first consulted me in 1861. This patient had then been confined to her room, and almost to her bed for ten years. She had been treated for spinal disease by some practitioners, and for irritable uterus by others. Of course, she had taken large quantities of medicine; while leeches, blisters, setons, &c., had been freely used. The recumbent posture had been maintained because of the pain (it was said to be "agony") caused by sitting up, and not for any supposed paralytic condition. On examination I found every part of her body healthy with the exception of the uterus, which was retroflexed. By replacing this organ, and by the use of galvanism to the long inactive muscles, a cure was effected; but the greatest patience was needed to get her from her bed to the sofa, from the sofa to the chair, from the chair to crutches, and so on until at the end of three months she could walk out in the open air. Some of these cases can be cured in a much shorter time; so that every now and then the public is gratified by hearing of some wonderful empiric, who has restored a case of paralysis to health simply by the command—"Rise up and walk." As, however, each example of hysteria varies in regard to important mental peculiarities, so there is no one remedy

* *Bed Case: its History and Treatment.* Boston, 1860.

applicable to all.   Frequently too, caution is needed lest the patient should determine not to get well.*

Treatment.—During a paroxysm the patient's dress is to be loosened; she must be prevented from injuring herself; and she should be surrounded by cool air. Smelling salts may also be applied to the nostrils; while if she can swallow, a draught containing a drachm of the ammoniated tincture of valerian, or of the

---

* The reader will find a good example of this variety of hysteria in Mrs. Oliphant's *Life of Edward Irving*, vol. ii. Appendix A. London, 1862. The patient describes her cure in a letter to a friend, the principal points in which are the following. She says,—"My dear Christian Friend,—I received yours of the 22nd on Friday last, and take up my pen with pleasure to inform you of the particulars of the Lord's gracious dealings with me. . . . . . I transcribe you a copy of facts, which by the wish of my dearest Father I have written out for the perusal of our Christian friends: it is a plain detail of facts from the commencement of my illness. In the month of November 1822, having for some months been in a bad state of health. it pleased God to visit me with a hip disease. Perfect rest was recommended by the late Mr. Pearson of Golden-square. . . . . This was the last application; and in September 1828, I returned home as unable to walk as when leaving: once or twice the attempt was made, but produced much pain. From this time no means have been used excepting constant confinement to the couch. Within these few weeks, even on the very day in which Jesus so manifested His Almighty power, I had attempted to walk; scarcely could I put one foot before the other, the limbs trembled very much. Thus it continued till the 20th October 1830, when a kind friend, who had seen me about two months before, had been led by God to pray earnestly for my recovery. . . . Sitting near me, we talked of his relatives and of the death of his brother. . . . . . After asking some questions respecting the disease, he added,—'It is melancholy to see a person so constantly confined.' I answered, 'It is sent in mercy.' 'Do you think so?' Do you think the same mercy could restore you?' God gave me faith, and I answered, 'Yes.' 'Do you believe Jesus could heal, as in old times?' 'Yes.' 'Do you believe that it is only unbelief that prevents it?' 'Yes.' 'Do you believe that Jesus could heal you at this very time?' 'Yes.' (Between these questions he was evidently engaged in prayer.) 'Then,' he added, 'get up and walk to your family.' He then had hold of my hand. He prayed to God to glorify the name of Jesus. I rose from my couch quite strong. God took away all my pains, and we walked down stairs. Dear Mr. G. prayed most fervently, 'Lord have mercy upon us! Christ have mercy upon us!' Having been down a short time, finding my handkerchief left on the couch, taking the candle I fetched it. The next day I walked more than a quarter of a mile, and on Sunday from the Episcopal Jew's Chapel, a distance of one mile and a quarter. . . . . It is material to add that my legs, the flesh of which was loose and flabby, feeling them in a short time after I walked down, were firm as those of a person in full health. The back, which was curved, is now perfectly straight. My collarbones have been pronounced by a surgeon to be in quite a natural state, whereas one of them was before much enlarged. I must tell you that my mind had not been at all occupied with those events which had taken place in Scotland; indeed, all I had heard concerning them was that a young person had been restored in answer to prayer: this was, perhaps, five or six months back. I had heard of nothing since, and can with truth say my mind had never been led to the contemplation of such subjects. I had not the least idea that my dear friend was offering up prayer in my behalf, for he did not say so till after the mighty work was wrought. . . . . . ELIZABETH FANCOURT."

fetid spirit of ammonia, can frequently be administered with benefit. When the apparent insensibility continues, the sudden and free application of cold water to the head and face will probably cut it short. Many a " fit-case," carried into the hospital on a stretcher, may have the use of her limbs (and the tongue also) immediately restored, by holding her head under the water-tap for a few seconds. ⟨U ⋀⋅⋅⋅ ⋅⋅ ⋅⋅⋅ ⋅⋅ ⋅⋅

In the other forms of hysteria the general health must be attended to, the bowels kept freely open, the plunge or sponge or shower bath daily used, and ferruginous tonics administered where there is a state of anæmia. When the catamenia are unnatural, the treatment must have reference to the nature of the particular disorder. Thus if too abundant, astringents and the cold hip bath, to the water of which alum or bay-salt should be added, ought to be employed : if scanty, the flow should be encouraged by aloetic purgatives, different preparations of iron with small doses of strychnia, and the warm bath. The compound decoction of aloes and the compound iron mixture—half an ounce of each—taken twice or thrice daily, will form an excellent medicine in such cases ; especially if a pill made of four grains of the compound assafœtida pill and a quarter of a grain of extract of nux vomica, be given with each dose. For hysterical aphonia, galvanism is often very useful. A mild induced current of galvanic electricity should be applied by means of moistened conductors; the poles being directed partially to the inferior laryngeal nerve, and partially over the crico-thyroid muscle since it plays an important part in the formation of the voice. In hyperæsthesia of the muscles, hot cataplasms, iodine liniment, warm baths, and a mild electric current, are the means to be tried; while in anæsthesia a cure can often be effected, by making a stronger current of electricity traverse the insensible muscles daily for some ten or fifteen minutes at a time. As in other cases of hysteria, so in these varieties, one or more of the preparations of assafœtida (F. 86, 89), of valerian (F. 87, 93), of zinc (F. 410), of quinine (F. 379, 411), of steel (F. 380, 394, 401), or of phosphorus (F. 405, 417, 419), &c., will every now and then be found serviceable. But it is a great mistake, on the other hand, to prescribe nauseous drugs as a matter of routine. In many instances more good will be done without than with physic ; provided the physician is sufficiently painstaking, and has sufficient sympathy with his patient to try and guide her aright.

The patient's diet should be regulated ; nourishing food being necessary, milk or cocoa displacing tea and coffee, and often a moderate quantity of wine or beer being allowed. Hot rooms and evening parties are to be proscribed ; stays can sometimes be advantageously dispenséd with, the spinal muscles being strengthened by bathing and friction ; while daily exercise is to be taken in the open air. And then, lastly, it is of the greatest importance that while the value of self-control is inculcated, healthy mental occupation and recreation should be afforded. Indeed without these latter, a permanent cure is not to be expected; for amongst the most frequent causes of hysterical affections we must count the want of proper employment for the mind and bodily energy.

XV. CATALEPSY.—ECSTACY.

These wonderful diseases are very rare, but they undoubtedly do happen occasionally. Nervous and hysterical women are most likely to suffer from them. They are not dangerous; although repeated attacks impair the intellect. They more frequently have their origin in strong mental emotion, than from any other source.

By a fit of *catalepsy* [Καταλαμβάνω = to restrain, or hold firmly] is implied a more or less complete suppression of sensation and volition; the patient remaining rigid during the attack, and in the same position in which she happens to be at the commencement, or in which she may be placed during its continuance. The seizure may last only a few minutes, or several hours, or even one or two days. On recovery, which is generally instantaneous and as if from a deep sleep, there may be momentary surprise and embarrassment but no recollection of what has occurred. Very rarely these cases terminate in apoplexy or insanity; or they may be connected with chronic softening, or with tumour of the brain.

"Absence of mind" is a slight form of catalepsy. Dr. Laycock well remarks, that "in *brown study* or reverie, the eye is fixed by a muscular action analogous to the cataleptic; and not the eye only, for a limb, or the whole body, will remain in the same position for many minutes, the senses themselves being in deep abstraction from surrounding objects."* With some individuals a cataleptic state may be induced by strongly fixing the attention on one object for a short time. The mental faculties get tired; there is diminished nervous influence or force; and persons so affected then believe that they are unable to move, cannot see, &c., until the so-called *mesmeriser* grants them permission. Examples of this state are also seen in animals,—as in birds and rabbits *fascinated* by the glaring eyes of the serpent.

Owing to the death-like condition which this disease may produce, cataleptics have been buried alive. Such an occurrence is scarcely likely to occur in our own country, where an interval of five or six days is allowed to elapse between death and interment.

An interesting report of a well-marked case of catalepsy, which was admitted into St. George's Hospital, has been published by Mr. Thomas Jones.† The patient was a male, aged 60, who for a

* *A Treatise on the Nervous Diseases of Women,* p. 316. London, 1840.
† *British Medical Journal,* p. 585. 6 June 1863.

fortnight had experienced much mental suffering owing to the sudden death of his wife.   He was always very excitable, but his previous health had been good.   Two or three days before the attack there were hallucinations of vision and hearing.   Then, while engaged in plastering, he became suddenly seized with tetanic rigidity of all the muscles, which caused him to be fixed in the position he was in at the moment.   Subsequently the limbs retained any position in which they were placed ; there was partial loss of consciousness ; and the duration of the fit was twenty-two hours.   The recovery was good.

An account of an endemic cataleptic disorder prevalent at Billingshausen, near Würzburg, has been published by Dr. Vogt.*   The population consists of 356 individuals, who are Protestants although living among Catholic neighbours.   They are small, feeble, and plain-featured.   "There is no poverty—the poorest man in the place is the minister."   About half the inhabitants, males as well as females, are affected ; being known as the *starren* (stiffened ones).   Without any premonitory symptoms, the patient suddenly falls down.   The aspect becomes death-like, the face pale, the eyes fixedly directed to one point with their axes converging, the lips closed and protruded, and the fingers semiflexed.   Attempts to speak result in short and unintelligible sounds.   The muscular system is alone affected : the senses and intellect remain uninterfered with.   The attack lasts from one to five minutes ; and its occurrence appears to be favoured by cold.   The long-prevailing system of intermarriages may be the cause.

Such of the Abyssinian unmarried women as lead dissolute and irregular lives are said to be especially liable to two diseases—the *Bouda* and *Zar*.   The former shows itself by a series of severe paroxysms of a cataleptic character.   The latter is evidently a variety of hysteria ; and according to the Rev. H. A. Stern it has this peculiar feature, that during the violence of the attack the patient imitates the sharp and discordant growl of the leopard.   "To expel the *Zar*, a conjuror, as in the *Bouda* complaint, was formerly considered indispensable ; but by dint of perseverance, the medical faculty of the country, to their infinite satisfaction, have at length made the happy discovery that a sound application of the whip is quite as potent an antidote against this evil as the necromancer's spell."†

In what is termed *ecstacy* ["Εκστασις, from 'Εξίστημι = to put a person out of his natural state] the condition is of an analogous kind. The patient is insensible to all external impressions, but is absorbed in the contemplation of some imaginary object.   The eyes are im-

---

* *Würzburger Medicinische Zeitschrift*, Band iv. p. 163.   1863.—*Half-Yearly Abstract of the Medical Sciences*, vol. xxxix, p. 81.   London, 1864.
† *Wanderings among the Falashas in Abyssinia*, p. 160.   By the Rev. Henry A. Stern.   London, 1862.

movably fixed; but impassioned sentences, fervent prayers, psalms and hymns are uttered or sung with great expression. The religious fanatic, by encouraging some predominant idea, falls into a state resembling the incipient stage of monomania. The "gift of unknown tongues" was mostly manifested by nervous women; who were not impostors, but simply diseased. Faith, imagination, perverted religious enthusiasm, erotic excitement, and an irresistible propensity to imitation, will explain the case of the convulsionaries of St. Medard over the grave of the Abbé Pâris. And so also with the victims of tarantism, the dancing mania, &c.

A similar plan of *treatment* to that recommended in hysteria must be relied upon for the repression of these emotional disorders. Remembering that most kinds of enthusiasm are contagious, it is usually advisable to isolate those that are afflicted. This advice should be particularly acted upon in the case of young persons at school.

XVI. CHOREA.

Chorea [Χορεία = a dancing or jumping; from Χορὸς = a dance accompanied with singing], or St. Vitus's dance, is characterized by irregular, tremulous, and often ludicrous actions of the voluntary muscles, especially of those of the face and limbs; there being incomplete subserviency of the muscles of this class to the will. In consequence of these jerking movements the disease has been quaintly designated "insanity of the muscles."

Causes, &c.—Chorea may last from one week to several months; the average duration in uncomplicated cases, under the use of tonics and good food, being about four weeks. It is often complicated with hysteria. The general health is usually below the normal standard from the commencement; while it deteriorates more and more as the disease gains ground. Fright appears to be the most frequent cause; blows or falls seem sometimes to have induced it; and the occurrence of the disease from irregular dentition, or from the irritation of intestinal worms, has long been noticed. It has by some, moreover, been attributed to onanism; while deranged uterine function is occasionally the apparent cause. Some of the worst cases that have been recorded have occurred during gestation, especially in women pregnant for the first time. I believe, too, that the children of nervous and hysterical women are more likely to be afflicted by it than others. Although most common in girls, yet boys from eight to sixteen years old not unfrequently suffer from it. The deaths from chorea registered in England in 1866 were $\frac{\text{Males } 20}{\text{Females } 43} = 63$; of which number 36 were above five years of age and under twenty.

Symptoms.—This disorder occurs most frequently in young girls between the age of six and sixteen; while it may be either of a mild or severe type. It begins generally with occasional clonic spasms of the muscles of the face; which somewhat distort the features so that the child seems to be making slight grimaces for fun or mischief. By degrees, all or almost all the voluntary muscles become affected. The child finds it almost impossible to keep quiet, though the movements are to some extent under the control of the will; while there is a constant restlessness of the hands and arms, and even of the legs. One half of the body is generally more affected than the other; while in a few cases the movements are entirely confined to one side—*hemichorea*. Moreover, the twistings and contortions of the features become more constant and distressing; the articulation gets impeded, so that the speech is indistinct; while all the shifting motions are most severe when the child is conscious of being watched. If the patient be asked to put out her tongue, she is unable to do so for some moments; but at last suddenly thrusts it out, and as suddenly withdraws it. If she be told to walk, she advances in a jumping manner, by fits and starts, dragging her leg rather than lifting it, and alternately halting and hopping. She cannot even sit still : her shoulders writhe about, she picks her dress, and shuffles or scrapes the floor with her feet. During sleep these irregular actions almost invariably cease. The disease must be present in a very severe form indeed, for it to prove an exception to this rule. All the time these symptoms are steadily progressing, the general health fails. The circulation becomes languid, as is evidenced by the cold hands and feet, and the liability to chilblains; while the blood gets poor as is shown by the pallor of the surface, and the puffiness about the ankles.

Supposing this disorder runs its course still further, endocarditis or pericarditis may supervene. Sometimes there is merely functional disturbance of the heart, with an anæmic murmur audible at the base. In other instances a loud bruit is detected at the apex; the origin of which has by several observers been thought to be due to choreic contractions of the musculi papillares, causing valvular imperfection and regurgitation. This explanation if correct, which it probably is not, can only apply to some cases; since the murmur not unfrequently remains permanent.

When an attack of chorea is of long continuance, the memory gets impaired, and the temper irritable; while often the countenance assumes a vacant appearance bordering on fatuity, and some imbecility of mind becomes manifest. The functions of the stomach and bowels are also frequently deranged; the appetite is irregular; the abdomen is swollen and hard; and there is often constipation. The urine is of high specific gravity, especially when the choreic movements are very active; a condition due, according to Dr. Todd, to the increased waste of tissue consequent on the disturbed state of the muscles and nerves. There is also very commonly an excess of urates; while now and then sugar has been detected. As the case gradually improves, the specific gravity of the urine diminishes. Moreover, all the symptoms cease on the termination of the disease; which is seldom fatal, or even dangerous, unless it merges into organic disease of the nervous centres, or of the heart, or into epilepsy.

Pathology.—As the appearances found after death are usually slight and by no means uniform, physicians have not agreed as to the pathology of chorea. Several observers regard it as a disease the essence of which is perverted nervous function. Others believe that the blood is primarily affected. There seems to be some obscure connexion between chorea and rheumatism; the latter disorder occasionally preceding the former, now and then accompanying it, sometimes following it, and perhaps even alternating with it. Numerous cases have been recorded in which morbid conditions of the heart and pericardium, of a rheumatic as well as of a non-rheumatic character, have given rise to choreic symptoms. Hence the latter have been supposed, by some authorities, to be produced through the irritation of the spinal cord by minute embolic particles which have been washed off the valves of a rheumatic heart. According to Dr. Hughlings Jackson it is probable that chorea occurs frequently from embolism of the minute vessels supplying the corpus striatum and neighbouring convolutions; the mechanical interference with the blood-supply causing an excitable ill-nourished nerve-tissue. In some instances of fatal chorea, the brain has been found congested; in others, there has been serous effusion under the arachnoid and into the ventricles; while in others again, a softened state of a portion of the brain, or of the spinal cord, or of both, has been detected. Moreover, occasionally the disorder would seem to have been connected with symptoms of mental imbecility.

Treatment.—Where medical treatment is called for, the only plan to be recommended consists in regulating the bowels, subduing irritation, and strengthening the system. For this purpose, the employment of cathartics of a stimulating nature is usually necessary, such as calomel and jalap; or, where worms are suspected, the oil of turpentine. A combination of tonic or antispasmodic medicines with purgatives, is often found to be serviceable. The three great remedies, however, are the tepid shower or douche bath, steel, and plenty of good nourishing food. As regards the bath, it should be employed every morning on the patient's rising; the temperature of the water varying with the season, and the reaction produced. Occasionally, a warm sulphur bath three or four times a week is to be preferred to the foregoing. With respect to the steel, different preparations have been recommended. Perhaps one of the best is the saccharated carbonate of iron, given in doses varying from five to twenty grains, mixed with treacle. The syrup of the iodide, or the ammonio-citrate, or the tincture of the perchloride of iron may, however, be used almost as advantageously. The combination of steel and arsenic (F. 399), or of steel and zinc (F. 414), or of steel and phosphate of lime, &c. (Chemical Food, F. 405) is to be preferred in some cases; especially in such as are of a severe and obstinate character. Cod liver oil is generally useful, administered simultaneously with tonics. Arsenic alone will sometimes effect a cure where steel fails (F. 52); and so will the sulphate or phosphate of zinc. I have likewise found much benefit in certain well-marked cases from the hypophosphite of soda or lime with bark (F. 419). The diet must be nutritious, with plenty of milk, and a proper allowance of claret or port or tokay or beer; exercise in the fresh air is to be freely allowed; and while amusement or occupation does good, yet mental excitement ought to be guarded against.

Where the choreic movements are so violent as to be the cause of exhaustion and continued sleeplessness, the aspect of affairs gets more alarming. Under these circumstances, opium is useless. It may be given until the pupils are contracted to the size of a pin's point, without lessening the irregular movements. Indeed, some of the most violent cases I have seen, have been those where this drug has been employed. The action of henbane is sometimes favourable, provided it be given in sufficient doses (from two fluid drachms to half an ounce of the tincture, for adults). Belladonna does good, particularly in combination with the henbane. Conium is also a valuable remedy; the officinal juice being the best preparation. The extract of Calabar bean in doses varying from $\frac{1}{18}$ to $\frac{1}{4}$ grain, every three or four hours, may be tried. These failing, the patient had better be put to sleep by some anæsthetic; a mixture of pure chloroform and ether (F. 313) being decidedly the best. The sleep will often be prolonged and rendered more refreshing by giving from ten to forty or sixty minims of the spirit of ether, in camphor water, by the mouth, just before the inhalation.

A choreic child should hardly be allowed to mix very freely with other children. For in the first place, it is cruel to expose the infirmity; and secondly, the effects of the principle of imitation are so remarkable in the young, that the disease may spread to the healthy. Falstaff's words have a wider application than he intended. "It is certain," says Sir John, "that either wise bearing, or ignorant carriage, is caught, as men take diseases, one of another: therefore, let men take heed of their company."

The employment of gymnastic exercises has been strongly recommended. In a memoir submitted to the French Academy of Sciences, M. Blache states, that he has treated by these exercises alone, or by these in combination with other measures, such as sulphur baths, 108 patients—84 girls and 24 boys. In 102 the cure was completed, on an average, in 39 days; in the remaining six, in 122 days. These figures prove very little; inasmuch as numerous cases can be cured in five or six weeks by moral control and nourishing food, without any other treatment whatever. Nevertheless, a system of gymnastics or of drilling may often be made supplementary to the tonic and other remedies with considerable advantage.

When chorea occurs during pregnancy it is sometimes so violent (especially in primiparous women) that the intellect becomes affected and the patient's life greatly endangered. To preserve the latter it may be necessary to induce abortion; taking care not to postpone this proceeding until the exhaustion is so great as to allow of little hope of restoration.

XVII. TETANUS.

The term Tetanus [Τείνω = to bend, or strain] is used to denote an acute disease, the principal feature of which is a long-continued and painful contraction or spasm of a certain number of the voluntary muscles. The rigidity of the muscles being continuous, we say that there is *tonic spasm* or *spastic contraction;* these terms being employed in contradistinction to the *clonic spasms* of convulsions, in which there is a state of alternate contraction and relaxation.

The *causes* of tetanus are chiefly exposure to cold and damp, and bodily injuries—particularly lacerated wounds. Foreign bodies in wounds such as bullets &c., pus confined under fasciæ, and sudden vicissitudes of temperature, are powerful causes. When due to cold, or when arising spontaneously it is termed *idiopathic;* when the result of wounds, *traumatic* tetanus. In idiopathic tetanus recovery may be hoped for; while in the traumatic form almost every case proves fatal. Taking both varieties into the calculation, it may be said that death is most likely to occur between the third and fifth days of the disease.

During the late American war the cases of traumatic tetanus which occurred look rather numerous in proportion to the total number of the wounded. On the registers, revised up to the 30 September 1865, it is shown that there are included 363 examples of tetanus in 87,822 cases of gunshot wounds and other injuries.* Of the 363 reported cases, 336 ended fatally; while the disease was of a chronic form in 23 out of the 27 recoveries. The majority of the patients were treated by the free use of opium, with stimulants and concentrated nourishment. Chloroform inhalations, subcutaneous injections of morphia and atropia, cathartics, quinine, cannabis indica, bromide of potassium, strychnia, belladonna, aconite, blisters, ice to the spine, and turpentine stupes were also among the remedies employed. The value of nicotine, curara, and the Calabar bean was not tested. This is to be regretted, as according to Demme, out of 22 cases of traumatic tetanus treated by curara 8 recovered.

The *symptoms* usually set in suddenly, the muscles of the jaws

* *Reports on the Extent and Nature of the Materials available for the preparation of a Medical and Surgical History of the Rebellion.* Circular No. 6, pp. 6 and 41. Philadelphia, 1865.

and throat being commonly the first affected. The patient complains that he has taken cold, and says that he feels as if he had got a sore throat and stiff neck ; but the stiffness and uneasiness soon increase, and extend to the root of the tongue causing difficulty in swallowing. The temporal and masseter muscles gradually get involved, and *locked-jaw* or *trismus* [Τρίζω = to gnash with the teeth] occurs. When the disease proceeds, the remaining muscles of the face, those of the trunk, and lastly those of the extremities, become implicated. The spasm never entirely ceases, except in some cases during sleep; but it is aggravated every quarter of an hour or so, the increased cramp lasting for a few minutes, and then partially subsiding. Where the strong muscles of the back are most affected, they bend the body into the shape of an arch, so that the patient rests upon his head and heels, a condition known as *opisthotonos* ["Οπισθε = backwards + τείνω = to bend]. When, on the contrary, the body is bent forwards by the strong contraction of the muscles of the neck and abdomen, the affection is termed *emprosthotonos* ["Εμπροσθεν = forwards + τείνω]. Again, if the muscles are affected laterally, so that the body is curved sideways, this state has been designated *pleurosthotonos* [Πλευρόθεν = from the side + τείνω], or *tetanus lateralis.* The symptoms produced by a poisonous dose of strychnia resemble those caused by tetanus.

The suffering caused by the tetanic spasms is absolutely frightful to contemplate. The face becomes deadly pale, and the brows get contracted ; the skin covering the forehead is corrugated ; the eyes are fixed and prominent—sometimes suffused with tears ; while the nostrils are dilated, the corners of the mouth drawn back, the teeth exposed, and the features fixed in a sort of grin— the *risus sardonicus.* The respirations are performed with difficulty and anguish ; severe pain is felt at the sternum ; and there is great thirst, but the agony is increased by attempts at deglutition. The pulse, too, is feeble and frequent ; the skin is covered with perspiration ; and the patient cannot sleep, or if he dozes it is only for a few minutes at a time. Yet with all this suffering, the intellect remains clear and unaffected. Death at length ends the agony, the release being due partly to suffocation and partly to exhaustion.

There is a peculiar form of this affection called *Trismus nascentium,* that occurs in young infants about the second week after birth, and which is very fatal. It is exceedingly rare in this country ; though some eighty years since, when the Dublin Lying-in Hospital was badly ventilated, it proved one of the most prominent causes of the infantile mortality in that institution. Tetanus infantum is still common in the West Indies, where it sometimes seems to rage as an epidemic. When prevalent, great care ought to be taken to guard the new-born child from cold or foul air, improper feeding, imperfect cleansing, and from retention of the meconium ; while attention should also be paid to prevent improper management of the remains of the umbilical cord by the nurse.

In dividing the funis at birth, not more than two inches should be left attached to the umbilicus.

With regard to the *morbid anatomy* of tetanus very little that is certain is as yet known.   Mr. J. Lockhart Clarke in describing the condition of the spinal cords in six cases, says that in every one there was more or less congestion of the bloodvessels; together with definite, and frequently extensive, lesions of structure. These lesions consisted of disintegrations of tissue in different stages of progress, from a state of mere softening to one of perfect fluidity; accompanied by certain exudations and extensive effusions of blood.   They were found chiefly in the gray substance; which was, moreover, in many places, strangely altered in shape—unsymmetrical on the opposite sides, or partially fused with the adjacent white column in a common softened mass.   Although lesions of this kind existed in one form or other in every region of the cord, they were absent in some places; nor did they ever for long together maintain the same size or appearance, but were constantly and alternately increasing or disappearing at short intervals. These lesions in tetanus are similar in character to those which Mr. Lockhart Clarke has discovered in the spinal cords of many cases of paralysis in which there has been no spasm.   Hence it follows that the former disease, in regard to its morbid anatomy, differs from the latter only in being associated with a morbid condition or injury of some of the peripheral nerves.   " It would therefore appear that this condition or injury of the peripheral nerves is the determining cause of the phenomena, and that the spasms of tetanus depend on the conjoint operation of two separate causes.   First, on an abnormally excitable state of the grey nerve-tissue of the cord, induced by the hyperæmic and morbid state of its bloodvessels, with the exudations and disintegrations resulting therefrom.   This state of the cord may be either an extension of a similar state along the injured nerves from the periphery, or may result from reflex action on its bloodvessels excited by those nerves.   Secondly, that the spasms depend on the persistent irritation of the peripheral nerves, by which the exalted excitability of the cord is aroused; and thus the cause which at first induced in the cord its morbid susceptibility to reflex action is the same which is subsequently the source of that irritation by which the reflex action is excited."*

The *treatment* is commonly empirical, and generally—it must be confessed—useless.   Since the publication of the fifth edition of this work, however, some very encouraging success has followed the employment of the ordeal bean of Calabar.   The officinal extractum physostigmatis is the best preparation for use; the dose varying from $\frac{1}{16}$ to $\frac{1}{4}$ grain for ordinary purposes.   But in the disease under consideration much larger quantities are needed; and at least one-fourth of a grain should be given every hour until an effect is produced.   If injected subcutaneously, the dose may

* *Medico-Chirurgical Transactions*, vol. xlviii. p. 263.   London, 1865.

consist of one-third of a grain in eight or ten minims of water, every two or three hours. Directly there is any feeling of sinking, stimulants and essence of beef must be given.

The Calabar bean failing, or not being indicated in any particular case, what is to be done? There are four remedies on which, it seems to me, some little reliance can be placed—viz., belladonna, chloroform, quinine, and wine. Opium has never been found to do any good; and it is now rendered probable that the use of it is objectionable, since this drug produces a state of congestion and polar excitement of the spinal cord somewhat similar to that caused by strychnine. Opium is known to contract the unstriped muscular fibre of the sphincter of the pupil, and perhaps also some of the voluntary or striped muscles of other parts. Belladonna and tobacco, and less powerfully henbane and hemlock, dilate the pupil and relax the voluntary muscles. Belladonna may be applied to the spine locally, smearing the extract well over this part; while it can also be administered internally, in doses of half a grain or one grain with two grains of quinine every four hours. The patient might also be kept under the influence of chloroform for very many hours: indeed I would not mind trying its use for one or more entire days, provided no symptoms (such as a failing pulse) to forbid it, arose during its operation. Under the influence of this anæsthetic the pulse falls to its natural standard, the respiration becomes easy, and all indication of suffering subsides; but as soon as the remedy is suspended, the fatal symptoms again begin to show themselves. With regard to quinine, from three to five grains may be given every four or six hours, either by the mouth or rectum or subcutaneously.

Considering that the action of woorara is antagonistic to the effects of the artificial tetanus of strychnia, it was hoped that this agent might prove useful in traumatic and idiopathic tetanus. It has now been used by inoculation in several cases; but the result, on the whole, has been unfavourable. Mr. Spencer Wells has suggested that, as the specimens of the extract brought to this country vary in strength, in future trials it would be as well to use a solution of the active principle of woorara—the alkaloid curarina. Further experiments are perhaps desirable before giving up this medicine. Again, a severe example of traumatic tetanus was successfully treated with nicotine by Mr. Tufnell in March 1862. Fifty-six drops (one or two for each dose) were administered in six days; each drop being equivalent to 23·3 grains of Virginian Cavendish tobacco. The Rev. Professor Haughton had previously met with successful cases from the employment of this agent.

There are a few other points worthy of recollection. Thus, if deglutition be difficult, enemata must be used. The inhalation of pure oxygen gas, diluted with about three times its volume of air, will often afford relief and prove agreeable to the patient's feelings (F. 370). Any bronchial irritation which may be produced by the gas will cease on discontinuing its use. I should also be inclined to try the prolonged application of ice to the spine.   Some practitioners recommend the frequent use of the warm bath, while others prefer the cold douche ; but neither appears to have been of much utility.   A few authorities have faith in conium when applied locally and taken internally ; while cures have followed the exhibition of aconite.   Remembering the supposed toxic origin of the disease, it might be worth while to see the effect of the sulphite of soda or magnesia (F. 48), other remedies failing.   Purgatives will generally be necessary ; full doses of calomel and jalap, repeated until the bowels have been thoroughly evacuated, being as efficient as any other medicine of the class of aperients.   Finally, it may save valuable time to remember that bloodletting, blisters, mercury, antimony, colchicum, large doses of assafœtida, turpentine, digitalis, musk, iron, hydrocyanic acid, and the extract of Indian hemp, have all been repeatedly employed, and as often caused disappointment.

XVIII. SLEEP AND SLEEPLESSNESS.

The necessity for *sleep* is apparent in all animals.   In the very young, while the functions of nutrition are most active and the waste of the system is small, the whole time is occupied in eating and sleeping.   During adult life, about one-third of the twenty-four hours is passed in repose.   In old age, when the nutritive operations are carried on with less vigour, more sleep is needed, to allow of the system being spared as much as possible.

Sleep may be said to be especially the rest of the nervous centres.   Repose is necessary for repair and nutrition.   Not that these processes occur only during sleep, but for their perfection sleep is required.   Sleep, in short, aids all those processes by which the nutrition of the different organs is effected.   Even in the heart's action there is a period of repose.   It is true that the rest after each pulsation is short ; but the total amount in the twenty-four hours becomes considerable.   In the same way if we analyse the act of respiration and separate it into three portions, one will be seen to be devoted to inspiration, one to expiration, and the third to a pause.   Hence, during eight hours of the twenty-four the muscles of the thorax and the lungs are in a state of rest.

Sleep is preceded by a softly approaching languor and welcome drowsiness ; during which the emotions and mental sensations are gradually lulled into forgetfulness.   The eyelids become heavy and droop ; and then little by little the senses of sight, hearing, and touch fail in succession.   With the limbs semiflexed and yielding to lassitude, the voluntary movements cease.   The eyes are turned upward, the pupils are contracted, the respiration and circulation get slow, consciousness has become imperceptibly abolished, and there is deep calm sleep.   From the time of this occurring until complete awakening, there is seldom one continuous state of repose. There are unquestionably periods of more or less imperfect slumber, when movements are performed under the influence of external impressions. Thus we seldom awake in the same position in which sleep came on, though there may be no consciousness of any change having been made. According to Sir Henry Holland, sleep, " in the most general and correct sense of the term, must be regarded not as one single state, but a succession of states in constant variation :—this variation consisting, not only in different degrees in which the same sense or faculty is submitted to it, but also in the different proportions in which these several powers are under its influence at the same time."* Man requires about eight hours of sleep ; and should not, as a rule, have less, if he would duly repair the waste which has arisen from active occupation. Numerous individuals do with five or six hours, even for a considerable term ; but I am inclined to think that many such enjoy snatches of slumber at odd times which they fail to reckon. Students working for an examination will often restrict themselves to five hours nightly for a few weeks ; but they subsequently make up for the deficiency by passing nine and ten hours in bed for three or four weeks afterwards. Doubtless, however, habit and temperament control us much in this respect.

Many physiologists have thought that venous pressure upon the encephalon was the cause of sleep. But the evidence in favour of this hypothesis breaks down upon a close examination. It has been argued that because coma is undoubtedly the result of congestion and pressure, so sleep must own the same cause ; but the fact is that the two conditions are in no way identical. The general inactivity of the brain during slumber is better accounted for on the supposition that there is a withdrawal of blood from the cerebral tissues, rather than an increased quantity. Dr. Pierquin observed in 1821, in one of the hospitals of Montpelier, a female patient, part of whose skull and dura mater had been destroyed by disease. The brain was perfectly motionless when she was in a dreamless sleep. When slightly agitated by dreams, there was elevation of the brain : when the dreams were vivid, the brain protruded through the opening in the skull, forming a cerebral hernia. The same phenomena were seen when she was perfectly awake, if engaged in active thought or sprightly conversation. Blumenbach has also mentioned cases in which, portions of the skull having been lost, he witnessed a sinking of the brain during sleep and a swelling with blood when the patient awoke. Dr. Alexander Fleming, while preparing a lecture on the action of narcotics, conceived the idea of trying the effect of compressing the carotid arteries with the fingers, on the functions of the brain. In several experiments made on himself and others it was found, that complete unconsciousness continued so long as the pressure was kept up. " A soft humming in the ears is heard ; a sense of tingling steals

* *Chapters on Mental Physiology.* Second Edition, p. 15. London, 1858.

over the body, and in a few seconds complete unconsciousness and insensibility supervene, and continue so long as the pressure is maintained."[*] Dr. Fleming also adds that the period of profound sleep never lasted more than fifteen seconds, although these seconds seemed like hours. In order positively to determine the condition of the cerebral circulation during sleep, Mr. Durham resorted to an ingenious experiment.[†] A dog having been chloroformed, a portion of bone the size of a shilling was removed from the parietal region of the skull, and the subjacent dura mater partially cut away. The part of the brain thus exposed appeared inclined to protrude. The large veins over its surface were distended, and the smaller vessels of the pia mater seemed full of dark-coloured blood; while there was no appreciable difference in colour between the arteries and veins. The longer the exhibition of the chloroform was continued, the more distended did the veins become. But as the deep anæsthesia passed off, the animal fell into a comparatively natural sleep. As he did so, the surface of the brain became pale, and sank rather below the level of the bone; the veins were no longer distended; a few small vessels containing arterial blood could be seen; and many previously congested vessels were now hardly distinguishable. After a time the dog was roused; and then the brain again rose, the pia mater became more injected, the cerebral surface assumed a bright red colour, and the veins and arteries appeared full of blood. After feeding, the animal again was allowed to sleep: the bloodvessels resumed their former dimensions and appearance, and the surface of the brain became pale as before. From his experiments Mr. Durham concludes,—the pressure of distended veins on the brain is not the cause of sleep: during sleep the brain is comparatively bloodless, and the rapidity of the circulation diminished: the blood derived from the brain during sleep is distributed to the alimentary and execretory organs: whatever tends to increase the activity of the cerebral circulation favours wakefulness.

Dr. Parkes points out the difficulty of ascertaining the effect of sleep on the urine, owing to the impossibility of eliminating the effect of other influences. According to some observers sleep diminishes this excretion. But the result of experiments performed by Dr. Böcker on his own person has been to show that all the urinary ingredients are increased during slumber, with the exception of the uric acid, phosphoric acid, and the fireproof salts. The increase in the sulphuric acid was slight, that in the urea very great. The decrease in the uric acid was considerable, in the phosphoric acid very great. "This would seem to show,"

[*] *On the Induction of Sleep and Anæsthesia by compression of the Carotids.* "The British and Foreign Medico-Chirurgical Review," vol. xv. p. 529. London, 1855.
[†] *The Physiology of Sleep.* "Guy's Hospital Reports." Third Series, vol. vi. p. 153. London, 1860.

says Dr. Parkes, "that the disintegration of nervous tissue is lessened during sleep."[*]

Heat creates drowsiness, and severe cold does the same. A hearty meal generally predisposes to it. A morbid disposition to sleep is a symptom of imperfect nutrition and degeneration of nervous tissue. Such a tendency is often the precursor of apoplexy; or it may be due to renal disease, with imperfect elimination of urea; or it will arise from alcoholic intoxication; or it can be caused by anæmia generally. The circulation of imperfectly oxygenated blood through the brain also causes narcosis, as is seen in those diseases which interfere with the process of respiration. A remarkable example of prolonged sleep, probably owing to anæmia and faulty nutrition of brain, has been published by Dr. J. Ward Cousins. The chief points in the report are these :—J. C., a farmer, ætat. 44, has been subject at intervals during the last twenty years to attacks of deep and prolonged sleep. The disorder began in 1842, or 1843, after getting very wet and suffering from a severe cold, and continued nearly a year. It returned in 1848 after catching cold, and persisted for nearly eighteen months. He was then free until the commencement of a long attack on 19 May 1860; since which time he has not slept naturally. He retires to bed at night soon after ten o'clock, and almost immediately falls into a profound sleep, from which all attempts at rousing him have failed. His appearance remains natural while asleep; but his face and ears are pale, feet often cold and livid, respiration scarcely perceptible, pulse slow, and feeble, &c. He awakes suddenly, and always seems refreshed. The longest period he has ever passed in profound sleep is five days and five nights. He has frequently slept three and four days, but the average is nearly two days. He is awake about four or five hours out of the forty-eight. During these sleeps he does not dream; the contents of the bowel and bladder are always retained; and on awaking his first question is,—"How long have I slept?" Lately he has looked pale and lost flesh. In 1848 he suffered frequently from spasmodic trismus, but has not done so since.[†] At this point Dr. Cousins' connexion with the case seems to have ceased; and I am indebted to Dr. Gimson for having kindly favoured me with the subsequent history. The attacks of profound sleep continued to recur. Thus, from between 11 and 12 p.m. on 2 January 1866, J. C. slept until 2 p.m. on the 6th. At midnight on 4 February he went to sleep and did not wake until 4 p.m. on the 8th; going off again about 11 p.m., sleeping until the 11th, when he remained awake for nine

---

[*] The Composition of the Urine in Health and Disease, and under the Action of Remedies, p. 91. London, 1860.

[†] Medical Times and Gazette, p. 396. London, 18 April 1863. The same history is published by Dr. Gimson, British Medical Journal, p. 616, 13 June 1863. The reader will also find the notes of some half-dozen anomalous cases of this nature in The Philosophy of Sleep, by Robert Macnish, p. 215. Glasgow, 1830.

hours, and then sleeping again for nearly four days. With the exception of five hours he slept from the 16 to the 26 of February. In March he slept from 10 p.m. on the 9th, until 4 p.m. on the 15th. No food was taken during any of these sleeps, nor was urine or motion passed. He died on the 23 December 1866. At the necroscopy the head only was examined. The skull was well formed; the bones were thin. The calvarium was readily separated from the dura mater. This membrane was normal, except over the anterior portion of the right hemisphere, where it appeared thickened and adherent to the pia mater. The brain substance was healthy. Indeed nothing at all abnormal could be observed beyond a varicose condition of the vessels of the choroid plexus; these vessels being not only dilated, but bulging in knots about the size of hemp seeds. The body generally was pale and wasted; while the rigor mortis was extreme 48 hours after death.

Insomnia or *sleeplessness* not only often forms one of the premonitory symptoms of insanity, but when persistent is a prominent cause of lunacy. Wakefulness is commonly present in mania, greatly aggravating the disease. Sometimes the insane are afraid to sleep because of the frightful dreams and visions which they experience; but often the desire for repose seems banished. All exciting passions have a tendency to prevent sleep; and many acute diseases, in their early stages especially, act in the same way. In some cases of jaundice there is sleeplessness; while others are characterized by excessive drowsiness. Probably, the greater the amount of blood poisoning, the greater the disposition to somnolence. Dyspepsia is a fertile source of restlessness; and so is the use of strong tea and coffee. Mental anxiety, with doubt or uncertainty as to the result of some important action of life, will cause morbid wakefulness; though grief and sorrow, especially if irremediable, produce sleep by the nervous exhaustion they have brought about. So also bodily suffering frightens " Nature's soft nurse;" while the ill effects of disease of the heart or large vessels are often aggravated by imperfect and disturbed sleep. And lastly, women of a nervous excitable temperament are often annoyed by an inability to obtain sound repose during pregnancy; or they may suffer from complete insomnia after delivery. In the latter case, the practitioner must be on his guard, lest puerperal mania supervene.

It is difficult to say for what length of time a person might exist without sleep. Dr. Forbes Winslow quotes the following case, which seems to have occurred in 1859 :* — A Chinese merchant, convicted of murdering his wife, was sentenced to die by being deprived of sleep. The condemned was placed in prison under the care of three of the police guard. The latter relieved each other every alternate hour, and they prevented the prisoner from falling asleep night or day. He thus lived nineteen days

* *On Obscure Diseases of the Brain, and Disorders of the Mind.* Second Note, p. 580. London, 1861.

without any repose. At the commencement of the eighth day he implored the authorities to grant him the blessing of being strangulated, guillotined, burned to death, drowned, garotted, shot, quartered, blown up with gunpowder, or put to death in any conceivable way which their humanity or ferocity could suggest.

The need for sleep is as great as that for nourishment; the suffering which ensues upon enforced wakefulness being only equalled by that caused through the want of water. At that disgusting exhibition on the Place de Grève, Paris, in March 1757, when Damiens (condemned as a regicide to be torn asunder by four horses) was tortured in a barbarous manner prior to execution, he remarked just before death that the deprivation of sleep had been the greatest of all his torments. The story goes that the French general Pichegru, while being tracked by the police of Buonaparte, gave 30,000 francs for a night's sleep; this sum, however, being insufficient to secure safe repose, for on that very night he was betrayed and given up. Again, amongst the fearful iniquities of the "Ordeal" and "Torture," the system of Marsiglio was highly commended. This consisted in keeping the victim from sleep for forty hours; upon which practice Farinacci jocosely remarked, that a hundred martyrs exposed to it would become confessors to a man.

To secure repose which may be refreshing and renovating to both mind and body in cases where there is unnatural wakefulness, a proper amount of exercise should be taken; the diet ought to be digestible, and especially such as will not favour the production of flatulence or acidity; and no tea or coffee must be allowed in the after-part of the day. In many cases I have seen benefit from the dinner being taken at half-past one or two o'clock in the afternoon, as was the old-fashioned custom, while a light supper has been enjoyed about an hour before bedtime; the good effect being due to the stomach attracting blood to perform its work in digesting food, and so lessening the amount to circulate through the brain. The reading of exciting works of fiction late in the evening is to be prohibited; and everything that is possible should be done to prevent the normal functions of the brain from being in any degree exaggerated during the day. The patient had better retire to rest at an early and regular hour; the apartment should be quiet, and proper means taken to have it well ventilated; and if the weather be at all chilly, a fire can often be kept up during the night with great advantage. Although a very low temperature predisposes to somnolence, yet I am sure that the moderate degree of cold which we have for six or eight months in this country has quite the reverse effect with many delicate individuals. The bed should consist of a mattress, without too many blankets; the pillows ought to be firm and high, so as to support the head well; and no curtains or hangings are to be permitted.

If attention to these simple rules fails to produce the desired effect, one or other of the following different plans may be practised perhaps somewhat empirically.   For example, Bacon used to indulge in a posset of strong ale, to subdue the activity of his mind, before going to bed ; and following this suggestion I have frequently seen a good result. particularly where there has been any debility, from a tumblerful of port-wine negus, or of mulled claret, or of hot elder wine, or of white-wine whey, being taken the last thing at night.   In other instances, where the skin has been hot and dry, a glass of cold water has appeared to be useful. So, again, the employment of a bath for about three or five minutes, at a temperature varying from 90° to 96° F., just before getting into bed often affords relief : as does also a rapid sponging of the body with tepid water.   Sometimes the use of a warm foot bath (at a temperature of 100° Fahr.), or of a hot water bottle in the bed, acts favourably, by drawing the blood from the brain to the extremities.   I have read somewhere, that it is a frequent practice in Kashmir for mothers to put their children to sleep by exposing their heads to a small stream of cold water for a couple of hours ; a practice which can only act by inducing cerebral anæmia.

When any physical cause for the wakefulness is discovered, it must of necessity be removed.   Thus, if the bowels are constipated, or if the excretions are unhealthy, laxatives and alteratives will be required.   Patients afflicted with heartburn should take three or four bismuth lozenges on retiring to rest.   If there be headache, a rag dipped in cold water will be useful ; while in some acute diseases the application of a bladder containing ice to the scalp may be advised.   These measures failing, all kinds of mental labour or excitement during the day must be greatly lessened, and to a considerable extent replaced by physical exertion.   Attempts may be made to get into "the land of Nod," while comfortably seated in an easy chair.   Recourse can likewise be had to sedatives ; for although the primary influence of these agents may be exciting, yet their secondary action is undoubtedly narcotic.   At first perhaps, henbane, hop, Indian hemp, or conium, had better be tried, since they neither affect the head nor confine the bowels.   But not unfrequently stronger drugs will be needed.   And then one-sixth or a quarter of a grain of morphia, with some spirit of chloroform ; or half a grain of extract of opium, with a quarter of a grain of extract of belladonna, and four grains of hyoscyamus ; or twenty drops of the liquid extract of opium, with the spirit of ether,— either of these may be prescribed.   Frequently I have found the exhibition of opiate enemata, or suppositories, or subcutaneous injections, preferable to the use of opium or morphia by the mouth. In insomnia due to nervous irritability, large doses of bromide of potassium (twenty or thirty grains at bed-time) are to be recommended ; one of the effects of this drug being probably to lessen the quantity of blood in the nervous centres, and so to cause drowsiness.

There can be no doubt that the manœuvres employed by mesmerists will induce sleep, when practised on certain susceptible persons.   In properly selected cases, there is no objection to the physician resorting therefore to this remedy. "For my own part," remarks Dugald Stewart, "it appears to me, that the general conclusions established by Mesmer's practice, with respect to the physical effects of the principle of Imitation and of the faculty of Imagination (more particularly in cases where they co-operate together), are incomparably more curious than if he had actually succeeded in ascertaining the existence of his boasted fluid.   Nor can I see any good reason why a physician, who admits the efficacy of the *moral* agents employed by Mesmer, should, in the exercise of his profession, scruple to copy whatever processes are necessary for subjecting them to his command, any more than he would hesitate about employing a new *physical* agent, such as electricity or galvanism."* Similar in its results to mesmerism, is hypnotism [from Ὕπνος = sleep + terminal ισμὸς], which Mr. Braid believes is capable of effecting more good than can be accomplished by the ordinary mesmerising processes. This gentleman says,—" My usual mode of inducing the sleep is to hold any small bright object about ten or twelve inches above the middle of the forehead, so as to require a slight exertion of the attention to enable the patient to maintain a steady, fixed gaze on the object ; the subject being either comfortably seated or standing, stillness being enjoined, and the patient requested to engage his attention, as much as possible, on the single act of looking at the object, and yield to the tendency to sleep which will steal over him during this apparently simple process.   I generally use my lancet case, held between the thumb and first two fingers of the left hand ; but any other small bright object will answer the purpose.   In the course of about three or four minutes, if the eyelids do not close of themselves, the first two fingers of the right hand, extended and a little separated, may be quickly, or with a tremulous motion, carried towards the eyes, so as to cause the patient involuntarily to close the eyelids, which, if he is highly susceptible, will either remain rigidly closed, or assume a vibratory motion—the eyes being turned up, with, in the latter case, a little of the white of the eye visible through the partially closed eyelids.   If the patient is not highly susceptible, he will open his eyes, in which case request him to gaze at the object, &c., as at first ; and, if they do not remain closed after a second trial, desire him to allow them to remain shut after you have closed them, and then endeavour to fix his attention on muscular effort, by elevating the arms if standing, or both arms and legs if seated, which must be done quietly, as if you wished to suggest the idea of muscular action without breaking the abstraction, or concentrative state of mind, the induction of which is the real origin and essence of all which follows."†

---

* *The Collected Works of Dugald Stewart, F.R.S., &c.*   Edited by Sir W. Hamilton, vol. iv. p. 167.   Edinburgh, 1854.
† *Magic, Witchcraft, Animal Magnetism, Hypnotism, and Electro-Biology.* Third Edition, p. 57.   London, 1852.

Before concluding these remarks a few words must be said on *dreams, somnambulism,* and *nightmare.* With regard to the first, it is most probable that dreams only occur during imperfect sleep, when there is partial or uncontrolled activity of the nervous centres. They are most common towards the morning, as consciousness is gradually returning. Many dreams are forgotten, especially those which are followed by sound sleep; just as the rambling talk of a patient slightly under the influence of chloroform is not remembered, if the inhalation be continued until complete anæsthesia ensues. The nature of the dream may be suggested by external circumstances; and although it will often consist of contradictory and grotesque or horrible elements, yet occasionally it presents a logical sequence of events free from exaggeration. In the words of Ben Jonson, there are "dreams that have honey and dreams that have stings." Disturbed and frightful dreams are sometimes the precursors of cerebral softening, apoplexy, insanity, tubercular meningitis, and epilepsy. Children are commonly alarmed by their dreams; the goblins and scarecrows having their origin in uneasiness from teething, a loaded bladder, irritation of the bowels, &c.

The somnambulist dreams and carries out his conceit. His movements appear to have the precision of one awake, because he is familiar with the objects and actions which he pictures to himself. The phenomena of somnambulism vary from simple talking or crying, to the performance of various actions as if the senses were in full activity and under the control of the understanding.

In nightmare or incubus [from *Incubo* = to lie upon] there are generally apparitions, horrible or ludicrous, with always a distressing consciousness of inability to move. It may arise from the presence of indigestible food in the stomach, or from pressure upon this organ, or from flatulence with acid secretions. The suffering usually commences with a disagreeable vision, and the sleeper attempts to escape from some imaginary danger. Then he experiences a sense of suffocation, which increases until there is an imperfect consciousness that he is in bed. But still there continues the tormenting oppression from the weight on the chest, which keeps him lying on his back; and he feels unable to inflate his lungs. The oppressed breathing becomes most painful; palpitations of the heart set in; attempts are made to move the arms, but it is found impossible to do so; and the countenance assumes a ghastly expression, with the eyes half-open. Within a minute or two the power of volition returns; and then, the patient accustomed to these attacks, immediately and thoroughly rouses himself, fearful lest the horrid paroxysm should recur.

Spasmodic contraction of the diaphragm and intercostal muscles has been assigned as the proximate cause of nightmare. Dr. Hodgkin, himself a sufferer, attempted to analyse the symptoms. The chief point he succeeded in making out was, that the involuntary movements of respiration appeared to be suspended, whilst the chest seemed to be passively collapsing. Following up the indications derived from this observation, he found that most speedy relief was obtained from so moving the arms that the pectoral muscles might elevate the ribs; and he consequently begged that whenever he appeared to be under the influence of an attack, one of his arms might be worked like the handle of a pump.* In cases where the seizure is apt to return on the same night, it may be warded off by an antacid draught (a little soda and ammonia in water), or by two or three bismuth or bicarbonate of soda lozenges. Of course, heavy suppers, and food likely to induce dyspepsia (especially malt liquors), should be rigidly avoided.

XIX. HYPOCHONDRIASIS.

The hypochondriac disorder [from Ὑποχονδριακὸς = affected in the viscera under the false ribs,—because such affection was regarded as the cause of melancholy], or the *vapours*, or the *spleen*, has received attention from the healers of the sick, whether priests or physicians, since the days of Hippocrates. The ancients imagined that the morbid sensations characteristic of this affection had their origin about the pyloric orifice of the stomach, or in the mesentery, or the liver, or the spleen. The followers of Galen maintained that the melancholy symptoms were due to black bile; a view which was held until Willis, in 1676, insisted that they were caused by the action of unhealthy splenic blood on the nervous system. Subsequently, more and more stress was laid upon the neurotic character of the affection; though it is scarcely half a century since the propriety of regarding " low spirits " as a nervous disease was generally determined.

Hypochondriasis may be said to consist prominently of an exaggerated egoism. With mental depression there is frequently functional derangement (occasionally structural disease) of certain organs, especially of those connected with the nutritive processes; these derangements occurring either primarily or secondarily to the erroneous action of the mind. The hypochondriac is ever writhing under the petty despotism of an imaginary evil. He fulfils all his duties naturally, and generally with amiability, for a season; but he is morbidly sensitive of the opinions and actions of other men, while he is also constantly tormenting himself by dwelling upon his own miserable condition. There is an unceasing dread of the existence of internal disease; with the fear either of impending insanity or of death. To the same extent that hysteria is peculiar to the female, so hypochondriasis is the special affliction of the male sex.

This disorder may vary in degree, just as individuals of different constitutions and temperaments possess a variable amount of

* *British Medical Journal*, p. 501. London, 16 May 1863.

control over the feelings and faculties of the mind. Doubtless education has also a considerable amount of influence in this respect. And it is not an extravagant assertion to say, that he who is commonly called a strong-minded man may shake off a real indisposition, to which another person, less happily constituted, will succumb; so remarkable is the power of the mind over the body. To believe firmly in one's ability and power of endurance to accomplish some great end, goes a long way towards attaining it. There is probably nothing which a sensible and persevering man may legitimately covet, that he cannot obtain; if only he determine to take the necessary steps. The influence of the will over even the involuntary muscles is sometimes extraordinary, as many remarkable cases attest. Thus, Celsus speaks of a priest who could separate himself from his senses when he chose, and lie like a man void of life and sense. Cardan used to boast of being able to do the same. But the most surprising example of this kind is the well-known case of Colonel Townshend related by Dr. George Cheyne.* The very essence of hypochondriasis, however, is a

* The quaint description given by this author of his patient's unnatural skill runs thus:—"*Colonel Townshend*, a Gentleman of excellent Natural Parts, and of great *Honour* and *Integrity*, had for many years been afflicted with a *Nephritic* Complaint, attended with constant *Vomitings*, which had made his Life painful and miserable. Dureing the whole time of his *Illness*, he had observed the strictest *Regimen*, living on the softest Vegetables and lightest *Animal Foods*, drinking *Asses Milk* daily, even in the Camp: and for common Drink *Bristol* Water, which the Summer before his death, he had drunk on the *Spot*. But his Illness increasing and his Strength decaying, he came from *Bristol* to *Bath* in a Litter, in Autumn, and lay at the *Bell-Inn*. Dr. *Baynard* (who is since dead) and *I* were called to him, and attended him twice a Day for about the Space of a Week, but his *Vomitings* continuing still incessant, and obstinate against all Remedies, we despaired of his *Recovery*. While he was in this Condition he sent for us early one Morning: we waited on him, with Mr. *Skrine* his Apothecary (since dead also); we found his *Senses* clear, and his *Mind* calm, his Nurse and several Servants were about him. He had made his *Will* and settled his Affairs. He told us, he had sent for us to give him some Account of an *odd Sensation* he had for some Time observed and felt in himself: which was, that composing himself, he could *die* or expire when he pleased, and yet by an *Effort*, or some how he could come to Life again, which it seems he had sometimes tried before he had sent for *us*. We heard this with *Surprize*, but as it was not to be accounted for from now *common Principles*, we could hardly believe the *Fact* as he related it, much less give any Account of it: unless he should please to make the *Experiment* before us, which we were unwilling he should do, lest, in his weak Condition, he might carry it too far. He continued to talk very distinctly and sensibly above a Quarter of an Hour about this (to Him) surprising *Sensation*, and insisted so much on our seeing the *Trial* made, that we were at last forced to comply. We all *three* felt his pulse first: it was distinct, tho' small and *threedy*: and his *Heart* had its usual Beating. He composed himself on his Back, and lay in a still posture some time: while *I* held his right Hand, Dr. *Baynard* laid his Hand on his *Heart*, and Mr. *Skrine* held a clean Looking-Glass to his Mouth. I found his *Pulse* sink gradually, till at last I could not feel any, by the most exact and nice Touch. Dr. *Baynard* could not feel the least motion in his *Heart*, nor Mr. *Skrine* the least Soil of Breath on the bright *Mirror* he held to his Mouth; then each of us by *Turns* examin'd his

want of resolution,—an inability to resist "thick-coming fancies." This morbid condition is a gigantic evil, the rock on which many an amiable man's happiness has been wrecked. It may seem hard to say so, but the affection is often the offspring of selfishness and indolence. At the same time there is sometimes associated with it bodily disease; although the injurious influences of this, as well as the symptoms it gives rise to, are greatly exaggerated. The most frequent of these affections belong to the stomach, liver, right side of the heart, large vessels, and urinary organs. In most instances the circulation is languid, and cold feet are particularly complained of. While therefore, on the one hand, care must be taken not to overlook the existence of organic disease, when present; so, on the other, it ought to be remembered that there is generally only a simulation of some serious malady, with functional disturbance of the viscus to which the attention is morbidly directed. Moreover, occasionally the organic affection is slight. Thus, some remarkable cases of long-standing hypochondriasis have fallen under my observation, where the only disease discoverable after careful and repeated examination has been in the teeth. And in such, no

Arm, Heart, and *Breath,* but could not by the nicest *Scrutiny* discover the least *Symptom* of *Life* in him. We reasoned a long Time about this odd *Appearance* as well as we could, and all of us judging it inexplicable and unaccountable, and finding he still continued in that Condition, we began to conclude that he had indeed carried the *Experiment* too far, and at last were satisfied he was actually dead, and were just ready to leave him. This continued about half an Hour. By Nine o'Clock in the Morning in autumn, as we were going away, we observed some Motion about the Body, and upon Examination found his *Pulse* and the *Motion* of his *Heart* gradually returning; he began to *breath* gently and speak softly: we were all astonish'd to the last Degree at this unexpected Change, and after some further Conversation with him, and among ourselves, went away fully satisfy'd as to all the Particulars of this Fact, but confounded and puzled, and not able to form any rational *Scheme* that might account for it. He afterwards called for his *Attorney,* added a *Codicil* to his *Will,* settled Legacies on his Servants, received the *Sacrament,* and calmly and composedly expir'd about five or six o'Clock that Evening. Next Day he was opened (as he had ordered): his Body was the soundest and best made I had ever seen; his *Lungs* were fair, large, and sound, his *Heart* big and strong, and his *Intestines* sweet and clean; his *Stomach* was of a due Proportion, the *Coats* sound and thick, and the villous *Membrane* quite entire. But when we came to examine the Kidneys, tho' the *left* was perfectly sound and of a just *Size,* the *right* was about four Times as big, distended like a blown *Bladder,* and yielding as if full of Pap; he having often pass'd a *Wheyish* Liquor after his Urine, during his Illness. Upon opening this *Kidney,* we found it quite full of a white *Chalky* Matter, like *Plaster of Paris,* and all the fleshy substance dissolved and worn away, by what I called a *Nephritick Cancer.* This had been the Source of all his Misery; and the *symptomatick* Vomitings from the Irritation on the consentient *Nerves* had quite starved and worn him down. I have narrated the *Facts,* as I saw and observed them deliberately and distinctly, and shall leave to the *Philosophick Reader* to make what Inferences he thinks fit; the Truth of the material Circumstances I will warrant."—*The English Malady: or a Treatise of Nervous Diseases of all Kinds, as Spleen, Vapours, Lowness of Spirits, Hypochondriacal and Hysterical Distempers, &c.,* p. 307. London, 1733.

real or permanent benefit has arisen from treatment until the foul stumps or carious organs have been all extracted.

No station in life gives immunity to attacks of hypochondriasis. But perhaps the most frequently affected are such as have been accustomed to an active life; yet who, having retired to enjoy the fruits of their industry, get oppressed with ennui, having no other means of employing themselves than that which they have thrown up. So also those who, from their social position, have not been brought up to any occupation, suffer greatly; those accustomed to sedentary pursuits, who neglect to take the exercise necessary for maintaining the healthy mind in the sound body; and those again who over-work the mind, or who have any prolonged mental anxiety, or who have imperfectly recovered from a tedious and prostrating sickness. The dejection, slight at first, gradually becomes extreme. Poor Cowper, writing to congratulate a friend on his recovery from severe disease, says,—" Your illness has indeed been a sad one, causing, no doubt, great distress to yourself, and considerable anxiety to your relatives and friends. But, oh! what are your *bodily* sufferings, acute as they undoubtedly were, to the unceasing *mental* torture I suffer from *a fever of the mind?*" Under such suffering it is hardly surprising that men have attempted suicide, as indeed Cowper did;[*] believing with the Son of Sirach, that—" Death is better than a bitter life or continual sickness."

Reading men at the Universities are not uncommonly tormented with great depression of spirits. Sometimes this is connected with spermatorrhœa, of which more will be said on a future page; often the conscience is over-sensitive, and the importance of becoming distinguished is exaggerated; frequently the strain produced by excessive mental labour, with the fear of ungratified ambition, is the only cause; but above all, I would attribute the mischief to the very imperfect way in which our youths are educated at the various public and other schools. That the supervision by the masters over the teaching of the boys is often of such a desultory and sluggish character that the latter need only learn just as much or as little as they please, is merely a part of that vicious system which leaves the cultivation of the bodily strength entirely to chance. There surely ought to be no necessity for insisting at the present day, that the employment and improvement of the physical powers require to be encouraged and carefully supervised; and that as with the mental studies, there is a proper process to be used. Far from being an advocate for those violent athletic exercises in which one youth is pitted against another, I am strongly inclined to condemn them. What I really desire to see is a methodical system of drill and exercise fitted to produce a sound constitution in the average boy. To secure this, every school

---

[*] The description of this attempt, as given by the poet himself, is of special interest to the psychological student. It is too long for quotation, and will not bear curtailment.—See *The Poetical Works of William Cowper.* Edited by Robert Bell, vol. i. p. 25. London, 1854.

ought to have a well-fitted gymnasium, attendance and work in which should be as regular and systematic as in the class room. Not that any compulsion would be necessary; for undoubtedly one part of a clever teacher's business would be to prevent the young plucky gymnasts from performing too venturesome feats before they were sufficiently prepared.

Entertaining these views my treatment of hypochondriasis may be imagined. In these cases, as in others of a similar kind, I have seen the greatest benefit from recommending young men to go through a modified system of physical training.* By this practice the invalid not only relieves his weary mind at the time; but, while bringing the various muscles and tissues into play he obtains general vigour, energy of body, buoyancy of spirits, a power of self-command, and, in short, that happy, desirable feeling which constitutes perfect health. The first rule in following such a course of treatment is to obtain natural, quiet sleep; to procure which the bed should be free from drapery, while it ought to be placed in a good-sized room—not in such cupboards as one sees at some colleges. There must be sufficient, but not too much clothing; while a hair mattress is serviceable, a feather bed being only fit for an effeminate milksop. The feet are to be kept warm, and the head cool. If there be restlessness, it may be relieved by a tepid sitz-bath a few minutes before retiring for the night; or in any case, the skin ought to be briskly rubbed with a coarse towel. From eight to nine hours of sleep will be needed. Then, on rising, a cold or tepid sponge bath had better be employed; unless sea bathing or a plunge in the river can be enjoyed, with a good swim for five minutes. The hair is to be kept short, and the teeth are to be well cleaned night and morning; and while flannel is to be worn next the skin during the day, only a cotton shirt must be slept in.—In having recourse to dumb-bell exercise, the best authorities recommend that the weight of the dumb-bells should be in proportion to that of the individual using them as pounds to stones. Thus, a man of ten stone will select instruments each weighing five pounds. Their use gives flexibility and tone to the muscles, and promotes general activity.—For club exercise, wooden bats are to be selected about two feet in length, and each having a weight of from three to nine pounds, according to the strength of the individual.—When rowing men are in training for a race, it is advantageous for them to take walking and running exercise in the fresh morning air. Running judiciously practised, is especially useful; since by it the man gains both muscular and respiratory power. But it is important that too much be not attempted at first: the speed should be increased very

* No man should be allowed to go into anything like severe training whose weight is not in due proportion to his height, and whose vital capacity is not normal (see tables in section on Phthisis). Moreover, his chest ought to have the minimum girth of 36 inches, and there must be no tendency to tubercular phthisis, either hereditary or acquired.

gradually and only as power is gained to permit of the requisite pace without distress.—For either running or walking, woollen socks of a proper size are to be worn. The boots or shoes ought not to be new; their upper leathers are to be light, while the soles should be double and water-tight; and care must be taken that there is sufficient length and breadth in the tread, as well as across the toes. It is simply from inattention to points like these that men get tender feet, sore shins, and blistered heels. On commencing a pedestrian tour, a short journey is to be taken the first day; the novice gradually increasing the distance until he can accomplish his twenty or five-and-twenty miles a day. The rate should be about three miles an hour; allowing regular intervals for rest and meals. A good bracing air is to be selected, remembering that the athletes of ancient Rome were trained in localities reputed to be the most healthy in the country. A party of three congenial friends will be all that is desirable; for desultory practice soon ends in disgust, and who can find more than two companions with whom he is likely to happily end a tour of some weeks' duration? And lastly, the diet ought to consist of stale bread or dry toast and fresh butter; black tea, with half milk; oatmeal porridge, if liked; white fish, mutton chops, steaks, roast beef and mutton, poultry, game, lightly-cooked eggs, light suet puddings, potatoes, watercresses, &c. Pure bitter ale or table beer, without spirits, will be necessary; or the invigorating Hungarian, French, or German wines may be substituted for malt liquors. All made dishes and rich sauces and pastry ought to be excluded. Breakfast had better be taken at eight o'clock, dinner at two, and supper at half-past seven or eight. There should be complete rest on the Sundays. And each one of the party is to remember the motto of training,—" Soberness, temperance, and chastity."

In concluding these remarks, the reader may look for some information as to the drugs which are useful in conquering hypochondriasis. But on this head I would rather give a word or two of caution, than a long list of useless remedies. In the first place, all purgative medicines are injurious. The action of the bowels must be maintained by exercise and diet. Secondly, narcotics and sedatives only increase the mischief, and check the secretions. In some of the books on training which I have seen, sweating liquors are recommended containing opium in such doses as can only produce a violent sick headache for four-and-twenty hours after being taken. Thirdly, tonics are seldom of more than temporary benefit. If there be anæmia, however, some preparation of steel may be given; or if there be great depression of the nervous system, the hypophosphite of soda and bark (F. 419) may be tried, or the nitro-hydrochloric acid with small doses of strychnia (F. 378). Cod liver oil will prove serviceable, when the hypochondriac is below his normal weight. Yet the chief point is for the practitioner to inspire his patient with confidence: failing to accomplish this, all else will be unprofitable. Though the sufferer neglect to attend to the necessary rules, nevertheless—as old Burton says, " It behoves a good physician not to leave him helpless.   But most part they offend in that other extreme, they prescribe too much physic, and tire out their bodies with continual potions, to no purpose."*   The physician of the present day, however, ought not to render himself amenable to this censure.

XX. NEUROMA.

By the term Neuroma [Νεῦρον = a nerve] is designated a tumour connected with a nerve. The growth may be solid or cystic; the former being the most frequent.   The solid growths are of a fibrous nature, consisting of dense plastic matter, implicating the neurilemma and nerve-fibres.   Occasionally the nerve-fibres are merely spread over or around the tumour, without being involved in its texture.

Neuromatous tumours sometimes form spontaneously, in which case they are generally single and very painful; it being remarkable that the suffering is much less when there are several tumours on the same or on an adjoining nerve, than when there is only one.   They are also an occasional result of a wound or other injury; and thus they are apt to be produced on the extremities of nerves after amputation.

Every now and then small cancerous masses become deposited in the course of a nerve, and thus simulate the disease under consideration.   But true neuroma is of a benign nature.   So again the presence of a painful subcutaneous tubercle may lead to an incorrect diagnosis.   These little bodies, however, are situated immediately beneath the skin, are seldom larger than a pea, and are formed of dense fibro-cartilage; while although sometimes very sensitive to the touch, they are rarely as painful as the tumours developed in the nerves.

Idiopathic neuromatous growths vary in size from a barleycorn to a good-sized melon.   They occur most frequently on the spinal nerves, the branches of the ganglionic system being very rarely affected.   Their growth is steady but slow.   They are of an oval or oblong form, the long axis corresponding with the direction of the nerve to which they are connected.   They may be due occasionally to neuritis, but often no appreciable cause can be detected. A single growth is frequently the origin of agonizing darting pain; which is increased by any attempt to move the tumour in the direction of the nerve.   Neuroma has been the antecedent of epilepsy in several recorded cases.   In the only instance of nerve-tumour which has fallen under my own observation it produced severe hypochondriasis.

In traumatic neuroma the growth is generally single; and is

* *The Anatomy of Melancholy.* Tegg's Edition, p. 301. London, 1845.

the source of paroxysmal pains of great severity, often comparable to a galvanic shock.   Complete division of a nerve seems especially to produce this variety; in which case the tumour is solid, not invested by the neurilemma, and is destitute of any distinct capsule.

No mode of treatment proves effectual but excision.   The only question for consideration is whether the growth should be carefully dissected out, or the neuroma and its corresponding portions of nerve be excised.   Dr. Robert W. Smith, in his excellent monograph on this disease, remarks that "the annals of surgery furnish numerous instances in which the excision of the neuroma, along with the corresponding portion of the nerve, has been followed by complete and permanent sucess. . . . . . Experience has further established that neither sensibility nor the power of voluntary motion are, of necessity, ultimately lost in consequence of the excision of even several inches of some of the largest nerves in the body."*   This latter observation can hardly be correct, though a fair allowance be made for the looseness of the phrase "several inches."   But allowing that there is an element of truth in it, conceding as I do that simple division of a nerve will often be followed by restoration of nervous power in the course of three or four weeks, and that even a small portion of a nerve may be removed without ultimate detriment, yet there must always be an element of doubt about the result.   Moreover, where a portion of nerve-tissue (say from one fourth to half an inch) has been cut away, some four or five or more months will elapse before sensibility and motion are restored to the parts supplied by it.   Consequently, when possible, the neuromatous tumour should be dissected out; or, if complete excision be resorted to, the two ends of the divided nerve had better be brought into apposition by a suture.   After the removal of a neuroma from the median nerve at the middle part of the arm, and the excision of the nerve itself to the extent of about two-thirds of an inch, M. Nelaton united the two cut ends by a suture.   No ill-result followed, and at the end of forty-three hours there was a return of sensibility and motion.   Supposing there are several neuromatous tumours, it will be very unwise to interfere with them.

XXI. NEURITIS.

Inflammation of a Nerve, or Neuritis [Νεῦρον = a nerve + terminal -itis], is an affection which seldom comes under the notice of the physician.   For although it can perhaps arise spontaneously in gouty or rheumatic subjects, yet it is much more frequently

* On the Pathology, Diagnosis, and Treatment of Neuroma, p. 7.   Dublin, 1849.

due to a bruise or wound, or to inclusion of some branch by a ligature in taking up a wounded artery.

The neurilemma is the tissue usually affected. The sciatic nerve is more frequently attacked than any other; and next, the branches of the brachial plexus. The special symptom of this disorder is severe and darting and remittent pain, extending along the trunk of the nerve and its ramifications. The constitutional disturbance varies according to the size of the inflamed nerve; but there is generally more or less fever, with great restlessness at night. In chronic cases, the symptoms are those of neuralgia.

The chief remedies in gouty or rheumatic neuritis, are iodide of potassium and colchicum and aconite. In all cases, the affected part must be kept very quiet; while it ought to be freely covered with belladonna and water dressing, or with linseed poultices containing the extract of poppies. The chronic form usually yields sooner to quinine than to any other drug.

XXII. NEURALGIA.

1. **INTRODUCTION.**—The pains which occur in the course of disease may be divided into two varieties: *i.e.*, into those occurring at the seat of mischief—as pain in the breast from cancer of the mamma, pain in a joint from inflammation of the synovial membrane, pain in the sciatic nerve from disease of the neurilemma, intercostal neuralgia from herpes of the same side; and those referred to parts not actually the seat of morbid action—as pain over the eyebrow from decayed teeth, pain through the shoulder from disease of the liver, pain down the left arm from angina pectoris, pain darting along the little finger from striking the ulnar nerve at the elbow, pain in the knee from disease of the hip, pain in the heel from disease of the bladder, and pain about the foot from piles or from stricture of the urethra, &c.

Neuralgia [Νεῦρον = a nerve + ἄλγος = suffering] consists of violent pain in the trunk or branches of a nerve, occurring in paroxysms, at regular or irregular intervals: frequently there are nocturnal exacerbations. It may attack the nerves of the head, trunk, or extremities; the subcutaneous nerves of these parts suffering the most frequently.

2. **VARIETIES.**—When the branches of the fifth pair of nerves are the seat of the pain, we call the disease *neuralgia faciei* or *tic douloureux*; when certain nerves about the head—*hemicrania*; when the sciatic nerve—*sciatica*. There are authorities who consider that *angina pectoris* is a neuralgic affection of some of the cardiac nerves; and *gastrodynia* a similar disease of the nerves of the stomach. The pain in dysmenorrhœa is at times neuralgic.

a. Tic Douloureux, or facial neuralgia, may affect either of the three chief branches of the fifth pair of nerves. Where the pain depends upon a morbid condition of the first or ophthalmic branch, the frontal ramification of it (the supra-orbital nerve) is that most frequently attacked; the suffering being referred chiefly to the tissues of the forehead. Supposing that the second or superior maxillary branch is the seat of the complaint, the infra-orbital nerve will be one of the most commonly affected; the symptoms consisting of excruciating pain shooting over the cheek, lower eyelid, alæ of the nose, and upper lip. Tic douloureux of the third or inferior maxillary branch is generally confined to the inferior dental nerve, especially to that portion of it which emerges from the mental foramen and extends to the lower lip. The pain is referrible to the lower lip, the alveolar process, the teeth, the chin, and the side of the tongue.

Whichever nerve may suffer, the torture is almost always confined to one-half of the face. The right infra-orbital nerve is the most frequent seat of this disease. The pain comes on usually very gradually—perhaps as a momentary twinge; yet soon it increases in severity, gets lancinating and burning, and often becomes excessive and intolerable. I have seen the most horrible sufferings induced; and until I became aware of the value of chloroform, have often been unable to afford relief. Not unfrequently the attack is preceded by nausea with derangement of the digestive organs, sometimes by dyspnœa, and occasionally by slight rigors followed by heat : oft-times there is no harbinger of any kind.

Facial neuralgia can be produced by many different conditions. Thus, it may arise from general debility, owing to simple anæmia or renal disease; from disease of the bones of the face; or from some tumour or other organic disease of the brain. Frequently the affection can only be regarded as a product of hysteria in an irritable constitution; sometimes it is intermittent and periodical, appearing to be due to the poison of malaria; in many cases it seems to be dependent on disordered digestive organs; while in not a few it cannot be traced to its real source.

But of all the causes of tic douloureux I believe none to be so frequent as some morbid condition of the teeth.* The disease

---

* The importance of investigating the state of the mouth in all cases of neuralgia about the face and head, headache, deafness, amaurosis, facial paralysis, epilepsy, abscess of the antrum, and hypochondriasis cannot be too strongly insisted upon. The teeth are divided into incisors, canines, bicuspids or premolars, and molars. A representation of the number of the different kinds of teeth in both jaws by means of symbols, constitutes what is called a " dental formula." The number and nature of the permanent teeth of man are thus expressed in the convenient signs put forward by Professor Owen :—

$$i. \frac{2-2}{2-2}; \ c. \frac{1-1}{1-1}; \ p. \frac{2-2}{2-2}; \ m. \frac{3-3}{3-3} = 32.$$

The formula for the deciduous, temporary, or milk teeth is as follows,—

$$d \ i. \frac{2-2}{2-2}; \ d \ c. \frac{1-1}{1-1}; \ d \ m. \frac{2-2}{2-2} = 20.$$

affecting these organs may be of the nature of caries, or necrosis, or exostosis of the roots ; or of inflammation or exposure of the dentinal pulp ; or of disease of the periosteum with suppuration. Even the presence of supernumerary teeth, with over-crowding of the jaw, will induce headache or tic douloureux in sensitive subjects. In all cases of neuralgia, therefore, the mouth should be carefully examined, so that any decayed teeth or stumps may be extracted. And it is important to remember that the pain may have its origin in the dental branches of the superior maxillary nerve (the second division of the fifth), without there being any toothache ; a point which is frequently incomprehensible to the patient, especially to the one who is unwilling to be convinced. Moreover it does not follow that there is no organic disease, because the neuralgia assumes a periodical form. Many cases have been recorded where some nerve in one of the extremities has been irritated by a tumour or an aneurism, and yet the paroxysms of pain have occurred with all the regularity of an ague; oft-times ceasing for a long interval, but generally returning again and again until the cause has been removed. Where exostosis takes place in apparently sound teeth, it will be difficult to fix upon the source of the suffering ; though frequently there is sufficient tenderness about the gum to remove all doubt. An extraordinary example of dental exostosis has been related by Mr. Fox :* A young lady, scarcely twenty years of age, had suffered for more than a year from deep-seated pains in the face, teeth, and gums. The pain had gradually extended to all the teeth ; and one by one those of the lower jaw, with the exception of the four incisors, had been removed. During this time every kind of treatment had been resorted to, without any alleviation. When Mr. Fox saw her she was only able to take fluid nourishment, the teeth of the upper jaw being so tender that the slightest touch caused extreme pain. There was a constant flow of saliva from the mouth ; while the sight of one eye was affected, and the lids had been closed for two months. The first molar of the upper jaw, on the side of the affected eye, was extracted. The fangs of this tooth were much enlarged and the periosteum thickened : its removal gave relief, and in two days the eye could be naturally opened. The relief, however, was partial ; and a perfect cure was only ultimately effected by removing all the teeth.—Mr. Tomes† mentions the case of a lady who had suffered from tic douloureux for some years. The crowns of the teeth were sound : nevertheless when extracted, the fangs were found to be enlarged from exostosis. The disease was not cured until the whole of the teeth in the upper jaw had been removed.—And lastly, Mr. Catlin‡ has recorded the

* *The Natural History and Diseases of the Human Teeth.* Second Edition, part ii. p. 45. London, 1814.
† *A System of Dental Surgery,* p. 441. London, 1859.
‡ *The Teeth in Health and Disease.* By Robert Thomas Hulme, F.L.S. &c., p. 211. London, 1864.

very singular instance of a lady who consulted him concerning a diseased right molar. For three months she had suffered acute pains in the tooth, ear, and side of the neck. When he saw her she had been deaf for four days. The inflamed tooth was extracted, and hearing returned within an hour after the operation.

In a person liable to neuralgia, the paroxysms of suffering are induced by very trifling causes; a slight current of air, a sudden jar or shake, or anything which reminds the patient of his malady, frequently sufficing to bring them on. The pains often prevent all attempts even at repose. When the sufferer is once asleep, however, the rest is sound and undisturbed; since the pains—as pointed out by Sir B. Brodie—are suspended by sleep.

β. *Hemicrania* ["Ημισυς = half + κρανίον = the skull] is merely headache affecting one side of the brow and forehead. It is often attended with sickness, and more frequently results from debility than from any other cause. Occasionally its attacks are periodical, coming on at a certain hour every day. It has been called *Sun-pain*, from the circumstance that at times it continues only so long as the sun is above the horizon.

γ. *Sciatica* ['Ισχίον = the hip] consists of acute pain following the course of the great sciatic nerve; extending therefore from the sciatic notch down the posterior surface of the thigh to the popliteal space, and frequently along the nerves of the leg to the foot. It very often results from pressure upon some part of the nerve, such as can be produced by intestinal accumulations, or by simple or malignant uterine tumours. Now and then too, this disorder arises from inflammation; sometimes from over-fatigue, and exposure to cold and wet; and occasionally from rheumatism. Puerperal women (especially those of a rheumatic or gouty diathesis) not uncommonly suffer from sciatica; the nocturnal exacerbations of pain quite preventing sleep, and exhausting the patient. Usually one limb only is affected, examples of bilateral suffering being uncommon. The muscles feel stiff, and as if their action were impeded; so that the patient is obliged to limp along with the aid of a stick. The duration of an attack of sciatica varies from a few weeks to several months; the middle period of life, from forty to sixty, is most obnoxious to it; and occasionally seizures of it alternate with other rheumatic or neuralgic affections.

3. TREATMENT.—In the treatment of neuralgia, it is obvious that our first efforts must be directed to the removal of the cause. So long as this remains we may relieve, but not remove, the effect. The state of the health will have to be looked to. It may be laid down as an axiom that this is always below par. Aperients will perhaps be needed, but they are to be of a mild kind, such as we possess in the various preparations of aloes (F. 155). Of course any accumulations in the rectum or colon are to be removed by more active purgatives and enemata (F. 190). Then the constitutional

debility ought to be corrected by a nourishing diet. I generally forbid the use of tea and coffee; but allow plenty of milk, raw eggs, animal food twice daily, with a regulated amount of malt liquor or some alcoholic stimulant. Cod liver oil is almost as necessary as good food,—in point of fact it is an excellent food. Warm clothing should be recommended, and especially the use of flannel next the skin. In sciatica, chamois-leather drawers often prove very comfortable. The employment of a salt warm or tepid bath every morning, followed by friction, will be beneficial.

Ferruginous tonics frequently prove of great value. Dr. Elliotson says, that "in all cases of neuralgia, whether exquisite or not, unaccompanied by inflammation, or evident existing cause, iron is the best remedy. The officinal hydrated peroxide may therefore be given in from five to thirty grain doses two or three times a day, with an occasional aperient. Quinine and steel (F. 380), or the reduced iron (F. 394), can also be recommended. When there are symptoms of disorder of the digestive organs, pepsine (F. 420), or rhubarb and ipecacuanha (F. 179), are indicated. If there be nausea or heartburn, antacids (F. 63, 65) often give great relief. Cases associated with rheumatism will derive benefit from iodide of potassium, aconite, arnica, actea racemosa, colchicum, and occasionally from turpentine, &c.; while those in which the attacks are periodic can generally be cured by full doses of quinine (F. 379, 383), or by minute doses of arsenic with bark, zinc, &c. (F. 52, 381, 399).

The efficiency of the valerianate of ammonia as a remedy for neuralgia, has been urged by many practitioners, though I must confess it has greatly disappointed my expectations. From ten to eighteen or twenty grains of this salt may be given, in two ounces of infusion of orange peel or calumba, thrice daily (F. 410). No stronger proof of the intense suffering which is produced by neuralgia could be given than is instanced by the fact that patients will take this most nauseous draught for weeks, if it only afford them moderate relief. From time to time I have seen benefit produced by the chloride of ammonium; thirty grains of which should be administered every hour in plenty of water, while the paroxysm is on. If after the fourth dose there be no diminution of the suffering, it will be useless to persevere. As soon as the pain is relieved, the dose can be reduced to fifteen grains three times a day.

With regard to the treatment of sciatica, mercury or iodide of potassium will be needed if there be any symptoms of a syphilitic taint; active purgatives, especially croton oil (F. 168, 191), where we fear the existence of faecal accumulations; and steel, with cod liver oil (F. 389), if there be general debility. In two or three cases where I could detect no cause for the disease, a cure has been effected by the sulphate of soda and steel (F. 181), with the use twice a week of a sulphur or hot air bath.

Certain topical expedients have been proposed. Division of the affected nerve is an unreasonable operation, which can rarely, if ever, be of lasting service. Supposing there is a tumour or foreign body pressing upon the nerve, it ought to be removed; or any portion of necrosed bone that may be the cause of the suffering must be taken away. In facial neuralgia, the extraction of carious teeth, &c., as already dwelt upon, will repeatedly effect a cure. An irritable condition of the dental nerves, which I believe to be the cause of much suffering, can be remedied in men by the cultivation of the moustache and beard. A clergyman who looked forward to his winter attack of bronchitis as a matter of course, not only destroyed the susceptibility to this foe by throwing away his shaving brush and razors, but gave me great praise for having also completely cured his frequent pains and aches about the jaws by my recommendation. Again, wherever the neuralgia may be seated, belladonna, veratria, aconite, or opium (F. 297, 304), applied to the affected part, will often at least palliate the suffering; while, in some instances, the cuticle can be removed by a blister, and the part dusted over with one or two grains of morphia mixed with the same quantity of white sugar. A small portion of an ointment, made by mixing one or even two grains of aconitine with sixty grains of lard (F. 296), may be cautiously smeared over the track of the painful nerve once or twice a day. Narcotic injections into the subcutaneous areolar tissue are now very commonly employed. Morphia with atropine forms, perhaps, the best compound, since it allays pain without causing sickness (F. 314); while as much relief is given by using this hypodermic method at a distance from the seat of pain, as by practising it at the neuralgic part. To inject the solution, a graduated syringe having a sharp perforated nozzle ought to be used. From time to time, however, cases are met with where the agony is intensified by any preparation of opium. Of this I am certain, having particularly noticed the harm I have temporarily done by opium and morphia given by the month or subcutaneously. In all such instances, I now find no remedy so valuable as a mixture of atropine and arsenic (gr. $\frac{1}{40}$ of the former, with gr. $\frac{1}{50}$ of the latter, in five minims of water) used hypodermically. Once or twice quinine has been used in place of the arsenic, but the latter has seemed most useful. So also warm baths, or hot douches of medicated water, or douches of hot and cold water alternately, will often be useful; though if the pain be of a burning character the patient will voluntarily apply cold water constantly, and will refuse to adopt any other practice. Yet in these cases, repeated blistering of the heated part, taking care to keep the surface sore for a time, will often have an admirable effect. Shampooing, the parts being very gently kneaded at first until they acquire a certain amount of tone, can be tried. And then, where there is no disease of the nervous centres, and where the affected nerve is not irritated by inflammation or by the pressure of some morbid growth, the use of a continuous current of galvanic electricity (such as can be obtained from one of Pulvermacher's chains) may diminish the morbid exaltation of sensibility, and so lead to a cure.

Not unfrequently the practitioner will be summoned to give some mitigation of suffering at once, without any reference to a cure. When the pain is on severely—when the patient is racked with torture, no agent produces such instantaneous relief as ether or chloroform (F. 313) ; the inhalation of one of which remedies, or of the two combined, should be permitted until complete insensibility is produced. On many occasions it will be found advisable to give fifty or sixty drops of the spirit of ether in water, or in brandy and water, just before the respiration of the vapour is commenced ; or a large dose of quinine (from 5 to 20 grains) may be administered, provided there are no symptoms indicative of cerebral or cardiac disease. The ease thus induced generally continues long after recovery from the immediate effects of the inhalation. For the relief of a violent attack, however, it is often advisable to inject subcutaneously, while the patient is under the influence of the anæsthetic, a dose of morphia and atropine, or of atropine and arsenic, or of atropine and quinine, where none of this last drug has previously been given by the mouth.

PART V.

DISEASES OF THE ORGANS OF RESPIRATION AND CIRCULATION.

I. CATARRH.

CATARRH [from Καταρρέω = to flow down little by little] consists of an acute or subacute inflammation of the mucous membrane of some part of the air-passages. It is called *coryza* [Κάρα = the head + ζέω = to boil], or *nasal catarrh*, if it affect the Schneiderian membrane of the nose ; *gravedo* [*Gravis* = heavy], if the frontal sinuses suffer ; *laryngeal catarrh*, when the larynx is involved ; and *bronchial catarrh* when the stress of the disease falls upon the trachea and bronchial tubes.

Catarrh is the commonest of diseases. It arises not from mere cold, but from too sudden a change of atmosphere, or from exposure to wet, &c., when the strength is exhausted. Sudden vicissitudes of temperature are not dangerous; for in the use of the Turkish bath a cold douche is commonly employed after leaving the sudatorium, while Dr. Currie and others have related many cases of fever, scarlatina, &c., which have been beneficially treated by cold affusion during the hot stage. The application of cold is only dangerous when the heated body, exhausted by exercise, is rapidly parting with its caloric. Under other circumstances, the glowing system can react upon the cold, and convert it into a strengthening rather than a depressing agent; but the frame which is quickly cooling after having been over warmed is not in a condition to react, and hence the application of cold increases the depression.

The *symptoms* of catarrh chiefly consist of lassitude, pains in the limbs, aching of the back, and a sense of tightness across the forehead ; these effects being quickly succeeded by excessive discharge from the nostrils, profuse lachrymation, hoarseness and sore throat, furred tongue, more or less feverishness, thirst with loss of appetite, and a quick pulse. An eruption of herpes also appears upon the lips ; and perhaps most frequently about the angles, or the middle, of the lower lip. At the end of some forty-eight hours these symptoms begin to subside ; or the disease passes into a more severe affection, such as acute tonsillitis, bronchitis, pneumonia, &c.

Attacks of catarrh are apt to recur, on slight causes, in many susceptible subjects. Occasionally the disease appears to get chronic, but this seldom happens when the system is strong. As the mischief leaves the mucous membrane of the nostrils, the trachea or bronchi may become affected. When this happens, the feverish symptoms get aggravated; while a frequent irritating cough results. Moreover, in catarrhal inflammation of the trachea there is often dysphagia; which at times is so severe for a day or two as to give rise to suspicions of grave disease. But independently of the fact that the pain soon ceases under simple treatment, there is an absence of all the usual symptoms of stricture of the œsophagus, aneurism, cancer, &c. The uneasiness is only felt during coughing or at the moment of deglutition, whether the substance passing consist of food or merely of saliva; and it is often referred by the patient to the top of the sternum. It is probably due to the stretching of the inflamed windpipe which takes place at the time of swallowing. There is commonly dysphonia, sometimes complete aphonia, in these cases.

Dr. Hyde Salter has suggested that the symptoms of catarrh depend upon a specific animal poison; and that they are attributable either to the material presence of this poison circulating in the blood, or to the irritation which it produces in those organs which are its constituted eliminants. The arrest of the function of the skin from exposure to cold throws back into the circulation that which ought to have been eliminated as the cutaneous excretion; and this either by itself, or by ulterior changes which it gives rise to in the blood, induces a condition of toxæmia. The vicarious emunctory for the correction of this state of blood poisoning, by the elimination of the material for whose excretion the skin has been temporarily rendered unequal through cold, is the respiratory mucous membrane; and the principal local symptoms—coryza, tonsillitis, bronchitis—depend upon the vascular changes in this membrane induced by such exceptional excretory function, and possibly by the irritation of the poison materially present thereat. So long as the blood is thus contaminated, the fever symptoms persist; while its depuration is immediately attended by their abatement.

No one applies to a doctor to cure a simple cold. Every man acts as his own physician, and judiciously amuses himself with slops, putting his feet in hot water, and perhaps by taking a few doses of James's powder; the disease meanwhile running its course, and in three or four days exhausting itself. Doubtless the cure can sometimes be expedited by a mild aperient in the morning after a ten-grain dose of Dover's powder has been taken at bedtime; or possibly by the administration of a few saline draughts (F. 348). A hot air or vapour bath may often do good. In some persons, an opiate at bedtime (fifteen or twenty minims of the liquid extract of opium, with one or two drops of chloroform), will cut short a catarrh; while in others, a good dinner, and two or three extra glasses of wine, may have the same effect.   In coryza, an immediate cure is said to result from the inhalation of iodine vapour, every three or four minutes for an hour; each inhalation lasting one minute, and being accomplished by merely holding in the warm hands a bottle of the tincture under the nose. Dr. C. J. B. Williams assures us that any cold can be cured in forty-eight hours or less by almost total abstinence from liquids; but it is a practice which in all probability very few have adopted, though it was originally recommended about one hundred and forty years ago by Dr. Richard Lower.

II. CHRONIC INFLAMMATION OF THE NOSTRILS.

Chronic inflammation of the nostrils, or ozæna ["Οζη = a stench], or rhinorrhœa ['Ρὶν = the nose + ῥέω = to flow,] is attended with heat and stiffness of the nose, tumefaction of the Schneiderian membrane, and an offensive sanious or muco-purulent discharge.

Causes.—This disease may result from repeated or long-continued attacks of acute inflammation, or of common catarrh; being especially apt to do so in such as are of a delicate constitution. It may also be a consequence of the strumous or gouty diathesis, when it is generally associated with disordered digestive organs. And again it not uncommonly depends upon a syphilitic taint.

Diagnosis.—In every case of ozæna the nostrils should be examined with a probe and a nasal speculum, to be certain that the symptoms are not dependent on any impediment (as a foreign body, piece of necrosed bone, or a polypus) to the free discharge of the nasal mucus; since if this secretion be allowed to accumulate, it soon putrefies and excites troublesome inflammation.

It is astonishing what extraordinary substances children sometimes push into the nasal fossæ.   Shells, cherry stones, pebbles, beans, pieces of slate pencil, &c., have been removed by me, after they had been causing an offensive discharge for months.

Rhinoliths ['Ρὶν = the nose + λίθος = a stone] sometimes form in the nasal cavities; these concretions consisting of the phosphate and carbonate of lime, magnesia, and mucus.   A portion of necrosed bone, or some foreign body introduced from without, usually forms the nucleus.   In a rhinolith which I extracted in 1862, the nucleus consisted of a shell; and the patient assured me that this must have been introduced at least thirty years previously.

Abscess of the septum will also give rise to an offensive purulent discharge, which may continue for some time in strumous subjects.   It almost always causes perforation of the septum.

Where there is a polypus, the necessity for its complete removal is to be remembered. Even after perfect extirpation, a gelatinous growth of this kind often forms again and again.

Where the cause of the symptoms is obscure, the posterior recesses of the nostrils ought to be examined by the rhinoscope; so that the condition of the turbinated bones, or the seat of any tumefaction or ulceration, or the glistening form of a polypus, may be reflected in the little glass or steel mirror after it has been passed to the back of the pharynx with its bright surface turned upwards. The throat is to be illuminated by the reflector fixed on the practitioner's forehead; the mirror throwing the rays of light upwards and forwards into the posterior nares, while it receives the reflection of this region. Like the practice of laryngoscopy careful manipulation is necessary to obtain a good image.

Symptoms.—The symptoms of ozæna vary somewhat according to the cause. Usually they come on insidiously with the indications of an ordinary cold; there being especially great uneasiness or "stuffiness" in the nose, owing to the thickened mucous membrane impeding the passage of the air. A portion of the Schneiderian or pituitary membrane may even swell, so as to look like a polypus on a superficial examination. There will be also frontal headache, cough, general weakness, and much mental depression; but the most troublesome symptom consists of a profuse and mephitic muco-purulent discharge. Sometimes this discharge is quite purulent; while it is generally tinged with blood if there be any ulcer on the mucous membrane. Large solid flakes of fibrin or of hardened mucus occasionally come away. The smell from these crusts, owing to the rapidity with which they decompose before they are expelled from the nasal fossæ, is so very offensive and taints the breath to such an extent, that the patient is unable to go into any society. He becomes even an object of disgust to himself; and if medicine should fail to give relief, he gets miserable and desponding, has a complete want of appetite, loses flesh and strength, and passes wretched restless nights. When the disease has continued some time, the septum of the nose often gets eaten through; or the spongy bones become implicated, and there is troublesome caries or necrosis. This is especially likely to happen when the system has been long tainted with the poison of syphilis.

Occasionally the symptoms in ozæna are very slight. The patient (most probably a strumous subject) is merely annoyed by an uneasy feeling in the nose, and especially by finding that whenever he uses his handkerchief he brings away thin mucus stained with blood. Advice is seldom sought until this has continued some time; and it is then perceived on examination, that a circular hole with abraded margins, perhaps large enough to admit a goose-quill, has been eaten through the septum nasi. The hole never closes. These cases are in no way connected with any venereal taint.

Treatment.—The remedies must be local and constitutional.

Remembering that the fetor of the discharge results, in part at least, from the decomposition of the retained mucus, we shall take care to have the nostril frequently and effectually syringed with warm water; to which some alum or zinc, or a solution of permanganate of potash (gr. 5—20 to a pint of water), or a small portion of chloride of zinc (gr. 12 to water fl. oz. 16), can often be very advantageously added.   I have seen cases where a large syringe has had to be used for half an hour at a time, in order completely to dislodge the inspissated matter; for unless the whole is removed no relief will be given.   To moderate the secretion subsequently, the nitrate of mercury ointment (one part to four or six of lard) should be applied up the nostril by means of a camel's-hair pencil every night; or the glycerine of carbolic acid can be tried in the same way every eight or twelve hours.   Atomised medicated fluids (F. 262) also do good service in these cases. Powders of subnitrate of bismuth, of chlorate of potash and sugar (thirty grains and half an ounce), or of red oxide of mercury and sugar (five grains and half an ounce), sniffed up the nostril twice or thrice daily, have been recommended by M. Trousseau and others; but they are less efficacious than injections where there is hardened mucus, while it is not always that we can get them thoroughly applied.   Tannic acid used as a snuff, as well as the high-dried Scotch snuff itself, will sometimes destroy small mucous polypi, possibly by causing them to shrivel up and degenerate.

Supposing the case to be one of catarrhal ozæna, in addition to injections or snuffs' attention ought to be paid to the digestive organs; and then such tonics as quinine and iron, the nitro-hydrochloric acid and bark, steel with arsenic, cod liver oil, and a nourishing diet, will prove the most appropriate constitutional remedies.   A few doses of blue pill and rhubarb may be needed.

In strumous cases I have found most benefit from the iodide of iron and cod liver oil, or from iodine and arsenic, together with the frequent injection of warm water.   The inhalation of steam, medicated either with iodine (F. 259), or creasote (F. 261), or turpentine (F. 260), is very useful.   Change of air, especially to a bracing part of the coast, often does great good.

The treatment of syphilitic ozæna is locally the same as for the other forms; while the constitutional remedies are those of secondary syphilis generally.   The mercurial vapour bath (F. 131) proves especially useful in these instances.

III. APHONIA.

Aphonia ['A = priv. + φωνή = the voice] is found to vary in degree from a slight impairment of the voice to complete dumbness. The loss may be temporary or permanent; and it may be due to functional disorder, or to structural change in the muscles and other tissues of the larynx and glottis. Occasionally there is disease in the nervous centres producing spasms or paralysis of the muscles which act on the vocal cords.

Of the *functional* variety, aphonia from hysteria and debility may be selected as the type. The diagnosis of this form is for the most part easy enough, since it is generally allied with other symptoms indicative of its nature. In women the uterine functions are usually disturbed, irritation of one or both ovaries being often present. Sometimes there is amenorrhœa, sometimes menorrhagia; but the former is more frequent than the latter. Leucorrhœa is commonly complained of. Now and then there is chlorosis.

The patient usually speaks in a whisper for days together. Then the power of the voice returns, but there are generally many relapses. In a fashionable school, where the studies were principally devoted to the so-called accomplishments, three out of eight of the pupils suffered from occasional attacks of aphonia. In two of the cases the disease was hysterical, the mind exercising some influence upon the laryngeal nerves, such as is seen in loss of voice from any sudden or violent emotion. But in the third instance the affection was simply feigned; the young lady being capricious and wayward, though in good health. Galvanism, moral influence, and ferruginous tonics cured all the patients; enabling the victims, to become the masters, of their nerves.

Aphonia from fright or shock may occur in men as well as in women. Deputy Inspector-General Longmore has related an interesting example of complete loss of speech from nervous shock.* The chief points in the case are as follow :—A stout healthy soldier of the Dragoon Guards was struck just below the centre of the lower lip, by a small matchlock-ball weighing nearly one ounce, during a charge of his regiment at the action of Pal-i-chou near Pekin, on the 21st September 1860. The bullet penetrated the tissues; carried away part of the alveolar process and four teeth on the left side; travelled downwards behind the symphysis, clearing away the origins of the genio-hyo-glossi muscles in its passage; and became lodged in the soft textures of the floor of the mouth, behind the frænum linguæ. The power of articulation was immediately lost. The ball was extracted from within the mouth on the twenty-third day. On examination at Fort Pitt, soon after his return home, the inferior maxillary bone was found a little thickened at the seat of injury. The tongue was somewhat wasted, and its movements rather limited; but there was no evidence of muscular paralysis, and no impairment of taste or sensation. Subsequently to his discharge from the service he was watched, but the dumbness continued. At the end of July 1862, thirteen months after becoming a pensioner, he suddenly recovered his speech while in a state of

---

* *Statistical, Sanitary, and Medical Reports for the Year* 1861. Army Medical Department, p. 461. London, 1863.

excitement, during an altercation in a public-house. Dr. Aitken attributed the loss of speech in this case to the injury of the insertions of the genio-hyo-glossi muscles, and to the probable disturbance of the ninth pair of nerves by the inflammation excited. Mr. Longmore objects to this view, on the ground that if it were correct the power of articulation should have been recovered gradually, as the injured parts were restored to health. He attributes the dumbness to the nervous shock ; classing it with those cases of temporary aphonia that occur from hysteria, fright, &c., and in which the recovery is often sudden.

When hysterical or any form of functional aphonia is of long continuance, the vocal cords may become flaccid or powerless, just as happens after severe loss of blood, an acute attack of fever, diphtheria, &c. Many examples of debility or paralysis of the adductor muscles of the vocal cords, so that on attempted phonation the cords could not be approximated, have been reported by Dr. Morell Mackenzie.* Dr. Althaus has related the case of a woman, aged thirty, who had lost her voice two months before he saw her in May 1862. An examination by the laryngoscope showed a paralytic condition of both vocal cords, which were perfectly motionless, while between them a considerable cleft was visible. After two trials of Faradization, the patient could speak again, though only in a hoarse whisper. The laryngoscope then showed that the right vocal cord had to a great extent recovered, and that it approached the middle line when an endeavour was made to pronounce a long "ah." By further treatment, the left vocal cord was also restored to its normal condition, and the voice entirely recovered.†

The chief causes of *organic* aphonia are inflammation, serous infiltration, or ulceration of the mucous membrane about the vocal cords ; the pressure of morbid growths in or near the larynx ; and tubercular or other disease of the lungs. The diagnosis of the first two sets of causes is readily made by the laryngoscope ; the best method of employing this instrument being well detailed by Sir George Duncan Gibb,‡ from whose practical and interesting volume I have derived much information. The laryngoscope consists of a little mirror attached to a flexible metallic stem, which is fixed into a handle of wood or ivory. It varies in size from three or four lines to an inch and a half in diameter ; and is of

---

* *Hoarseness, Loss of Voice, and Stridulous Breathing, in relation to Nervo-Muscular Affections of the Larynx.* Second Edition, p. 3. London. 1868.

† *On Paralysis, Neuralgia, and other Affections of the Nervous System, &c.* Third Edition, p. 154. London, 1864.

‡ *On Diseases of the Throat and Windpipe, as reflected by the Laryngoscope, &c.* Second Edition, p. 445 to 456. London, 1864.—The work of Dr. Morell Mackenzie (*The Use of the Laryngoscope in Diseases of the Throat,* London, 1865) likewise contains full and valuable instructions on all matters appertaining to Laryngoscopy.

a circular, oval, elliptical, or quadrangular form. Glass are better than steel mirrors, according to most authorities. Before introducing the laryngeal mirror into the mouth it should be gently warmed over a spirit lamp, and the temperature estimated by applying the back of the plate to the cheek. The throat is to be illuminated by means of a light thrown into it from a reflecting surface; a proceeding which is accomplished by wearing a large ophthalmoscopic mirror before the right eye, between the two eyes, or on the forehead. I have always used the latter, and been well satisfied with it; though it is not a matter of much moment which form is selected. The attachment of the mirror by a ball-and-socket joint to a large spectacle-frame, the forehead band, or the mouth-piece of Czermak, permits of its movement in any necessary direction. The light to be employed for reflection may be natural or artificial; the former comprising day and sunlight, and the latter a good moderator lamp or an argand gas lamp, with a plated mirror at the back of the cylindrical glass chimney. In sunlight the patient has his back to the window, and the rays being received in the reflector are thence conveyed to the laryngeal mirror. But, as a rule, artificial light is the best; and the mode of proceeding is then as follows:—The patient is to sit erect, with the lamp near his left elbow. His head can be supported on a kind of photographer's rest, if deemed advisable. The mouth ought to be on a level with the nose or eyes of the operator, the flame of the lamp being on a line with the operator's eyes. The position being rendered comfortable, the patient is to protrude his tongue, and with his handkerchief to firmly hold it outwards and downwards; at the same time opening his mouth as wide as possible, and reclining the head a little upwards. The proper focal distance being ascertained by movements of the head forwards, the operator introduces the warmed laryngeal mirror with the right hand, or with his left if he would keep the right free for applying remedies or instruments; gently placing the mirror against the middle of the soft palate and uvula, without touching the tongue or back of the pharynx. The handle of the mirror is to be well kept to the left side of the patient's mouth out of the light, the patient breathing quietly as usual. The back of the tongue with its large follicles first comes into view: then the hollow space between it and the anterior or glossal surface of the epiglottis; next the apex and laryngeal surface of the epiglottis; and then the interior of the larynx, in which is seen an extremely moveable antero-posterior fissure, bounded by two brilliant pearly borders, that palpitate with surprising rapidity. This last is the glottis; being formed by the inferior thyro-arytenoid ligaments or true vocal cords, in contradistinction to the false cords which are above the glottis and are formed by the superior thyro-arytenoid ligaments or muscles. Beyond the glottis the trachea is seen; the rings of which are distinctly visible far down, even to the bifurcation, during deep inspiration.   In cases where the throat and fauces are unusually irritable a few whiffs of chloroform will some-times relieve this condition.   Dr. Morell Mackenzie says he has found the best effects result from sucking ice for some ten minutes before the mirror is to be introduced.   Other physicians have advised about ten grains of the bromide of ammonium to be ad-ministered thrice daily, for a couple of days prior to the investiga-tion; inasmuch as this agent seems to deaden the sensibility of the mucous membrane.   My own throat is so sensitive that I have only once been able to practise autolaryngoscopy, and this was after taking the iodide of potassium for some days.   But usually the first-named salt is preferable to the latter.

In connexion with this subject it only remains to notice that for the cure of inflammation and ulceration about the cords the best application (by means of a curved brush) is that recommended by Sir G. D. Gibb; viz. from forty to eighty grains of the crystals of nitrate of silver to the ounce of distilled water.   Scarificators are employed for œdema of the glottis, curved forceps for the extraction of foreign bodies, and the wire écraseur for the removal of polypi or other growths.   The inhalation of atomised fluids (F. 262) will prove most serviceable in some instances.

Tubercular disease of the lungs, with deposits in the larynx, causing aphonia is hopeless.   The loss of voice only occurs to-wards the end of the affection, and may be considered as indicat-ing a quickly fatal termination.   Aphonia at times, however, occurs in phthisis merely from debility; there being no disease whatever in the windpipe.   In such, properly directed treatment will be useful. The laryngoscope will show the nature of the case.

Disease of the brain affecting the pneumogastric nerve may cause paralysis of the muscles of the larynx, on the normal action of which the tension and position of the vocal cords depends. The aphonia thus resulting could never be mistaken for that failure of articulate language (aphemia or aphasia) which is the consequence of disease in the cerebral hemisphere—the seat of mind.   A few years ago, I saw at Millbank a prisoner who was completely dumb and had been so for some months, in consequence (as he believed) of a blow on the back part of the head from a policeman's truncheon. His mind was healthy and active. He had no difficulty in express-ing his wishes and ideas in writing. Such was his intelligence indeed, that by some practitioners this man had been deemed a clever malingerer; though I felt convinced from his general ap-pearance and symptoms that the suspicion was unjust. To remove all doubt, however, he was put carefully but fully under the in-fluence of chloroform; in the conviction that as the anæsthetic effect passed off he would betray himself, if the aphonia were feigned, before perfect consciousness returned.   But though he evidently strived to talk, he merely uttered a few guttural sounds, something like those produced by a deaf mute when excited. The laryngoscope was not then in daily use as it is now, or doubtless paralysis of the vocal cords might have been detected.

The difference between aphonia and aphasia (see p. 379) may perhaps be clearly illustrated by what is seen in the case of a man with a cut throat, and comparing the effects with those which result from an aneurism of the cervical portion of the internal carotid artery on the left side. In the case of the cut throat, supposing the trachea to be opened below the glottis, the voice disappears—there is aphonia. There will be no aphasia or loss of the faculty of speech —no mental defect. The man with the wound in his windpipe may in fact speak, and were he deaf he might doubtless imagine that his voice was audible. But there is no voice simply because the current of air which should play on the vocal cords does not reach them. Close the wound artificially, and then there will be both speech and voice. Now in the other instance, the aneurism of the left internal carotid necessitates the application of a ligature to the common carotid. Thus a considerable supply of blood must be cut off from the brain, and especially from that part supplied by the anterior and middle cerebral arteries. The balance cannot be perfectly restored by any compensating enlargement of other vessels. As a consequence of the defective nutrition, softening by and by takes place of the posterior part of the third left frontal convolution; and if this be the convolution of articulate language, as M. Broca maintains, aphasia or cerebral speechlessness must result. The organs of the voice are healthy enough, but the mental faculty of speech has gone for ever.

IV. DYSPHONIA CLERICORUM.

Dysphonia [from $\Delta\nu\varsigma$ = difficulty or pain + $\phi\omega\nu\dot{\eta}$ = the voice] clericorum, or clergyman's sore throat, is frequently a nervous complaint; being unattended, at least in its early stages, by any organic lesion, but consisting rather of hyperæsthesia or irritability of the investing membrane of the fauces. Subsequently, however, a series of important morbid changes takes place. These are chiefly congestion, inflammation, or relaxation of the mucous membrane; enlargement of the tonsils; elongation of the uvula; with irritation, inflammation, morbid deposit, and ulceration of the mucous follicles about the isthmus faucium. Dr. Horace Green of New York has described this affection, when far advanced, as consisting of a diseased condition of the glandular follicles of the mucous membrane of the throat and windpipe; commencing usually in the mucous follicles of the isthmus of the fauces and of the upper portion of the pharyngeal membrane; and extending by continuity until the glandulæ of the epiglottis, larynx, and trachea are extensively involved in the morbid action.   He calls it *follicular disease of the pharyngo-laryngeal membrane.*

Symptoms.—These principally consist of an uneasy sensation in the upper part of the throat, with continued inclination to swallow ; as if there were some obstacle in the œsophagus which could be removed by deglutition.   The patient also makes frequent attempts to clear the throat of phlegm by coughing, hawking, and spitting : he will point to the larynx, too, as being the seat of pain.   At the same time the voice undergoes an alteration ; there being loss of power, and hoarseness—sometimes complete aphonia, especially towards the evening.   On examining the throat and fauces, we shall find these parts presenting an unhealthy, slightly raw, or granular appearance ; the mucous follicles may be visible, sometimes filled with a yellowish substance ; and a viscid muco-purulent secretion will be seen adhering to the palate, as well as to the edge of the velum pendulum palati.

This sore throat either exists alone, or it may accompany or follow laryngitis, bronchitis, or phthisis.   Clergymen, barristers, public speakers, actors, singers, &c., are most liable to it.

Treatment.—In its early stages, when merely a nervous affection, the treatment is resolved into the use of tonics, especially iron and quinine ; cold plunge or shower baths or sea bathing; together with temporary change of scene and occupation.   Where the disease is further advanced, a combination of internal with local remedies will be necessary.   Iodide of potassium (F. 31), iodide of iron (F. 32), iodide or bromide of ammonium (F. 37, 38), small doses of perchloride of mercury (F. 27), phosphate of zinc (F. 414), strychnia and steel (F. 408), steel and chlorate of potash (F. 402), quinine with iron and arsenic (F. 381), phosphoric acid with nux vomica and bark (F. 376), and cod liver oil (F. 389), will prove the most efficacious remedies.

The local treatment consists in the application of a solution of nitrate of silver (from forty to sixty grains of the crystals to the ounce of distilled water) to the diseased parts, and even to the interior of the larynx.   This is effected by means of an angular brush, or of a whalebone probang about ten inches long, having a piece of fine sponge, the size of a pistol-bullet, attached to its extremity. The difficulty of introducing the sponge or probang between the lips of the glottis is greatly lessened by employing the laryngeal mirror ; with which the instrument can be seen to enter the larynx. One of the methods of using the sponge is described somewhat thus by Dr. Hughes Bennett :—The patient being seated in a chair and exposed to a good light, the practitioner stands on the right side and depresses the tongue with a spatula held in the left hand. Holding the probang with the sponge saturated with the solution in the right hand, this instrument ought to be passed carefully over the upper surface of the spatula exactly in the median plane, until it is above or immediately behind the epiglottis.   The patient should now be told to inspire; and as he does so, the tongue must be dragged slightly forwards with the spatula, and the probang thrust downwards and forwards by a movement which causes the right arm to be elevated, and the hand to be brought almost in contact with the patient's face. The operation of course requires dexterity, since the rima glottidis is narrow, and unless the sponge comes fairly down upon it, the aperture is readily missed. The passage of the sponge into the proper channel may be determined by the sensation of overcoming a constriction, which is experienced when it is momentarily embraced by the rima, as well as by the spasm and harsh expiration that it occasions.* When recourse is had to the laryngoscope, the patient draws his tongue forwards and holds it tightly. Then, the operator taking the mirror fixed in its handle with his left hand, introduces the sponge with his right, and guides it by the aid of the reflected image (see p. 520).—The application, however made, will be required about every other day for two or three weeks.

If it be thought preferable, as it usually must be, to disperse a minutely-divided and misty shower of some medicated solution over the diseased surfaces, recourse may be had to one of the many excellent instruments now in use for the inhalation of medicated fluids reduced to the form of spray. This practice first attracted attention in 1858, when Sales-Giron constructed his " Pulvérisateur portatif des liquides médicamenteux." Some years previously, however, Mr. Tompson had published an account of his very ingenious " Hydro-pneumatic inhaler ;" an instrument consisting of a bellows worked by the foot, a glass cylinder or flask traversed by sixteen capillary tubes, an adjusting apparatus, and a nozzle furnished with a screw-cap for the enclosure of a plate of fine silver-wire gauze. The fault of this apparatus is its clumsiness. Hence it must be superseded by such as Bergson's hand-ball spray producer ; which has the merit of simplicity and cheapness, and from which the tubes sold by perfumers for pulverizing scents have been adapted. Siegle's atomizer as modified by Krohne and Sesemann, in which the fluid is forced forwards by steam instead of wind, is a most serviceable instrument. The " traveller's atomizer," made according to the suggestions of Dr. Beigel, can also be strongly recommended. The drug to be chosen will depend on the symptoms, but generally an astringent (F. 262) is needed. Gibb's laryngeal injector, or hand atomizer, can be employed when it is desirable to apply a shower of spray to the larynx alone, without allow-

---

* The mistake of trusting to these sensations is well illustrated in the Report of the Commission of the New York Academy of Medicine, appointed to inquire into this subject :—" We witnessed in cases 11 and 21 the fallacy of Dr. Horace Green's opinion as to the success of his experiment, though based on so large an experience. In both instances, whilst positive that he had successfully passed the instrument (an elastic tube) into the trachea, *the patient vomited through the tube,* and thus demonstrated his error." This of course happened before the laryngoscope had come into vogue.

ing it to be inhaled. This instrument consists of a ribbed india rubber ball, a curved silver tube having a small circular disc near its terminal end, and screwed to this disc a capsular bulb of platinum with very minute perforations. This injector answers admirably for applying one or two drops of a solution of nitrate of silver to the interior of the larynx.

To prevent a recurrence of follicular disease the throat should be properly covered ; no protection being more efficient than that with which man is naturally provided. Hence the beard ought to be allowed to grow. Moreover, every working man requires one day's rest in seven. The conscientious clergyman, whose duties are as toilsome as those of the mechanic or day labourer, should make a rule of taking a thorough holiday on every Monday. In obstinate cases, a winter at the Undercliff (F. 434), or at Torquay (F. 436), at Pau (F. 443), at Malaga (F. 445), or at Algiers (F. 451), may be strongly recommended.

When the tonsils remain enlarged and indurated (as they often do after this form of sore throat, as well as after repeated attacks of tonsillitis) various astringent gargles and inhalations, preparations of iodine, and the solid nitrate of silver have been long employed. A piece of pyrethrum (Pellitory of Spain) chewed slowly, is occasionally useful in relieving relaxation of the tonsils. Nevertheless, not unfrequently permanent and effectual relief will only be obtained by the excision of one or both of these glands. Mr. Harvey has condemned this practice, and has stated that removal of the tonsils interferes with the development of the genital organs. I have seen, however, so much benefit from the operation, without any bad results, that I cannot but doubt the correctness of Mr. Harvey's views.

V. CROUP.

Croup (*trachealia, tracheitis*, or *cynanche* trachealis*) will be best defined as an acute inflammatory disease of the trachea, or often of the glottis and larynx and trachea ; the fever and inflammation being accompanied by the exudation of false membranes upon the affected mucous surfaces.

Croup is a disease of early life ; most cases of it occurring during the second year of childhood. Some families seem more predisposed to it than others. Male children are rather more obnoxious to it than female ; while when an attack has been gone through, there is a liability to a recurrence of the disease at any time up to puberty. The inflammation is often complicated with bronchitis or pneumonia. It may end fatally from exhaustion, suffocation, convulsions, or the formation of a clot in the heart.

---

* From Κύων = a dog + άγχω = to strangle ; because dogs were supposed to be especially liable to sore-throat.

Symptoms.—In the incipient stage the symptoms are those of a common cold—such as slight fever, cough, hoarseness, drowsiness, suffusion of the eyes, and running at the nose. There is usually more or less fretfulness. In some few instances, the child clutches or rubs its larynx, as if there were an uneasy sensation there; or there may be a slight hesitation in swallowing, as in simple sore-throat. If we examine the fauces, however, no traces of disease will be detected; and if we resort to auscultation or percussion, the chest will be found healthy.

At the end of twenty-four or thirty-six hours the second or developed stage sets in. The child is suddenly awoke, almost invariably during the night, by a sensation of suffocation; together with a peculiar acute and dry and ringing brassy cough, and hurried breathing. He is agitated and alarmed, and wants to sit up or leave his bed; his face becomes slightly swelled and flushed; and his eyes are suffused and bloodshot. Each inspiration now becomes prolonged; while it is attended with a characteristic crowing noise, readily recognised when once it has been heard. These distinctive coughs, and the difficult and crowing inspirations, probably continue to recur in paroxysms, through the remainder of the night; while the little sufferer continually changes his position, in the vain attempt to find that relief which is denied to him. As the morning dawns, however, there is a slight remission of the symptoms, and a short slumber will probably be obtained. But the improvement is transitory: the disease advances, the fever increases, the voice becomes more hoarse, the paroxysms of cough get more frequent, and the breathing is more difficult and hurried. There is also great thirst, the tongue is coated with a thick fur, the pulse gets quicker and harder, and the child becomes very irritable and restless. It is now very commonly noticed that the hand seizes the larynx as if to remove some obstruction; or the fingers are thrust into the mouth as if to drag away the cause of suffering. Then the arms are thrown wildly about, and all covering tossed aside; the countenance becomes flushed, and at times almost livid; while as each paroxysm of cough comes on, and as the dyspnœa becomes urgent, the head is thrown back as far as possible in order to increase the capacity of the windpipe. Through the whole progress of the disease exacerbations are observed to take place at night, with remissions in the morning. The cough is unattended by expectoration, and each fit of coughing is usually followed by a paroxysm of dyspnœa. The act of speaking seems to increase the suffering, for the child only whispers or often refuses to utter a word. The bowels are constipated. There is seldom any sickness. And although the appetite for food is quite lost, there is a constant desire for drink; notwithstanding that deglutition sometimes appears to cause pain.

As the disease advances towards the third stage or that of collapse—or of threatened suffocation, the intermissions between the paroxysms grow shorter, so that there is scarcely any remission ; the cough gets more difficult, less audible, suppressed, and strangulating ; the voice is nearly or quite abolished ; the croupal respiration is permanent ; and every now and then suffocation seems imminent.   Moreover there is drowsiness, which soon becomes extreme though the sleep is uneasy ; for the child starts and wakes in terror and grasps convulsively at any object near him. If no relief be given by the expectoration of the muco-purulent matter or of the membranous exudation obstructing the larynx and trachea, very alarming effects follow.   The skin becomes cold and covered with clammy sweats ; the pulse gets very frequent, feeble, and intermitting ; the respiration grows more difficult and accompanied with a hissing noise ; the movements of the larynx are forcible and incessant ; while the head is thrown back, the alæ nasi are rapidly dilated and contracted, the eyes are dull and sunken, and the complexion is livid.   The countenance is also expressive of the greatest agony.   At the end of about twelve or eighteen hours the child dies with signs of convulsive suffocation, or it sinks exhausted into a state of coma from which death ultimately relieves it.

The practice of auscultation in the second and third stages, yields information as to the amount of air entering the lungs, and the extension or not of the inflammation to the bronchial tubes and lungs.   When the obstruction to the entrance of the air is great, the inspiratory murmur may be quite imperceptible in the smaller bronchi, except during an unusually deep inspiration after a fit of coughing : at the same time there is healthy resonance on percussion.   According to Barth and Roger,* a kind of vibrating murmur or *tremblotement* can be heard over the larynx or trachea, when the false membrane has become partially detached and is floating ; but this murmur is in reality seldom to be detected. Should bronchitis supervene, we shall find the sonorous rhonchus indicative of it, masked in some degree by the croupy noise in the trachea ; and such will likewise be the case with regard to the small crepitation of pneumonia.   But in the latter case there will be impaired resonance on percussion over the inflamed portions of lung.

The *duration* of the disease varies according to the violence of the inflammation and the strength of the patient : the average time is from two to six days, a fatal issue being most common on the fourth day.   Occasionally, however, the morbid action runs a very rapid course.   Thus, Professor Gölis of Vienna relates the case of a healthy little boy, aged four years ; who—going into the open air on an extremely cold day—was attacked with croup, which proved fatal in fourteen hours.†

Morbid Anatomy.—The mucous membrane of the larynx and

* *Traité pratique d'Auscultation.*   Second Edition, p. 261.   Paris, 1844.
† *Tractatus de rite cognoscendâ et sanandâ Anginâ membranaceâ.* Obs. iv., p. 141.   Viennæ, 1813.

trachea and bronchial tubes is generally found inflamed, red or livid, congested, and swollen. Sometimes there are abrasions or ulcerations; while very frequently there is a layer of viscid muco-purulent matter, or more commonly an exudation of false membrane. This membrane is found more frequently in the larynx than in the trachea, and in both structures more often than in the bronchial tubes. On the Continent frequently, although very rarely in this country, the exudation is also found on the velum palati, and about the fauces and pharynx. It generally presents the appearance of a thin but rather firm layer; it is unorganized; and consists of either coagulated albumen or of fibrin, but most probably of the former. Signs of pneumonia are not unusual. Care must be taken not to confound the symptoms and appearances due to pulmonic congestion arising from the suffocative influence of croup with those which result from inflammatory action.

Pathology.—From the foregoing it seems evident that this disease consists of inflammation of the mucous membrane, exciting spasmodic action in the larynx and trachea, and giving rise to a peculiar product—a pseudo-membranous secretion. The result is imperfect aëration of the blood; for the access of air to the minute vessels is impeded by the spasm, as well as by the extension and accumulation of the croupal productions.

The question as to whether the inflammation is of a simple kind, or dependent upon the presence of some specific poison in the system—as is the case with the eruptive fevers &c., has been entertained but not satisfactorily answered. My own views are certainly in favour of the latter opinion, and for these reasons:—The second attacks of croup are (as a rule) much less severe than the first, because the susceptibility of the system to the action of the poison is partly exhausted, just as is seen in the practice of syphilisation: the occasional prevalence of the disease in an epidemic form seems to indicate a particular agent as its cause: when laryngitis is excited in children by some poisonous irritant, or by drinking boiling water from the spout of a tea-kettle, the results are very different; and false membranes are not exuded, even though the inflammation extend to the trachea. Cases of croup though rare in the adult sometimes occur; but the symptoms are different from those of simple laryngitis, and they do not as often yield to the same treatment—*i.e.*, to making an artificial opening into the windpipe—which sometimes cures the latter. Again, if laryngitis be artificially produced in the lower animals, false membranes are not exuded; though croup (identical in its phenomena and organic changes with the disease in the human subject) does spontaneously occur in them, as is seen in lambs, calves, puppies, cats, and in chickens—constituting the "pip." The latter especially often prevails epidemically in a farmyard, and produces a large mortality.

Complications of Croup.—One of the most dangerous complications is with cynanche maligna, as is sometimes seen when croup occurs during the course of scarlatina anginosa. The exudation thrown out from the inflamed surface, forms a pellicle which covers the fauces and extends down the pharynx as well as down the air-passages : occasionally the pellicular exudation is only produced in patches, giving rise to an appearance of thin sloughs. Some authorities have thought that croupal inflammation might originate in tonsillitis, the disease extending over the fauces, as well as down the pharynx and larynx ; but I have seen nothing which would lead me to coincide with this view. Occasionally croup is complicated with aphthous ulcerations about the mouth and palate : this is seen when the disease occurs in feeble subjects, who have been previously suffering from disordered states of the alimentary canal. Where croup supervenes upon measles or small-pox or erysipelas, the inflammatory fever assumes a low type, convulsions are frequent, the difficulty of respiration is excessive, and the paroxysms of suffocation are extreme. Lastly, the croupal inflammation of the larynx and trachea, may extend to the bronchial tubes, and thence to the substance of the lungs—pneumonia; a complication which in almost all cases terminates fatally.

Diagnosis.—The manner of the onset, the hoarseness or loss of· voice, the dry ringing cough, the early severity of the symptoms, the exacerbations and remissions, the croupal inspirations, the inflammatory fever, the heaving of the thorax, and the motions of the larynx and trachea, distinguish this disease from every other. It can indeed only be confounded with true laryngitis. But this latter affection occurs in adults, very rarely in children, except as associated with croup ; laryngitis causes a fixed burning pain in the larynx increased by any examination; it does not give rise to the exudation of false membranes ; and when prolonged it ends in suppuration, or ulceration. The diagnosis between croup and spasm of the glottis is very simple : for in the latter there is an absence of fever and of the peculiar cough, the intermissions between the fits of suffocation are complete, and there are general convulsions with spasmodic contractions of the toes and thumbs during the seizure.

Prognosis.—Croup may terminate in—(1) Recovery. This result can be expected in mild forms, when the respiration is comparatively quiet during the intervals between the paroxysms of cough ; when the cough is loose, and followed by the expectoration of muco-purulent matter, or of fragments of the membranous exudation ; when there is a gentle perspiration over the skin ; when the disease is uncomplicated ; and when it is not attended with great prostration of the vital powers. (2) The disease may pass into some other malady, or excite additional disease,—thus materially increasing the danger. In addition to the obstruction of the respiration produced by the exudation of croup, this affection tends to give rise to spasmodic closure of the glottis ; the fits of suffocation which result always leading to great pulmonary congestion, as well as to a marked disposition to consecutive disturbance. The extension of the inflammation to the bronchi and to the substance of the lungs is a very unfavourable event ; producing lividity of the face, great drowsiness, cold clammy sweats, great frequency of pulse, and suffocating paroxysms of cough with very short intermissions. What is called laryngeal or tracheal consumption will perhaps result from croup ; a condition characterized by pain in the larynx, suffocating cough, spasmodic attacks of dyspnœa, muco-purulent expectoration, and hectic fever,—coming on after the subsidence of the acute symptoms, and perhaps just as a successful termination is about to be prognosticated.   Or, the active signs of croup may be subsiding, and suddenly a relapse take place, owing to the aggravation of the slight inflammatory action which remained unsubdued.   This tendency to a relapse must make our prognosis guarded for the two or three weeks during which it exists, in all instances ; but particularly in weakly and irritable children.   Lastly, congestion of the brain, giving rise to the effusion of serum into the ventricles, convulsions, &c., may be an indirect consequence of croup.   Dr. Copland and others have met with instances of hydrocephalus following the disease, but they are not common.   (3) In the greater number of cases it is to be feared, this disease ends fatally.   Much danger is to be apprehended where the symptoms progress to the third stage ; where the fever, from the first, is intense ; where the attacks of dyspnœa are very severe ; where the cough is not followed by expectoration ; where the pulse is very frequent, small, and irregular ; and where the countenance becomes livid, the eyes sunken, the features contracted, the tongue dark, and the lips covered with sordes,—all symptoms indicative of great exhaustion.

The mortality from croup is very great, for probably rather more than half of the children attacked die.   If we take twelve cases of death from various diseases during childhood, we shall find that about one is owing to croup.   The fatal cases of this disease in England, during 1866, amounted to $\frac{\text{Males } 2706}{\text{Females } 2462} = 5168$; of which number 4533 were under 5 years of age.   In a large number of the unfavourable cases death seems to take place from asphyxia ; while in some instances it certainly appears due to a deposit of fibrin in the heart.   After death from acute croup, Dr. Richardson has more than once found the cavity of the right auricle filled with a fibrinous concretion ; which must have been formed during life, as the masses of fibrin were grooved by the currents of blood passing over them from the inferior and superior venæ cavæ.   With such cases death begins at the heart ; the dyspnœa being caused by the want of blood in the pulmonic capillaries.   The lips are slightly blue, the body is pale, and the pulse irregular ; while the heart-beats are feeble and quick and irregular.   The sounds are muffled, and sometimes there will be a bruit.   The respiratory murmur is everywhere audible ; and frequently there are signs of emphysema.

When in croup death is going to happen from suffocation, auscultation and percussion give evidence of the existence of congestion of the lungs, but never of emphysema; while the body becomes of a dark hue, there are convulsive muscular movements, the heart-sounds are clear, and the pulse gets very feeble.

Causes.—Croup is more frequent in cold, damp, changeable climates, than in warm regions: hence it is common in the north-west countries of Europe, but almost unknown in the south. It is also most prevalent in low moist localities; during the winter and in the early spring months; and especially perhaps after the long continuance of heavy rains with east or north-east winds.

Children of a nervous and sanguine temperament seem more disposed to the disease than others. When it occurs during the first twelve months of life it is seen most frequently in weakly infants brought up by hand; and boys are more liable to it than girls, perhaps (though this is very doubtful) because they are more exposed to its exciting causes. Some authors imagine that an hereditary tendency to croup often exists; others, that the disease is infectious: the only support, however, to these opinions is derived from the circumstance that two or more children in the same family are often seized with it, forgetting that they have been placed under the same circumstances as regards the exciting causes. There is but little doubt, that though croup usually occurs as a sporadic disease, yet it sometimes prevails as an epidemic; and perhaps it did so more in former times than in the present day.

As regards the immediate or exciting causes of croup (the foregoing must be regarded more as predisposing causes) very little is positively known. Still it is probable that habitual exposure of the neck and throat to cold, insufficient clothing, and such circumstances as induce common catarrh and bronchitis in the adult, will under certain conditions give rise to it.

Treatment.—In no disease, perhaps, is it more necessary to be prompt and cautious and unwearying in our attendance. Even where an attack of croup is merely apprehended in a child having a catarrh and slight rough or ringing cough, we should carefully watch the patient, place it in a warm bath for some ten minutes, confine it to bed, keep the air of the apartment moist by the evaporation of boiling water, allow only a milk diet, and order frequently-repeated draughts of a saline mixture containing small doses of ipecacuanha wine with spirit of nitrous ether.

When the inflammatory action is established, there are three remedies on which all authorities teach us to rely—viz., blood-letting, tartarated antimony, and mercury. Perhaps there is no infantile disorder which is so surely and early recognised by practitioners, and so zealously and perseveringly treated on this plan, as croup; for mistakes in diagnosis are very rare, and errors in treatment are seldom committed,—supposing that the authorities are correct. The question may well be asked then,—How is it that the disease is so fatal? I believe, from my own experience, because the chief remedies are not only inappropriate but mischievous.

Every physician knows that when he is summoned to a consultation on a case of croup, he is sure to find that the sufferer has been either leeched or blistered; and he probably is informed that *in spite* of the loss of blood the inflammation has increased. It never strikes the practitioner that he should say—"in consequence of;" yet it would probably be nearer the truth. I would strongly urge then, that this plan of indiscriminate bleeding be discontinued; and at the same time would recommend that even antimony and mercury be administered very cautiously, if at all. Blisters never have any other than an injurious effect.

But if we are not to bleed or blister in a severe case of croup, what are we to do? Well, in the first place, the little patient is to be confined to bed, and to be clothed in flannel. The air of the room is to be kept warm and moist. If our visit be paid at the onset of the disease, the inflammatory action can sometimes be arrested by hot fomentations alone—as recommended by Dr. Lehmann and successfully practised by Dr. Graves. A sponge, the size of a large fist, dipped in water as hot as the hand can bear, must be gently squeezed half dry and instantly applied beneath the little sufferer's chin so as to cover the larynx; the temperature being maintained by re-soaking it every two or three minutes. A steady perseverance in this plan for twenty or thirty minutes produces vivid redness of the skin over the whole surface of the throat; while under the influence of this soothing topical treatment, a gentle perspiration breaks out—to be encouraged by warm diluents. A notable diminution also takes place in the cough, hoarseness, huskiness of voice, dyspnœa, restlessness, &c.; while frequently a sound sleep is enjoyed, from which the patient awakes nearly well. Supposing that this amelioration does not take place, very little time has been lost, and we must resort to emetics—a most valuable class of remedies. The ipecacuanha wine (in doses varying from one fluid drachm to two drachms, according to the age) should be given every fifteen minutes until free vomiting has been induced; while unless the breathing is relieved, a dose sufficient to keep up the nausea may be repeated every three or four hours until decided ease is afforded. When this is obtained, great benefit will result from the administration every two hours of a draught containing one or two grains of iodide of potassium, some aromatic spirit of ammonia, a little senega, and any aromatic water. Some broth or beef tea ought to be given repeatedly; together with sweetened tea containing half milk, cocoa or chocolate made with milk, and melted calf's foot jelly or any agreeable demulcent drink. At the same time that this plan is pursued, the temperature of the body is to be taken by a thermometer placed under the armpit, or with care under the tongue; and if (as it usually is in the first and second stages) the degree of heat be above the normal standard, a warm bath ought to be administered, and the patient immersed in it up to the chin for fifteen or thirty minutes, according to the effect produced.   It is of course clear, that a patient having a temperature of 104° or 105° Fahr., must part rapidly with some of this heat, if placed in water warmed only to 98° or 100°; unless as fast as the heat is given off it be regenerated.   This bath is not only cooling, but sedative : it may be repeated twice or thrice in the twenty-four hours, but only under the personal superintendence of the practitioner.   To avoid alarming the child, the bath ought not to be prepared in its presence; and when brought into the sick-room the top of it should be covered with a blanket, on which the patient can then be placed and slowly lowered into the water. A piece of wood or some toy may be floated on the surface, to engage the attention of the little sufferer.

In order to prevent the formation of false membranes, some physicians assert that mercurial inunction should be had recourse to from the commencement of the severe symptoms; thirty, or even sixty grains, of the unguentum hydrargyri being gently rubbed in every four or six hours.   The practitioner must use his own judgment as to the employment of this agent.   No harm can arise from calomel given at the onset as a purgative, in doses of two, three, or four grains; but I have no faith whatever in the power of mercury to control croupal inflammation, and believe that its frequent administration is very injurious.—During the latter stages of the disease, it will be necessary to support the powers of life by the exhibition of the yolk of a raw egg beaten up in tea, and good broth or beef tea ; while wine, or a few drops of aromatic spirits of ammonia, or brandy with milk or water, should be frequently repeated.   A mixture of ammonia and ether (F. 364) often gives temporary strength, and acts as a restraint upon the formation of blood clots.   The inhalation of oxygen, from a gasometer charged with equal parts of common air and oxygen gas, has been recommended when asphyxia threatens ; and certainly this remedy appears deserving of a trial, though no opportunity of testing its value has fallen in my way.   I have, however, administered the peroxide of hydrogen (F. 370); but the effect has only been of a negative character—it seemed to be neither beneficial nor injurious.

According to M. Küchenmeister of Dresden, diphtheritic membranes are rapidly dissolved in lime water.   Pieces of these membranes put into lime water break up in from ten to fifteen minutes.   M. Biermer, Professor of Clinical Medicine in the University of Berne, confirms this statement.   In a bad case of croup this latter gentleman effected a cure by the use of hot pulverised atomised ?) lime water.   The inhalations softened and detached the exudations.   M. Küchenmeister also successfully treated a case of diphtheritic pharyngo-laryngitis by lime water inhalations ; and Dr. Brauser cured one of croup in the same way. There are also other drugs (F. 262), and even plain warm water, which may be fairly tried in the form of spray.

Can we do any good by tracheotomy ?   This is a question the consideration of which must force itself upon every practitioner treating either a case of croup, or one of diphtheria, or one of laryngitis, &c. Looking at the pathology of the disease now under consideration, remembering that the inflammation frequently extends into the bronchial tubes, that the serous dyspnœa for the most part arises from the albuminous exudation obstructing the trachea and bronchi, and that tracheotomy when performed in croup has a tendency to induce bronchitis or pneumonia,—remembering these points, there appears to be much less chance of a favourable issue than may be expected from the same proceeding in laryngitis. Moreover, if the sufferer appears to be dying from syncope (from some obstruction about the heart) then tracheotomy will be useless ; for there has probably been a deposition of fibrin in the right auricle or ventricle, and we can only trust to the administration of ammonia with other restoratives. Yet granting all this, it must still be remembered that making an opening into the trachea is sometimes the only proceeding which can be of any avail to prevent immediate asphyxia ; while not only does it directly prolong life by the admission of air, but it affords time for the disease to run through its several stages with more or less hope of its terminating favourably. The strong advocate for this surgical proceeding was M. Trousseau ; who during four years operated twenty-four times in private practice with fourteen cures, and two hundred and sixteen times at the Hôpital des Enfans Malades with only forty-seven recoveries. Many of the latter patients, however, were in a miserable condition before being seen. My former colleague Dr. Conway Evans says—" The operation of tracheotomy for the relief of croup has been many times performed in this country, and in at least *ten* cases with the most signal success ; life having been saved when the patient had been literally almost at the last gasp."* Mr. Henry Smith is also a strong advocate for this operation ; and he tells me that when it fails to save life, it still affords great temporary relief. The truth of this observation will be apparent to every practitioner who may have had the opportunity of comparing the very painful death which results from gradual suffocation, with the easy sinking of fatal exhaustion.

To bring these remarks to a practical issue I would therefore say, that if the predominant symptoms are those of asphyxia—if the air does not freely enter the lungs at each inspiration, tracheotomy is the remedy ; this proceeding being resorted to as soon as the false membranes appear to be causing obstruction, instead of deferring it as a last resource. The operation should be performed slowly and cautiously and deliberately, so as especially to avoid wounding large vessels ; either pure chloroform or chloroform and ether (F. 313) ought decidedly to be used, unless the child's consciousness have been already destroyed by the circulation of non-oxygenated blood ; the external incision is to be large enough for

* *Edinburgh Medical Journal*, vol. v. p. 416. November 1859.

the operator to see what he is about; the double bivalve cannula must be employed, taking care not to have it too small; and before thrusting the scalpel into the trachea, this tube should be fixed and drawn forwards by means of a sharp hook inserted into it.   As soon as the rings of the trachea are divided the child coughs violently, mucus and shreds of false membrane are expelled through the opening, and the air rushes out with a characteristic shrill and hissing noise.   If any pieces of false membrane bulge out of the wound, they should be gently withdrawn.   The outside shield or tube is to be introduced, taking care that it really does enter the trachea; and then the inner tube is easily passed through this valvular cannula.   With adults it may possibly be best to open the larynx by dividing the crico-thyroid membrane; but in children the larynx is too small to admit the tube, and therefore tracheotomy will have to be performed through the upper rings of the trachea.   Dr. Marshall Hall suggested that when the operation has to be performed before instruments can be procured, it may be done with a simple pair of pointed scissors.   The integument, being taken up horizontally by the thumb and finger of the left hand, is to be divided longitudinally by the scissors; these should then be promptly forced into the trachea, to the proper depth, and opened horizontally to the just extent; the scissors must be then turned, being kept in their place, and opened in the direction longitudinally.   The operator has thus made, in little more than a moment of time, an opening through which the patient may breathe until further appliances can be obtained.   Life or death depends meanwhile upon keeping a steady hold of the instrument. But most decidedly such a rough proceeding as this, full of danger, can only be justified by the peril of immediate death from suffocation.   In whatever way the operation may be performed, when completed the most urgent thing to attend to is the feeding of the child; for, under the influence of abstinence, the absorption of external miasmata as well as of the vicious secretions fabricated within the body is favoured, and the power of resistance is enfeebled.   Milk, eggs, chocolate, and broths form the most suitable diet.   Then also, I am convinced that medicines had better be abandoned; the air of the apartment is to be kept warm and moist; and the patient's neck should be lightly enveloped in a large piece of muslin, or in a very thin fomentation flannel.

Every now and then it happens after the operation that there is a difficulty with deglutition; fluids especially passing through the glottis, and penetrating down the trachea to the bronchi.   The irritating effect thus set up makes it most difficult to persuade the child to take nourishment.   The best means of remedying this is to avoid liquid diet, giving solid or semi-solid substances; at the same time allaying thirst by a little cold water just before or long after the repast, so as to avoid exciting vomiting.   The inconvenience usually commences three or four days after the operation, and rarely continues longer than from the tenth to the twelfth day. It might be thought that the larynx, which thus permits liquid aliments to pass, would allow the passage of the air also; but it is not so, for if we remove the cannula, the natural passage will be found insufficient. M. Archambault, who has paid much attention to this complication, believes that it results from the child having by the use of the tracheal tube lost the habit of moving the muscles which close the larynx, in harmony with those which propel the food; and he has found it advantageous to temporarily close the tube with the finger during the attempt at deglutition, the child then being obliged to bring the laryngeal muscles into action, and the harmony becoming re-established. This stratagem, however, often fails.

Finally, the removal of the cannula and the definitive closure of the wound require attention. This instrument can seldom be dispensed with before the sixth day, and sometimes not till the twelfth or fourteenth; but usually about the end of the first week we shall be justified in taking it out with great care, provided that for a day or two previously the child has been able to breathe for a time with the tube obstructed by the finger or any easily-fitting plug. The young patient, however, having become accustomed to breathe by the artificial aperture may be seized with a paroxysm of fear and difficult respiration on the first removal. There will possibly be some obstruction of the larynx, by slightly adherent false membranes, mucus, or tumefaction; and the laryngeal muscles may have somewhat lost the power of harmoniously contracting. Yet the difficulty of breathing usually soon disappears if the child can be kept quiet; and, according to the degree in which the laryngeal passage seems re-established, the wound can be strapped with court plaster, or left for a day longer covered with ointment or lint. Supposing the air does not pass easily through the chink of the glottis, the cannula and tube ought to be replaced and retained until they can be removed without any dyspnœa occurring. When healthy respiration is re-established, the opening in the trachea usually becomes closed in four or five days, and the external wound heals soon after.

VI. DIPHTHERIA.

Diphtheria (Διφθέρα, a skin or membrane) may be described as an epidemic sore-throat of great severity, due to toxæmia; being attended with much prostration, and characterized by the exudation of false membranes on the tonsils and adjacent parts. When it does not end fatally, it is often temporarily followed by an alteration in the voice, partial paralysis of the muscles of deglutition, weakness of the upper extremities, anæmia, and impaired vision.

From the writings of old physicians it appears certain that this disease prevailed extensively at different times in the sixteenth, seventeenth, and eighteenth centuries. In France an epidemic broke out in 1818, which was described by Bretonneau, under the name of Diphthérite, in Mémoires communicated to the Académie Royale de Médecine in 1821. About the same time also, some sporadic cases seem to have occurred in Scotland, and a few in England. English physicians, however, paid only slight attention to the subject until the outbreak of the epidemic at Boulogne, in January 1855. In this country the first cases of the last epidemic were observed in the middle of the year 1856 ; and it has continued more or less prevalent in different parts of England up to the present time.

Prior to an outbreak of diphtheria in any locality throat affections have often been noticed to be unusually prevalent.

Pathology.—Diphtheria is a specific blood disease, which runs a rapid course. Its anatomical character is a spreading inflammation of the fauces and œsophagus and respiratory tract, with the exudation of lymph. In some instances (nasal diphtheria) the mucous membrane of the nasal fossæ is alone affected ; recovery or death occuring before the morbid action has extended through the posterior nares to the pharynx. The lymphatic glands of the neck often become swollen and tender, especially in strumous subjects.

Where the cases recover, some remarkable nervous affections are apt to supervene ; consisting of impaired or perverted sensibility, with progressive paralysis of the muscles of the tongue, fauces, pharynx, neck, trunk, or one of the extremities. These secondary nerve affections occur after mild as well as after severe attacks ; while generally a few days of convalescence intervene between the two series of phenomena. During the year 1860 there occurred 210 cases of diphtheria at the Paris Hôpital des Enfans, and paralytic symptoms followed in 31 of them. The proportion was most likely greater ; inasmuch as several of the children were removed from the hospital prior to the time at which consecutive paralysis is usually developed, while others died before this period arrived. M. Roger believes that the ratio generally may be considered as one in three or four. These secondary paralyses are as rare in the other acute diseases of children as they are common in diphtheria. Thus, in the same year and place, among 61 cases of angina simplex, 12 of typhoid fever, 33 of rubeola, 12 of scarlatina, 4 of variola, and 24 of pneumonia, not an instance of secondary paralysis occurred ; and the like negative results were observed in M. Blache's wards.

Diphtheria and scarlatina sometimes occur as epidemics in the same district, while occasionally they coexist in one individual. Hence some have thought that diphtheria was only scarlatina without any eruption ; and they have pointed to the facts that in modified scarlet fever there is now and then an exudation slightly resembling the diphtheritic membrane, while albuminuria sometimes is present in both diseases. Further investigation shows, however, that these affections are distinct from each other, although there may be some analogy between them.   Thus, an attack of the exanthematous fever, while it confers immunity to a second assault, does not afford any protection against diphtheria.   A person may suffer from the latter disease more than once, the last seizure being as violent as the first ; relapses are not very uncommon ; and the larynx is often affected, though it is never involved in scarlet fever.   Furthermore, albuminuria occurs only during convalescence from scarlet fever ; while when it takes place in the epidemic sore throat, it may be found on the first or second day of the disease.   And then, lastly there is a marked difference between the sequelæ of the two affections.

Diphtheritic affections now and then appear sporadically, they often seem to be endemic, while they are also epidemic and contagious (not infectious).   Bretonneau asserts, from the consideration of innumerable facts, that those who attend patients with diphtheria cannot contract it, unless the diphtheritic secretion, in the liquid or pulverulent state, is placed in contact with a mucous membrane, or with a part of the skin denuded of epidermis.   Diphtheria attacks both sexes, at all ages, though children seem to be especially obnoxious to it ; it is probably most fatal to the poor, or such as reside in damp situations and in badly drained houses ; while spring and autumn appear to be the seasons when its ravages are greatest.

Symptoms.—Diphtheria sets in very gradually, with feelings of depression and muscular debility, headache, nausea, slight diarrhœa, chilliness, and drowsiness.   Many hours before the throat is actually sore a sense of stiffness in the neck is complained of.   Then the tonsils become rather dark-coloured and swollen, and the glands about the angles of the lower jaw get tender ;   while as the low inflammatory action proceeds, it involves the velum, uvula, posterior part of the pharynx, &c., and perhaps causes painful or difficult deglutition.   With regard to the small word " perhaps " just employed, it is meant that the amount of pain in the throat affords no criterion as to the extent of the constitutional disease ; for in not a few instances there is less general discomfort and local suffering than in simple acute tonsillitis, while in many of the fatal cases there has been little more than a feeling of uneasiness.

It is probable that at this stage resolution of the inflammation may in some instances take place, and the patient be soon restored to health.   More commonly, however, the characteristic feature of the disease now becomes manifested, and a plastic fibrinous material is effused.   This exudation commences in the nasal fossæ, or on the soft palate, or on one tonsil, or on the back of the pharynx, in the form of small ash-coloured specks ; these spots by their enlargement and coalescence forming patches of considerable size.   As the disease spreads, the false membrane increases in thickness and in extent ; it usually becomes firmly attached to the mucous tissue beneath ; and if it be forcibly removed a new patch will be produced by the end of a few hours.   But if the exudation be cast off naturally, then either no new false membrane is formed, or only one which is much more filmy than the first. The exudation has been compared to wet parchment, or to damp and dirty wash-leather. It may spread forwards to the cheek and gums, upwards into the nares, downwards into the œsophagus, and even through the glottis into the larynx and trachea; and when it begins to separate and decompose, the patient's breath is rendered most offensive. Probably, the browner or blacker the colour of the pellicle and the more dense its texture, the greater is the danger. As the lymphy deposit is cast off, we shall either have ulceration, sloughing, or gangrene of the mucous coat; or this tissue will gradually assume a healthy appearance. And lastly, true diphtheritic membranes may form on abraded cutaneous surfaces,* on the conjunctiva, on the vaginal mucous coat, or on the lining membrane of the rectum; giving rise to a general morbid state very likely to be misinterpreted, unless the possibility of this occurrence be remembered.

The general symptoms may be rather slight, especially at first. Perhaps there is only a sense of weariness or dejection. In other instances the prostration is extreme, and there is considerable restlessness. Pain may be almost wanting. There is only moderate pyrexia, though the skin may be dry and harsh; the pulse is neither sharp nor hard, but it increases in rapidity as the depression becomes greater; while the tongue is clean or only slightly furred, the tonsils are much swollen, the saliva perhaps dribbles from the mouth, the breath is fetid, and there is a disinclination to move even to take drink or food. Then there may be great dysphagia, or the throat will even be much affected without any difficulty in swallowing. There are frequently attacks of hæmorrhage from the nose, fauces, or bronchi. Sometimes there is purpura, now and then an erythematous rash, once in a way typhoid-looking rose spots, and occasionally sudamina; while in many severe instances there is found, from an early stage, albuminuria with fibrinous

---

* One of the worst cases of diphtheria which I have seen occurred in this way:—Three or four members of a family at Peckham were affected with diphtheria towards the end of 1866. They were tenderly nursed by their mother, who remained free from the disease. But just as the patients were convalescent, this lady imagined that she was going to have an attack of bronchitis; and without speaking to the practitioner who was in daily attendance, thought she would cure herself. She therefore applied a large blister over the sternum,—such a blister as only an amateur physician knows how to make use of. In a few days the raw surface thus produced was found freely covered with an ash-coloured diphtheritic membrane; and the disease spreading, the whole front of the chest, including both breasts, became attacked. When I saw her in consultation with Dr. Griffith and Mr. Philps on the eighth day of the disease, she had also two diphtheritic ulcers on the soft palate, one being of the size of a shilling. Her extremities were cold; the pulse was extremely weak; and the stomach was very irritable, so that food and medicines had been retained with difficulty. Milk, cream, brandy, ice, and pills of quinine with reduced iron were ordered. But all proved useless. She died about 25 hours afterwards, viz., on the 29 November.

casts of the tubes.—Death may happen from hæmorrhage, gangrene, slow exhaustion, or from asphyxia—when the larynx and trachea are affected; the mental powers generally retaining their full vigour till the last. There have been many instances where a fatal termination has taken place very suddenly; and as I believe, from the deposition of fibrin within the heart or in one of the large vessels, and not from syncope as has commonly been stated.

In cases of recovery, the convalescence is often very slow. There may be anæmia for many weeks; the voice is left impaired, owing to paralysis of the soft palate; sometimes the power of deglutition is not thoroughly regained for several months, the difficulty of swallowing liquids especially remaining; while the muscles of the neck are not unfrequently paralysed, so that the head cannot be properly supported, or the muscles of the arm may be powerless, or there may be paraplegia, or very rarely there is hemiplegia (see p. 449). Enfeebled action of the heart is often a source of anxiety. With the diminution of motor power, there is commonly lessened sensibility. Defective vision is occasionally complained of, owing probably to paralysis of the ciliary muscle, and consequent loss of adjusting power; a condition which is to be remedied by the use of a low convex glass. In addition, I have seen more than once intense neuralgia as a sequela of diphtheria.

If the diphtheritic exudation be examined microscopically, it will be found to consist of molecular particles, epithelium, pus cells, and blood corpuscles. Fibrillæ are but very rarely seen. The oïdium albicans can occasionally be detected; but the occurrence of this fungus is only exceptional, and when the membrane has begun to undergo an acid putrefaction. So also the leptothrix buccalis may be discovered, but it is also often found in the buccal mucus of healthy persons.

Prognosis.—On several grounds this is a very grave disease. Death not unfrequently happens, even within thirty-six hours, from the intensity of the general disorder—the blood poisoning; or at a later period, from the severity of its local effects, or from the occurrence of some complication. A patient will apparently be doing well at the end of five or six days from the onset, and the pulse will be moderately good, yet in a few hours the exudative inflammation may extend to the larynx and rapidly cause asphyxia. If this danger be escaped, there is the fear of thrombosis, of uræmia, or of fatal innervation. Pyæmia has also occurred, from the absorption of sanious matter produced by the putrid sloughs. Generally speaking, the following symptoms are especially alarming:—albuminuria, suppression of urine, epistaxis, a very frequent pulse, a very slow pulse, delirium, somnolence, and dyspnœa.

The duration of diphtheria may be stated as commonly from three to twelve or fourteen days.—For the number of deaths registered as due to this disease in the seven years 1860-66, see the table at page 271.

Treatment.—Every one who has witnessed much of diphtheria must feel that remedies of a supporting kind are those which alone give any promise of being useful. There is no specific for this disease; and all that we can reasonably hope to accomplish is to guide the patient safely through it. From the beginning, the sick room must be kept clean and wholesome; sulphurous acid gas (F. 74), or carbolic acid, or some other disinfectant being employed, if needed. It will also be as well to see that the atmosphere of the house is not being tainted by effluvia from the drains and dust-bin, and such-like fruitful sources of mischief.

With regard to *local treatment*, it must be recollected that external applications to the throat are injurious or useless; leeches and blisters being only powerful for mischief, while fomentations or poultices fail to give any relief. If the case be seen within a few hours of the commencement of the symptoms, relief may be afforded by allowing the inhalation of acid vapour (two or three ounces of vinegar to the pint of boiling water). Then as the peculiar pellicle begins to show itself, we shall perhaps do good by painting the fauces gently with the tincture of the perchloride of iron, or with turpentine and glycerine mixed in equal proportions; or we can employ a gargle of one or two drachms of the tincture of perchloride of iron with seven of sweetened water, or one of the permanganate of potash (from one to two fluid ounces of the official solution, or four to eight grains of the salt, to eight ounces of water). The atomized spray of the officinal sulphurous acid (F. 262) is in my estimation a very valuable remedy in these cases; while it is so grateful to the patient that I have known its use asked for every few hours. Dr. Greenhow has very properly remonstrated against the severe topical applications which have been resorted to: —"I am sure much mischief has been produced by its indiscriminate use, especially by the frequent tearing away of the exudation by probangs, or similar contrivances for the application of nitrate of silver, or of strong caustic solutions. Observing that removal of the exudation, and the application of remedies to the subjacent surface, neither shortened the duration nor sensibly modified the progress of the complaint, but that the false membrane rarely failed to be renewed in a few hours, I very soon discontinued this rough local medication to the tender and already enfeebled mucous membrane."*

As to the *general remedies*, I believe that when the patient is seen early it may be advantageous to give an emetic of ipecacuanha and ammonia (F. 233); following up its action by a free allowance of some alkaline drink (F. 356, 360). But if the patient be depressed, if there be a manifest tendency to hæmorrhage, or if the urine contain any albumen, I at once order the tincture of the perchloride of iron, as was first recommended by Dr. Heslop of

* *On Diphtheria.* By Edward H. Greenhow, M.D. &c. p. 263. London, 1860.

Birmingham; and very frequently it has seemed advantageous to combine it with quinine (F. 380). Where the formation of fibrinous clots (thrombosis) is feared, ammonia and bark (F. 371), with or without opium, ought to be prescribed in the place of the steel. Possibly the peroxide of hydrogen, or some other preparation of oxygen (F. 370), might have a beneficial influence. Dr. Wade of Birmingham strongly recommends iodide of potassium, believing that it eliminates the poison from the system; with which object he gives two, three, or four grains, with five or ten grains of chlorate of potash, every two or three hours. My own belief is, however, that chlorate of potash in bark, without iodide of potassium, is preferable. But whatever medicine be selected, only limited confidence is to be placed on its efficacy. Simultaneously, pure milk and strong beef tea are to be systematically given, port wine should be administered, and a raw egg with cream or brandy and water (F. 17) is to be ordered twice or thrice in the twenty-four hours. Sometimes iced champagne proves very grateful to the patient's feelings: frequently a good draught of bitter ale, or lemonade or spring water, or not rarely a tumblerful of milk will be prefered; either of these drinks being beneficial if wished for. Considerable benefit usually arises from constantly sucking small pieces of ice; in the same way that pure water is valuable as a diluent, especially by greatly increasing the action of the kidneys. Moreover, the use of ice is valuable in allaying vomiting, when the stomach is irritable; its power in this respect being aided by the application of sinapisms to the epigastrium. Directly there is great depression, brandy in often repeated doses must be trusted to; and in such instances I think it better not to give any other alcoholic stimulant.

Under all circumstances the patient is to be kept in bed, and especially in the recumbent position. It frequently seems advantageous to have him clothed in flannel. The air of the apartment should be warm (70° F.) and moist; the latter being effected by keeping a pot of boiling water on the fire, through the lid of which a long curved tube has been fixed so as to allow the free end to project a few inches above the mantelpiece.

Many physicians begin the treatment of every case with an aperient, but I have seen no advantage from this practice. Of course the bowels can be acted upon, if necessary; but I always prefer a mild cathartic like castor oil, to an active dose of calomel and jalap.—If the secretion of urine be scanty, large and hot linseed poultices, with an occasional sinapism, ought to be applied over the loins, changing them every two hours.—Where the exudation is obstructing the larynx, a stimulating emetic will possibly cause its expulsion; but this failing, tracheotomy may be demanded to prevent suffocation and save life. A most unequivocal example of the value of this operation is related by Sir William Jenner. He says:—"There is not a shadow of a doubt on my mind that he (Dr. C.) would have been dead in two minutes, had his larynx not been opened at the moment it was by Mr. Quain. I never saw any one so manifestly brought back from the threshold of death. His complexion had that bluish pallor that precedes immediate dissolution. My hand was on his wrist. I felt his pulse failing under my finger, until at last it was imperceptible. His eyes closed, and his diaphragm was making those convulsive contractions which indicate that respiration is about to cease, when the knife entered the larynx, and the air was drawn by what really seemed the last effort of the diaphragm into the lungs. The natural hue of his face returned; his pulse was again perceptible; his eyes opened; consciousness was restored; and the patient was alive again. He finally recovered."*—In not a few instances, the attacks of dyspnœa are only paroxysmal, with somewhat long intervals between them. In such, the repeated inhalation of chloroform and ether will prove most serviceable to the weary sufferer, and may render an operation unnecessary. But if tracheotomy be employed, the air-tube is to be opened with all the precautions detailed in the preceding section.—When there is great difficulty in swallowing, we must trust to enemata containing essence of beef, cream, port wine, quinine, and the tincture of the perchloride of iron; repeating the clyster every four or six hours, according to the rapidity with which absorption takes place.

Directly convalescence is safely established, nothing does so much good as change of air—particularly to the sea side. Furthermore, any remaining paralytic symptoms will be best treated by a generous diet and cod liver oil; supplemented by a good deal of rest, quinine and ferruginous tonics, small doses of strychnia or nux vomica, and local Faradisation.

VII. LARYNGITIS.

Cynanche laryngea, or laryngitis, is not happily a very common disease. In the greater proportion of cases in which it has occurred, the morbid action has proved fatal.

Cold and wet acting on unhealthy or enfeebled systems, are commonly the exciting *causes* of the inflammation. Speaking generally, the affection may be said to be peculiar to adults.

The *symptoms* of acute inflammation of the larynx are often at first obscure, as the disease may make its approach in an insidious manner. At the end of some hours, however, they are these:—Fever, redness of the fauces, pain referred to the pomum Adami, difficulty of breathing and of swallowing, considerable anxiety, with hoarseness or even complete loss of voice. There are frequent spasmodic exacerbations of these symptoms, causing distressing paroxysms of threatened suffocation. The inspirations are long

* *Diphtheria: its Symptoms and Treatment*, p. 75. London, 1861.

and attended with a peculiar wheezing sound, as if the air were drawn through a narrow reed. If there be any cough, it is harsh and brassy. The face becomes flushed, the eyes are protruded, the lips are swollen, the pulse is hard ; and unless relief be afforded, the distress gets greater and greater. The larynx and trachea move with excessive rapidity upwards and downwards, while all the muscles of respiration are brought into action, so that the chest heaves violently. The patient gasps for breath, and tries to get to the open window to obtain more air. He soon sinks into a drowsy and delirious state ; and then speedily dies suffocated, the chink of the rima glottidis becoming closed from the swelling of the mucous membrane lining it, or from the effusion of serum into the adjacent connective tissue.

In many instances the act of swallowing is attended with so much suffering that nutrient enemata have to be employed. As in dysphagia from some other causes liquids are swallowed with greater difficulty than solids. There is considerable mental distress, until the sensibility gets blunted in consequence of the imperfect oxygenation of the blood.

The inflammation is often of very limited extent: the distress and danger are entirely owing to its situation. To avert the peril our *treatment* must be promptly carried out. The patient is to be closely watched, kept very quiet, and not allowed to talk. The air of his room is to be made warm and moist ; while if the apartment be too large to do this effectually, the bed can be covered with curtains making it to resemble a tent. He should frequently inhale the steam of simple boiling water, or of that which is medicated by hydrocyanic acid with a little spirit of chloroform (F. 261), or the spray of a solution of belladonna (F. 262) : in the intervals of doing so, it will prove advantageous for him to wear a home-made woollen respirator. But directly it is evident that the remedies are not acting favourably, that the general distress is increasing, and that the blood is not being thoroughly oxygenated, the trachea must be opened. Mr. Porter* has well remarked that tracheotomy allows the organ in which the diseased action is situated perfect repose ; it removes the danger of the lungs becoming congested and engorged ; it frees the patient from those terrible paroxysms of spasmodic suffocation ; and in short it takes the place of all other treatment, which, besides being injurious from loss of time, *is often in itself positively detrimental.* He quotes, also, the opinion of the late Sir William Lawrence, that "bleeding, blistering, and the usual means for subduing inflammation, are here found totally inefficacious." Is it not then a matter for regret that many still recommend the adoption of the antiphlogistic practice, and bid us persevere with it ; the usual argument amounting to this, that because all the cases have not died under such a plan, therefore there is every

* *Observations on the Surgical Pathology of the Larynx and Trachea, &c. &c.* pp. 86, 143. London, 1837.

ground for encouragement.   Moreover, the administration of mercury proves equally unavailing in checking either the inflammation
or the effusion ; unless indeed, the disease be dependent upon the
poison of syphilis, in which case calomel with opium should be
given, and mercurial vapour baths employed, so as rapidly to influence the system.   After opening the air-tube, the patient's
strength will have to be supported by milk, beef tea, and wine or
brandy, if there be—as there usually is—much depression.

Œdema of the glottis will sometimes arise from other causes
besides inflammation, and produce the same effects as laryngitis.
It is often due to the action of boiling water, or of some strong
mineral acid, or of one of the alkalies, taken accidentally into the
mouth ; either of these corrosives producing sudden contraction of
the muscles of the pharynx and larynx, whereby it is expelled
through the nostrils and mouth to the great injury of all the
tissues over which it passes.   The case is different when a caustic
poison is voluntarily employed ; inasmuch as the individual bent on
suicide is prepared to make the necessary effort for swallowing the
fluid, which quickly passes into the stomach without injuring the
larynx.   Then the poison of erysipelas may likewise give rise to œdema
glottidis, the inflammation either having its onset in the fauces and
larynx, or extending to these parts from the face.   To favour the
subsidence of the tumefaction, we may (if the symptoms be not
urgent) sponge the epiglottis and cavity of the larynx with a solution of the crystals of nitrate of silver, sixty grains to the ounce, as
recommended by Dr. Horace Green.   Scarifying the œdematous
swelling, with the object of permitting the escape of the effused
fluid, has been adopted with success.   But these plans failing or
appearing inapplicable, laryngotomy or tracheotomy becomes our
only resource.   Yet it is necessary before proposing the operation
to be positive as to the diagnosis.   For example, a patient in King's
College Hospital with renal disease and general anasarca, had considerable dyspnœa.   Œdema of the glottis being thought to be the
cause, the necessity for tracheotomy was discussed.   An examination with the laryngoscope demonstrated, however, that no such
condition as was suspected existed ; while it proved that there was
no disease in the larynx to account for the dyspnœa.

The larynx is also prone to suffer from *chronic* disease.   Thus,
chronic inflammation and ulceration, owing to the deposit of tubercle,
are not uncommon in cases of pulmonary consumption ; a species of
tuberculosis being consequently known as *phthisis laryngea*.   So too,
the membrane lining the laryngeal cartilages often becomes
thickened and ulcerated in secondary syphilis,—*syphilitic laryngitis*.
The ulcers are probably the result of the breaking down of gummata ; they may cause considerable loss of substance, destroying
perhaps the vocal cords, epiglottis, &c. ; but they are amenable to
treatment by iodide of potassium and the inhalation of atomized

fluids (F. 262), especially of the perchloride of mercury. Again, *fibrous tumours, polypi, warty growths,* and *epithelial cancers,* all of variable size, may arise from different parts of the larynx, and cause great impediment to the entrance and exit of air. The first systematic account of these growths was published by Ehrmann ;* but their diagnosis has been very much facilitated since then by the use of the laryngoscope. They are frequently attached to one or other of the vocal cords, or just above their level. All such tumours have been repeatedly removed with success by the écraseur. Even in epithelial cancer seated about the vocal cords, the growth may be excised. The removal is to be effected through the upper aperture of the larynx, if the tumour be pedunculated ; or by an incision through the trachea, in the median line of the neck, when the growth is sessile with its broadest diameter on the floor of the ventricle. In cases of non-malignant disease, a permanent cure will be effected. With respect to cancer, we can reasonably hope to afford much relief; for although the disease is almost certain to return, yet life will probably be prolonged for some months by the operation.

VIII. FOREIGN BODIES IN THE AIR PASSAGES.

The number and variety of articles which may enter the air tubes, and give rise to severe or fatal mischief are very remarkable. The most frequent substances which do so are seeds of all kinds, beans, peas, cherry stones, pieces of hard wood, buttons, pins, small coins, marbles, pebbles, teeth, bits of slate pencil, beads, screws and nails, portions of bone, and ears of corn. The size of these articles is often such that it would seem almost impossible they could have passed through the chink of the glottis; yet they have done so. Thus, to select only a few examples, Dr. Mott has recorded an instance in which a child, barely eleven months old, inhaled a black shawl-pin two inches long, with a head nearly as large as a small marble.† At Königsburg in Germany, the larynx of a goose became impacted in the windpipe of a boy twelve years old.‡ M. Bérard had to perform tracheotomy on a boy not quite seven years old, to remove a marble eight lines in diameter.§ And Sir William Fergusson has had to resort to the same operation to extract a plum stone from the trachea of a girl seven years of age.||
When the extraneous substance is of an animal or vegetable nature, it is apt to swell considerably owing to its imbibing moisture ;

* *Histoire des Polypes du Larynx.* Par C. H. Ehrmann. Strasbourg, 1850.
† *New Hampshire Journal of Medicine,* p. 197. April, 1852.
‡ *London Medical Gazette,* vol. xi. p. 559. 1850.
§ *Archives Générales de Médecine.* 2nd series, tom. ii. p. 125. Paris, 1833.
|| *A System of Practical Surgery.* Third edition, p. 648. London, 1852.

so that a small bean or pea has been known to increase to thrice its size in a few days. In a few fortunate cases the material has become softened and broken up, permitting of its expulsion piecemeal: when retained, as it usually is, the foreign body becomes incrusted with mucus, or with lymph, or even with a few grains of carbonate or phosphate of lime. The substance either gets lodged in one of the ventricles of the larynx, or it becomes fixed between the chordæ vocales, or it may be arrested in the trachea, or it will descend into one of the bronchial tubes—especially into the right.

Symptoms.—The entrance of the foreign body usually occurs during a strong and sudden inspiration; it immediately gives rise to a violent spasmodic cough, dyspnœa, and a sense of impending suffocation; and sometimes it even causes sudden death by arresting the respiration. After a few minutes, the violence of the first symptoms usually abates for a time; the cough and dyspnœa returning at variable intervals. Sometimes the calm lasts for many hours; usually it is short—of twenty or thirty minutes' duration. The subsequent symptoms will depend upon the situation in which the foreign body is retained. Thus, if it remain in the *larynx*, there will usually be violent, harassing, and suffocative cough; perhaps loss of voice, or inability to speak above a whisper; probably pain in swallowing, with tenderness over the part; and noisy hissing respiration, with more or less dyspnœa. When the substance descends below the larynx, it is seldom retained in the trachea, but passes on into *one of the bronchial tubes*—in the great majority of instances into the right, being directed to this by the bronchial septum. If, under these circumstances, auscultation and percussion be practised, it will be found that air does not enter the obstructed lung at all, or, where the obstruction is only partial, that it fills the lung incompletely. Hence there will be a complete loss or a diminution of resonance on percussion, with diminution or absence of the respiratory murmur on auscultation. The foreign body not unfrequently *plays up and down the trachea*, under the influence of fits of coughing. This change in position gives rise to severe spasmodic attacks of dyspnœa; a peculiar sensation of movement appreciable by the patient; and a sound of motion detected by auscultation, as well as possibly to a flapping or valve-like sound produced by the foreign body being forced against the rima glottidis in expiration.

Supposing that the substance is not expelled or removed, the patient will be liable to be suffocated at any moment from the foreign body pressing up into the larynx under the influence of a fit of coughing; or if he escape this risk, there is the fear of inflammation with all its dangers. After the subsidence of the immediate symptoms, the foreign body sometimes gives rise to no appreciable inconvenience for many weeks or months. Louis relates such an instance, where the patient did not (after the first few minutes) experience a bad symptom for twelve months, at the end of which time he coughed up a cherry stone followed by such copious expectoration that he died from exhaustion in three days.* Dr. Condie attended a child who continued free from all symptoms of disease for a week, after the first symptoms had subsided : pneumonia then set in, which ended fatally on the fifth day, when a large bead was found obstructing the right bronchus.†

Occasionally death occurs during the act of vomiting, owing to some of the ejected matters lodging against the rima glottidis, or even passing down the windpipe. Thus, Corvisart being desirous of exercising a close supervision of the clinical wards at La Charité, visited them one evening unexpectedly. The steward, who had been indulging in a hearty meal, was taken by surprise and became sick ; but making a violent effort to repress the vomiting, he fell to the ground and expired. On examining the body, the larynx, trachea, and bronchial tubes were found filled with half-digested food.‡

Diagnosis.—The symptoms set up by extraneous bodies in the respiratory organs may be imitated by different diseases. But before mentioning these it should be remembered, that if the foreign substance be entangled in the ventricles, or between the vocal cords, the use of the laryngoscope will not only enable the body to be seen, but must likewise show how and where it can best be seized so as to permit of extraction. Groping about in the dark therefore, under such circumstances, can no longer be justifiable. When the body has passed beyond the upper portion of the larynx the symptoms produced are to be distinguished from those of *croup*, by the state of the pulse and skin, which are rarely excited until the foreign substance has had time to give rise to inflammation ; by the difficulty of breathing existing during expiration, and not most severely during inspiration as in croup ; by the absence of the croupy character of voice ; and by the complete intermissions. The case will be known from *hooping cough* by the history, the want of the peculiar hoop, and by the absence of great dyspnœa during inspiration. The diagnosis from *spasm of the glottis* is to be made by considering the history, and by the non-existence of any auscultatory signs. And lastly, the symptoms will be proved not to be owing to *the impaction of extraneous substances in the pharynx and œsophagus*, by examining these passages with the finger and probang. The want of this latter precaution has proved fatal :—Thus, a man while eating, was seized with symptoms of suffocation and difficult deglutition ; the trachea was opened ; but as nothing could be found it was concluded that the sub-

---

* *Memoir on Bronchotomy*, in *Memoirs of the Royal Paris Academy of Surgery*. Translated by Ottley, p. 277. London, 1848.
† *Diseases of Children*. Third edition. p. 366. Philadelphia, 1850.
‡ *Laennec on Diseases of the Chest*. Translated by Forbes. Fourth edition, p. 131. London, 1834.

stance had descended into one of the bronchial tubes, until after death the surgeon was surprised at discovering it fixed in the œsophagus.

There will, however, be but little difficulty in forming a correct diagnosis in the majority of cases, if the history be carefully attended to. For example, suppose a healthy individual "has been playing with a grain of corn, bean, pebble, or similar body, and has been suddenly seized with symptoms of suffocation, violent spasmodic cough, lividity of the face, pain in the upper part of the windpipe, and partial insensibility, the presumption will be strong, that the substance, whatever it may have been, has slipped into the air-passages, and is the immediate and only cause of the suffering which the surgeon has been sent for to relieve. The presumption will be converted almost into positive certainty if the person was just previously in the enjoyment of good health; if he was romping, jumping, or laughing at the moment of the accident, with the substance, perhaps, in his mouth, or while attempting to throw it into that cavity; and especially, if the symptoms, after having been interrupted for a few minutes, continue to recur, with their former, or even with increased intensity, at longer or shorter intervals."*

Pathological Effects.—The most common is inflammation of the mucous membrane, perhaps going on to ulceration: the latter effect is generally confined to the tissues in contact with the extraneous substance. The normal secretion of mucus is always increased; while frequently the fluid becomes muco-purulent, and in some instances the bronchi have been found loaded with it. When the foreign matter is retained in one of the bronchial tubes, it may produce pulmonary collapse if it completely obstruct the tube; or inflammation of the corresponding lung may be set up, giving rise to all the ordinary symptoms of pneumonia. Abscesses also form at the seat of obstruction. In a few instances pulmonary emphysema has been induced; in others, pleurisy leading to effusion; and in a very small number, inflammation of the heart and its investing serous membrane. Mr. Herbert Mayo has recorded a case in which a boy twelve years old died in consequence of the inhalation of an ear of rye: pulmonary irritation with the most fetid expectoration followed, and hectic fever set in which proved fatal. On dissection the extraneous body was discovered in an abscess common to the lung and liver; the latter gland having become involved by the extension of the inflammation through the diaphragm.†

Treatment.—The foreign substance is sometimes spontaneously expelled, especially during a paroxysm of cough and dyspnœa. This has occurred when the patient has been laid upon a bed with his head hanging over the edge; and in a few instances when he has

* *A Practical Treatise on Foreign Bodies in the Air Passages.* By S. D. Gross, M.D. &c. p. 90. Philadelphia, 1854.
† *Outlines of Pathology,* p. 506. London, 1836.

been in the erect posture. The time at which this fortunate termination can be hoped for is variable : it may happen a few minutes after the accident, or months subsequently. Dr. Webster has recorded an instance where a cherry stone was expelled sixty-eight days after its introduction, and the patient recovered after having suffered from pneumonia, abscess, and hectic fever.* Sir Thomas Watson refers to an instance where an ear of barley was spontaneously ejected seven years after the accident, and the patient (who had suffered from repeated attacks of hæmoptysis) got well.† In a few instances the substance has been got rid of by inverting the body, and smartly striking the back of the chest to dislodge the obstructing agent ; but the latter, on touching the glottis, gives rise to such severe spasm, that it very rarely passes out.

These facts have led practitioners to attempt the expulsion of extraneous substances by the use of medicines, especially by sternutatories and emetics ; but the anticipated result has so very rarely ensued, that the practice ought to be abolished, especially as it is not without danger and causes the loss of valuable time. Since then, no patient can be regarded as safe who has a foreign body in any portion of the windpipe, how is it to be got rid of ? When the body is fixed in the larynx so that it cannot be seen by the laryngoscope, laryngotomy should be performed as early as possible ; but when it has descended lower, and perhaps in all cases in young children, the trachea ought to be opened. The substance may be ejected through the glottis, or through the artificial opening, directly the latter is made ; but should this not take place, then the patient's body had better be inverted, and a few smart taps made to dislodge the substance. The inversion is not likely to be followed by any bad consequences, because the patient will breathe through the artificial opening ; and hence the coin, or bean, or whatever it may be, will not give rise to that severe spasm of the glottis which it would otherwise do. In the well-known case of Mr. Brunel, April 1843, in which a half-sovereign slipped through the chink of the glottis while this gentleman was amusing some children with conjuring tricks, all attempts to procure the expulsion of the coin by sloping his body downwards failed in consequence of the violent coughing that ensued. Three weeks after the accident, Sir Benjamin Brodie opened the trachea ; and it was tried to reach the coin with forceps, but without success. Sixteen days subsequently, the wound in the trachea having been kept in an open state, Mr. Brunel's body was inverted on a moveable hinged platform to which he had been firmly strapped. The back of the chest was then struck with the hand, two or three efforts to cough followed, the coin was felt to quit the bronchus, and immediately afterwards it struck against the upper incisor teeth and fell on the floor. Recovery took place without any drawback.

* The Lancet, vol. i. p. 802. London, 1830.
† Lectures on the Principles and Practice of Physic. Third edition, vol. ii. p. 225. London, 1848.

The question may properly be entertained whether the foreign body might not be discharged without opening the windpipe? In a case which was under the charge of Dr. Duncan of Edinburgh, shortly after the successful issue just related, a man who had got a shilling in his larynx was relieved of the intruder by being suddenly turned topsy-turvy, without any other operation. Usually, however, this proceeding causes most dangerous cough and dyspnœa. Possibly the spasm of the glottis might be overcome by the inhalation of chloroform, without opening the trachea; but I am not aware of any instance where such a plan has been tried. If, however, a surgeon determine to resort to it, he must be prepared to perform tracheotomy immediately, in case of the necessity arising.

When the extraneous body resists all efforts to remove it, the wound in the trachea should be kept open to favour its extrusion subsequently. Where the operation, however, is successful, the incision ought to be immediately closed by two or three interrupted sutures, or by strips of adhesive plaster.

IX. LARYNGISMUS STRIDULUS.

Laryngismus stridulus [from Λαρυγγίζω = to vociferate with all his might; *Strideo* = to make a hissing noise], infantile laryngismus, spurious croup, or child-crowing, is a spasmodic disease occurring in infants chiefly during the period of dentition—before the completion of the second year. The affection consists of a temporary or partial or complete closure of the rima glottidis, by which the entrance of air into the lungs is impeded or stopped. The deaths registered from this disease in England, during 1866, were $\frac{Males\ 195}{Females\ 105}$ = 300; of which total 168 were infants under one year of age.

Symptoms.—Infantile laryngismus is unattended by fever, almost its only symptom being the interruption of the breathing. The first seizure frequently occurs in the night; the child having been often apparently quite well when put to bed. Perhaps the attack is so slight, that after two or three crowing inspirations the little patient falls asleep again. In other instances, there may have been irritability and restlessness, perhaps disordered bowels, for a few days. Then the child is suddenly seized with dyspnœa, it struggles and kicks, is unable to inspire, and seems about to perish from suffocation. Presently the spasm gives way; air is drawn in through the chink of the glottis with a shrill whistling or crowing sound, and the paroxysm is over; sometimes to return shortly, or in a few hours, or not perhaps for several days. In severe forms, the symptoms may have more of an epileptic character; there being suspended breathing, turgidity of the veins of the neck, and carpopedal contractions. Now and then the child seems dead during these intervals of suspended respiration; until at the end of a couple of minutes or a few seconds longer there is a faint gasp, followed by thin stridulous breathing. There is, however, much fear of death really happening during one of these paroxysms.

Pathology.—This affection was carefully investigated by Dr. Ley, who attributed it to pressure made by enlarged glands in the neck or chest upon the recurrent nerve, or upon some part of the eighth pair of nerves. The pressure subverts the exact antagonism by which the glottis is automatically and involuntarily kept open, and allows its margins to come together; thus occasioning the dyspnœa and peculiar kind of inspiration so much resembling that of croup. It was reserved for Dr. Marshall Hall, however, to give the immediate explanation of the phenomena of this disease, by showing that it is to be attributed to some source of irritation producing reflex spasm—to an excitation of the true spinal excitomotory system. It *originates* says Dr. Marshall Hall, in—

1. *a.* The *trifacial nerve* in teething.
   b. The *pneumogastric,* in over or improperly fed infants.
   c. The *spinal nerves,* in constipation, intestinal disorder, or catharsis.

These *act* through the medium of—

2. The *spinal marrow,* and—
3. *a.* The *inferior* or *recurrent laryngeal,* the constrictor of the larynx.
   b. The *intercostals* and *diaphragmatic,* the motors of respiration.

Functional disorders of the brain, cerebral ramollissement, apoplexy, a rachitic state of the bones of the skull, organic disease of the cervical portion of the spinal cord, and scrofulous adenitis, have all been regarded as possible causes of infantile laryngismus.

Treatment.—During the paroxysm the treatment should be the same as that employed in resuscitating still-born children. Hot water to the lower parts of the body, with cold affusion to the head and face; slapping the chest and nates; exposure to a current of cold air; the gentle inhalation of chloroform; and artificial respiration if necessary, taking care to draw the tongue well forwards. The vapour of ether or ammonia can also be applied to the nostrils; while, as a last resource, tracheotomy ought to be performed.

The subsequent remedies must consist of mild purgatives and anti-spasmodic tonics; and, above all, change of air. Belladonna, commencing with one sixth of a grain thrice daily, is sometimes useful; while its efficacy may be augmented by combining the bromide of potassium or of ammonium with it, or the sulphate of zinc in gradually increasing doses. The diet ought to be very simple: a child at the breast should not be otherwise fed, but the practitioner should make sure that the milk is good. Many of the diseases of infants are caused by the silly obstinacy of some mothers, who are only happy when overloading the stomachs of their children.

X. BRONCHITIS.

Inflammation of the mucous membrane of the bronchial tubes is one of the most common of the pulmonary diseases which come under the notice of the practitioner. Bronchitis [from Βρόγχος = the windpipe; terminal -*itis*] may be acute or chronic; and one or both lungs may be affected throughout, or only a portion of these organs—usually the upper lobes.

The fatality of bronchitis in England is much greater than is commonly believed. The deaths registered from it, as compared with those due to phthisis and pneumonia, are as follows:—

	1860.	1861.	1862.	1863.	1864.	1865.	1866.
Bronchitis .	32,347 .	30,986 .	32,526 .	32,025 .	38,969 .	36,428 .	41,334
Pneumonia	25,264 .	22,914 .	23,713 .	24,181 .	24,470 .	22,489 .	25,155
Phthisis . .	51,024 .	51,931 .	50,962 .	51,072 .	53,046 .	53,734 .	55,714

For the estimated population in these years, as well as for the total number of deaths from all causes, reference should be made to the section (p. 271) on the eruptive fevers.

1. **ACUTE BRONCHITIS.**—This is a dangerous disorder; partly owing to the way in which it interferes with the due oxygenation of the blood, and in some measure because of the frequency with which the inflammatory action spreads to the capillary bronchi as well as to the vesicular texture of the lungs. The danger, however, principally exists amongst the young and old. Thus, of the 41,334 deaths registered from bronchitis in 1866, those occurring in children under 5 years of age were $\frac{\text{Males } 8812}{\text{Females } 7493} = 16,305$; the number for infants under 1 year being 11,754. Then, from 5 to 45 years we find only $\frac{\text{Males } 1663}{\text{Females } 1605} = 3268$ fatal cases; while during the next 40 years (45 to 85) they reach to 20,781.

Symptoms.—The chief symptoms consist of fever, a sense of tightness or constriction about the chest, sternal pain or tenderness, hurried respiration with wheezing, severe cough, and expectoration —at first of a viscid glairy mucus which subsequently becomes purulent. The pulse is frequent and often weak; the temperature in the axilla varies from 99·5 to 102°; the tongue is furred and foul; and there is headache, together with lassitude, sickness, and often much mental uneasiness or even great anxiety.

Inflammation of the larger and medium-sized tubes is attended by less severe symptoms, and is much less destructive to life than *general and capillary bronchitis,* in which all the ramifications of the bronchi are affected. This latter form of the disease is chiefly seen in the very young and old, being rare in adults : while it is readily recognised by its tendency to produce asphyxia; by the paroxysmal attacks of dyspnœa [$\Delta v\varsigma$ = difficulty + $\pi v\acute{\epsilon}\omega$ = to breathe], or of orthopnœa [$\text{O}\rho\theta\grave{o}\varsigma$ = erect + $\pi v\acute{\epsilon}\omega$]; as well as by the congestion of the surface of the body, the perpetual cough, and the extreme general restlessness. The patient is obliged to sit up in bed; the urine is scanty, deep-coloured, of high specific gravity, and sometimes slightly albuminous; the skin is clammy; the pulse is regular but feeble, and from 120 to 150; the prostration rapidly increases, and we may have anasarca of the feet and legs; while in fatal cases there will soon be somnolence, muttering delirium, coma, and death. That severe suffering, not uncommonly ending in the destruction of life, should thus result, is only what we might expect; for to congest and thicken the lining mucous membrane of the capillary bronchia, and then to coat it with viscid mucus, is virtually to completely occlude these air-passages.

From time to time it happens during the progress of a case of bronchitis, that one or more of the tubes become choked up with the viscid phlegm; and we have, as the result, *pulmonary collapse*, a portion of the lung being emptied of air. Thus, supposing a plug to form in one of the bronchi, the lung beyond it in expiration soon forces out the air by the side of the foreign body; but each inspiration draws the obnoxious substance towards a narrower part of the tube, which it seems effectually to cork up. The consequence is, that as each succeeding expiration expels the air retained behind the obstacle, while none is inspired to take its place, the sacs or vesicles must collapse. Then the collapsed portion of the pulmonary tissue becomes condensed; this condensation having been formerly considered as due to inflammation, whence it was termed *lobular pneumonia*. One frequent result of the collapse is the production of vesicular emphysema; so that the loss of function in the airless part of the lung is compensated for by an increase of volume in the non-obstructed portion.

On practising *auscultation* in the early stage of acute bronchitis, two *dry* sounds will generally be heard—viz., *rhonchus* and *sibilus*; both of which indicate that the air-tubes are partially narrowed, owing to the mucous membrane lining them being dry and tumid. Rhonchus in itself need give us no anxiety, as it belongs entirely to the larger divisions of the bronchial tubes; sibilus, on the contrary, bespeaks more danger, since it denotes that the smaller air-tubes and vesicles are affected. After a time, the inflamed mucous membrane begins to pour out fluid—a viscid, transparent, tenacious mucus is exhaled; this constituting the second stage of the inflammation. Two very different sounds to those just noticed are then to be detected—viz., *large crepitation* and *small crepitation*, or, as they are often called, the *moist* sounds. As the air passes through the bronchial tubes it gets mixed, as it were, with the mucous secretion, so that numerous air-bubbles keep forming and bursting. When this occurs in the larger branches, it gives rise to large crepitation; when in the smaller, to small crepitation. We have therefore rhonchus and large crepitation as, respectively, the dry and moist sounds of the larger air passages; sibilus and small crepitation as those of the smaller branches.——On practising *percussion*, no appreciable alteration in the resonance of the chest will usually be discoverable; bronchitis in this respect offering a marked difference to the dulness which is present in pneumonia. If the lungs, however, are acutely emphysematous, there will be increased resonance; while if there be collapse of a large portion of the pulmonary tissue from the obstruction produced by the pressure of an enlarged bronchial gland upon a tube, or from the choking-up of the latter with inspissated mucus, the percussion-note will be dull.

The occurrence of *bronchitis during childhood* is always to be dreaded; inasmuch as the disease has a twofold source of danger —pulmonary collapse and capillary bronchitis. For the production of the first, little is needed beyond a copious secretion of viscid mucus with sufficient debility to prevent its expectoration, and so allow of its choking up some of the smaller bronchi. Should this occur, we shall find that the difficulty of breathing increases, without any exacerbation of the fever; and that where there was previously resonance on percussion there is substituted dulness and bronchial respiration. If this condition be mistaken for pneumonia, and venesection and leeches and antimony be resorted to, the severity of the symptoms will be increased and possibly a fatal result induced; while on the contrary, under the early influence of stimulants and rubefacient liniments, relief may often be speedily given. The second element of peril—capillary bronchitis—is that in which the smaller air-tubes become intensely inflamed, this inflammation quickly ending in a copious secretion of pus. This severe and often fatal affection may not only result from an extension of the inflammation of the larger air-tubes; but, in infants especially, it may also occur primarily. It chiefly produces great acceleration of the breathing, so that the respirations are repeated from thirty to forty times in a minute; distressing and frequent cough; great anxiety of countenance with frequent flushings; heaviness of the eyes with injection of the conjunctivæ; extreme restlessness; and great frequency with weakness of pulse. The diagnosis is not free from difficulty, for the symptoms bear a striking resemblance to those of pneumonia: and it is by no means easy to practise percussion or auscultation, in the alarmed and restless child. If we succeed in doing so, however, we shall obtain a natural degree of resonance on percussion; while with the ear to the chest we shall detect a sub-crepitant râle, a moist sound which is larger than the small crepitation of pneumonia, and yet smaller than the large crepitation of simple bronchitis. There is often also, rhonchus and sibilus; all these being best heard at the back and bases of the lungs. In favourable cases, these sounds are gradually replaced by large crepitation and the vesicular murmur;

while the general disturbance subsides. On the contrary, where death is about to happen, the face assumes a livid hue, the cough becomes smothered, the respiration more laboured, and there is great drowsiness. Then for a few hours the sufferings appear lessened, unless under the influence of a paroxysm of dyspnœa, and the child quietly dies.

Prognosis.—In the bronchitis of adults, when relief is not afforded by the copious expectoration, or by remedies, the disease assumes a very dangerous character. The strength becomes much reduced, signs of great pulmonary congestion ensue, and symptoms of partial asphyxia often follow that soon end in death. With favourable cases, however, the affection begins to decline between the fourth and eighth day, and shortly either entirely subsides, or passes into the chronic form. Probably from one-half to three-fourths of those attacked with capillary bronchitis die between the sixth and tenth days of the disease.

Treatment.—The patient is to be confined to his bed. The temperature of the room may vary from 65° F. to 70°; and it is usually beneficial to have the air moist, as recommended when speaking of diphtheria. Beef tea, milk arrowroot or gruel or corn flour, tea with milk, and a mucilaginous drink (F. 19) ought to be allowed; while if there be indications of debility, white wine whey (F. 10) will prove a good restorative. An agreeable demulcent drink can also be made with sarsaparilla, squills, and barley water (F. 238).

Then, after a brisk purgative, a saline mixture containing ipecacuanha or squills (F. 348) should be prescribed; or, if there be any depression, a stimulating expectorant (F. 235) must be ordered. Gentle counter-irritation to the front of the chest by dry cupping, turpentine stupes, or sinapisms, will also prove valuable. Should the phlegm appear to accumulate in the bronchial tubes, an emetic (F. 231, 233) will readily remove it; or warm water inhaled as spray (F. 262) will suffice to do so, at the same time that the application is grateful. When Physician to the Farringdon Dispensary, where the patients were very poor, I was in the constant habit of successfully treating acute bronchitis from the commencement with stimulating expectorants (ammonia, squills, and senega being the chief ingredients in the prescription), good beef tea, the inhalation of the steam of hot water, and counter-irritation by means of rubefacient liniments or turpentine stupes. Opium, cautiously given, often affords relief for the night; though it is not to be employed if there be any indications that the blood is insufficiently aërated—if the complexion be dusky or bluish.

The treatment of bronchitis in children ought to be subordinate to the degree of inflammatory action, and the strength and constitution of the patient; regard being likewise paid to the fact of the disease being primary, or of its setting in secondarily to some other affection—as measles, hooping cough, &c. As in the adult, simple bronchitis in the young often ceases after a few days without medicine. But with the latter, great care is needed to guard against the occurrence of pulmonary collapse; and so the child is to be kept in a warm and comfortable atmosphere, to be allowed plenty of milk and broths and demulcent drinks, and to be daily watched. In acute cases, the chief remedies are ammonia and ipecacuanha and senega; with linseed poultices to the chest, and occasionally sinapisms or somewhat irritating liniments. If pulmonary collapse take place, a stimulating emetic may be given once; followed by a warm bath, good beef tea, milk or cream, and wine or ammonia with ether. And then after all forms of the disease, a nourishing diet with plenty of milk, ammonia and bark, cod liver oil, and a pure air to breathe, will form the necessary treatment during convalescence. Where the debility is great, port wine will be serviceable; while if there be any difficulty in insuring the digestion of the cod liver oil, this agent may well be introduced into the system by freely rubbing the thoracic and abdominal walls with it twice or thrice in each twenty-four hours.

2. CHRONIC BRONCHITIS.—Chronic inflammation of the bronchial tubes is very common, particularly in advanced life. The first attack usually occurs during the winter. The disease has a great tendency to recur again and again: some people indeed, seem to be scarcely ever free from it. The slighter forms are indicated only by habitual cough, more or less shortness of breath, and copious expectoration; these symptoms being always aggravated by exposure to cold and wet, or by bad living. The physical signs of chronic bronchitis are, chiefly, slightly impaired resonance on percussion, especially low down posteriorly; while the vesicular murmur is feebly heard, and is mingled with rhonchus and sibilus and moist crepitation. The majority of " winter coughs " in old people are examples of bronchial inflammation of a low lingering kind. After repeated attacks many of these cases end fatally somewhat suddenly. They are apt to become complicated with valvular disease of the heart, or with contracted gouty kidneys; dropsy and albuminuria setting in. Chronic bronchitis arises idiopathically, or it may follow an acute attack. The morbid action is often associated with other pulmonary lesions. A general dilatation of the bronchi, especially of the finer tubes, occasionally results from this disease, as well as from hooping cough; this dilatation keeping up, for a time, excessive and fetid muco-purulent secretion—bronchorrhœa. Chronic bronchitis is seldom fatal in itself; but it is often the indirect cause of death by leading to other diseases.

There is a peculiar and severe form of this disorder, occurring in aged people, which deserves notice. It has been described as *peripneumonia notha* (bastard peripneumony), or *catarrhus senilis,* or *subacute bronchitis;* and it really consists of a subacute attack of general or capillary inflammation of the tubes. In these cases there is often only the appearance of a violent catarrh, with more or less severe dyspnœa, and an excessive secretion of opaque frothy mucus loaded with pus cells and columnar epithelium (visible with a ¼-inch object glass). The symptoms are frequently much relieved by remedies which cause a free and copious expectoration : an emetic of ipecacuanha with a little ammonia oft-times has a marvellously good and speedy effect. Now and then it happens that insufficient care is taken at the onset ; the feverish and catarrhal phenomena being possibly at first very moderate, and apparently unimportant. But after a few days these symptoms suddenly become considerable : there is the orthopnœa and tendency to asphyxia already noticed ; we find a rapid pulse with hurried respiration ; the urine is scanty and perhaps albuminous ; great prostration soon sets in ; and a fatal event occurs so quickly, that it is probably unexpected. Capillary bronchitis sometimes proves fatal by the accumulated mucus, which the patient has not the power to expel, causing suffocation ; while in other instances deficient oxygenation of the blood leads to coma.

Plastic bronchitis is a rare form of bronchial disease, characterized by the formation of solid or tubular concretions of exudation-matter within the bronchial tubes. It is a disorder which runs its course very slowly. The chief symptom is the occasional expectoration of casts of the tubes ; very little suffering being caused by the bringing up of small fragments, while the expectoration of moulds of notable size is usually preceded by dyspnœa, dry cough, and not unfrequently by hæmoptysis. Sometimes the hæmoptysis is the first symptom ; the concretions being detached, but not expelled, from the bronchi. The bleeding frightens the patient, and perhaps is really abundant. In exceptional instances there may be slight aneurismal or some other form of acute hæmorrhage into the tubes, the casts consisting of decolorized coagulated blood. Suspended in water, the branching appearance presented by these fibrinous moulds explains their nature.

Cases of plastic bronchitis not uncommonly last for years ; the patients having troublesome seizures, attended with the peculiar expectoration, every few weeks or months. Medical treatment seems to have no permanent effect upon this disease ; but I believe that the prolonged use of the carbonate of ammonia will prove more useful than the employment of most other drugs. Where there is hæmorrhage, however, we must trust at the time to gallic acid or turpentine or iron-alum, with perfect quiet. Over-active femedies, especially of an alterative or depressing nature, will only be productive of great mischief. In fact, the symptoms show the need for simple nourishing food, with cod liver oil. Sea air can also be recommended.

Bronchitis occurring secondarily in blood diseases is not uncommon, though often very troublesome. Thus, *typhoid bronchitis* not very unfrequently occurs during typhoid fever ; in severe cases greatly aggravating the danger of this disease. We may also have *gouty* or *rheumatic bronchitis*, only to be cured by the relief of the constitutional disorder. Rare cases have been observed where attacks of gout and bronchitis have seemed to alternate ; the latter subsiding on the development of a smart fit of the former.   So again, persons poisoned to the second, or to the tertiary degree, by syphilis, are apt to suffer from *syphilitic bronchitis ;* giving rise to troublesome substernal pain or sense of constriction, more or less cough and dyspnœa, slight muco-purulent expectoration, night sweats, great debility, and wasting.   Iodine spray inhalations (F. 262) are useful in these cases, in conjunction with anti-syphilitic remedies.   It should be remembered, moreover, that occasionally this last variety of bronchitis assumes the acute form ; while from time to time instances are met with where ulcerations of the mucous membrane of the bronchi are set up.   Under these circumstances disintegrated gummata will usually be found ; so that these cases are more properly to be regarded as instances of syphilitic phthisis.

Severe examples of all varieties of chronic bronchitis, when accompanied by abundant offensive expectoration, are apt to be mistaken for cases of gangrene of the lung, or for phthisis ; especially if there be also dilatation of the bronchi.   Professed consumption-curers often commit the latter error in diagnosis ; and then vaunt their very ordinary as extraordinary cures.

The *treatment* of chronic bronchitis obviously depends very much upon the age and constitution of the patient.   The cases which have fallen under my own observation have been most benefited by various stimulating expectorants, such as combinations of ammonia, senega, ipecacuanha, conium, spirit of chloroform, squills, and ether (F. 235, 237, 239, 243, 245) ; by tonics (F. 371, 375, 386) ; by cod liver oil, milk, and good nourishing food ; and by the moderate use of wine, or some other stimulant.—When the disease is due to the poison of syphilis, it will be most readily cured by iodide of potassium and the compound calomel pill.—If the patient be gouty or rheumatic, colchicum and iodide of potassium often work wonders.—In mechanical bronchitis, from fifteen to twenty grains of larch or Venice turpentine (Terebinthina laricea) made into pills with liquorice powder, and administered thrice daily, frequently prove of great service.—Supposing there to be any difficulty in throwing off the muco-purulent secretion, we shall do most good with ammonia, squills, spirit of chloroform, and spirit of ether or of nitrous ether.   Sometimes an emetic of ipecacuanha acts most favourably in these cases ; guarded with a dose of the aromatic spirit of ammonia lest it should cause much depression.

The inhalation of simple vapour is generally useful.   Where the secretion is excessive, turpentine or creasote (F. 260) inhalation may deserve trial ; or these remedies in the form of spray (F. 262) can be had recourse to with almost certain profit.   Counter-irritation by sinapisms, turpentine stupes, or rubefacient liniments, will give great relief ; while flying blisters frequently do good.   Patients often subsequently derive advantage from covering the chest with a large warm or chalybeate plaster.   And finally, susceptible subjects may ward off bronchial attacks by wearing the pneumoclime of Mr. Jeffreys, when in the open air at night or during unfavourable weather; although this instrument would seldom be required by men, if they did but allow the protecting medium which they naturally possess to grow freely. I am sure that I have again and again witnessed the most marked benefit arise in what are called "weak chested" individuals, from a cultivation of the moustache and beard.

XI. BRONCHIECTASIS.

Dilatation of the bronchial tubes, or bronchiectasis, was first described by Laennec, about the year 1818; when he showed how this organic lesion had previously been overlooked both by the anatomist and the practitioner.

The *dilatation may be uniform*, disturbing the calibre of one or more tubes for a variable length; or it will be *saccular*, consisting of one or several sacculated or bead-like dilatations, affecting particular points of one or more tubes, and giving rise to the appearance of cavities. The structure of the walls of the dilated parts is altered. Thus, their mucous lining becomes villous and ultimately ulcerated when the natural secretion cannot be thoroughly got rid of; so that it accumulates and decomposes, and sets up much irritation. Then, the muscular and elastic coats are found to have wasted, their elements having undergone a granular degeneration. The mucus in the bronchiectases is generally abundant; but it may either be natural in character, or thick and of a grey-yellow tinge, or inspissated and very fetid from decomposition. It is not improbable that the peculiar smell of the sputa depends upon their decomposition producing butyric and acetic acids, ammonia, and sulphuretted hydrogen.

The *condition of the lung tissue surrounding the dilatations* has been better described by Dr. Grainger Stewart than by any other writer that I am acquainted with.[*] He shows that there are various states:—(1) The lung tissue may be unaltered; being found soft, spongy, and crepitant. (2) It will be collapsed or atrophied. There is neither a spongy, nor an indurated condition. The atrophy is sometimes so extensive that nought remains in the affected part save dilated bronchi. (3) The pulmonary tissue is densely consolidated, constituting what some observers have called cirrhosis, and others fibroid degeneration of the lung. Under these circumstances it is said, that with occlusion of the air-cells there is also a marked increase of the fibrous tissue; a condition believed by Sir Dominic Corrigan to be identical with cirrhosis of the liver. (4) The surrounding lung tissue forms an

[*] *On Dilatation of the Bronchi, or Bronchiectasis*, p. 9. Edinburgh, 1867. This essay originally appeared in the *Edinburgh Medical Journal*, pp. 39-58. July 1867.

abscess, in the centre of which the thin walls of the dilated bronchus can be seen.   And (5) the walls of the bronchi and the surrounding lung tissue are destroyed by gangrenous inflammation.   M. Briquet first drew attention to this variety of pulmonary gangrene, and his observations have since been confirmed by others.   His chief conclusions are, that there is a form of dilatation of the bronchi in which the extremities of the tubes are dilated in sacs, which may be with or without dilatation of other parts of the bronchial tree ; and that these dilated extremities are liable to gangrenous destruction independently of gangrene elsewhere.

Very different opinions have been promulgated as to the *cause* of these dilatations.   Laennec believed that they were only met with in cases of chronic mucous catarrh ; a temporary dilatation resulting from a voluminous sputum, and being rendered permanent by the successive secretion and stagnation of similar ones.   This mechanical explanation was disputed by Andral with regard to one form of bronchiectasis, which he believed was the result of a vital hypertrophy.   And so conflicting views have prevailed according to the skill with which they have been advocated ; the theories of Sir Dominic Corrigan, Professor Gairdner, and Dr. Stokes having been the most extensively adopted.   After examining these, and considering the conclusions deducible from his own observations, Dr. Grainger Stewart believes that the essential element in these cases is atrophy of the bronchial wall ; so that the thinned and weakened tissue readily yields to the pressure of air, just as the force of the blood will produce an aneurismal tumour when the middle coat of an artery becomes weakened.   Moreover, the enfeebled and dilated bronchi encourage the accumulation of mucus ; while this decomposing secretion leads to irritation and inflammation of the mucous membrane, the growth of villous processes from it, the formation of increased connective tissue in the walls, irritation of the cartilages, and frequently to consolidation of the surrounding lung with abscess or gangrene.

The *symptoms* by which this morbid condition can be recognised in its early stages are not very distinct.   The general history is that the patient has caught a violent cold, that this has been followed by a frequent spasmodic cough, that there has been considerable expectoration, and that the sputum has been occasionally tinged with blood.   Advice has been had without as much relief being obtained as was hoped for.   Hence, the patient requires a consultation ; or he enters the hospital.   His chief complaints are then, a progressive loss of strength ; more or less dyspnœa on exertion ; a moist cough, which comes on in paroxysms ; an offensive odour about the breath and body generally ; and especially an abundant expectoration of greyish nummular sputa, occasionally mingled with fragments of fibrin which have been moulded in some of the bronchi so as to form casts, but always possessing a most fetid odour.   This fetor is distinct from that met with in gangrene ;

while when concentrated it is most disgusting. It is due to the retention and decomposition of the thick mucous or puriform secretion
from the walls of the bronchiectases; this secretion being occasionally so abundant that a pint or even more may be expectorated in
the twenty-four hours.   The temperature of the body is not raised
above the healthy standard.

The *physical signs* vary according to the extent of the dilatations, the amount of their contents, and the state of the surrounding lung. Obviously, percussion will elicit a more resonant sound
than natural if the dilatation be near the surface of the lung and
empty; but no clear note can be obtained if the tube be well
surrounded with condensed pulmonary tissue.   On auscultation,
coarse mucous rhonchus is heard; this being generally most distinct about the lower lobes.   Sometimes there is distinct gurgling,
exactly like that which is heard in a tubercular cavity.   To prevent any error in diagnosis it should be remembered that these
sounds in bronchiectasis are usually detected over the middle and
lower parts of the lungs, the apices being healthy; the phenomena
occasionally disappearing as the dilatations are emptied by a copious
expectoration, and then returning. In tubercular disease the upper
lobes are, as a rule, those first attacked; while the physical signs
are much more constant.

The *treatment* must first be directed to maintaining the general
health by nourishing food and cod liver oil.   Then, to diminishing
the secretion from the bronchial mucous membrane by such remedies as the compound tincture of benzoin, balsam and tincture of tolu,
or turpentine; by counter-irritation to the chest walls with the
liniment of iodine or croton oil, or the officinal blistering liquid
(liquor epispasticus); and especially by the inhalation of atomised
fluids containing alum, or tannic acid, or turpentine, or creasote
(F. 262).   And lastly, to keeping the bronchiectases as empty as
possible, so as to prevent the decomposition of the secretions;
which is to be effected by such expectorants as squill or ipecacuanha, and the use of creasote vapour.

XII. HAY ASTHMA.

This peculiar disease (commonly known as *hay asthma, hay
fever,* or *summer catarrh*) may perhaps be best described as a severe
catarrh frequently having asthmatic symptoms superadded.   The
conjunctival, nasal, faucial, and bronchial mucous membranes are
each affected; so that the patient has all the suffering often experienced from an aggravated common cold.   There is headache,
which is often severe; together with suffusion of the eyes, sneezing, irritation of the nose and fauces, and a dry harassing cough.
Then at intervals there will be experienced paroxysmal attacks

o o 2

of asthma, lasting for two or three hours; the dyspnœa being sometimes so urgent, that the patient has the most distressing sensations of impending suffocation.

Hay asthma is not a very common disorder. It probably arises from the inhalation of the pungent aroma of spring grass and hay (*Anthoxanthum odoratum*); or from the perfume of the *Nardus stricta* when in flower, a grass which is abundant in many grazing fields, for cattle will not eat it. Exposure to the emanations of *ipecacuanha powder* will produce it in impressible individuals. Dr. Pirrie says that a disorder analogous to hay asthma prevails in some parts of the United States where the rose is largely cultivated, and that it is known by the name of *rose fever* or *rose catarrh*. This gentleman also believes that hay fever is seldom, if ever, due to the same noxious agents which are always the causes of hay asthma. Thus, whereas the latter is the consequence of the action of the powder of flowering grasses or other vegetable irritants; the former is to be attributed, more or less directly, to exposure to an excess of solar heat, aided in many instances by intensity of light. Commenting on the histories of what he therefore proposes to call " summer fever" instead of " hay fever," Dr. Pirrie attempts to prove the correctness of his views by asking for attention to the condition under which some attacks originally supervene; their persistence after removal from the sphere of supposed contraction; the evident increase and decrease of the symptoms with a rise and fall of temperature; the manifest and oft-expressed aggravation of general as well as local suffering after exposure to strong light, or to a burning sun; the strong likeness of many of the features of the popularly termed hay fever to those constituting some of the after-effects of grave disorders commonly ascribed to solar heat or high temperature; and the induction of a like train of phenomena in some persons by heated air where no vegetation exists. Whether the mischievous effects of great heat and intensity of light are favoured by any unusual telluric or atmospheric conditions—as by an unusual amount of ozone, is uncertain. Dr. Pirrie seems, however, to think that the electricity of the atmosphere and the sun's rays may have some influence in the induction and maintenance of the disorder.

Supposing that an ordinary case of hay asthma be allowed to run its course without medical treatment, it will probably have a duration of three or four weeks. The disorder may, however, usually be cut short by removal from the cause: a visit to the sea side is often effectual. In some instances the susceptibility to the disease has been destroyed by the use of quinine and iron, or of arsenic, or of nux vomica; in combination with such hygienic management as is calculated to give tone to the nervous system. During the attack, relief can be obtained from antispasmodics like the tincture of lobelia (F. 88); ammonia and sumbul, or valerian, and assafœtida (F. 86, 87, 95); belladonna, ether, and iodide of potássium (F. 31); Indian hemp and ether (F. 337); or from stramonium, conium, opium, camphor, colchicum in gouty subjects, &c. A trial of creasote inhalations (F. 260) once or twice daily, as recommended by Dr. Walshe, may be resorted to. The inhalation of steam medicated with carbolic acid, or with turpentine, might do good. An anæsthetic composed of equal parts of pure chloroform and ether may be employed for moderating the asthmatic paroxysm. For this purpose too, few agents are more valuable than tobacco; inasmuch as directly the nausea and collapse caused by smoking set in, the sense of suffocation will pass off and the patient be enabled to forget his sufferings in sleep.

XIII. INFLUENZA.

Influenza [from the Italian, *Influénza ;* because the phenomena were thought to be due to the influence of the stars], or epidemic catarrhal fever, or in France "la grippe," is an epidemic disorder attended with great depression, chilliness, running from the eyes and nose, frontal headache, cough, restlessness, and fever.

Influenza arises at various periods from some peculiar condition or contamination of the atmosphere. The first visitation of it in this country, of which we have a trustworthy description, was that of 1510. The poisonous influence, whatever its nature may be, wings its way with greater celerity than the speed of human intercourse; while its progress seems uninfluenced by the season of the year, it is said to travel from east to west, and it seldom stays in one district more than six or seven weeks. Some visitations have proved more severe than others : one in 1782, which extended over the whole of Europe, was very fatal. Dr. Southwood Smith said that when the influenza broke out in London in 1847, it spread in a single day over every part of the metropolis, and affected upwards of 500,000 persons.

Symptoms.—The chief symptoms presented by this somewhat mysterious affection are heat and dryness of the skin, urgent frontal headache, coryza, sneezing, tenderness of the fauces, hoarseness, harassing cough, shortness of breath, pains in the back and limbs, perverted taste, and disorders of the stomach. There are, in addition, all the signs of nervous and muscular prostration, such as an uncommon degree of languor and debility and dejection of spirits. Occasionally the danger is much increased by the setting-in of acute bronchitis, capillary inflammation, or even of pneumonia.—The suddenness and rapidity with which the fever occurs are very remarkable. This disease is more fatal to elderly than to other persons. In favourable cases it runs its course in rather less than a week ; often terminating in an attack of diarrhœa, or in profuse sweating or diuresis, and merely leaving great feebleness.

Diagnosis.—Influenza differs from a common cold in its greater severity, and especially in the amount of prostration to which it gives rise. Between the reception of the poison and the commencement of the symptoms, there is a period of incubation ; but as to the duration of this we know nothing, since in some well-observed cases it has appeared to be only ten or twelve hours, while in other instances it has been as many days. The *prognosis* is favourable as a general rule. The deaths amongst persons under forty years of age were very small indeed, in all the epidemics ; but frequently amongst the aged, the mortality has been large.

Treatment.—About the treatment there can be no mistake. The patient had better be kept in bed, and barley water with nourishing broths must be administered. In mild cases no drugs are needed. If the catarrhal symptoms become urgent, ten grains of the compound ipecacuanha powder may be given at night ; or a mixture should be ordered containing Indian sarsaparilla with infusion of linseed (F. 241), or one of spirit of ether and senega and camphorated tincture of opium (F. 235). A sinapism applied to the chest, together with the inhalation of the steam of hot water, may be necessary. A vapour or hot air bath would in many instances give great relief. When prostration is the predominant symptom, stimulants are to be freely resorted to ; such as wine, ammonia, or even brandy. Milk and raw eggs help to give strength. The subsequent debility will be most quickly removed by tonics— especially by bark and phosphoric acid (F. 376), or quinine and iron (F. 380). Great good always accrues from a few days' holiday in the country.

XIV. HOOPING COUGH.

Pertussis [from *Per* = very + *tussis* = a cough], or hooping cough, is an infectious disease ; rarely occurring more than once in the same individual ; attended with more or less fever, and vomiting ; and accompanied at first by catarrh, and subsequently by a peculiar hard and convulsive cough which occurs in paroxysms at uncertain intervals. Its duration varies from three or four weeks to as many months. It is especially a disease of childhood.

Pathology.—Hooping cough appears to depend upon some peculiar poison, communicated through the atmosphere, which affects and irritates the pneumogastric or vagus nerve. The disease is now and then epidemic.

The bronchial glands are occasionally found enlarged after death. In many cases also, structural changes have been detected in the air-passages, or in some portion of the alimentary canal. Collapse of one or more of the lobes of the lungs seems to be a frequent cause of death. A general dilatation of the bronchi has now and then been found; the finer tubes being usually most affected, because their structure is entirely membranous without any plates of cartilage to strengthen them. This dilatation probably results from the violent inspiratory efforts which cause the hoop. Sir George Duncan Gibb has pointed out that in many cases the urine is saccharine (*pertussal glucosuria*), the quantity of sugar being usually small, and often consisting of a mere trace.

Symptoms.—At the commencement (after a latent period of perhaps six days) the poison produces a simple febrile stage of eight, ten, or twenty days' duration; this stage being sometimes accompanied, but generally followed, by severe attacks of coughing. The little child is seldom confined to his bed; though he is restless from the coryza, oppression of the chest, and heat of the skin. When the fever begins to remit at about the end of ten days, the cough changes its character; becoming convulsive and prolonged, assuming its peculiar shrill sound or hoop, and being followed by expectoration or vomiting of ropy mucus. As the severity of the cough increases, the paroxysms assume a suffocative character which terrify the patient. The vessels of the head, neck, and face become congested and swollen during each attack; the eyes appear as if starting from their sockets; the nose may bleed; and frequently the contents of the bladder and rectum are discharged involuntarily. Prior to the commencement of each fit the sufferer has a kind of warning, and he runs to his nurse for protection. The series of coughs or expiratory efforts are so powerful, and expel the air so largely from the lungs, that the patient seems on the point of being suffocated; until a long-protracted inspiratory act follows, the rush of air through the contracted glottis causing the characteristic crowing or hooping noise. As Dr. Todd was in the habit of teaching, this is the signal of the child's safety. Directly the fit, which bears some analogy to laryngismus stridulus, is over, the child regains his courage, soon appears well, and returns to his amusements; while even if it end in an attack of vomiting, there is a craving for food immediately afterwards, and he asks for something to eat. Where the fits of coughing are very severe they are occasionally followed by hæmorrhage from the mouth as well as from the nose, while sometimes there is even bleeding from the ears. In this latter case, rupture of the membrane of the tympanum has happened, deafness resulting in the affected ear unless the laceration completely heals. Ecchymosis of the conjunctivæ, from the giving way of one or more small subconjunctival vessels, is far from a rare occurrence. The frequency with which the paroxysms of cough recur varies: there may be only two or three in the day, or as many in an hour. The cough is usually most severe at night, and the first manifestation of improvement is a decrease in these nocturnal exacerbations. Then the paroxysms become altogether less severe as well as less frequent, until at the end of an uncertain time no symptom remains of the disease.   Under the influence of exposure to cold, or of improper food, however, the cough may return with all its former violence ; so that for several weeks after apparent recovery great care will be needed.

The duration of hooping cough is very variable, some cases being susceptible of cure in a fortnight or three weeks, while others continue troublesome for several months.   When the disease comes on in the autumnal or winter quarters, I believe it to be more obstinate than when it sets in during the spring or summer.

Complications.—Hooping cough does not always run its course in the comparatively simple manner just described.   Sometimes it supervenes upon other disease.   Thus, it may come on during convalescence from measles, and not only give rise by itself to dangerous symptoms, but very likely become complicated with bronchitis or pneumonia,—or with some cerebral affection.   These complications may occur in any case ; and inasmuch as they are very troublesome and not unfrequently dangerous, they demand a brief notice.

(1) Hooping cough *complicated with bronchitis or pneumonia*—is met with most frequently during the cold months of winter or spring. Unless the inflammation is severe, it will only be noticed in the commencement that the child is feverish and that the breathing is accelerated in the intervals between the paroxysms of cough; that the expectoration is opaque and glairy ; and that the cough is less constantly followed by vomiting than in simple pertussis. But as the morbid action progresses, the constitutional disturbance becomes great, the respiration difficult and quick, the pulse frequent, the fever burning, and the general signs of bronchitis or of pneumonia get fully developed ; while if auscultation be practised the diagnosis will not be difficult, with one exception.   We are indebted to Dr. Alderson, and subsequently to Dr. Graily Hewitt, for distinctly pointing out that when hooping cough proves fatal, it generally does so not by giving rise to pneumonia as has been thought, but by inducing catarrhal inflammation of the bronchial tubes, attended with collapse of a portion of the lungs.   This airless state of a part of the lung has also been found in young children from other causes besides hooping cough ; as well as in adults, as has been already mentioned in the remarks on bronchitis (see Sections X. and XVII. of this Part).   Pulmonary collapse, however, is not by any means necessarily fatal unless it prove extensive, or be badly treated by lowering measures : it is a condition which especially calls for the free employment of stimulating expectorants, wine, and as strong liquid nourishment as can be digested.

(2) Hooping cough *associated with convulsions, congestion of the brain, or with hydrocephalus*—is not uncommon, especially in infants about the period of dentition.   In these, convulsions of various forms, spasm of the glottis, screaming, &c., are of frequent occur-

rence, and are indicative of cerebral irritation. Congestion of the brain, owing to the return of the blood from this organ being interrupted during the paroxysms of cough, may be very slight and temporary, or excessive : in the latter case it will perhaps lead to inflammation of the membranes, or to the effusion of serum into the ventricles, or even to softening of some of the central parts. "In all cases of pertussis," says Dr. Copland, "when chills, followed by burning heat of the surface; pains of the head, with obscure redness of the conjunctiva; a fixed, brilliant, dry, and peculiar appearance of the eye; unusual redness or pallor of the face; very torpid bowels with morbid excretions; irritability of stomach independently of the fits of cough; aversion from light or noise; heaviness or drowsiness and languor; grinding of the teeth; or sudden starting or shocks of the body in sleep; rolling or tossing back the head, and piercing screams are observed, then irritation of the brain or its membranes, which will soon pass into organic change and effusion, is manifestly present, whether there be convulsions or not. When stupor or unconsciousness has come on, with one arm waving in the air, or tossed over the head, whilst the other is paralysed, a farther advanced state of disease than mere inflammatory irritation, or softening or effusion, may be inferred."*

(3) Hooping cough *may be complicated with disordered conditions of the bowels*—as indicated by a loaded tongue, foul breath, loss of appetite, a tumid abdomen, and offensive unnatural evacuations. If these symptoms continue for some time unrelieved, the chronic irritation of the digestive mucous surface gives rise to a remittent febrile disorder; in which the attacks of cough become more frequent, the breathing gets oppressed and hurried, the child's aspect becomes peculiar, and it is constantly picking its nose and lips. There is also increasing emaciation, and febrile exacerbations and remissions are observed twice in the twenty-four hours. Should the disorder proceed further still, serous effusion into the ventricles of the brain may take place, or disease of the mesenteric glands will be very likely to result.

Diagnosis.—This can only be at all difficult, when (as is sometimes the case) the characteristic hoop is wanting. Even then, the paroxysmal nature of the cough, the tendency to transitory attacks of retching, the character of the expectoration, the intervals of complete relief, and the evidence of a tendency to cerebral congestion during the convulsive attacks will serve to mark the affection.

Prognosis.—In simple cases a favourable opinion may always be given, unless the cough be very violent, the intervals of relief short and imperfect, the breathing hurried, the rest at night much disturbed, and the appetite very bad. With regard to the different complications it should be remembered, that they often make their approach very insidiously; that they are the more to be feared, the

* *A Dictionary of Practical Medicine.*   Article—" Hooping Cough,"
vol. ii. p. 239. London, 1858.

younger the child; that they are especially dangerous at the period of dentition; and that they are more alarming in such children as have strumous or consumptive parents.   Moreover, pulmonary complications are very apt to ensue when hooping cough occurs during convalescence from measles or scarlatina.   And then, finally, all kinds of cerebral symptoms, severe nocturnal exacerbations, fever and dyspnœa during the intervals, and difficult and scanty expectoration after the fits of coughing, are signs of danger.   The mortality of hooping cough is larger in female than in male children; and the colder the season of the year, the greater the fatality.   During 1866 the deaths in England from this disease were 15,764; of which number $\frac{\text{Males 6893}}{\text{Females 8345}} = 15,238$ were children under 5 years of age.

Treatment.—To describe all the remedies that have been proposed for the cure of this affection, either by orthodox physicians or dangerous amateurs, would occupy several pages; but as the majority of the " specifics" are worthless, such a labour is unnecessary.

The object of our treatment must be to keep the disease simple, to prevent other affections from complicating it; for since it arises from a particular contagion, as small-pox and scarlet fever do, so it has a tendency to run a certain course uncontrolled by art.   In mild cases very little management is required.   The patient should be warmly clothed, kept in-doors, fed with light nourishing food, and allowed to drink freely of some sweetened mucilaginous fluid.   No medicine need be administered internally; but the spine may be rubbed every night with belladonna and soap liniment in the proportion of two drachms to twenty-two, or with a mixture of equal parts of tincture of belladonna, glycerine, and camphor liniment.

With regard to the more severe forms of the disease, emetics (F. 231) are often very beneficial, especially if their use be followed by mild sedative expectorants, such as the tincture of squills and camphorated tincture of opium; or by a mixture of ammonia and ipecacuanha and senega (F. 235).   As in all diseases, blood-letting has been recommended by some physicians.   But I think it is impossible not to see that this affection, instead of being an inflammatory, is rather a spasmodic complaint; and consequently on this ground alone it may be positively asserted that antiphlogistic measures can wisely be discarded.   The patient must be kept from cold air, in an apartment having a temperature of about 65° or 68° Fahr.; he ought to be clothed in flannel; while the general nutrition should be maintained by food easily to be assimilated, such as fish, milk, light suet puddings, and new-laid eggs.   The chest can be sponged, back and front, once or twice a day with cold salt water; and embrocations containing sedatives may be afterwards used to the same part.   The best drugs are those known as tonics and antispasmodics—such as some salt of zinc, bark, quinine, morphia, aconite, belladonna, conium, hydrocyanic acid, assafœtida, camphor, spirit of ether, and chloroform.   It need hardly be mentioned that the greatest caution will be necessary in the use of most of these remedies, that they should be given in minute doses, and that their effects ought to be narrowly watched. A favourite practice with me is to order the sulphate of zinc, in gradually increasing doses, thrice daily; to give a mixture of ammonia, ether (or spirit of chloroform), morphia, and hydrocyanic acid, which shall be administered occasionally, as the frequency of the paroxysms may demand; and to have the spine well rubbed, night and morning, with an embrocation made of two parts of belladonna liniment, two of chloroform liniment, and twenty of camphor or soap liniment.

Dr. Fuller speaks very highly of the use of sulphate of zinc and belladonna (F. 92); under the influence of which remedies, given in increasing and large doses, he says the hoop rarely lasts more than twenty-one days, while it sometimes subsides in ten. In out-patient hospital practice I was generally disappointed with this treatment; but there are many reasons why too much reliance should not be placed upon results thus obtained.

Sir G. D. Gibb states that nitric acid (F. 91) is a specific. This remedy was first recommended by Dr. Arnold, of Montreal, several years ago. There are other practitioners who also think highly of it; but as they rarely seem to trust to it alone, the value to be attached to their opinions cannot be easily estimated. Certainly, in my hands nitric acid has not acted in any degree to the favourable extent that was expected from all that had been urged in its favour.—Dr. George Harley has found the bromide of ammonium useful, possibly owing to its peculiar anæsthetic effect upon the nerves of the larynx and pharynx. The dose is from two grains thrice daily for an infant, up to twelve grains for older children.— In many instances great benefit will be produced by sponging the fauces and glottis with a solution of nitrate of silver, (twenty grains to the ounce of distilled water).—Where the secretion from the bronchial tubes is excessive, it should be checked by astringents; as, for example, by alum, sulphate of zinc, small doses of sulphuric acid and infusion of bark, or gallic acid.—When there is much debility the solution of raw beef (F. 2), aided with good milk, small quantities of brandy, and perhaps a few drops of tincture of cinchona, will prove most serviceable.—And lastly, supposing the case becomes chronic, a cure may be effected by ferruginous tonics, cod liver oil, and change of air—particularly by removal to the sea side.

XV. ASTHMA.

Asthma [from 'Ασθμάζω = to gasp for breath] should be defined as essentially a nervous disease; the phenomena which it presents being dependent upon tonic contraction of the circular muscular fibres of the bronchial tubes. The paroxysms can be induced by direct or reflex mechanism,—or in other words, the stimulus to contraction may be central, in the medulla oblongata ; or it will be in the pulmonary or gastric portion of the pneumogastric, or in some other portion of the nervous system besides the vagus, and being transmitted to the medulla oblongata by incident, may be thence reflected by motor filaments.

Symptoms.—A fit of asthma is either preceded by headache and sleepiness, or by various digestive or other disturbances, or it occurs suddenly without any warning. The patient awakes two or three hours after midnight with a sensation of suffocation or constriction about the chest ; the dyspnœa gradually increasing until a fearful and most painful struggle for breath sets in. Various postures are assumed to facilitate the attempts at emptying and filling the lungs : the patient stands erect, or leans his head forwards on his hands on some piece of furniture, or holds himself up at the open window where he will remain almost for hours gasping for air. The chest is distended to its utmost limit, inspiration and expiration are performed with the greatest difficulty, and there is evidently some serious obstruction to the entrance and exit of air. If we auscult the thorax no normal respiratory murmur is audible ; but we hear sibilant rhonchi, loud wheezing, or shrill whistlings. For inasmuch as the varying calibre of the tubes, due to the muscular contraction, causes the air in them to be thrown into vibrations, so we of course have musical sounds of greater or less intensity according to the size of the constricted bronchi. The pulse is small and feeble ; the eyes are staring ; and the countenance is anxious. The skin gets cold (the temperature often falling to 82° Fahr.) and clammy from deficient oxygenation, while it may subsequently become bathed in a hot sweat owing to the fatigue produced by the respiratory efforts. The patient's whole appearance is most distressing, so much so that he seems to bystanders who are unacquainted with the character of his disease to be dying ; while he is either irritable at his prolonged suffering, or he looks beseechingly at the attendant for relief from his intense misery. Then, after a certain lapse of time, varying from two or three to thirty-six or even more hours, comes a remission. Cough ensues, and with the cough expectoration of little pellets of mucus ; and soon the paroxysm ceases, to allow the sufferer to fall into the long-desired sleep.

When the attack has been prolonged, the intercostal muscles, as well as all those brought into play by the act of respiration, ache continuously for two or three days after the fit has ceased. The patient commonly says that he feels sore all over. There is indeed genuine myalgia, produced by the enormous exertion which has been made to lessen the distress occasioned by the urgent dyspnœa.

Dr. Sidney Ringer has examined the urine in one case of spasmodic asthma. He found a remarkable diminution of the urea and the chloride of sodium, in the hours immediately succeeding the attack. There was, therefore, either a considerable arrest of formation or of elimination; most probably of the former. After four hours the urea rose to its former amount; while the chloride of sodium was increased beyond it.*

During the interval which elapses between one asthmatic paroxysm and the next, the patient very often enjoys moderately good health, and has his breathing quiet and free. Most asthmatics however, are thin and characteristically round-shouldered; they have an anxious appearance of countenance, the cheeks are hollow, and the voice is rather hoarse ; while there is habitually a slight cough. The length of the interval varies greatly in different cases; but not unfrequently the attacks are periodic, whether the time of recurrence be once in twenty-four hours, or once a week, or once a month, or once in twelve months. In one of the most trouble- some cases (though there was no organic disease) which have come under my notice, the paroxysm always came on every morning at 1 o'clock ; the dyspnœa continuing just as regularly for two hours. Thinking that this periodicity might be due to some par- ticular stage in the function of digestion, the patient was advised to discontinue taking supper, but no alteration was induced in the disease. In a second remarkable instance, a fit of asthma can always be produced by a dose of opium in any form or quantity ; a drug which unfortunately often seems demanded by other severe symptoms due to intestinal disease. On two or three occasions also the asthmatic attack has merged into one of catalepsy ; this state lasting for a few hours. Then again, with another asthmatic, habit has something to do with the attacks. Thus, he is generally well in London, yet being fond of Brighton tries to stay there some weeks in each year. But if, on the first night of sleeping away from town he experience an attack, a paroxysm is sure to recur nightly, until he is compelled to return ; whereas if this night be safely passed over, he may continue his sea side residence for weeks without any fear. As a rule, according to my experience, the bracing air of Brighton and similar localities is seldom favour- able to asthmatics. They, indeed, are often much more comfort- able in districts which are less healthy—particularly at night. A professional friend instead of adopting the common plan of getting a partial holiday for a few weeks by sleeping out of town, reverses the practice; inasmuch as he leaves London in the morning to spend his day in the country, returning home every evening to his bed. Dr. Salter† mentions somewhat similar cases ; while this gentleman also points out the capriciousness of asthma, one patient being better in a crowded city than in the country, another being benefited by a bracing air and injured by a relaxing climate, a third preferring the winter months to the autumnal, while again there are other instances where it is just the reverse of all this.

---

* *The Composition of the Urine, in Health and Disease, and under the Action of Remedies.* By Edmund A. Parkes, M.D. &c., p. 319. London, 1860.
† *On Asthma: its Pathology and Treatment*, pp. 230-261. London, 1860.

Asthma is more common in men than in women; it is often hereditary; and it sets in at any time of life, though most frequently about the middle period. It may be uncomplicated,— that is to say, in all other respects the sufferer is perfectly healthy, there being no lesion of the brain, lungs, heart, stomach, or other organs; or it may be complicated with, or indeed symptomatic of, some disorder like chronic bronchitis, heart disease, ovarian or uterine disorder, a morbid state of the nervous system, &c. The first form is sometimes known as *idiopathic* or *spasmodic*, the second as *symptomatic* or *organic* asthma.

Causes.—The fact that the tendency to asthma may be hereditary has just been mentioned; but it must be remembered that often no influence of this kind can be discovered. Again, this affection will sometimes be owing to some organic disease within the chest, while frequently no such cause can be detected.

The paroxysm may be directly due to an irritant inspired into the air-passages, such as dust, cold air, certain vapours, and emanations from hay or ipecacuanha or mustard. Any preparation of opium will provoke an attack in certain constitutions. The influence of particular atmospheric or climatic conditions is well known; though we are unable to explain why one asthmatic should be unable to sleep in a smoky and dirty city, while another can live nowhere else. Improper food, or an excessive quantity, or meals taken at certain particular times (*e.g.*, late suppers) may originate a fit. Sausages, kidneys, pork, cold boiled beef and pickles, toasted cheese and porter, &c., freely partaken of at night, have had the credit in cases which I have seen of starting off the attack. So again, the cause may be some irritation applied to parts of the body remote from the chest; as was observed in a patient of Dr. Chowne's, where the application of cold to the instep at once induced the fit. And lastly, mental emotion— fear, disappointment, anger, &c., may originate it.

I have very little doubt, moreover, that a tendency to asthmatic paroxysms may be kept up by skin diseases, as well as by affections of the stomach and intestines; though I am not as certain about these disorders acting as causes in the first instance. It has seemed to me that asthmatics are unusually liable to cutaneous eruptions.

Prognosis.—Spasmodic asthma very rarely, if ever, directly destroys life; and even many who are subject to it live to a good old age, perhaps for the reason that they are obliged to take great care of themselves. Moreover, a complete cure occasionally takes place; though, as a rule, when an attack has once occurred, the chances are in favour of there being many repetitions of it.

The disease is nevertheless a very serious one; partly because of the distress it entails, though chiefly in consequence of the morbid pulmonary and cardiac conditions which it sometimes induces. The principal of these are congestion of the lungs, emphysema, and hypertrophy with dilatation of the right side of the heart;

which conditions mostly arise in consequence of the repeated obstruction to the circulation of the blood through the pulmonary capillaries, impeding the action of the right side of the heart. When either of these complications has become thoroughly established, the asthmatic passes but a poor time with it. Indeed, his life is gradually rendered more and more miserable by cough, abundant expectoration, orthopnœa, venous regurgitation, œdema, and cyanosis; until at length, after a long period of ill-health, the circulation of venous blood produces somnolence and coma, which are soon followed by a welcome death.

Treatment.—Under this head must be considered the measures necessary to relieve the paroxysm, and those which should be employed in the hope of preventing or delaying its recurrence.

(1) *During the paroxysm* we first have to try to remove the exciting cause; as by giving an emetic when the stomach contains an undigested meal, or administering an enema if a loaded rectum seem to be the source of the irritation. Then our efforts ought to be directed towards relaxing the bronchial spasm, and for this purpose we resort to the use of sedatives. Frequently I have found that the latter object has been admirably fulfilled by a large dose of *iodide of potassium* (ten or even twenty grains), combined with some aromatic spirit of ammonia and spirit of ether and tincture of belladonna. *Tobacco* may be employed as a depressant or as a sedative, and in either way it often effects good. To those who are unaccustomed to smoking, a pipe of Latakia, (which is quite strong enough for the purpose) soon produces exhaustion; while directly the feeling of nausea and collapse comes on, the attack of asthma ceases. As a sedative, tobacco is more uncertain, though it will perhaps prove useful if taken when a fit seems impending. *Chloroform* is invaluable in many instances, while in others it does harm; and such is also the case with the vapour of *ether* (F. 313). The latter possesses this advantage, that with proper directions it may be entrusted to the patient's wife or nurse for administration, after it has been found to have a favourable effect. Moreover, it rarely nauseates patients so much as the prolonged use of chloroform frequently does; while to many it is, from the first, more agreeable. It will seldom be necessary to produce complete insensibility, and when there is any blueness of the surface it can never be advisable to do so. The inhalation of a mixture of equal parts of chloroform and ether is not only attended with less depression than when chloroform simply is used, and with less excitement than when pure ether is employed, but it has also seemed to be useful where neither agent alone has answered. While the patient is under the influence of the anæsthetic I have used, with great advantage, subcutaneous injections of atropine, or of morphia, or of a combination of both (F. 314); of course avoiding the morphia where the use of opium is known to have the effect of causing an attack. *Stramonium*, or Thornapple, acts like a charm with certain asthmatics, a few whiffs of

a pipe filled with it, or of a cigar, giving relief; but, in other cases it is quite worthless.   Care must be taken to get the drug good, while it may be remembered that the seeds are much more powerful than the leaves and stalk cut up.   The fumes of the *Datura Tatula*, obtained by smoking cigars made of this plant, act in a similar way to those of the Datura Stramonium.   The *Cigares Anti-Asthmatiques de Mr. Joy*, are occasionally very efficacious.   I do not know their composition; but imagine they may be made of bibulous paper soaked in an arsenical solution of nitrate of potash, flavoured with tobacco.   *Nitre-paper fumes* (the fumes of burning filtering or blotting paper which has been soaked in a saturated solution of nitrate of potash and dried) affords much alleviation in many cases of uncomplicated asthma.   And lastly, there are instances where palliation is soonest obtained from a *stimulant*, as a glass of whisky or brandy toddy, or a cup of very strong coffee. I am told that the poor of Perth often stop an attack with a noggin of whisky; but a paroxysm thus starts off the propensity to drink, which is sometimes only checked when the sufferer has pawned all that he possesses.

(2) Our *treatment in the interval* ought to be directed to improving the general health by prescribing tonics, a regular mode of life, and the use of the cold shower or sponge bath; to laying down rules as to diet, so as to obviate attacks of dyspepsia; to so ordering the times of the various meals that the process of digestion may be finished before bedtime; and to choosing a climate, the opposite to that in which the fits come on—as London air for those who are worst in the country, and the reverse.

Where there is a relaxed condition of the mucous membrane about the fauces, and the expectoration is copious, *tannin* or *catechu lozenges* prove useful.   When the digestion is weak, benefit will often be derived from the *nitro-hydrochloric acid* (F. 378) with *pepsine* (F. 420) at the meals.   In many instances, where the cause is obscure, the *iodide of potassium* (F. 31) certainly works wonders. While the fourth edition of this work was in the press I was trying this remedy, but had not then had sufficient experience to justify my recommending it.   Since then it has seemed to effect a complete cure in several well-marked cases, while it has proved beneficial in many others; so that I am inclined to think there is no single remedy which can compete with it.   This drug requires to be persevered with for some weeks; the patient being watched, lest it impoverish the blood and produce purpura, or boils, or even a carbuncle.   Directly any hæmorrhagic spots appear, however, all may be made to go well by temporarily substituting quinine, or nitric acid and bark.   *Arsenic* is another medicine which at times seems to exert a favourable influence.   The peasants of Styria and Hungary who eat this metal find that it strengthens their lungs, or they say it does so.   When an extremely clever gentleman buys a showy cob at a horse fair, upon his own responsibility, he not unfrequently finds himself possessed of "a shotten piper,"—a broken-winded animal whose failing has been concealed by a generous dose of shot and tallow. The "coper," who has gone off quietly at the conclusion of the bargain, has probably administered the remedy, on the mechanical principle that it will prevent "a rising of the lights;" but scientific witnesses affirm that the arsenic in the shot is the effective agent, this medicine being good for the wind of horses, greyhounds, and sporting dogs. Whether, on this view, arsenic is likely to be serviceable in asthma is deserving of consideration. As far as my own experience goes I can only say that in cases where patients have simultaneously suffered from lepra and asthma, arsenic has done great good. But whether the benefit has been owing to the remedy itself, or has only arisen secondarily from the cure of the skin disease, must at present remain a matter of doubt. Dr. Beigel, however, remarks that the inhalation of spray medicated with from five to ten minims of the arsenical solution (F. 262), has rapidly succeeded in curing inveterate cases of asthma after the failure of other remedies.

In conclusion, if there be constipation during any plan of treatment, a mild aperient should be given at bed-time,—such as five grains of compound rhubarb pill with the same quantity of extract of conium. The inhalation of oxygen gas might (as suggested by Dr. Goolden and others) do good in some instances ; or the peroxide of hydrogen (F. 370) would perhaps afford temporary ease; or possibly the respiration of compressed air (long since recommended by Sir John Sinclair and others) would give relief in similar cases, by affording the system an excess of oxygen. Without condemning these remedies I am bound to confess, however, that disappointment has been the usual result of my trying them. As regards blisters to the spine and nucha, galvanism, issues, the administration of strychnia, &c., it need only be said that the obvious theoretical objections to these agents have not been overcome, so far as I know, by any practical experience of their utility; although they are not unfrequently recommended.

XVI. EMPHYSEMA.

The diseases of the lung thus denominated are of two kinds. One consists essentially of enlargement of the air-cells, atrophy of their walls, and obliteration of their vessels : this is called *vesicular* or *pulmonary* emphysema ['Εμφυσάω = to inflate]. When, on the other hand, there is infiltration of the air into the interlobular connective tissue, or into the sub-pleural connective tissues, the disease is known as *interlobular* emphysema. Both forms give rise to habitual shortness of breath, with occasional severe paroxysms of asthma; in many instances they lead to disease of the right cavities of the heart, with venous congestion and dropsy; while they are at all times very distressing complaints, and quite unfit the sufferer for any active occupation.

Vesicular emphysema may affect one lung, or both, or only a part of each—especially the anterior edges and the apices. The increase in the size of the air-cells necessarily diminishes the contractility of the yellow elastic fibrous tissue of their walls; which tissue, on being long overstretched, is unable to recover its tone. Then the walls become perforated, small oval openings resulting; the perforations gradually increasing in size. As the disease progresses there is a complete wasting of the partitions between the sacs; so that two or three or more form one cavity, which may project from the surface of lung like a bladder. The dilated air-vesicles, in partial emphysema, are not found in those parts of the lung where there is evidence of pre-existing bronchitis, but in the opposite portions.

According to Professor Gairdner,* vesicular emphysema is of mechanical origin, is produced by the inspiration force, and is essentially a compensatory dilatation of the air-cells, implying that a portion of the lung is non-expansible; hence the foundation of the disease may be bronchitis, pulmonary collapse, asthma, &c. Some discussion has since arisen as to whether the extra strain upon the cells really occurs from the pressure of the air during inspiration or expiration; and it seems probable that although a certain amount of dilatation may be determined by inspiration, yet—as Sir William Jenner† has shown—the most efficient cause is the pressure of the air contained in the lung brought to bear upon the inner surface of the air-cells by the expiratory efforts.

Dr. Waters recognises and defines three forms of pulmonary vesicular emphysema.‡ The first, or *partial lobular emphysema*, exists usually with the second form, and consists of small patches of dilated air-sacs especially along the margins of the lobes. These patches involve a few air-sacs only, they elevate the pleura, and they are sometimes found along the margin of the base of the lung looking like a row of beads. The second form, or *lobular emphysema*, is the most common. It involves one or more lobules in different parts of the lung; but is particularly seen at the margin of the base, at the anterior border, and at the apex. This kind is often met with in phthisis, and in those disorders of the respiratory organs which are accompanied by violent cough. The third form, or *lobar emphysema*, is by far the most formidable; often destroying life at an early period. There is an emphysematous condition of the whole pulmonary tissue of a lobe, or of one lung, or of both lungs. The dilatation of the air-cells comes on insidiously, but progresses

* *British and Foreign Medico-Chirurgical Review*, vol. xi. p. 469. London, 1853.
† *Medico-Chirurgical Transactions*, vol. xl. p. 25. London, 1857.
‡ *On Diseases of the Chest, &c.*, p. 109. London and Liverpool, 1868.

steadily; while as the distension increases the walls of the cells get thinner and thinner, until they become perforated and broken down. This disease is constitutional—the result of some degenerative process, the exact nature of which is uncertain. Dr. Rainey and Dr. C. J. B. Williams have expressed the opinion that it is a fatty degeneration of the lung-tissue which brings about the atrophy and rupture of the cells; while Sir William Jenner regards the change as a fibrous degeneration—the consequence of an exudation of lymph from the capillaries, when they have been the seat of slight long-continued congestion. These conclusions are disputed by Dr. Waters; who admits the constitutional nature of the disease, but has not been able to trace the precise kind of degeneration. Still he believes, that the most important feature in it is a malnutrition of the lung-tissue; and this is the point to be borne in mind, since it necessarily influences the question of treatment. Dr. Waters founds his view on these facts,—the emphysema may reach a high degree of development without any previous history of long-standing cough; the disease is sometimes hereditary; the uniform manner in which the whole of both lungs is occasionally attacked; and the way in which the disease is influenced by those remedies that act beneficially in other cases attended with degeneration of tissue. These are certainly strong corroborative circumstances. It is further considered that the distension is not brought about by expiratory efforts, but by inspiration; the abnormally weak lung-tissue giving way under the influence of a pressure, which in a state of health it would be able to resist. Hence, the primary step in the disease is a degeneration of lung-tissue, and the mechanical distension a secondary consequence.

The prominent symptom of emphysema is dyspnœa; which is much increased upon any exertion, and is aggravated by cold and damp. There is also a feeble cough, difficult expectoration of frothy sputa, a dusky appearance of the countenance, weakness of the voice, a stooping gait, loss of flesh with strength, a lowered temperature of the body, constipation, a weak and slow pulse, a sense of oppression about the chest, and a diminished frequency of the respirations. The physical signs of this disease consist of unnatural clearness and resonance on percussion; while only a very indistinct vesicular murmur is heard on auscultation. Occasionally a moist râle will be detected, like the sub-crepitant rattle of bronchitis. The heart's sounds are merely feebly audible, and this organ is often displaced; while if only one lung be affected there will be cardiac displacement to the opposite side, or if both be involved we shall have displacement downwards and to the right. The diseased side of the thorax is always more prominent and rounder than the healthy one. Thus, as regards percussion and auscultation, emphysema affords results the reverse of other affections: the disease consisting, as it were, of a superabundance of air which does not pass away, there is more resonance, but less sound in the air-passage—less respiratory murmur. It can only be confounded with pneumothorax; but it may be distinguished by remembering that this latter disease merely affects one side of the chest, that the percussion note is much more tympanitic, and that the site over which the resonance is obtained is considerably more extensive than in emphysema.

The affections more frequently associated with emphysema than any others are the following :—*Asthma*, the most distressing seizures of which usually occur in the night, and which probably is due to irritation from pulmonary congestion setting up reflex paroxysmal contractions of the muscular fibres of the bronchi. In some cases asthma is the primary disease, producing the emphysema. *Bronchitis* often occurs where there is emphysema. The inflammation may cause death by the excessive secretion of muco-purulent fluid accumulating in the bronchi, and so leading to slow suffocation. Not uncommonly, a fatal termination is due to the formation of fibrinous clots in the cavities of the heart, or in the commencement of the aorta or pulmonary artery. *Affections of the heart ;* hypertrophy, with dilatation of the ventricles, being the most common.

With respect to treatment, we can, for the most part, only attempt to give relief by an invigorating diet, rest, warm clothing, and attention to the digestive organs; as well as by the occasional use of tonics and antispasmodics. Amongst the former drugs, quinine and iron are the most useful (F. 380); or if the digestion be weak, steel and pepsine (F. 394) at the meals, may be preferable. Strychnia has failed to be of any service. Cod liver oil ought also to be administered. Amongst the latter remedies, ammonia, ether, hydrocyanic acid, sumbul, &c. (F. 85, 86, 95) are the most promising. The ethereal tincture of lobelia has been recommended, and so has the Indian hemp. Stramonium may also be smoked; or the camphor cigarettes of M. Raspail can be tried. Sometimes I have seen a preparation of oxygen (F. 370) give relief. Occasionally the vapour of chloroform is of great temporary service.

A warm climate is often very beneficial to sufferers from this affection; the dyspnœa being always most urgent in cold weather. Mr. Jeffrey's pneumoclime (respirator) can generally be worn with advantage, during unfavourable states of the atmosphere. If Sir William Jenner's theory be correct, we must, as he shows, moderate the violence of the expiratory actions in persons disposed to emphysema; and not allow them to follow toilsome occupations (such as carrying or pushing heavy weights) which necessitate expiratory efforts with a closed glottis.

The management of all the secondary affections requires to be conducted with caution; for if lowering measures are employed, the patient's safety will be much jeopardised. In bronchitis more especially ammonia does much good; inasmuch as it aids the expectoration of the fluid which is apt to produce apnœa if allowed to accumulate in the air-tubes, while it also diminishes the chance of thrombosis. Nourishing food, milk, and moderate quantities of alcoholic stimulants will also be needed.

Interlobular emphysema consists of an infiltration or collection of air in the connective tissue between the different lobules.   It is generally produced by the sudden rupture of some air-cells in consequence of violent strain or effort. Hence it may be caused by forcing or bearing-down at stool, by the expulsive pains of parturition, by repeated fits of coughing, and so on. On examining several fatal cases of hooping cough, M. Guillot found extensive sub-pleural emphysema; in a few instances emphysema of the areolar tissue of the mediastinum, and even of the neck, being also present.

This affection is not to be diagnosed by any certain signs during life. Every now and then it is associated with vesicular emphysema; it is frequently very limited; while when unusually extensive, it can at once give rise to fatal asphyxia.

XVII. CONDENSATION OF THE LUNG.

Condensation of the lung may result from pneumonia, from phthisis, from cancerous deposit, or from the exudation and infiltration of a syphilitic material into the pulmonary tissue; as well as from pressure exerted on the lung by fluid poured out in pleurisy, by enlarged bronchial glands, and by aneurismal or other intra-thoracic tumours. A small tube, or even a main bronchus, will thus become so obstructed that air cannot pass; and as a consequence there results collapse of that portion of the lung to which the compressed bronchus leads.

But in the present section the foregoing cases have not to be dealt with. We have now to consider that particular variety of pulmonary condensation, which is owing to collapse of the air-cells from the plugging-up (generally by a thick tenacious secretion) of a bronchial tube. This form has been variously designated as *disseminated lobular pneumonia*, or *marginal pneumonia*, or *carnification*, or *pulmonary collapse*. The same condition is sometimes met with in new born infants, from congenital non-expansion of the air-cells, being known as *atelectasis* of the lungs. Hence it will be convenient to speak of these two sets of cases separately, under the heads of *acquired* and *congenital* pulmonary condensation.

In *acquired* pulmonary collapse, the margin of the lung, or an irregular portion of one lobe, or an entire lobe, or even the whole of the organ is found involved. The obstruction may be owing to an increase in the secretion of the mucous membrane, with inability to cough it up; and therefore it not unfrequently occurs in bronchitis and hooping cough, especially in feeble subjects. Or, the secretion being natural in quantity, is expelled with such great difficulty (owing to old age or general debility) that an accumulation takes place in the central or some other part of the lung, and then acts like a plug.   In either case, it can be readily understood that a portion of tenacious mucus at the bifurcation of a bronchus will play like a valve; at every expiration permitting of the escape of air, but falling close on the opening at each inspiration so as to prevent ingress.   Consequently the vesicles beyond the obstruction gradually become emptied of air, and then collapse; this condition causing more or less severe dyspnœa, in proportion to the extent of lung affected.   The physical signs of collapse ought to consist of decided dulness on percussion, with an absence of the respiratory murmur over the affected parts.   Where, however, the morbid condition has been of some duration, the signs are apt to be masked by the occurrence of a kind of compensatory emphysematous distension of those portions of lung anterior to the obstruction.

The indications for treatment are sufficiently obvious.   Instead of inflammation we have general debility with deficient inspiratory power.   Hence stimulating expectorants (more particularly ipecacuanha and ammonia), tonics, and restorative food are the remedies to be employed.

Congenital non-expansion of the air-cells is met with in weakly infants.   Some portions of the lungs (especially the lower edge of the upper and lower lobes, and the middle lobe of the right lung) are liable to remain solid and unaërated, giving rise to the condition known as *atelectasis* ['Ατελὴς = imperfect + ἔκτασις = expansion].   An infant thus affected looks as if it had only been born to die speedily.   It is often jaundiced; it utters a weak whimper or cry; it can scarcely suck; it remains very feeble and drowsy; the surface is cold and slightly livid; and the chest is but partially dilated by the imperfect respiratory movements.   After the lapse of a few days, or possibly weeks, the child either gradually becomes stronger, the paroxysms of dyspnœa materially lessen, and good health is ultimately obtained; or, in less fortunate cases, the symptoms increase, convulsions occur, and death ends the sufferings.   To avoid this latter termination we must keep the infant wrapped up in flannel or cotton wool, in a warm room; while it should be so placed, on a firm pillow, that the respiratory act may be impeded as little as possible.   Stimulating oily liniments can be rubbed over the back and front of the chest, and along the spine.   Ether with ammonia, or port wine with a few drops of tincture of bark, ought to be administered every few hours.   If the air-tubes appear to be obstructed by mucus, an occasional mild emetic of ipecacuanha may serve to remove it.   And then, if the exhaustion be too great to admit of attempts at sucking, the mother's milk must be drawn off, and feeding with a spoon had recourse to.

XVIII. ŒDEMA OF THE LUNGS.

The effusion of a clear watery fluid, or of a sanguinolent serum, into the pulmonary tissue is known as œdema of the lungs.   It is a secondary affection of some consequence; since it may give rise to considerable suffering, while it often hastens death when connected with general dropsy. The fluid is probably exuded from the pulmonary vessels into the air-sacs and their partitions; as well as into the connective tissue around the bronchi, vessels, and lobules.

Œdema of the lungs may come on secondarily in Bright's disease, in valvular and other affections of the heart, and in general dropsy, &c. The suffocative dyspnœa which sometimes sets in suddenly during the progress of the eruptive fevers and other acute diseases, is probably due to this condition. Its symptoms are equivocal. Dyspnœa, slight cough, tightness or a sense of oppression about the chest, and the expectoration of a watery fluid can only lead to a suspicion that there is pulmonary œdema. In some cases the expectoration is copious, colourless, frothy, and not very consistent; presenting an appearance compared by Laennec to that of white of egg dissolved in an equal part of water. Both lungs are generally equally affected. By percussion, a duller note than natural will usually be obtained. On auscultation, more or less moist crepitation can be detected.

The remedies needed will be those for the primary affection. Perhaps diuretics, with as much simple nourishment as can be assimilated, may prove serviceable. Tonics can seldom be borne by themselves; but in combination with drugs to act on the kidneys and skin they sometimes do good for a short time.

Further observations on the extravasation of blood into the air-sacs of the lungs (the so-called *pulmonary apoplexy*) are unnecessary after what has been said in Part I, section 7, sub-section 6.

XIX. PLEURISY.

Pleuritis, or pleurisy, are terms applied to inflammation of the pleura—the serous membrane investing the lungs and lining the cavity of the thorax. The disease will run either an acute or a chronic course; while one side only is usually affected, though occasionally we have double or bilateral pleurisy. Uncomplicated cases very rarely end fatally.

Causes.—The most common causes of pleurisy, in subjects suffering from some morbid condition of the blood, are exposure to cold and wet, sitting or sleeping in damp clothes, &c. I do not believe, however, that any amount of cold by itself, will produce the disease in a healthy individual. It may prove the exciting, but not the essential cause of the inflammation. The statement has been made that in the greater number of cases of pleurisy on the right side, the inflammation depends on the pre-existence of tubercle in the lung; while pleurisy of the left side is usually independent of this cause.   In cancer of the female breast pleurisy often occurs secondarily, either from the irritation of the pleura by a deposit of cancer beneath it ; or in some instances probably, as Dr. Walsh suggests, by the sub-inflammatory action on the confines of the diseased gland extending through the intervening tissues to the pleura.   During the progress of continued fever, of an eruptive fever (especially measles), and of Bright's disease, an attack may set in. And, lastly, mechanical injuries will excite inflammation of this serous membrane. Thus the jagged ends of a fractured rib often give rise to it ; while if they also wound the pulmonary pleura, air will escape from the lung into the pleural cavity.

Symptoms.—This disorder is ushered in with chilliness or slight rigors.   Then follows fever, and an acute lancinating pain in the side, called a stitch ; which pain is commonly seated below the nipple, over the antero-lateral attachment of the diaphragm.   It is aggravated by the expansion of the lung in inspiration, by coughing, by lying on the affected side, and by pressure.   There is also a short harsh cough, the skin remains hot and dry, the cheeks are flushed, the pulse is hard and quick, the respirations are slightly increased in frequency, there is anxiety with considerable restlessness, while the urine is rather scanty and high coloured.   The temperature of the body gradually rises to perhaps 103° ; but it probably never attains the height it acquires in pneumonia, and it usually falls with much more rapidity to 99°·5, and thence to the normal standard.

When we listen to the painful part of the chest at this period, we shall hear the dry inflamed membranes—the pulmonary and costal pleuræ—rubbing against each other, and producing a *friction sound ;* or if the hand be placed on the corresponding part of the thorax, this rubbing may be distinctly felt.   But the sound soon ceases : either the inflammation terminates in resolution, and the two surfaces of the pleura regain their natural moisture and smoothness ; or, the roughened and inflamed surfaces get adherent, the lymph which has been exuded forming a pseudo-areolar tissue ; or they become separated by the effusion of serum, and a kind of dropsy results, known as HYDROTHORAX ["Υδωρ = water + θώραξ = the chest].   If the pleurisy have been severe, the effusion becomes excessive (it may vary from a very few ounces to several pints) ; and the fluid accumulating in the sac of the pleura compresses the yielding lung, suspends its functions, displaces the heart, and somewhat distends the thoracic parietes.

When the pleuritic inflammation ends in suppuration, and the pus accumulates in the cavity of the chest, we have what is called EMPYEMA ['Εν = within + πύον = pus] ; a termination which is much more frequent in men than in women.   Some practitioners speak of true and false empyema : the first form being that in which the pus is secreted by the pleura ; while the second is that in which the pus finds its way into the cavity of the thorax from the rupture of an abscess of the lung.   Now and then the pus forms a bulging tumour in one of the intercostal spaces; fluctuation generally being appreciable to the touch. Where the swelling is on the left side, a pulsation synchronous with the heart's beat may perhaps be observed. A careful examination will prevent "pulsating empyema" from being mistaken for an aneurism; since the tumour diminishes and increases with each inspiration and expiration, while there is neither an aneurismal thrill nor bruit. Nevertheless, if it be determined to evacuate the matter, a grooved needle should be introduced, as a precautionary measure, before using the bistoury. Occasionally ulceration takes place in the costal pleura and gradually extends through the muscles, or a portion of the rib becomes carious, and an aperture is formed externally; through which channel (a *parietal fistula*) pus continues to be discharged for a long time in cases of chronic pleurisy. On the other hand, the pulmonary pleura may be perforated, and an opening take place into the air-tubes; which opening, when it fails to close after the evacuation of the fluid by the bronchi, is known as a *bronchial fistula*. The matter thus evacuated is usually most offensive.

Whether the matter effused consist of serum, or of serum mixed with blood (as in hydrothorax occurring in a scorbutic subject), or of pus, we shall find, on listening to the chest, that the respiratory murmur is diminished in proportion to the quantity of fluid thrown out. Where this is excessive and the lung is compressed backwards—flattened almost against the spinal column, no vesicular breathing at all will be heard; but instead we shall detect the air passing into the larger bronchial tubes, the condensed lung and the layer of fluid acting as conductors of sound. We then say that *bronchial respiration*, and *bronchial voice* or *bronchophony*, exist. The bronchophony may be accompanied by a tremulous noise, resembling the bleating of a goat; it is then termed *ægophony*. If the lung be completely compressed, so that air cannot enter even the bronchial tubes, then no sounds of any kind will be heard; but on the healthy side the respiration will be more distinct than natural—will be *puerile*. There must also be dulness on percussion all over the affected side, if the pleura be full of fluid : if it be only partially filled, we can sometimes judge of the quantity by placing the patient in different attitudes ; for since the liquid will gravitate to the most dependent part of the cavity, so it necessarily carries the dull sound with it. The exceptions to this rule which may be met with, consist of cases where there is solid exudation-matter as well as fluid; for if the pleura be coated with a thick pulpy substance, there will evidently be dulness on percussion in whatever posture the patient may be placed. We shall often more decidedly be able to judge of the amount of the effusion by noticing the dyspnœa which the patient suffers from ; inasmuch as this will, of course, be most urgent when the lung is most compressed. At the same time, also, the sufferer is commonly unable any longer to lie on the sound side ; for the simple reason that the movements of the healthy lung are then impeded by the superincumbent weight of the dropsical pleura. The pain, moreover, no longer prevents his lying on the diseased side. If we measure the two halves of the chest, the side containing the effusion will be found the largest : we must remember, however, that in many persons the right half of the chest is naturally rather larger than the left. In making an ocular examination of the affected side, it will be discovered enlarged ; the intercostal muscles are seen inactive, and the spaces quite obliterated or even bulging if the secretion be copious ; there is marked fulness of the infra-clavicular region ; and the shoulder is depressed. From some inexplicable cause, pleuritic effusion occurs most frequently on the left side.

After a time the symptoms often begin to decrease, and absorption of the effused fluid fortunately commences. Supposing the lung to be bound down by adhesions, it will not be able to expand in proportion to the absorption of the fluid. The affected side consequently shrinks inwards, and instead of any longer remaining larger than the sound one, will become smaller.

With one form of the disease, known as *latent pleurisy*, there may be neither pain, cough, nor dyspnœa ; and yet effusion may go on until one half of the chest becomes filled with fluid, as shown by the physical signs.

The presence of air in the pleura will occasionally be found to be due to other circumstances than the injury produced by a broken rib. Thus it may arise from an external wound ; as well as from ulceration owing to the extension of a tubercular cavity. When the pleura contains air alone, we say there is PNEUMOTHORAX [Πνεῦμα = air + θώραξ = the chest] ; when, as generally happens, there is a liquid with the air, we call the disease PNEUMOTHORAX WITH EFFUSION. The physical signs of pneumothorax are abnormal resonance on percussion, and loss or indistinctness of the respiratory murmur on auscultation. The patient's breathing, cough, and voice, give rise to a ringing metallic noise like that produced by blowing obliquely into an empty flask, and hence called *amphoric resonance*. When there is also liquid with the air, we obtain in addition (especially on practising succussion) a sound known as *metallic tinkling ;* which some authorities believe to result from a drop of fluid falling from the upper part of the cavity and causing a little splash, but which is in all probability simply due to the bursting of an air-bubble in a confined cavity with firm walls.

Diagnosis.—The distinction between pleurisy and pleurodynia (pain in the muscles of the thorax) is rendered so easy by attention to the foregoing description of the symptoms, that nothing more need be added. Malignant disease of the lung or pleura is more likely than any other affection to be mistaken for empyema ; since in both of these instances there has generally been pleurisy, while in both there may be displacement of the heart, dulness on percussion, absence of respiratory murmur, inability to lie on the sound side, and œdematous enlargement of the affected side. Again, empyema of the right pleura is not always easily diagnosed from enlargement of the liver; but the difficulty will be lessened by noticing that in the latter there is no intercostal paralysis, there is resonance on percussing the middle and upper parts of the chest, the force of the respiratory murmur in the postero-inferior portion of the chest is much greater than the dulness would lead us to anticipate, and the heart is displaced upwards instead of laterally.

Prognosis. — Simple unilateral pleurisy always terminates favourably. Even when it is bilateral, or when it occurs during the progress of some chronic ailment—as Bright's disease, tuberculosis, cancer, &c., it is not often the immediate cause of death.

Treatment.—The indications for the treatment of pleurisy are first, to subdue the inflammation; and, secondly, to promote the removal of its products. To obtain these results the sufferer is to be kept very quiet in bed; while in order to prevent undue friction at the inflamed part, he should be cautioned against talking or taking full inspirations. The application of a fine flannel bandage round the chest, may sometimes be serviceable by lessening the movements of the ribs. As in all probability, the more the patient is lowered, the more severe will be the results of the inflammation, I would advise the practitioner not to resort to general bleeding; but rather to trust to the administration of diaphoretics (F. 211, 212), with opium to relieve the pain. Locally, no measures give greater relief than large and very hot and moist linseed poultices, covered with the extracts of poppies and belladonna (F. 297); or the use of poppy-head fomentations may be recommended, provided they can be sedulously applied. Some practitioners prefer the employment of sinapisms or turpentine stupes, but they have often the disadvantage of irritating the patient. When the pain is very severe, the removal of three or four ounces of blood by cupping will possibly give relief sooner than any other proceeding, by unloading the congested vessels. The same effect can be brought about by the application of half-a-dozen leeches. But even before taking away this small quantity of blood, in subjects disposed to weakness, it will be better to try the effect of the medicated poultices or fomentations; proceedings which I constantly resort to with the greatest advantage. If the practitioner have faith in the powers of mercury to control inflammation, he will administer calomel and opium; though it is very doubtful if the calomel can exercise the slightest beneficial influence. The bowels must be kept open by purgatives, if necessary. The diet should consist of gruel, arrowroot, plenty of milk, eggs, light puddings, and good broths; while cooling refreshing drinks are to be freely allowed.

If these means prove insufficient and effusion take place, we must then endeavour to promote absorption. The patient had better be kept on a moderate diet, free from stimulants; a succession of flying blisters ought to be applied to the diseased side, or the action of the absorbents may be increased by sinapisms, or friction with the ointment of red iodide of mercury can be tried; and purgatives as well as diuretics are to be administered. The iodide of potassium (F. 31), will often be useful; or a combination of squills, digitalis, and blue pill (F. 28), has been highly recommended. Very often, however, mercury in any shape administered internally does harm; and especially if the effusion be due to chronic pleurisy, or if there be any tubercular or cancerous deposit. In such cases the compound tincture of iodine, or the iodide of iron, or cod liver oil, are more likely to forward our views.   .

When the foregoing remedies fail, tapping the thorax so as to let the fluid out has been resorted to, and on many occasions with success.   The opinions of physicians vary widely as to the propriety of performing this operation.* My own impression is, that as a general rule it ought not to be performed unless the effusion is excessive; nor until proper attempts to procure absorption have been adopted.   In any instance, if we felt satisfied that the pleura was full of pus an operation should be performed; but I know not how it can be decided whether such is the case, or whether the effusion is only of the nature of a serous fluid.   The question is always a very important one, for if tapping be determined on it is by no means to be left as a last resource; inasmuch as if deferred too long, irremediable mischief takes place in the lung. Thus, ulceration of the pulmonary tissue may take place and extend until a large bronchus is opened; through which the contents of the pleural sac will pass upwards to the trachea and so be expelled. An opening thus formed, closes only for a time. The pleura goes on secreting pus, and at the end of a few days this is again brought up as before.   So matters go on until death perhaps occurs.   In other instances too, the lung becomes carnified, and deprived for ever of its power of expanding; while the pleura continuing to secrete fluid, bands are formed between the pulmonary and costal portions which lead to future contractions of the chest. Supposing

* This discrepancy can scarcely be better illustrated, or less satisfactorily accounted for, than by the following facts.   Drs. Hughes and Addison were both physicians at the same time to Guy's Hospital.   The former (*Guy's Hospital Reports*, Second Series, vol. ii. p. 48. London, 1844) speaks in high terms of the good which he has seen effected by tapping the chest in numerous cases, and the facility with which it may be performed. The latter gentleman (*Lancet*, 17 November 1855) says he believes, from the numerous cases seen every year at Guy's Hospital, that paracentesis thoracis is one of the worst and most deceiving operations in general practice. A serous cavity, he thinks, is almost invariably changed into a cavity pouring out purulent matter by the first operation; and the thick, leather-like, false membranes lining the pleura soon make the operation one of very great difficulty and danger.   Nature herself, if assisted by proper remedies, will often remove serous effusions from the pleura; but if once interfered with by instrumental assistance, the amount of pus separated from the system is almost incredible, and beyond her power to get rid of.   Cases are mentioned of twelve and fourteen pints of purulent matter drawn from the chest, but its production is very possibly due to the first opening made in the pleura.

it is decided to resort to paracentesis, it will be as well to commence by making an exploratory puncture with a grooved needle ; when if fluid issue, a trocar and cannula may be introduced. The best position for the puncture is probably the intercostal space between the fifth and sixth true ribs, at or somewhat anterior to the digitations of the serratus magnus muscle ; provided of course, that the lung is not fixed to this part by adhesions and that no good reason exists (such as the pointing of the tumour) for selecting a different spot. It will probably be better to remove all the fluid. If serum come out, the orifice should be closed and healed : if pus escape, the aperture may be enlarged and kept open by a piece of catheter, or an india-rubber drainage tube. When this tube is employed, two openings have to be made, as recommended by Dr. Goodfellow and Mr. Campbell de Morgan. The operation is a simple one, as performed by the latter gentleman. A puncture with a trocar, or a simple incision, is to be made into the cavity of the chest at the usual place (between the fifth and sixth, or sixth and seventh ribs) or indeed in any convenient situation. A firm long iron probe, somewhat bent, is then passed through the opening, and directed towards the lower and back part of the cavity—the lower the better. If the end of the probe be pressed against the inside of the thoracic walls, it may be distinguished from the outside through the intercostal space—perhaps obscurely, owing to the thickness and toughness of the false membrane within. The lowest site in which the probe can be felt having been selected, an incision is made upon its end, which is then pushed out of the opening thus formed. A strong piece of waxed twine is passed into the eye of the probe, and drawn through the two openings ; and the drainage-tube, perforated at short intervals, being firmly tied to one end, is then pulled through by means of the twine. The ends of the tube are fastened together, and the operation is completed. The pus drains away through the perforations. The admission of air through the tube, or through the cannula of the trocar, into the pleura does no harm, for it becomes spontaneously removed in a few hours. It must be remembered that the intercostal artery has been wounded in the operation of tapping, giving rise to serious hæmothorax [Αἷμα – blood + Θώραξ = the chest] ; an accident which may be best avoided by keeping free of the borders of the ribs.

Where the dyspnœa has been very urgent in some examples of pneumothorax, it has been found necessary to puncture the pleural cavity with a grooved needle, to let the air escape. Such cases, however, are very exceptional.

XX. PNEUMONIA.

Pneumonia, or more correctly pneumonitis [from Πνεύμων – the lung + the terminal -itis], or acute inflammation of the substance of the lung, is a serious disorder, though its fatality has been diminished by our improved practice. The disease is commonly ushered in by restlessness with general febrile disturbance. At the end of from one to three days there are rigors; soon followed by nausea, cough, pain in the side, distressed breathing, a pulse reaching to 140 or even 160 beats in the minute, burning heat of skin, thirst, loss of appetite, prostration, headache, and sometimes transient delirium. Frequently, no notice is taken of the primary restlessness; so that the patient describes the succession of his symptoms as shivering, fever, cough, and breathlessness.

Each case of pneumonia may be said to consist of four degrees or stages—viz., first, that of congestion of the pulmonary membrane, with dryness; secondly, that of engorgement or splenization; thirdly, that of red hepatization; and fourthly, that of grey hepatization, or purulent infiltration. In each stage there is, speaking summarily, fever; the temperature rising towards the end of the first day to 101° or even 102°·5, and gradually increasing until the fifth or sixth day when it will probably be as high as 105° Fahr. Next we have more or less pain in some part of the chest—most severe at the commencement; together with accelerated and oppressed breathing. There is great depression, with occasionally delirium. And then we find a very distressing cough, with expectoration of viscid and rust-coloured sputa; which unite into a mass so tenacious, that even inversion of the vessel in which it lies will not detach any portion. If these sputa be minutely examined, they will be found to consist chiefly of mucus, epithelium, exudation-matter, blood cells, and oil globules; the presence of sugar may sometimes be detected by Trommer's test; while there is also an excess of chloride of sodium. Moreover, as the blood contains an undue amount of fibrin, coagula may form in the right side of the heart or in the pulmonary arteries, and give rise to urgent dyspnoea or even to sudden death.

During the *first* stage, or that of *dryness of the pulmonary membrane*, there is no crepitation to be heard, but simply a harsh dry respiratory murmur. The percussion note is natural. The skin is hot and dry; the pulse and respirations are frequent; and there may be pain over the affected side. The duration of this stage does not exceed twenty-four hours.

The *second* stage, or that of *engorgement*, is that in which the air-cells of the affected part of the lung become loaded with blood or bloody serum. The inflamed portion of lung is of a dark-red colour externally, and on cutting into it a quantity of red and frothy serum escapes; while its appearance somewhat resembles the spleen, its elasticity and sponginess being diminished, though it will still float in water. If the chest be listened to when the lung is in this condition, we shall hear very fine crepitation; a sound which is known as *minute crepitation* or *crepitant rhonchus*. If a lock of one's own hair be rubbed between the finger and thumb close to the ear, a sound will be produced nearly resembling it. The natural respiratory or vesicular murmur is still heard mingled with this minute crepitation, especially at the beginning : as the inflammation advances, however, the healthy sound is quite displaced by the morbid one. Percussion also, at first, affords almost the natural resonance : gradually this becomes decidedly obscured.

Where the inflammation proceeds, it passes into the *third* degree, or that of *hepatization ;* in which the spongy character of the lung is quite lost, and the texture becomes hard and solid—resembling the cut surface of the liver, whence it is said to be hepatized. If we now practise auscultation, neither the minute crepitation nor the vesicular murmur will be any longer perceptible. *Bronchophony,* however, often exists, more particularly if the inflammation be seated near the upper part or in the vicinity of the root of the lungs ; and it is accompanied also by *bronchial respiration,* these sounds being conducted by the solidified lung. The resonance on percussion is dull over the whole of the affected part.

Advancing still further, we now have the *fourth* stage of pneumonia, or that of *grey hepatization,* or *purulent infiltration ;* which consists of diffused suppuration of the pulmonary tissue, parts of the lung remaining dense and impermeable. In many instances there is no true suppuration, the appearance of such a condition being simulated by liquefied exudation-matter. Circumscribed abscess of the lung is very uncommon ; but diffused suppuration is said to be a frequent consequence of inflammation of the pulmonary tissue. There are no physical signs by which this stage can be diagnosed, until part of the lung breaks down and the pus is expectorated : *large gurgling crepitation* will then be heard.

If the inflammation subside before the stage of purulent infiltration, as it fortunately often does, then the febrile disturbance decreases, the temperature drops towards its normal standard, the cough becomes less irritable, and the general distress mitigates. Still the frequency of the pulse, and the hurried breathing, continue until the lung begins to lose its solidity. The hepatized condition may, however, remain permanent ; though as a rule it will gradually pass away. In the latter case we shall find the air slowly re-entering the lung ; as will be indicated by a return of the minute crepitation, mingled with—and subsequently superseded by—the healthy vesicular murmur.

When the urine of a healthy person is treated with nitrate of silver,* after being acidulated with nitric acid, the copious precipitate of chloride of silver which is thrown down shows the

---

* Nitrate of silver, added to healthy urine, throws down a whitish precipitate, which consists of chloride and phosphate of silver. A few drops of nitric acid will dissolve the phosphate, leaving the insoluble chloride. The chloride of silver is readily soluble in a little ammonia. Nearly all the chlorine contained in the urine occurs as chloride of sodium.

presence of a considerable quantity of chlorides. In pneumonia, a normal amount of the chlorides may be found for the first day or two ; but the quantity gradually diminishes as the inflammation advances, until by the time hepatization is perfect they have entirely disappeared. As the hepatization recedes, so the chlorides reappear ; continuing to increase as convalescence favourably progresses. Dr. Redtenbacher further observed that the more intense the inflammation, the greater was the diminution in the chlorides ; while the rapidity or slowness of the decrease or increase was in constant relation to the rapid or slow course of the disease.   Dr. Beale, in confirming the important views of Redtenbacher, says— " There is reason to believe that the absence of the chloride of sodium from the urine during the stage of hepatization, depends upon the determination of this salt to the inflamed lung ; and that when resolution occurs, this force of attraction ceases, and whatever salt has been retained in the lung is re-absorbed, and appears in the urine in the usual way."*   It must be remembered, however, that a deficiency of chloride of sodium, or its total absence from the urine, is not peculiar to cases of pneumonia, nor even to acute inflammations generally. According to Neubauer and Vogel, the diminution depends chiefly upon the loss of appetite, and the saltless nature of the diet of the patients; in addition to which there are occasionally abstractions of chlorine from the blood, as in diarrhœa, exudations, and pneumonic sputa.

Occasionally, in depressed constitutions, as well as where the system is contaminated by syphilis, acute inflammation of the lung terminates in *diffused* or in *circumscribed gangrene*. Sphacelation may also arise from other conditions than pneumonia ; as, for example, from tubercle, cancer, hæmorrhage, the presence of morbid poisons in the blood, and disease of the brain causing perverted innervation of the lungs. It occasionally occurs in children after the eruptive fevers, or as an accompaniment of cancrum oris. The characteristic symptoms of such an occurrence are an intolerably fetid state of the breath, resembling the odour which proceeds from external gangrenous parts ; together with dyspnœa, and very great prostration. The physical signs are those of softening and excavation of the pulmonary tissue. The disease is usually more extensive and progresses more rapidly in diffused than in circumscribed gangrene. Unless the mortified portion be small, death will in all probability result.

During old age, as well as in some forms of insanity, an attack of pneumonia now and again runs its course and even ends fatally, before its presence has been suspected. I have seen one lung in an old woman 70 years of age quite solid from hepatization, and who died as it was said suddenly. For her pulse had not been above 90 for weeks before her death, her skin had not been unduly hot, and when she was quiet there had been no dyspnœa. No exami-

* *Medico-Chirurgical Transactions,* vol. xxxv. p. 375. London, 1852.

nation had been made of the chest during life, for the simple reason that no disease had been suspected there by her medical man. Similar cases are now and then met with in lunatic asylums.

Chronic pneumonia may occur as a sequel of the acute disease; or it can be set up by the irritation of gummata in advanced forms of syphilis. However produced, it now and then gives rise to persistent consolidation of a portion of the pulmonary tissue, which may be mistaken for solidification resulting from tubercular deposit. This error is the more likely to be made, seeing that the general symptoms are partly those of phthisis; such as weakness, emaciation, cough, pallor, a sense of oppression within the chest, and loss of appetite. Slight hæmoptysis occurs very rarely; while attacks of feverishness, of night sweats, and of diarrhœa are remarkable by their absence. Iodide of potassium and bark, or iodide of iron, or ammonia and bark, with cod liver oil or glycerine, and good diet, are the remedies to be trusted to.

With regard to the *pathology* of pneumonia it seems certain that the disease essentially consists of an exudation into the air-sacs themselves. There is no interstitial inflammation, as was long taught, because there is no connective tissue between the air-cells to get inflamed. The matters poured out from the vessels in the walls of the air-sacs consist of serum, lymph, and subsequently of purulent fluid. At the same time that the cell-cavities get thus loaded, the thin fibrous structure of their walls doubtless becomes infiltrated with exudation matter.

Whether the capillaries of the pulmonary artery, or those of the bronchial arteries, or both sets, are the vessels mainly affected in pneumonia, is a question which has not been positively determined. Dr. Waters has argued, that the branches of the pulmonary artery which constitute the pulmonary plexus are the nutrient vessels of the air-cells and the seat of inflammation in pneumonia; because although the bronchial arteries pass along the bronchial tubes and supply the structures of those tubes and the connective tissue of the lungs, yet they send no branches to the walls of the air-sacs, which are solely occupied by the plexus formed by the pulmonary artery. Dr. Morehead on the contrary has reasoned that if inflammation be an altered state of the nutritive processes of the affected part, then the capillaries immediately concerned in inflammation must be those which in their normal state circulate arterial blood for nutrition: that the blood which is a factor in inflammation, must be blood which normally is a factor in nutrition. It is maintained, therefore, that capillaries of the bronchial arteries are those immediately concerned in the nutrition of the air-cells, and therefore in pneumonia; chiefly for the reason that they are the nutrient vessels of the visceral pleura, of all the tissues of the bronchial tubes, the coats of the bloodvessels, the nerves and lymphatics, and the connecting areolar tissue of the lungs, as well as the seat of inflammation in visceral pleuritis and bronchitis.

Pneumonia may affect one lung or both; or, technically speaking, it may be double or single. The right lung suffers from inflammation nearly twice as often as the left: about once in eight cases both are affected. The lower lobes are more obnoxious to inflammation than the upper. The average duration of the disease when uncomplicated is about fourteen days: when complicated, not less than twenty-one days. Mild cases, unless subjected to heroic treatment, are often fairly convalescent on the ninth day. In fatal instances death occurs between the sixth and the twentieth days. Pneumonia destroyed life in 25,155 cases in England, during the year 1866 (see p. 554); the mortality being greatest in the winter quarters. Of this number of deaths those occurring in children under 5 years of age were no less than $\frac{\text{Males } 9584}{\text{Females } 7876} = 17,460$.

Pneumonia without a degree of bronchitis is probably never seen. It may happen with or without pleurisy. Supposing the pneumonia forms the chief disease, the double affection is termed *pleuro-pneumonia*; while when the pleurisy predominates, it is sometimes called *pneumo-pleuritis*.

The *treatment* of pneumonia remains to be considered. After what has been said, however, in speaking of the remedies for inflammation, only a few remarks are called for. Bleeding, tartar emetic, and mercury, are the agents on which we have been mainly taught to rely; but these remedies will, I feel convinced, do much more harm than good if applied to the treatment of inflammation of the lungs in the present day. It is the more necessary to insist upon this point, because some of our text-books still advocate depletion; although more than twenty years have elapsed since Dr. George W. Balfour showed very strikingly the good results obtained by Skoda at Vienna, while withholding all active medication from his pneumonic cases. In recommending the adoption of a very simple line of practice, therefore, I am only doing that which both my reading and experience have long taught me is much the best, not only for the ultimate safety of the patient, but even for diminishing the duration of the disease. I am quite alive to the argument that whereas our ancestors bled too much, we may fall into the opposite error, and bleed too little. But whatever may be said upon this head, it can only be replied, that the practitioner is advised not to have recourse to antiphlogistic remedies in the treatment of pneumonia, because it is firmly believed that no amount of venesection can remove the exudation which has taken place into the air-sacs; while the more the patient is weakened the greater will be the fear of our failing to restore him to health.

When the case is first seen, attention must be paid to the bowels, a dose of castor oil being given if necessary. The most perfect quiet in bed is then to be enjoined; the air of the sick-room being kept moist by the evaporation of boiling water, while the temperature should not be allowed to fall below 65° Fahr. From two to four fluid drachms of the liquor ammoniæ acetatis, freely diluted, may be given every three or four hours according to the action of the skin, with or without a few drops of the wine of colchicum ; while small doses of opium are also to be administered, if there be pain or restlessness. The vapour of chloroform can occasionally be used to relieve the cough and dyspnœa; but I have had no experience in the treatment by full inhalations repeated every three or four hours. When the patient's constitution is feeble, a draught containing an excess of ammonia, according to F. 212, is to be ordered. At the same time, large linseed poultices or poppy-head fomentations must be directed to be properly used over the affected side ; or if the pain be bad, recourse had better be had to turpentine stupes night and morning. All that is necessary besides is a light diet with a free supply of cold water ; together with milk, strong beef tea, and tea with milk. Moderate quantities of wine or brandy, somewhat in accordance with the patient's ordinary habits, may be prescribed as soon as there are any indications of greater weakness than can safely be borne. Where the crisis occurs by sweating or by diarrhœa, care must be taken not to check it unnecessarily; while during convalescence milk and cream, raw eggs, animal food, and wine may be allowed with discretion. Few tonics will then be more useful than ammonia and bark (F. 371); followed subsequently by quinine and steel (F. 380), with perhaps cod liver oil.

In some very severe cases the only question is how to keep the patient alive, until the exudation-matter occupying the air-cells becomes absorbed. Under these circumstances brandy is invaluable; but it must be freely administered,—possibly even to the extent of half an ounce every second hour, in milk or water or beef tea, for one or two days. The brandy and egg mixture (F. 17) does good. The essence of beef (F. 3) will also prove useful.

Should the inflammation end in *gangrene*, stimulants and tonics are then especially needed. When the odour of the breath is very offensive, the solution of chlorinated soda (F. 76) may be prescribed. Ammonia and bark, or chlorate of potash and steel, with cod liver oil, are valuable remedies. The inhalation of spray medicated with creasote or carbolic acid (F. 262), every eight or twelve hours, can be strongly advised. Dr. Skoda, of Vienna, has published several cases in which the symptoms gave way on the use of terebinthinate vapours and the free exhibition of quinine. The inhalations he used were made by pouring oil of turpentine on boiling water; the vapour being inspired for about fifteen minutes every two or three hours. Wine and nourishment in as large quantities as can be assimilated by the weakened digestive organs, will be required.

XXI. PHTHISIS.

The name of Phthisis [from $\Phi\theta\text{\'iω}$ = to waste away] has usually been regarded, until very recently, as synonymous with tubercular

disease of the lungs.   The time, however, seems now to have
arrived when it may advantageously be allowed that several diverse
affections, radically distinct from each other, should be included
under the common designation of phthisis, or pulmonary consumption.   Instead therefore of restricting these expressions to indicate
that morbid condition which arises from the deposit of tubercles in
the lungs, they ought to be employed as generic terms for those
pulmonary diseases which are characterized at first by progressive
condensation, and subsequently by suppurative degeneration with
excavation, of the affected portions of lung tissue; these local
changes being in some instances preceded, in others only followed,
by constitutional disease.

What then are the diseases which lead to ulceration and destruction of the lung tissue,—in other words, what are the varieties
of phthisis? Arranged in the inverse order of their importance, we
are at present justified in recognising the following :—

(1) *Hæmorrhagic* and *embolic* phthisis; in which there is cheesy
disorganization and disintegration of blood-clots (after pulmonary
extravasation), or of deposits produced by pulmonary emboli from
the liver or veins, as well as of those portions of lung tissue affected by the foreign matter.

(2) *Bronchial* and *pneumonic* phthisis; attended with ulceration
of the bronchi and air-sacs, as well as with cheesy degeneration
and disintegration of any bronchial or pneumonic exudations or
deposits which have occurred.   This variety should include those
cases hitherto described as forms of mechanical bronchitis; in
which the morbid action is set up by the inhalation of different
particles of matter that irritate the tubes and their terminal extremities—the air-sacs.   We have thus the so-called grinders' asthma,
or knife-grinders' rot; carbonaceous bronchitis, or black phthisis,
or miners' asthma, occurring in miners from the inhalation of the
lamp-smoke, and the inspiration of the carbonic acid gas formed
in the pits; millstone makers' phthisis observed in stonemasons
and others; and cotton pneumonia, or cotton phthisis, met with
amongst the operatives in cotton-mills.

(3) *Syphilitic* phthisis; being that condition in which there is
deposition or infiltration of gummatous matter through more or
less of the substance of the lungs, with subsequent cheesy degeneration.   It has already been shown that a chronic erythematous
inflammation of the mucous lining of the bronchi may occur as a
part of the constitutional lesions of syphilis.   But in the class of
cases now referred to, gummatous nodules are produced in the pulmonary substance; these deposits being at first very hard, though
subsequently undergoing a process of softening and decay.   Not
unfrequently this disease becomes associated with tuberculosis ;
so that in a case of phthisis, attended with nodes on the tibia and
other marks of syphilis, the conclusion must not be too readily
jumped at that a cure is to be effected by iodide of potassium and

such-like remedies. When small syphilomata exist alone, however, even though they have softened and produced little vomicæ,
attempts at cure can be hopefully made. That well-directed efforts
have been attended with success cannot be doubted, because the
cicatrices of healed cavities have been found after death has happened from other causes.

(4) *Fibroid* phthisis (described by some authors as cirrhosis of
the lung, interstitial pneumonia &c.) is usually that state in which
systemic disorder localizes itself, more or less completely, in one or
both lungs in the form of a fibroid exudation. Occasionally, perhaps, the disease is local,—confined to the lung. When of constitutional origin, the general affection may be due to rheumatism or
gout, syphilis, an unhealthy mode of life, abuse of alcoholic drinks
&c. Sometimes also, in addition to the pulmonary mischief, there is
a similar degeneration of the endocardium, liver, kidneys, capsule of
spleen, and other organs. The leading features of the lung mischief
are very characteristic ; this organ being found heavy and tough,
indurated and contracted, either by fibroid tissue or by a fibrogenous material involving dilated bronchi. Moreover, portions
but especially the inferior lobes, are invaded by cheesy deposits
and small cavities. The tough fibrogenous exudation is either
identical with amyloid substance, or nearly related to it. The pleura
is occasionally much thickened, having fibrous bands passing from
it into the lung tissue. The left lung is more frequently invaded
than the right ; but both will be involved more often than one.
The bronchial glands may be enlarged and indurated. Usually, the
disease progresses slowly. At times these cases are complicated
with tuberculosis ; a complication which appears to lengthen life
by delaying the disintegration of the tubercles. Death occurs from
exhaustion, or from some intercurrent attack of pleurisy or bronchitis or pneumonia, or even from hæmoptysis.

Perhaps the most instructive case of fibroid phthisis on record
is that reported by Dr. Andrew Clark.* The patient was the
subject of constitutional fibroid degeneration (fibrosis) ; which,
while affecting different textures, especially and destructively
localized itself in the left lung. The mischief in the latter appeared to commence about July 1867. The prominent symptoms
and signs were vomiting, prostration, paroxysmal cough, occasional
hæmoptysis, muco-purulent expectoration containing lung tissue,
œdema of the extremities, albuminuria, and intermitting diarrhœa.
The left chest-wall was unevenly depressed, and moved but slightly
on inspiration. Percussion tympanitic in supra-clavicular region :
breath sounds blowing ; resonance bronchophonic with echo.
From the second to the fifth rib, and from near the sternum

* *Transactions of the Clinical Society of London*, vol. i., p. 174. London,
1868. The student will also find an excellent essay on "Fibroid Degeneration
of the Lungs," by Dr. Henry G. Sutton, in the *Medico-Chirurgical Transactions*, vol. xlviii. p. 287. London, 1865.

to the posterior part of the axillary region, there was hard resistant dulness, with considerable contraction of the chest-wall.   In front of this region the inspiration was bronchial, and accompanied by moist subcrepitant râles ; expiration being dry, and not sensibly prolonged.   At two spots about the middle of the axillary region the breathing was cavernous and the voice pectoriloquous.   The inspiratory murmur over the lower part of the lung was harsh : fine dry crepitation was heard on forced inspiration.   While in the London Hospital, the condition varied but little.   Sometimes there was obstinate vomiting ; sometimes constipation, alternating with diarrhœa.   No evening fever : no night sweats.   Pulse never rose above 92, respiration above 26, temperature above 99 ; while until near the close of life the figures were considerably lower. Upon great restlessness followed increasing weakness ; then coma ; and on the 3rd December, death.   The necroscopy revealed, as had been predicted during life, fibroid disease of left lung, with dilated bronchi, cheesy deposits, and cavities arising from their disintegration ; enlargement (and waxy degeneration) of liver ; granular contraction (and some waxy change) of kidneys ; ulceration of the bowels ; enlargement of mesenteric glands ; and fibroid degeneration of, or deposit in, other organs and tissues.

(5) *Tubercular* phthisis, or pulmonary tuberculosis, is a destructive disease, attended by the growth and degeneration and disintegration of a lowly organized material called tubercle ; which material is the local manifestation of that general unhealthy condition of the system known as scrofula.   This, by far the most prevalent form of phthisis, is of such importance that it will be better to consider it in a separate section.

XXII. TUBERCULAR PHTHISIS.

Tubercular phthisis, or pulmonary tuberculosis, is a constitutional disease manifesting itself especially by certain very important and destructive changes in the lungs.   The morbid action may run an acute or chronic course.

The *acute* form is not often observed.   It commences suddenly with shivering, fever, rapid pulse, pain, cough, and dyspnœa ; soon there is hectic fever, with profuse sweating and diarrhœa ; there is rapid degeneration of the lung substance, so that small cavities form speedily ; the increasing emaciation becomes daily more perceptible ; and death may happen from exhaustion within as few a number of weeks as from three to twelve from the commencement of the disease.   Generally the tubercular deposit is spread all through the lungs ; while instead of being at first deposited in the upper lobes, it often begins in the middle and lower ones.   Acute pulmonary consumption now and then occurs as the sole morbid state. It may, however, set in during the progress of chronic phthisis ; or it occasionally proves the termination of some chronic malady, as was the case in a lady long under my care with pelvic abscess.

Chronic phthisis is that variety which is ordinarily met with; the symptoms, diagnosis, &c., of which will be presently detailed.

Pathology.—The origin and formation of tubercle have already been considered in the section on Scrofula with Tubercle (p. 144). It is only necessary to mention, therefore, that in phthisis the development of tubercle takes place in the interlobular connective tissue, in the air-cells themselves, and in the smaller bronchial tubes communicating with them; and that wherever a speck of this matter is formed, whether it be an exudation or a retrograde metamorphosis of pre-existing structures, it continues to increase by constant addition. In its hard state it is called crude tubercle. After a time, inflammation arises in the pulmonary substance surrounding the deposit, and suppuration occurs; the tubercular matter softening and breaking down, and at length being gradually expelled through the bronchi and trachea and mouth. Thus are left cavities or excavations of various sizes. Sometimes the cavities close and heal : more frequently tubercular matter continues to be deposited on their sides and in other parts of the lungs, until these organs become diseased to an extent incompatible with the continuance of life.

A more or less abundant deposit of tubercle is, at times, to be found in other organs as well as in the lungs. Thus, in many cases of pulmonary consumption, this material may be detected in the tissues of the intestinal canal, mesenteric glands, kidneys, peri-toneum, liver, spleen, bronchial glands, heart and pericardium, or of the nervous centres. Moreover, fatty degeneration of the liver is a frequent accompaniment of phthisis; while less commonly the muscular fibres of the heart, and the middle coat of the aorta or other vessels, are found in a similar state of deterioration.

Symptoms.—The general symptoms of tubercular phthisis are gradually increasing cough, hæmoptysis, debility, expectoration, loss of appetite and a dislike to fatty food, dyspepsia in some form or other, acceleration of the pulse, pyrexia, slight dyspnœa, loss of flesh, sweating, and diarrhœa. Weakness of the voice or hoarseness is not uncommon. A mark at the reflected edge of the gums, usually deeper in colour than the adjoining surface, and producing a festooned appearance by the accuracy with which it corresponds to the curve of the gingival border, was first observed by Dr. Theophilus Thompson to be very frequently present in these cases. A dull aching pain under the clavicles or scapulæ is often complained of, even when the amount of tubercle is small. Variously seated muscular pains are common; especially after any exertion which may be excessive in relation to the patient's powers. Sometimes, especially in males, the formation of an abscess by the side of the rectum, resulting in a fistula in ano, is one of the earliest symptoms; a complication which, when left alone, becomes highly injurious by lowering the general strength.

Pulmonary tuberculosis ordinarily sets in with a short dry cough, which the patient often refers to the trachea. It is doubtless due to tubercular deposit irritating the bronchial membrane; it may continue some time without being aggravated, or without the supervention of any other symptom; and each paroxysm is followed by the expulsion of a little thick semi-purulent expectoration. With other cases, the cough is loose, hollow, and less severe; being succeeded by a copious frothy phlegm, derived from the congested mucous membrane of the bronchi.

In about 50 per cent. of the cases, there is hæmoptysis; which, recurring at variable intervals, gives the patient the first unmistakeable intimation of the disease. It occurs much more frequently in the first, than in the second or third stages. The hæmorrhage varies in amount from one or two drachms to the same number of pints. It may indeed be so considerable as to kill directly or indirectly. Dr. Walshe states that his analysed series of 131 cases of phthisis furnishes but two examples of such mode of death. In one, death was direct from asphyxia, owing to the plugging of the trachea and bronchi with blood; in the other, it occurred from exhaustion at the end of five days.* Now and then the rupture of an aneurism of the pulmonary artery has been the source of the hæmorrhage. In a case which was under the care of Dr. Cotton at the Hospital for Consumption, and in which large quantities of blood were occasionally spat up for ten weeks before death, there was found in the left lung a tubercular cavity the size of a Tangierine orange, which was partially filled with the collapsed sac of an aneurism. This aneurism arose from one of the primary divisions of the left branch of the pulmonary artery; and prior to rupture must have been large enough to fill the vomica.

Among other symptoms the patient complains also of languor; slight exertion—ascending a hill or going upstairs—causes fatigue, hurries the breathing, and often gives rise to palpitation; the uterine functions are more or less disturbed in women; and the liver often becomes congested and tender. The tongue gets red and irritable; and aphthæ frequently form about the mouth and fauces. The mucous membranes of the bronchi, larynx, and pharynx are also very apt to become affected with a low form of inflammation; while occasionally tubercle is deposited in the sub-mucous tissue of these organs, leading to ulceration and even extensive destruction. The latter is, I believe, most likely to occur when the fauces are relaxed and the uvula elongated; since the constant cough and irritation then set up prevent all attempt at reparation. Sometimes, where the perspiration is abundant, the patient and friends are much annoyed by the ill-smelling feet of the former; a condition, however, which can be cured by soaking the feet in tepid salt-water night and morning, dusting them freely with powdered

* *On Diseases of the Lungs, Heart, and Aorta.* Second Edition, p. 505. London, 1854.

charcoal, and by wearing shoes with thin upper leathers and well open about the instep so as not to confine the transpiration. It is also remarkable that in some cases the nails become incurvated, while the ends of the fingers get a peculiar round or clubbed appearance. The latter is referred by M. Labalbary to the imperfectly arterialized state of the blood, and to venous stasis in parts furthest removed from the centre of the circulation; in consequence of which stagnation, tubercular matter is deposited from the blood. In cyanosis, the digital extremities sometimes assume the same character.

While the disease has been gradually progressing, the cough and expectoration have been increasing considerably. " The microscopical elements of phthisical sputa"—says Dr. Walshe—"are very numerous. First epithelium tesselated, cylindrical, and ciliated from the bronchial tubes; salivary fluid, and epithelium from the mouth. Secondly, blood-disks (even when no reddish tint exists to the naked eye), melanic cells and molecules, molecular fat, oil globules, and saline matter, crystalline and amorphous. Thirdly, exudation-matter in patches, exudation-cells, and pus-cells. Fourthly, fragments of pulmonary fibre, capillary vessel and nerve. Fifthly, dark molecular matter, soluble neither in ether nor in hydrochloric acid, and probably tuberculous,—and, in very rare cases, cells possessing the characters originally assigned by M. Lebert to those of tubercle : I have—at least occasionally— seen, in the opaque buff-coloured striæ of comparatively clear sputa, cells non-nucleated and more angular in outline than those of exudation-matter. Sixthly, the vibrio lineolar, and mycodermatous entophytes. Now the presence of fragments of tissue indicates breakage of the lung-substance, and may furnish its earliest evidence. The existence of tubercle-cells, if certain, is, of course, distinctive of phthisical disease. Otherwise, the characters enumerated have no precise diagnostic signification."* The plan hitherto adopted for finding pulmonary tissue has been to pick out from the sputum any portions which appear to be likely to contain elastic fibre. Dr. Fenwick advises, however, that the expectoration should be liquefied by boiling it with a solution of pure soda, and then placing the fluid in a conical-shaped glass; upon doing which every particle of elastic tissue falls to the bottom and can be removed and placed under the microscope, as is done in the examination of urinary deposits. In this way he has easily found $\frac{1}{100}$th part of a grain of pulmonary structure after it had been mixed in bronchial mucus; and he calculates that $\frac{1}{10000}$th to $\frac{1}{50000}$th part of a grain might be detected in any expectoration containing it.

As time goes on, the mischief proceeds. Hectic fever appears. There is a loss of all appetite, with thirst. The emaciation can be almost seen to advance daily. The hair gets thinned, and quantities fall off on brushing it. The debility quickly gets more marked; the

* *On the Diseases of the Lungs.* Third Edition, p. 447. London, 1860.

countenance becomes frequently flushed; and chilliness is complained of in the evening, while on awaking in the night or early morning the body is found bathed in a profuse sweat.   Moreover, in women, there is a total cessation of the catamenia ; a very discouraging indication of want of vital power.   The patient still continues to lose flesh ; until he looks as if nothing remained but skin and bone. An unmanageable diarrhœa (which is due either to disordered secretions, or to ulcerations of the mucous membrane of the ileum and colon) often sets in and greatly increases the debility ; while the urine is sometimes found to contain albumen, and occasionally minute quantities of sugar.   The lower limbs become painful and œdematous.   The cough and abundant sputa continue ; so that the sufferer is often unable to sleep for more than a few minutes at a time, owing to the necessity for expectorating.   Then the desire for a frequent change of position, the cramps in the legs, the attacks of pain about the loins, the difficulty of micturition, the utter prostration, and the ever present dyspnœa,—all these troubles tend to render the last few nights most distressing both to the patient and attendant relatives.   Death is looked forward to as the only available relief for the great misery ; and at this pass the sleep from which there is no awaking soon ends the scene, the mental faculties remaining clear until the last few hours.

In some cases perforation of the lung happens towards the close, and then the resulting pneumothorax greatly adds to the sufferings. As Dr. Scott Alison points out, perforation is a natural consequence of progressive excavation ; and were it not for the pleural adhesions, its occurrence would be almost unavoidable. This condition is readily recognised by the urgent dyspnœa which follows the formation of the aperture ; by the tympanitic percussion-note; and by the occurrence (not constantly) of amphoric respiration, and metallic tinkling.

During the progress of phthisis, as well as after its cure, the patient is liable to suffer from other diseases due to degeneration of tissue.   The kidneys are more frequently affected than other organs ; the morbid action consisting of fatty degeneration of the tubules.   Thus is produced that albuminous condition of urine which has just been said to be by no means uncommon.

Diagnosis.—The attempt has been made by Dr. E. Smith to show that before the deposition of tubercle in the lungs, there is an abnormal physical condition of these organs and of the body generally, which manifests itself by certain indications.   The physical signs of this so-called *pretubercular state* are very slight subclavicular dulness, diminished vesicular murmur, less forcible and deep inspiration, and flattening of the apices of the lungs.   If there are also symptoms of dyspepsia present, and certainly if there be likewise loss of weight, it seems to me that the evidence is in favour of tubercle having been actually deposited, rather than that it is only about to invade the lungs.

Many authors have divided the course of phthisis into three

stages; a plan which is convenient, to say the least. During the *first*—that in which tubercles become developed in the lungs— neither the local nor the general symptoms warrant us in positively announcing the presence of any other affection than severe catarrh. Directly there is any solidification, however, the respiratory sound during expiration becomes prolonged; an easily recognised sign of the earliest effect of tuberculisation, which was first taught by Dr. Jackson of Philadelphia. When the tubercles are deposited in considerable quantity, the infra- and supra-clavicular regions will be found flattened; while there can likewise be observed defective expansion of the upper and front part of the affected side of the chest. The sound on percussion will be dull; or it may be morbidly resonant if the deposit extend from the costal surface directly to the trachea or large bronchi. There will be harsh or tubular inspiration; the act of expiration will be prolonged, owing to impairment of the elasticity of the lungs; and *bronchial respiration* and *bronchophony* can be heard. A distinct bruit, synchronous with the systole of the heart, may sometimes be detected under one or both clavicles. Speaking from my own experience, I should say that this *subclavian murmur* was more frequently present on the left than on the right side. It may proceed from the left subclavian, the innominata, or from the pulmonary artery; and it is due to pressure exerted on the vessel from behind. Hence it is not distinctive of tubercular deposit in a crude state; though in practice it will be found that this is by far the most frequent cause, inasmuch as solidification of the lung's apex except from tubercle is rare.—In the *second* stage, the tubercles have increased both in number and size, so as to compress and obstruct the substance of the lung, and occasion dyspnœa; while they have also begun to soften and disintegrate. There is now marked depression of the infra- and supra-clavicular regions; the affected side is often contracted, owing to the destruction of the vesicular tissue by the pressure of the morbid material; there is a deficiency of movement; and there is a stooping rounded back. The dulness on percussion is usually decided; though the note elicited may be normal, if the amount of tubercle be small and well surrounded by slightly emphysematous lung. On practising auscultation, *large crepitation* (*liquid* or *mucous râle*) will be distinct, and in the sound lung *puerile breathing*.—In the *third* stage, the softened tubercles are eliminated: they make an opening for themselves through some of the surrounding or involved bronchi, and getting thus evacuated, they give rise to the formation of cavities. On inspection we observe a well-marked depression below the clavicle; the whole side is flattened and generally contracted; the intercostal spaces are much retracted; and the heart's impulse may be distinctly seen and felt to be most intense at a higher point than the normal one. Notwithstanding the existence of one large or of numerous small cavities, percussion almost invariably affords a dull sound; dulness existing even if the cavity (unless of great size) be empty, owing to the layer of lung forming the wall being dense and solid.   Auscultation now elicits a peculiar sound called *gurgling*, caused by the bubbling of air with the pus or mucus contained in the cavity.   Gurgling, it must be remembered, may also arise from that rare disease circum-scribed abscess of the lung, as well as from the mixture of air with liquid in a dilated bronchus affected with chronic inflammation. When the cavity contains little or no liquid, we hear *cavernous respiration ;* if it be large, *amphoric resonance* and *pectoriloquy* will also be distinguishable.

The *spirometer* is an instrument for measuring the volume of air expired from the lungs ; and as this volume is always diminished in each stage of phthisis we have a rough kind of aid to diagnosis, for which we are indebted to Dr. Hutchinson.   The quantity of air expired after the most complete inspiration is termed by this gentleman the *vital volume* or the *vital capacity.*   Now the vital capacity always increases with stature : it will also be slightly affected by weight, but not sufficiently, as a rule, to interfere with the correctness of the following table, which is intended to show the capacity in health and in the three stages of phthisis.   When the vital capacity is to be tested, the patient should loosen his vest, stand perfectly erect, take as deep an inspiration as possible, and then place the mouth-piece of the spirometer between his lips.   The observer having opened the tap, the patient empties his lungs, making the deepest possible expiration ; at the termi-nation of which the operator turns off the tap, thus confining the air in the receiver.   The receiver is then to be lightly depressed until the surfaces of the spirit in a bent tube on the outside of the instrument are on a level with each other, when the vital capacity may be read off from the scale.

Height.				Capacity in Health.	Capacity in Phthisis Pulmonalis.		
					1st Stage.	2nd Stage.	3rd Stage.
Ft. in.		Ft.	in.	Cub. in.	Cub. in.	Cub. in.	Cub. in.
5	0 to	5	1	174	117	99	82
5	1 ,,	5	2	182	122	102	86
5	2 ,,	5	3	190	127	108	89
5	3 ,,	5	4	198	133	113	93
5	4 ,,	5	5	206	138	117	97
5	5 ,,	5	6	214	143	122	100
5	6 ,,	5	7	222	149	127	104
5	7 ,,	5	8	230	154	131	108
5	8 ,,	5	9	238	159	136	112
5	9 ,,	5	10	246	165	140	116
5	10 ,,	5	11	254	170	145	119
5	11 ,,	6	0	262	176	149	123

This table reads thus :—A man whose height is between 5 ft. 7 in. and 5 ft. 8 in. should breathe in health 230 cubic inches : in the first stage of consumption this will be reduced to 154 ; in the second, to 131 ; and in the third, to 108 cubic inches.   It must not be forgotten that the vital capacity is temporarily decreased by great fatigue, want of sleep or food, an attack of fever or any lowering illness,—in short by whatever diminishes the power of the muscles of respiration. As these are all obvious causes of lessened force, so they need not make the practitioner attach less importance to the indications afforded by the spirometer in phthisis. They only show that certain precautions are necessary in drawing conclusions from the data obtained.

Another very early, and therefore highly important, sign of pulmonary consumption is *loss of weight*. A slow and gradual fall is more serious than a rapid and irregular diminution in weight; *a steady loss always precedes tuberculosis*. Dr. Hutchinson, from an examination of 2650 healthy men at the middle period of life, has deduced the following table :—

Exact Stature.		Mean Weight.		Weight increased by 7 per Cent.	
Ft.	in.	St. lbs.	lbs.	St. lbs.	lbs.
5	1	8 8 or	120	9 2 or	128
5	2	9 0 „	126	9 9 „	135
5	3	9 7 „	133	10 2 „	142
5	4	9 13 „	139	10 9 „	149
5	5	10 2 „	142	10 12 „	152
5	6	10 5 „	145	11 1 „	155
5	7	10 8 „	148	11 4 „	158
5	8	11 1 „	155	11 12 „	160
5	9	11 8 „	162	12 5 „	173
5	10	12 1 „	169	12 13 „	181
5	11	12 6 „	174	13 4 „	186
6	0	12 10 „	178	13 8 „	190

This reads :—A man of 5 ft. 8 in. should weigh, in his clothes, 11 st. 1 lb. or 155 lb. (14 lb. = 1 stone). He may exceed this by 7 per cent., and so attain 11 st. 12 lbs., or 166 lb., without affecting his vital capacity; though beyond this amount his respiration becomes diminished. According to M. Quetelet the average weight of the clothes at different ages is one-eighteenth of the total weight of the body, and one-twenty-fourth of that of the female.

In Dr. Robert Boyd's article on *Vital Statistics and Pathological Contributions*[*] it is mentioned that the mean height of 141 adult male paupers, measured by Dr. Hutchinson in the Marylebone workhouse, was a little more than 5 ft. 3 in. and their mean weight 134 lbs. The mean height of the male consumptive patients has been nearly 4 inches more, and their weight nearly one-third less. Hence it would appear that tall persons are most subject to consumption. Moreover, the immense loss of weight is in the muscular structure, the several tissues, and the framework; since Dr. Boyd shows that the internal organs were all heavier than the healthy standard.

Causes, &c.—Tubercular phthisis may be inherited or it may be acquired; but in no sense of the word can it be said to be contagious. Of 1000 histories collected by Dr. Cotton, at the Consumption Hospital, 367 cases were hereditarily predisposed;

* *The Edinburgh Medical and Surgical Journal*, vol. lxi. p. 290. 1844.

582 being males, and 418 females.   Until about the year 1790 it was generally believed that phthisis was contagious.   We find the earliest traces of this doctrine in the writings of Aristotle, who flourished B.C. 340.   Galen, who was born about the year A.D. 130, seems to have adopted the same view ; since he says that it is dangerous to pass the whole day with the consumptive. Lommius, about 1563, thought that the sputa were contagious. Dr. Richard Morton, regarded as an authority on this disease at the commencement of the seventeenth century, asserts that consumption may be communicated to a bedfellow like a malignant fever. Hoffmann, towards the close of the seventeenth century, taught that a natural predisposition to consumption might be called into action by attendance on a sufferer from consumption.   Morgagni, writing in 1760, accounts for his having made but few dissections of this disease by expressing his fears of its infectious nature ; while Portal, a few years later, hesitated to attend the autopsies of persons who had died from consumption.   Cullen, in 1777, had never seen a case in which phthisis had been communicated from one person to another ; though he would not assert that it is never contagious, especially in warm countries.   This opinion seems to have paved the way for the modified view that there is only contagion in extreme cases ; or, as Darwin said in 1793, between persons nearly connected.   And so the idea of infection seems gradually to have died out ; though Heberden in 1802 could not be convinced one way or the other.   In 1808 Portal's fears as to the dissection of examples of fatal phthisis had vanished ; and henceforth the idea of contagion was decidedly negatived.   Nevertheless, during the last ten years some few authors, while declaring against contagion, have maintained that a close and devoted attendance upon one affected with phthisis has appeared to be accompanied with danger ; while certain strong believers in non-contagion as a rule, have yet thought the disease might be transmitted by sexual intercourse or other intimate relations with an affected person.

The left lung suffers more frequently than the right : in Dr. Cotton's cases the left lung was affected in 455, the right in 384, and both were diseased in 161.   The apices and posterior parts of the upper lobes of the lungs are ordinarily the situations in which the deposit first takes place.   In some few instances, probably not more than one or two per cent., the development of tubercles begins at the base of the lung ; the deposit gradually extending upwards.   As these cases at the onset are apt to manifest the physical signs of pneumonia, especially persistent minute crepitation best heard about the angle of the scapula, and as there is steadily increasing dyspnœa with more or less fever, they have not unfrequently been erroneously treated.   To avoid this mistake it is only necessary to observe that the general symptoms are not those of inflammation, but of the very opposite character— of steadily increasing depression.

No period of life is exempt from this scourge. I have already shown that in the year 1866, considerably more than one-seventh of the whole number of deaths in England were due to scrofulous affections in some form or other; 55,714 of these, out of a total of 72,425, being registered as cases of phthisis. Insufficient and bad food, impure air, confinement, deficiency of light, long-continued grief, immoderate indulgence of the sensual passions, the poison of syphilis, and indeed whatever produces nervous exhaustion or impoverished blood, may be regarded as frequent causes. Its ordinary duration varies from about six to twenty-four months : it very rarely proves fatal in less than three months, unless indirectly from severe pneumonia or pleurisy.

Treatment.—This resolves itself into that necessary for the prevention of tubercular phthisis, and that to be adopted to stay its course when it has once developed itself. As regards prevention, I need only refer to the observations which have been made in the remarks on scrofula.

When the disease is present—when tubercles have become developed in the lungs, we must endeavour to *improve the general nutrition,* by attention to the quantity and quality of the food, by enjoining residence in a healthy climate (not necessarily a warm one), by ordering exercise in the open air, by taking care that the patient never sits or sleeps in a vitiated atmosphere, by advising warm clothing, by recommending daily tepid sponging with friction of the skin, and by the administration of cod liver oil. The patient's system should in no instance be lowered ; and even during those temporary exacerbations of fever which occur in the progress of every case, it will only be necessary to substitute salines and diuretics in the place of tonics, for a day or two, to speedily give relief. The irritation and weakness produced by fistula in ano are much more injurious than the simple operation of laying open the sinus with division of the sphincter, while the patient is under the influence of chloroform ; and consequently the old-fashioned rule of not interfering in these cases should be disregarded, especially if the lung disease be comparatively slight. On the same principle I have not hesitated to remove uterine polypi : while in one instance I even operated (23 March 1861) on a case of vesico-vaginal fistula, where the lungs contained tubercle ; the cure of the opening which resulted not only having been the means of relieving the sufferer from constant distress, but in all probability also of prolonging her life, for death did not take place until the 18th of June 1862.

As regards the *diet* in phthisis, only the most nutritious food ought to be allowed ; an animal diet being absolutely necessary, so long as the powers of the stomach and alimentary canal are sufficiently strong to digest and assimilate it. When the strength of the digestive organs fails, and when there is acidity of stomach, pepsine (F. 420) with the two principal daily meals should be ordered. Milk and cream are very nutritious, and so are raw eggs (F. 5, 15, 16). A mixture of cream and cherry brandy will perhaps be relished for a time. The addition of a teaspoonful of the saccharated solution of lime to a tumblerful of milk will often allow this fluid to pass uncoagulated into the duodenum, when it would not otherwise do so. A small allowance of brandy, or a moderate quantity of wine, or of good bitter ale, or of Scotch ale, or of Guinness's stout, may always be advantageously permitted. Too long an interval should not elapse between each meal; it being much better to take food rather frequently, instead of making one or two heavy meals in the day.

Change of air is an important element in the treatment. Speaking generally, phthisical patients require an elevated site upon a dry and porous soil. They should avoid all places that lie low. One special object in making a selection is to get a locality where daily exercise may be taken throughout the winter. If this can be obtained in the midst of beautiful scenery, so much the better. As a rule it must be recollected, however, that this change is to be resorted to only in the early stages and in chronic cases; for it is cruel to send patients away merely that they may die in a strange country. When softening of the tubercles has begun, it will generally be too late to expect much benefit; and certainly nought but mischief can ensue from depriving a sufferer of the comforts of home when extensive cavities are formed. Phthisical subjects sometimes imagine that change of climate is *the* remedy, instead of being only *one* of the steps which favour the accomplishment of a cure. Consequently such persons on leaving home should be cautioned to act with prudence; to avoid high living and over excitement; to take open-air exercise in moderation, and not to walk up high hills exposed to the sun's glare; to attend to the skin, and the proper action of the bowels; to wear flannel next the body, and to be provided with proper clothing so as to guard against sudden changes of temperature; and to keep regular and early hours, always being indoors between sun-set and sun-rise. Moreover, they are not to give up the use of such drugs as steel, cod liver oil, bark, &c., if these have been found beneficial at home.—The chief circumstances which render it advisable for a patient to return home, are—the persistence of diarrhœa or dysentery, increased debility, serious disturbance of the functions of the liver, or any symptoms of a disposition to ague. In women, change of climate often disorders the uterine functions; in which case it is especially necessary that any tendency to menorrhagia be checked, since it will otherwise form a serious complication. Even a leucorrhœal discharge is very weakening; and therefore attempts ought to be made to stop it by astringent injections.

Torquay (F. 436), the *Undercliff of the Isle of Wight* (F. 434), *Sandgate* (F. 431), *Hastings* (F. 432), and *Penzance* (F. 436), are places in our own country admirably adapted for the winter residence of those consumptive invalids who need a relaxing or sedative atmosphere. But if a more bracing air be suitable we may recommend *Brighton* (F. 432), *Southport* (F. 438), *Queenstown* (F. 440), or *the Western Coast of Scotland* (F. 441). Frequently a more complete change of climate is wished for by the patient, who longs for a clear atmosphere and a cloudless sky. We may then send him to *Mentone* (F. 443), *Cannes* (F. 443), *Ajaccio* (F. 444), *Malta* (F. 449), *Malaga* (F. 445), or to *Algiers* (F. 451). The mild and equable temperature of *Madeira* (F. 452) renders it a fitting residence for patients whose pulmonary disorder is aggravated by an irritable condition of the mucous membrane of the larynx and bronchi; while it is also useful for invalids threatened with consumption. The colony of *Natal* (F. 453) is particularly healthy, and is certainly deserving of trial. There are many phthisical invalids who are always worse in warm than in cold weather; and for such *St. Moritz* (F. 500), in the Engadine (a valley of Switzerland lying between two principal chains of the Rhætian Alps), might offer a good residence. During the winter of 1867-68, a few consumptives had the courage to remain at Samaden (a village in the same valley as St. Moritz, from which it is distant about four miles); and I believe they all derived much benefit from the stimulating and bracing air. The climate of *Canada* (F. 454) is salubrious; the great cold of the winter being mitigated by the dryness of the atmosphere and the absence of high winds. And, lastly, where a sea voyage is indicated I have found no change sc beneficial as a trip to *Australia* or *New Zealand* (F. 574), in a well-appointed vessel. While these recommendations were being first written (August 1864) I received a letter from a gentleman who reached New Plymouth on the 24 March 1864 in tolerable health. At the end of the summer of 1863, it had been necessary to remove him from Hastings in an invalid carriage; so shattered by a prolonged attack of hæmoptysis, that he could scarcely turn himself in bed. Had he remained in England during the inclement winter of 1863-64, I believe he would have died before its close. Yet he improved directly he got to sea by the end of November; and was able to be on deck for some hours every day during the voyage, suffering no inconvenience whatever until the provisions began to run short, and diarrhœa returned to a slight extent.

Since this case occurred I have known of other instances where great good has occurred from a similar voyage. Even the anticipation of the change from a dreary sick-room buoys up hope, and seems to renovate the system. And though a passage of some eighty days appears long, yet I have found patients wonderfully like Mr. Micawber; who, as he was about to go from London to Canterbury talked as if he were proceeding to the farthest limits of the earth, and when he went from England to Australia spoke as if he were taking a little trip across the Channel. As our old friend said,—" It's merely crossing. The distance is quite imaginary."

With respect to *drugs*, there are certain agents which must be especially mentioned. *Cod liver oil* (F. 389) is a most valuable remedy : it nourishes the body ; diminishes the cough, expectoration, sense of exhaustion, and night-sweats ; and, there is every reason to believe, checks the exudation of tubercular matter. In the beginning, a teaspoonful should be given twice or thrice daily, and gradually increased to a tablespoonful three or four times a day; remembering that it will be more easily digested if taken directly after the meals. If there be much acidity of stomach, the oil may be made into an emulsion with *lime water ;* or if it produce nausea and heartburn, then four or five grains of *pig's pepsine* in a pill can be given with each dose.   Dr. Horace Dobell has advised the use of *pancreatine*— the active principle of the pancreas—for aiding the digestion of all oleaginous and fatty substances, whether they be taken as food or medicine.   The dose is from six to eight grains, in water or ginger wine, taken directly after a meal.   I confess, however, that pancreatine has not appeared of as much service in my hands, as was anticipated from the eulogistic reports of others.   When there is great rapidity of the pulse, the ozonized oil, as recommended by Dr. Symes Thompson and his father, is deserving of trial ; for in twenty cases, in which it was administered by the former gentleman, the pulse was reduced more than twenty beats a minute in eleven, and to a less extent in seven of the remainder.   Where the stomach will not tolerate any form of cod liver oil, enemata containing it may be resorted to ; or this agent may be introduced into the system by inunction (F. 283), and by applying lint saturated with it to the chest.   Inunction with the best *sperm oil* has also proved rather useful in my hands.   *Cocoa nut oil*, especially in a mixture with the *citrate of iron and ammonia* (F. 391), merits a trial in these instances.   *Glycerine* is certainly very inferior in its effects to cod liver oil, while it often has the disadvantage of relaxing the bowels ; but it may at times, and in exceptional cases, be found efficacious.   The dose varies from one to four teaspoonfuls two or three times a day ; and it can either be given with some bitter infusion, or with the *syrup of iodide of iron*, or with the *tincture of perchloride of iron* (F. 392), or with *quinine, &c.*

The various preparations of *iron* (F. 380, 394, 397, 401, 403, 405, &c.) are very useful in many cases : especially during the second and third stages of the disease, provided there be neither hæmoptysis with a full pulse, nor pulmonary congestion.   Supposing the use of steel to be indicated where there is hæmorrhage from the lung or a tendency to it, no preparation will be found more useful than iron alum (F. 116).   *Iodine* and its compounds —especially the iodide of potassium—have been highly praised : the iodide of iron is the best preparation, though I have but little faith in it.   *Bark* is an excellent tonic ; and I have frequently seen much good from giving one or even two drachms of the compound tincture three or four times in the twenty-four hours.   The officinal liquid extract of yellow cinchona is an excellent prepara-

tion which can at times be borne well, when the tincture and
infusion give rise to headache. *Liquor potassæ* is often beneficial
in the early periods where the secretions are unduly acid, particularly if it be combined with bark (F. 373); but it is a less favourite
remedy with me than the *carbonate of ammonia* (F. 371). Dr. J. F.
Churchill regards *phosphorus* in certain combinations as a specific.
Without endorsing this extreme view, I am bound to say that the
hypophosphites of soda and lime (F. 419) have proved of great use
in some instances, particularly when the disease has been in an
early stage.   Whether simple alkaline remedies might not have
proved equally beneficial in these cases, I cannot determine ; for
having once put a phthisical patient on a plan under which his
symptoms are steadily ameliorated and his weight decidedly
increased, I am only too glad to leave well alone. When the cough
is severe, small doses of *opium* or *morphia*, frequently repeated, give
relief ; especially if the soothing effect be assisted by demulcent
drinks, decoction of Iceland moss, &c.   Sore lips, which irritate
the patient, are to be healed by *lip-salve* (F. 306), or by rubbing
them with the *glycerine of starch*, or by covering them with *gold-
beater's skin;* while aphthæ will best be remedied by painting the
sore patches with the *glycerine of borax.*   Where there is troublesome hæmoptysis, the *oil of turpentine* (min. x. every hour) at times
checks it ; or with greater confidence the *ammonio-sulphate of iron*
(F. 116), or *gallic acid* (F. 103) may be tried ; or the inhalation of
fine *spray medicated with tannic acid* (F. 262) is almost sure to be of
service.   Supposing the heart's action is irritable, it may be controlled by *hydrocyanic acid* with or without small doses of *digitalis*,
or by the tincture of *American wild-cherry* (F. 333).   If the night-
sweats weaken and annoy the patient, they will often be checked by
gallic acid, or by the *mineral acids with bark*, or especially by the *oxide
of zinc* in four or five-grain doses at bed-time ; or where it can be
digested, a dose of *cod liver oil* on port wine, taken directly after
supper, frequently succeeds. And then the diarrhœa, when urgent,
must be stopped by *catechu* (F. 97), *kino and logwood* (F. 108), the
officinal *compound kino powder*, the *enema of opium* of the British
Pharmacopœia or that of F. 113, *vegetable charcoal* (F. 98), *subnitrate of bismuth* (F. 112), *oxide of silver and opium* (F. 47), &c.
   Counter-irritation to the chest by dry-cupping, or the use of the
croton oil liniment (F. 303), or a succession of small blisters, or
frequent sinapisms, or turpentine stupes, or setons, or friction with
the officinal iodine liniment diluted with an equal proportion of
tincture of aconite, often gives relief.   In some instances, blisters
kept open for weeks with savine ointment or Albespeyre's plaster
(F. 208) have proved useful ; particularly where the tubercle is
near the surface, with adhesions between the and pulmonary costal
pleuræ.   When there is much laryngeal irritation, sponging the
epiglottis, back of the pharynx, and even the interior of the larynx,
with a strong solution of nitrate of silver, serves to ease the

breathing and to diminish the dysphagia; or this sponging can be supplanted by employing either an astringent or a sedative atomised fluid (F. 262) for inhalation, according to the indications manifested.

And lastly, it only remains to say that I am sceptical of good arising from the administration of pancreatine and pancreatic emulsion, naphtha, malt, sulphur, and common salt. Without any doubt, however, it is believed that in tubercular phthisis nought but mischief can result from the use of arsenic, oxalic acid, phosphate of lime, oxygen gas, daily emetics, excreta of reptiles, inhalations of chlorine, Turkish baths, frequent small bleedings, antimony, mercury, and colchicum—although each remedy has found an advocate.

XXIII. CANCER OF THE LUNG.

Pulmonary cancer, more commonly of the encephaloid than any other kind, is a rare disease. It may occur either as a partial or general infiltration, or as an encysted or non-encysted nodular deposit. Primary is more common by far than secondary cancer. One or both lungs can be attacked. In the secondary form, both lungs usually suffer: in the primary kind, the right lung appears to be much more obnoxious to the disease than the left. The lung mischief is generally associated with mediastinal cancer.

When the disease occurs *primarily*, the symptoms must obviously vary with the extent of the infiltration. There will, however, often be found—flattening of the affected side, impairment of the respiratory movements, and dulness on percussion. Moreover, pain, emaciation, night-sweats, failure of the powers of life, modifications of the voice, dyspnœa, cough, purulent expectoration—often mixed with blood and of a dark colour, dysphagia, and sometimes fetor of the breath, will be present. Chronic bronchitis also frequently complicates the disease.

With *secondary cancer* the symptoms are very obscure: indeed dyspnœa is often the only indication afforded during life. Both lungs are usually affected. In an example of cancerous infiltration of the penis, with secondary deposits in the lungs and elsewhere, the chief indication of pulmonary (cardiac?) mischief was that the man could not inhale chloroform without showing alarming symptoms of collapse. In the course of a month he died. On examination afterwards it was found that the whole penis was occupied by soft cancerous deposit; that there was a cancerous ulcer of the bladder; cancerous deposits in the lungs and bronchial glands; and that several of the bones were similarly affected. The heart was in a state of extreme fatty degeneration. The patient was in St. Bartholomew's Hospital under the care of Mr. Holmes Coote.

The weight of each lung in health is about 1¼ lbs., the right being rather heavier than the left. In cancer, without much apparent increase in bulk, the weight may rise to 5 or 6 lbs. Cancer and tubercle but rarely coexist. Isolated cancer of the pleura is of very uncommon occurrence. Dr. Walshe states that the mean duration of cancer of the lung may be estimated at 13·2 months; the longest time being 27 months, the shortest 3·5 months.

All varieties of pulmonary cancer manifest a tendency to soften : they are also liable to destructive inflammation, ending in suppuration or gangrene. Though the distress is great, the actual pain is not severe. Death occurs from asphyxia produced by the pressure of the disease, or from exhaustion, or from hæmorrhage, or from suppuration and gangrene involving the parenchyma of the lung.

As regards the treatment, we can only attempt to relieve the cough, dyspnœa, intercurrent complications, and other symptoms as they arise; while we try to support the strength as long as possible by nourishing food, cod liver oil, and stimulants.

XXIV. PERICARDITIS.

Pericarditis [Περὶ = about + καρδία = the heart; terminal -itis], or inflammation of the external fibro-serous covering of the heart, may be regarded as a local manifestation of constitutional disease, save in those few instances where it is the result of mechanical irritation or injury. The morbid action varies much in degree in different cases ; sometimes being so slight as to give rise to scarcely appreciable symptoms, while at other times both the local and general effects are most distressing.

Causes.—This disorder frequently arises from acute rheumatism, from the contaminated state of the blood produced by renal disease, from chorea, from damp and cold, and from mechanical injuries. As regards acute rheumatism, probably one case in nine or ten will be complicated with pericarditis : in Bright's disease the proportion will possibly be only one in eighteen or twenty. The tendency to cardiac complication in rheumatism diminishes with increase of age after fifteen. Dr. Ormerod reduces all cases of pericarditis to two classes :—1. Rheumatic pericarditis ; 2. Non-rheumatic pericarditis. In the first, the disease is always well-marked, it is associated with affections of the joints, women appear rather more subject to it than men, it is most common in the young and delicate, and it is rarely directly fatal. With respect to the second, the inflammation occurs at a later period of life, is most common in men, occurs most frequently in bad constitutions, and is very often the cause of death. Moreover, non-rheumatic pericarditis may be due to some local irritation, such as that set up by cancer, tubercle, incised wounds, the formation of a fistulous opening between a cavity in the lung and the pericardial sac, the extension of hepatic abscess through the diaphragm to the pericardium, &c.; or it will arise from a particular constitutional cause,—disease of the kidney, scurvy, typhoid fever, pleurisy, pneumonia, pyæmia, or one of the eruptive fevers.

Symptoms.—There is a considerable difference in the nature and degree of the symptoms; for while sometimes they are so slight that the disease escapes detection during life, in other cases they are strongly marked. When merely a slight exudation of fibrin has taken place, or when the serum thrown out has been rapidly absorbed and adhesions early effected, the patient may simply experience a feeling of fever and oppression; but where there is abundant effusion pressing upon the heart and embarrassing its movements, or where there is co-existent myocarditis, then both the local and general symptoms are rendered much more decided. Thus, in these latter instances, there will probably be high fever; pain referred to the region of the heart, often darting through to the left scapula, upwards to the left clavicle and shoulder, and down the arm; violent palpitation, the motions of the heart being tumultuous, and perceptible at a distance from the patient; irregularity of the pulse, usually with great frequency; hurried respiration; incapability of lying on the left side; strong pulsation of the carotids; anxiety of countenance; difficulty in swallowing; with frequently, noises in the ears, giddiness, and epistaxis. As the disease advances, there is extreme debility; with a perceptible dicrotism of the radial pulse, cough, suffocative paroxysms, occasionally a tendency to syncope, and œdema of the face and extremities. The heart's action also becomes much weaker, the impulse irregular and trembling, and the sounds get weakened and altered in character. In very severe cases, indications of disturbance of the nervous centres frequently show themselves; especially great restlessness, distortion of the features, tetanic spasms, and furious delirium.

The uncertainty of the general symptoms of pericarditis makes it all the more necessary that in every instance where the occurrence of this disease is feared, the physical signs which indicate its commencement should be carefully watched for. On practising auscultation we shall find, during the earliest stages, increased intensity of the natural sounds; while if endocarditis coexists, as it so frequently does, a loud systolic *bellows-murmur* will also be heard. Very early, too, a distinct *alternate rubbing* or a *to-and-fro sound*, as Sir Thomas Watson terms it, will be audible. The bellows-sound indicates fibrinous deposits in the texture as well as on the surface of the valves, from inflammation of the internal membrane of the heart—the endocardium—and it generally continues for life. The to and-fro sound is evidence of inflammation of the pericardium, and it commonly ceases in a few days, when either adhesion between the two roughened surfaces of the membrane takes place, or when effusion happens. Every now and again it will be noticed that the friction sound continues here and there audible, particularly about the base of the heart, though the effusion is copious. The exocardial friction-sound may so closely simulate endocardial murmur that it is sometimes difficult to distinguish between the two. Moreover, it is probable that a full development of the friction-sound can only take place when both divisions of the pericardium are the seat of plastic exudation.

Where serous effusion occurs, there will be a feebleness and deficiency of tone and force in the heart's sounds, probably owing to the deadening influence of the fluid surrounding the heart. There must also be increased dulness on percussion in the cardiac region; the dulness extending upwards to the level of the second rib or clavicle, though but little below the healthy limits. The dull region may also change its extent from day to day. Hypertrophy of the heart, as well as serous effusion, can produce præcordial bulging; though there may be a large quantity of fluid poured out without this bulging being present. In hypertrophy of the heart, the percussion-dulness is extended in all directions and remains stationary. In cases of effusion, also, it has been specially insisted upon that an undulatory or vermicular movement accompanies the cardiac impulse; but this motion has also been seen where no serous effusion existed—in enlargement of the heart, and in adherent pericardium. If the fluid does not become absorbed, we say that *hydro-pericardium* exists; a dropsical affection which sooner or later usually proves fatal. Only when the friction-sound is loud will it be sensible to the touch; since a more powerful rubbing is needed to produce a tactile than an audible phenomenon.

If we classify the physical signs of pericarditis, the arrangement will be as follows :—(1) Sensations of friction appreciable to the hand. (2) Friction-sounds: of short duration. (3) Extension of limit of cardiac dulness : not the consequence of œdema or congestion of the heart, but of the liquid effusion. (4) Valvular murmurs, where the endocardium is involved. (5) Signs of excitement or irritation of the heart. (6) Signs of loss of power or even paralysis of the heart.

Pathology and Morbid Anatomy.—The inflammation will occasionally end in resolution. More commonly there is effusion of serum, the quantity varying from a few ounces to three or four pints. Lymph may also be extravasated with or without the serum. This lymph oft-times forms a false membrane, covering the heart and lining the pericardial sac; the thickness of the exudation being variable but usually measuring some two or three lines, while it often presents a peculiar irregular or honeycomb appearance. And then, in cases occurring in depressed constitutions, the inflammatory action is very likely to end in the formation of pus; these instances of suppurative pericarditis generally ending fatally.

In severe cases, the muscular walls of the heart are very often involved in the morbid action. So also endocarditis frequently arises during the course of rheumatic pericarditis. White patches of lowly organized fibrin may be found after death, effused either into or upon the tissue of the pericardium, especially that part covering the right side of the heart. They are of no importance, and are probably due to the friction arising from the cardiac movements.

The sac of the pericardium is now and then obliterated owing to adhesions between its free surfaces; a condition which generally arises from inflammation of a chronic rather than of an acute character, occurring for the most part in strumous subjects. Occasionally there are only partial adhesions, obliterating the sac in parts; in such instances, the adhesions being most common at the base. Adherent pericardium is not unfrequently found with a healthy condition of the heart; but when there is an alteration in the muscular structure, the left side of the organ is by far the most frequently affected, the cavities being generally dilated, with hypertrophy of the walls. In a less number of examples of adherent pericardium, however, the heart has been found partially or entirely atrophied; this condition probably existing where the adhesions have been so thick as to compress the organ. Lastly, together with the adhesions there may be fatty degeneration of the heart's texture.

Prognosis.—Pericarditis, and especially the rheumatic variety, is not so much to be feared for its immediate danger, as for the traces of permanent injury which it leaves behind. The endocarditis that so frequently accompanies it, especially produces serious mischief to the valves of the heart. Hence an individual, after apparent recovery, seldom finds himself as strong or hearty as he was before the attack: he suffers occasionally from cough and shortness of breath, together with palpitations of the heart on moderate exertion. Sometimes the symptoms remain latent for a few years; that is to say, they are not appreciable to the patient, who flatters himself that he is free from all traces of his attack. But after a time (much shorter in those who have to work hard for their daily bread, than in the well-to-do members of society) the health begins to fail; the general weakness, difficulty of breathing, and palpitations return; dropsical symptoms set in; or perhaps an attack of inflammation takes place, and proves fatal.

Treatment.—In no disease was the lancet used with a more unsparing hand only a few years since, than in inflammation of the pericardium. More extended experience has proved to us, however, that this heroic and sure method—as it was deemed—of extinguishing the morbid action, is not only uncertain, but often very dangerous. Dr. Markham well says,—" Experience has also shown us that venesection has no *directly* beneficial influence over pericarditis; and that large bleedings are prejudicial, and therefore inadmissible in this disease. Nevertheless, that small bleedings are often of very great service *in relieving the congestions of the heart and lungs,* which so often arise as consequences of and coincidently with the pericarditis, is, I think, an undoubted fact."* Then we were also taught the great importance of rapidly getting the system under the influence of mercury after bleeding; but the

* *Diseases of the Heart; their Pathology, Diagnosis, and Treatment.* Second Edition, p. 45. London, 1860.

observations which have already been made (p. 112) upon this head render further remarks unnecessary here.

The treatment which was first advocated in the third edition of this work, published in 1857, and which I have since continued to adopt, is that practised by many for the relief of acute rheumatism, —the three principal remedies being the bicarbonate of potash in doses of thirty grains every two or three hours, opium in sufficient quantities to relieve pain and restlessness, and the vapour bath. Locally, poppy and chamomile fomentations, or very hot linseed poultices, are decidedly useful. From these agents I believe that I have seen the greatest benefit; and certainly in no instance have they been prejudicial. They give considerable relief to the patient's sufferings, without inducing debility; and they in no way complicate the symptoms. The quantity of opium which may be needed, will vary with the severity of the suffering; but usually full doses (perhaps one grain every three or four hours) are wanted. Now and then a single vapour bath suffices: in other cases it is necessary to repeat it daily, for three or four times. Alkaline drinks (F. 355, 356, 360) are also refreshing and do good. In most cases it will be necessary to administer a few doses of some purgative: the neutral salts (F. 141, 148, 150, 169) generally agree well. For pericarditis from a punctured wound, or that due to the extension of mischief from adjoining organs, any treatment beyond the administration of opium and the ordering of perfect rest, can only tend greatly to diminish the chances of recovery.

At the commencement of the attack the nourishment should be light, consisting of gruel, arrowroot, milk, and mutton broth. Directly the strength begins to fail, however, the diet must be made more strengthening; and soup, strong beef tea, and wine freely allowed. Dr. Stokes states that he is convinced patients are often lost from want of stimulation at the proper time; and he directs us to give support directly the pulse becomes feeble or intermittent, or the jugular veins appear turgid, or pallor and coldness of the surface set in, or a tendency to faint upon exertion is manifested. He says,—" It may be laid down as a general principle that there is no local inflammation whatever, the mere existence of which should prevent the use of wine, if circumstances require it. In two cases especially—namely, cerebritis and pericarditis, we find the greatest timidity in practice with respect to the use of wine. Yet even in the first case it may be required; and in the second its employment is imperative, when, as too often happens, excessive depletion has been resorted to."* Absolute repose of body and mind, in all cases, is important.

When the effusion into the pericardium is abundant, a large blister should be applied over the præcordia; or a succession of smaller blisters will perhaps answer the same purpose. The iodide of potassium (F. 31) has been advantageously administered to promote absorp-

* _The Diseases of the Heart and the Aorta_, p. 88. Dublin, 1854.

tion.   It has been proposed as a forlorn hope in obstinate hydro-pericardium, to remove the fluid by the introduction of a trocar and cannula.   M. Aran, Physician to the Hôpital St. Antoine at Paris, relates a case of pericarditis with copious effusion, in a young man aged 23, which he treated by an injection of iodine. The pericardium was punctured from below upwards, with a capillary trocar, in the fifth intercostal space, a little beneath the spot where the dulness on percussion was well marked : about twenty-eight ounces of a transparent reddish serum were removed.   A mixture formed of four drachms of tincture of iodine, fifteen grains of iodide of potassium, and an ounce and a half of water, was then injected without causing any pain ; a drachm or two being allowed to escape before closing the wound.   The fluid having reaccumulated the operation was performed a second time, at the end of twelve days, giving outlet to forty-nine ounces of a greenish-albuminous fluid ; a stronger injection then being employed, formed of equal parts (fl. drs. xij.) of tincture of iodine and water, with sixty grains of iodide of potassium.   The treatment was successful.*

XXV. ENDOCARDITIS.

Endocarditis [from Ἔνδον = within + καρδία = the heart ; terminal -itis], or inflammation of the whole or of a part of that delicate membrane which lines the interior of the heart and its valves, is of great interest to us as pathologists and physicians, owing to the severe organic diseases that so constantly spring from it.

Inflammation of the endocardium is most commonly associated with acute rheumatism.   Dr. Hope was of opinion that endocarditis more frequently occurs without pericarditis, than the latter without the former.   Dr. Stokes has come to a different conclusion, and he places these diseases in the following order of frequency :— 1. Acute pericarditis with endocarditis ; 2. Acute pericarditis without endocarditis ; and 3. Endocarditis without pericarditis.   It is certain, however, that endo-pericarditis is more frequently met with than simple endocarditis.

Symptoms.—In very severe instances the inflammation chiefly gives rise to a sense of oppression and uneasiness at the præcordial region ; while the patient prefers to lie on his back, and is restless and anxious.   There will be fever, with a small and feeble and intermittent pulse ; while there may be also cold sweats, oppressive dyspnœa, jactitation, and syncope.   Where the unhealthy process is only of limited extent, or when it assumes a chronic form, the symptoms are much milder and more obscure ; so that it not very unfrequently occurs during the progress of rheumatic fever

* The Lancet, p. 407.   London, 12 April 1856.

without being recognised. Nevertheless, the power of the disease is manifested by the structural changes which remain after apparent recovery. Endocarditis of the left is much more common than of the right side of the heart; while that part of the membrane which covers the valves and lines the orifices is most prone to become affected. The disease is seldom directly fatal; its remote effects being those so much to be dreaded.

Diagnosis.—Upon applying the hand to the chest in simple endocarditis, the action of the heart may appear to be violent; while sometimes a vibratory thrill will be felt. The patient himself may complain of the palpitations and irregular action, and feel alarmed. But it must be recollected that the inflammation may be progressing without causing pain, or any disturbance appreciable to the sufferer; while, on the other hand, these symptoms occasionally arise from simple irritability of the heart.

Percussion, it is said, often discovers an augmented extent of dulness in the præcordial region; this dulness being distinguished from that caused by pericardial effusion, by the beat of the heart appearing superficial instead of remote and distinct. But it is very doubtful if simple endocarditis can ever give rise to so much tumefaction or congestion of the walls of the heart, as to produce such an increased degree or extent of dulness as could be appreciated on making the usual examination.

Auscultation alone affords us any reliable information. On listening to the heart's sounds we shall usually detect a soft bellows-murmur, the most constant and characteristic of the phenomena of endocarditis. It is not always easy, however, where pericarditis exists to distinguish between an exocardial and an endocardial sound; while when it is certain that a valvular murmur is present, it may be perplexing to determine whether this is the consequence of old or recent mischief. Supposing that during the progress of an attack of rheumatism a murmur is found where none existed before, we of course cannot be wrong in diagnosing endocarditis; while we may with equal certainty infer that some fibrinous exudation into and upon the delicate lips of a valve has caused misshapement. If this exudation get indurated, it obstructs the orifice: if it weaken and pucker the valve, there will be regurgitation. When the murmur proves to be systolic, most distinct at the base and along the course of the aorta, and accompanied with a small pulse, it is significant of *aortic obstruction:* if systolic, most distinct at the apex, and with an irregular pulse, it is due to *mitral regurgitant disease.* A diastolic murmur, most distinct from the centre of the sternum (on a level with the third intercostal space) upwards towards the base, with a jerking pulse, is indicative of *aortic regurgitation;* while a diastolic murmur, most distinct from the fourth left intercostal space downward towards the apex, with an irregular small pulse, is the result of *mitral obstruction.* The murmurs of purely acute endocarditis are thus arranged in order

of frequency by Dr. Walshe :*—Aortic obstructive ; mitral regurgitant ; aortic regurgitant ; aortic obstructive and mitral regurgitant together ; aortic obstructive and regurgitant together.   Pulmonary systolic and diastolic murmurs are infinitely rare.   Dr.
Walshe has never observed acute obstructive mitral murmur, nor
acute regurgitant tricuspid murmur.

To recapitulate, the questions to be decided by auscultation are
these :—Is the abnormal sound exocardial or endocardial?   If the
latter, is the murmur old or recent?   Allowing it to be recent, is
it aortic or mitral ; or is there a double bruit owing to the valves
at both orifices being affected?   Primary disease of the pulmonic
and tricuspid valves is so very rare, that the consideration of such
need not here be allowed to complicate the points for scrutiny.
Then finally, is it obstructive or regurgitant disease ; or aortic obstructive and mitral regurgitant together ; or aortic obstructive
and regurgitant together?

For the further consideration of the physical signs, see the
section on *Diseases of the Valves of the Heart.*

Terminations.—The terminations of acute endocarditis are permanent valvular disease, with implication of the heart's substance,
and all their combined consequences.   Persistent valvular disease
leads to dilatation of the cavities ; the system loses tone, and the
blood becomes impoverished ; while after a variable interval dropsy
sets in.   Thenceforth the progress towards a fatal termination is
rapid, life rarely being prolonged beyond fifteen months from the
occurrence of dropsy.

When fibrinous deposits have taken place upon the valves, portions of the exudations may become detached and circulate with
the systemic blood until they get arrested in some artery where
they act as a plug, and so cut off the supply of blood to the part
(see p. 50).   Temporary paralysis is not very rare in heart disease,
and may arise from an embolus carried upwards in this manner ;
the power being restored if the collateral circulation is able afterwards to afford a due supply of blood, or if the mass of fibrin should
soften and break up so that the vessel once more becomes perme-
able.

Sometimes the fibrinous deposit sets up great irritation in the
tissue of the valves ; and then ulceration may take place, producing
perforation or a ragged condition of the edges.   The disorganizing
process will even extend to the chordæ tendineæ, breaking them
down and rendering them useless.   Dr. Ogle has given an account
of twenty-one cases of ulceration of the valves, which occurred in
St. George's Hospital.†   The report is very instructive, and
deserves a careful perusal.

* *The Diseases of the Heart and Great Vessels, including the Principles of
Physical Diagnosis.*   Third Edition, p. 248.   London, 1862.
† *Transactions of the Pathological Society of London.* Vol. ix. pp. 131-153.
London, 1858.

Treatment.—This must be conducted on the same principles as should guide the practitioner in the treatment of pericarditis. Owing, however, to the power of ammonia in preventing deposition of fibrin, it is very advisable to administer full doses of the carbonate or the aromatic spirit of this salt, from the commencement of the inflammation.

XXVI. MYOCARDITIS.

Myocarditis [from Μῦς = a muscle + καρδία = the heart; terminal -*itis*], carditis, or inflammation of the muscular substance of the heart, seldom occurs as a distinct affection ; being generally (if not always) combined with pericarditis, or with endocarditis, or with both. The morbid action, it is probable, extends from the investing or the lining membrane to the muscular substance ; though our present knowledge will not justify our denying that the starting-point of the inflammation may be in the muscular fibres themselves. The walls of the left ventricle seem to suffer more frequently than other parts of the heart. The results of myocarditis are induration of the muscular structure in consequence of the deposit of lymph ; the formation of abscesses ; aneurismal dilatation of the walls of the heart ; and perhaps, rupture.

Dr. Latham met with an almost unique case of universal carditis, in which there was effusion of pus generally throughout the cardiac fibres. The whole heart on being opened was seen to be deeply tinged with dark-coloured blood, while its substance was softened. Here and there, upon section of both ventricles, innumerable small points of pus oozed from among the muscular fibres. This was the result of most rapid and severe inflammation ; death having occurred after an illness of only two days.

The report of another notable instance of inflammation of the muscular substance of the heart has been published by Mr. Salter :*—In this case, the disease ran its course in seven weeks. It commenced with an acute pain in the left side of the chest ; which came on when the patient was walking, lasted a short time, and recurred about a week afterwards whilst he was using the same exercise. The pain subsequently became very frequent, and was induced by the slightest exertion. When Mr. Salter first saw him about a week before his death, there was orthopnœa, and an uneasy sensation or dull aching referred to the stomach and middle of the sternum. Venesection, calomel and opium, with counter-irritation were the means adopted to stay the disease ; but they were unavailing, and death took place. At the *post-mortem examination* the pericardium was found inflamed, especially in its diaphragmatic portion ; its vessels were distended, and spots

* *Medico-Chirurgical Transactions.* Vol. xxii. p. 72. London, 1839.

of ecchymosis were discovered beneath the serous membrane. The substance of the heart was moderately firm; but the left ventricle had almost entirely lost the colour of muscle, pus could be scraped from its surface, and in some parts there were cavities in the muscular substance like small abscesses.

The history of an example of acute inflammation of the muscular structure of the heart without any inflammation of the endocardium or pericardium, was detailed to the Fellows of the Royal Medico-Chirurgical Society by Dr. C. B. Radcliffe in 1865:—The patient was a strong middle aged man, a varnish maker by occupation. For six weeks he had suffered occasional attacks of sharp pains at the pit of the stomach, shooting thence into the left arm—attacks evidently of the nature of angina pectoris. He was well enough to follow his daily work, and to get about with little or no discomfort up to the day before his death. When first seen (27 July 1865), the indications pointed to a very weak heart. The pulse was extremely feeble and somewhat slow, but not irregular; hands cold and clammy; first sound of the heart absent; cardiac impulse against the walls of chest could not be felt; while the second sound of the heart could be only faintly heard, and several times was distinctly reduplicated. There were no morbid sounds of any kind. In the attempt to detect the cardiac impulse the patient winced, and complained of feeling sore at the part. On the following day, he was dying. Sitting awkwardly upon the edge of a chair by the side of the bed supported by his wife, he gasped out, " I must keep as I am, I dare not stir." He had been in this uncomfortable position for ten or twelve hours. His face was pale and ghastly, large beads of sweat stood out on the forehead, while his extremities were clammy and pale and cold. The pulse had failed : the breathing was shallow and gasping and attended with a rattle, of which the significance could not be mistaken. His mind was clear and collected ; he complained of sickness ; and said he knew that he was dying. At the *autopsy*, twenty-four hours after death, the heart was found dilated and flabby. The muscular structure of both ventricles, and in a lesser degree of both auricles, was soft and friable and almost black. It broke down readily under the finger like hepatized lung. As seen with the naked eye, it did not appear to be fatty, but there were considerable deposits of fat about the exterior of the heart. The pericardium, endocardium, and all the valves were quite healthy, and so also was the aorta. The left ventricle contained some loose and dark clots of semi-coagulated blood : in the right ventricle were some fibrinous but not discolorised clots adherent to the walls. Upon lifting up the heart by a portion of the right ventricle, the muscular structure broke down, and tore like wet paper by the weight of the heart itself. Unfortunately no microscopic examination was practicable.

There seems to be some reason for believing that the muscles of the heart may occasionally be affected with rheumatic inflammation, causing sudden paralysis of the organ and death. This occurrence will possibly explain those cases of acute rheumatism, where patients have been suddenly seized with severe pain in the cardiac region, suffocative dyspnœa, insensibility, convulsions, and death; and where afterwards no appearances have been detected on a careful examination of the body to account for the abrupt invasion of the fatal symptoms. It must not be overlooked, however, that possibly in some of these cases the fatal event may have been due to the formation of a coagulum in one of the large arteries.

XXVII. VALVULAR DISEASES OF THE HEART.

A few words on the normal sounds of the heart may not be out of place, before speaking of the valvular diseases of this organ. On practising auscultation over the cardiac region we can detect two sounds, very quickly following each other. They are succeeded by an appreciable period of silence. If the time occupied by the sounds and the pause be divided into fifths, we shall find the first sound occupying two-fifths, the second sound rather more than one-fifth, and the pause rather less than two-fifths. The *first sound*, sometimes called the systolic or inferior sound of the heart, should be listened to over the apex : it is dull, booming, and prolonged; and is coincident with the systole [Συστέλλω = to contract] of the ventricles, pulse of the arteries, diastole [Διαστέλλω = to dilate] of the auricles, and impulse of the apex against the thoracic parietes. The *second sound*, often termed the diastolic or superior sound, is best heard about the middle of the sternum : it is short, abrupt, and clear ; and is synchronous with the passive flow of blood from the auricles into the ventricles, the diastole of the ventricles, and the retrocession of the apex.

All physiologists agree in regarding the *second sound* of the heart as due to the brisk tension of the semilunar valves at the orifices of the aorta and pulmonary artery. The cause of the *first sound*, however, has long afforded a subject for controversy. By different eminent authorities it has been said to be due, entirely or partially, to the following :—The collision of the particles of blood with each other, and with the heart's parietes. The rush of blood through the narrowed openings of the great arteries. The impulse of the heart's apex against the thoracic walls. And the muscular bruit, produced by the contraction of the muscular fibres of the heart.

Now Dr. Halford believes that he has solved this delicate problem ; for he says his experiments demonstrate the fact that both sounds " depend upon the same cause, which is simply the vibration of the valves, produced by the backward pressure of the blood, first against the auriculo-ventricular, and secondly against the ventriculo-arterial valves." It may be questioned, however, whether this explanation is altogether satisfactory ; and whether the experiment by which he supports it—viz., exposing the heart of a living animal, and completely arresting the flow of blood through it—is not liable to mislead the student. For it is clear that if the circulation through the heart be arrested, none of the supposed causes of the first sound can act : there can then be no rush of blood through the arterial orifices, no impulse against the thoracic walls, no collision of the particles of blood with each other. I do not say that Dr. Halford's view is incorrect, because the more it is considered the more I am inclined to adopt it ; but I simply feel that the way he attempts to prove it is not convincing. Dr. Halford does not pretend to have originated this valvular theory, but to have finally confirmed it. In 1832 Dr. Billing taught that,—" the first sound is caused by the tension produced in shutting the auriculo-ventricular valves, and the second sound is caused by the tension produced in the shutting of the ventriculo-arterial valves." Putting together the evidence of Drs. Billing, Halford, Rouanet, Bryan, and others, it seems impossible to deny that the closure of the auriculo-ventricular valves is an important element in producing this first sound ; while it seems almost over-sceptical to doubt that it is the sole cause.

Causes and Effects of Valvular Disease.—Most of the alterations in the internal lining membrane of the heart result from inflammation, which gives rise to a deposit of lymph upon and beneath the serous membrane. The valves thus lose their beautiful thinness and transparency : they become thick and indurated, or puckered up, or adherent to each other or to the opposite walls of the channel. Independently of inflammation, the valves sometimes become covered with warty vegetations or excrescences, or they may be injured and lacerated, or they can be rendered inefficient by simple dilatation of the orifices which they guard, or they are found to be the seat of atheromatous or calcareous degeneration.

The *effects* are twofold : either to contract and narrow the orifice and so obstruct the passage of the blood—*valvular obstruction ;* or by puckering and shortening the valves, to make the orifice more or less patent, and hence permit of regurgitation of blood—*valvular insufficiency, regurgitant disease of valves,* &c. There may be only valvular obstruction or valvular insufficiency in any given case ; but often these conditions coexist.

Diagnosis.—In the diagnosis of the diseases under consideration attention must be directed, firstly, to the physical signs ; and secondly, to the chief functional symptoms.

1. The Physical Signs.—Physicians in all ages have very properly attached considerable importance to the rate and force at which the circulation is carried on. As a measure of these con-

ditions, as well as of the quantity of blood sent forth at each contraction of the heart, appeal is usually made to the *pulse* as felt
by the finger placed over the radial artery at the wrist.   Now
the pulse of the adult in health beats about 75 times in a minute,
and some considerable practice is needed to enable the observer to
appreciate the characters of each of these pulsations.   But if this
be true, how much more difficult must it be in disease, with a
pulsation frequently occupying less than half a second.   To remove this difficulty recourse has been had to mechanical appliances.   Vierordt was the first physiologist to invent an instrument
capable of conveying the impulse from an artery to a lever which
should mark the movement on a revolving cylinder of paper.   This
instrument is called a *sphygmograph*.   The traces made by it are
regular; and mark the extremes of dilatation and the number of
pulsations in a given time.   The misfortune is that its application
is difficult.   Hence, endeavours were made to produce a piece of
mechanism which could be easily used, and which should produce
a trace representing the shades of dilatation and contraction of
the vessels.   M. Marey has supplied this want; and his sphygmograph, substantially the one now used, accurately and minutely
records the movements of an elastic steel pad pressed upon the
artery.   By this instrument, placed upon the arm over the
radial artery, a trace can be procured on paper showing the form and
duration and regularity of the pulsations.   On examining such
a pulse-tracing it will be found to consist of a series of curves, each
of which corresponds to that succession of events which forms a
cardiac revolution, and which is known as a beat or pulsation.
Every pulsation is said to be composed of a line of ascent, a
summit, and a line of descent.   When the ventricles contract, all
the arteries suddenly expand, while a wave movement is propagated along the arterial system; this movement probably producing the line of *ascent*.   The more rapid the entry of blood into
the arteries, the more vertical will be the ascent of the lever of
the sphygmograph.   The *summit* of the pulsation corresponds
with the period when the afflux of blood into the artery and the
efflux are equal.   This period may be so brief that the summit
of the curve is only a point, or it may be more or less blunt as
happens when the heart is weak.   The line of *descent*, the most
important portion of the curve, is coeval with the diminution of
arterial pressure.   It is coincident with the time which intervenes
between the closure of the semilunar valves of the aorta and the
next ventricular systole.   This line varies in its obliquity in different cases; but it is likewise peculiar in being broken by two
undulations or notches showing that the pulse in health is registered as tricrotous, instead of dicrotous as taught by Marey and
those of his followers who thought there was only a single undulation.   The first undulation occurring soon after the summit of
the curve is called by Wolff the first incisure; the elevation

which succeeds being the first secondary wave or undulation. The
dicrotism of Marey is the great ascension; the notch (probably to
be known for the future as the aortic notch, since it is synchronous with the reflux of blood closing the aortic valves) which
precedes and separates it from the first secondary wave being the
great incisure. At the bottom of this great incisure there can
sometimes be seen a slight undulation, known as the second
secondary wave.

The diagnosis of organic disease of the heart by auscultation
and percussion is so comparatively simple and easy that any further
physical means of investigation may be deemed unnecessary. We
cannot afford, however, to dismiss any aids to the investigation of
disease; and hence it has been considered advisable to direct attention in the foregoing manner to the uses of the sphygmograph.
The few results which have been so far obtained by it in disorders
of the circulation will be noticed presently, as well as subsequently
when speaking of aortic aneurisms. The value of this instrument
in fever has been already (p. 232) described.

The average frequency of *respiration* in health, in a state of
mental and bodily rest, is 18 in the minute, in the adult; taking
the pulse at somewhere between 72 and 80. This ratio is not only
easily disturbed by disease, but also by mental emotion and other
agents. To show the extent to which the pulse-respiration ratio is
altered in disease, cases of fatty degeneration of the heart may be
instanced. Thus, in this condition the ratio will often be as 1 : 2,
with such numbers as $\frac{12}{18}$, or $\frac{20}{18}$. In most forms of embarrassed
cardiac action the respirations are unduly frequent. The difficulty
of breathing varies from the slightest dyspnœa to the most severe
orthopnœa. Often it is the principal source of suffering, preventing the sufferer from lying down, and giving rise to most restless
nights. In cases of heart disease where the victim is able to
pursue his ordinary avocations to a certain extent, any undue
exertion will often produce an attack of dyspnœa. This, however,
is seldom noisy, as it is when the bronchi or pneumogastrics are
pressed upon or irritated by an aortic aneurism.

The natural *sounds of the heart* are liable to be modified and
changed by disease, causing either sound or both to be accompanied
or to be supplanted by a noise which has been aptly compared to
the blowing of a pair of bellows: hence it is termed by us a *bellows-
murmur*, and by the French a *bruit de soufflet*. A bellows-murmur
may be harsh, or rough, or cooing, or whistling, or musical; but
these modifications are of little importance. For of whatever
nature, the important point to remember is, that this bruit is caused
either by the presence of obstructions (the consequence of disease
or malformation) which impede or break the free current of blood
through the heart and its great vessels—producing an *organic*
murmur; or else it is occasioned by a change in the composition of
the blood, or a clot in one of the heart's cavities—giving rise to an
inorganic, or *functional*, or *hæmic* murmur. Where the valves of

the heart are affected so that they act ineffectively, an organic bellows-murmur must result.

The arteries may also become the seat of murmurs. When the calibre of a vessel is much increased so that the direction of the blood-current is altered, or when the capacity is diminished so that there is increased friction of the blood against the coats ; when the coats of the artery are diseased, with or without aneurism ; and when there is some direct communication between an artery and a vein,—in all these cases an *organic* murmur results. An *inorganic* murmur is due either to altered composition of the blood, or to the formation of a clot in the vessel.

During the early stage of phthisis, a murmur (which, strictly speaking, can neither be referred to the organic nor inorganic class just described) may sometimes be detected under the left clavicle, owing probably (as before mentioned) to the pressure of the tubercles upon the left subclavian artery ; while not uncommonly a systolic bellows-sound is heard in the second left intercostal space over the pulmonary artery, the heart and the pulmonary artery being quite healthy. Moreover, displacement of the heart, owing to the pressure of pleuritic effusion, ascites, &c., may give rise to a loud murmur which does not disappear until the organ is restored to its natural position, by the removal of the fluid ; though it must be confessed that a bruit under these circumstances is a rare event, for I have frequently looked in vain for it when the heart has been pushed considerably upwards by the presence of an ovarian tumour, or by pregnancy advanced to the full term.

The loudness and distinctness of organic cardiac murmurs are not proportionate to the extent of disease causing them, for sometimes an exceedingly small vegetation on one of the valves will produce a very loud murmur. Dr. C. J. B. Williams had a man, thirty years old, under his care, in whom there was a very loud murmur following the second sound ; which murmur, though most distinct in the mid-sternum, was also heard in every part of the chest, in the arteries of the neck, and even slightly in the radial. The man caught typhus fever, from which he died ; and at the post-mortem examination it was found that the valves were all healthy except the aortic, while in these the only change was that one of them had the free margin neatly retroverted so as to leave a small smooth chink for regurgitation. The ventricles were also moderately enlarged and thickened.

The lining membrane, valves, and orifices of the left side of the heart are much more frequently diseased than those of the right ; so much so, that it is almost a question whether disease of the tricuspid or pulmonary valves can be accurately diagnosed. " Practically, in at least nineteen out of twenty cases," says Dr. Harvey, " the questions to be determined are, whether it be the mitral or the aortic valve that is diseased, or both ; and whether the disease be of the nature of valvular obstruction, or of valvular insufficiency, or both."* Diseases of the left side chiefly affect the arterial pulse, giving rise to irregularity and inequality; those of the right side affect the venous circulation, causing regurgitation into the jugular veins—a condition known as the venous pulse. Dropsy is more often connected with disease of the right than of the left cavities.

Disease of the *semilunar valves of the aorta* is not uncommon. When of sufficient duration, it will be found to have produced hypertrophy of the left ventricle; which hypertrophy may compensate for the obstruction or regurgitation caused by the aortic disease. Thus, the systemic circulation may be uninterfered with. Supposing that the affected valves diminish the aortic orifice during systole (or contraction) so as to prevent the blood from freely flowing out of the ventricle, a systolic bellows-sound will result. This can be best heard at the base of the heart, along the course of the thoracic aorta, up towards the right clavicle, and even in the carotids; the sound diminishing as the stethoscope is moved towards the apex of the heart. If the valves close imperfectly, permitting reflux of blood from the aorta, the morbid sound will be diastolic—will accompany the dilatation of the ventricle. The short, second sound of the heart will also be muffled and indistinct. Sometimes we have both these conditions of the aortic valves in the same case—aortic obstructive and regurgitant together; a double bruit or bellows-sound being then produced. The pulse of aortic disease is regular: in the regurgitant form it is often peculiar, being generally sudden and sharp, and without any prolonged swell of the artery; Dr. Hope calls it a jerking pulse. The sphygmographic traces of such a pulse are said to show certain peculiarities. There is a great amplitude of trace. The line of ascent is vertical. The curve usually presents a pointed summit. This vertical line of ascension and pointed summit are not peculiar, however, to aortic regurgitation; similar appearances being produced in functional disturbance from anæmia. But when the valvular incompetency is so great that there is free regurgitation, the descending line of the curve shows a sudden fall with an absence of dicrotism; the aortic notch being more or less suppressed, since the closure of the aortic valves which produces it is imperfect.

The *mitral valve* which guards the left auriculo-ventricular orifice, may become thickened or ossified; the effect of which is to prevent its closing the auricular orifice during systole, as well as to hinder its lying flat against the walls of the ventricle so as to allow the blood to pass freely out during the diastole. In such cases the orifice is almost rendered a permanent oval slit. A double bruit may perhaps be detected: the first, systolic, caused by the regurgitation of the blood from the ventricle into the auricle; the second, diastolic, and due to the impediment to the passage of the

* "Notes on Chronic Heart Disease." *Association Medical Journal,* p. 785. 1 September 1854.

blood from the auricle to the ventricle.   Such a double bruit is but rarely heard, however.   The murmur or murmurs can be best distinguished towards the apex of the heart, on the left.   Although mitral murmurs are often inaudible at the base of the heart, yet they can frequently be heard clearly behind—at the lower angle of the left scapula.   The pulse is irregular, and usually soft and frequent : the irregularity is clearly registered by the sphygmograph.   Palpation also often discovers a purring thrill.   Mitral disease, whether obstructive or regurgitant, interferes with the pulmonary circulation ; all the vessels concerned in which get enlarged, the lungs are constantly overloaded with blood as the circulation through them is sluggish, and hence there is lividity with a tendency to hæmorrhage into the air-sacs.   The right ventricle becomes hypertrophied and ultimately dilated ; and sooner or later there will be a condition of stasis in the systemic veins, persistent congestion of the liver and often of the kidneys, with jaundice and dropsy and albuminuria.

Following the plan of Dr. Harvey, the signs of disease of the aortic and mitral valves may be thus briefly tabulated :—

Bruit :—If *systolic*, and loudest at
    Base = Aortic *obstruction.*
    Apex = Mitral *insufficiency.*
Bruit :—If *diastolic* and loudest at
    Base = Aortic *insufficiency.*
    Apex = Mitral *obstruction.*
Pulse : If *regular*,
    Full or strong,   } = Aortic disease.
    Jerking, resilient,   }
Pulse : If *irregular*,
    Intermittent, unequal,   } = Mitral disease.
    Soft, small, weak,   }

The *semilunar valves of the pulmonary artery* are very rarely diseased ; so rarely that any organic alteration in them is a pathological curiosity.   When, however, a bellows-murmur can be traced from the middle of the left edge of the sternum up towards the left clavicle, and when this murmur cannot be heard in the subclavian or carotid arteries, we may assume that it originates at the orifice of the pulmonary artery.   The pulse remains unaltered.

The *tricuspid valve*, guarding the right auriculo-ventricular opening, is also but seldom found otherwise than healthy.   When diseased, the morbid condition will almost invariably exist in combination with aortic or mitral affection, or with both.   In dilatation of the right ventricle from mitral incompetency there may be tricuspid regurgitation without change of structure.   In such cases there may, or may not, be tricuspid murmur, occurring with that of mitral obstruction or regurgitation.   Turgescence, with pulsation of the jugular veins at every ventricular systole is present in those cases of tricuspid disease dependent on dilated right heart.

But whether the venous pulse is a symptom of tricuspid regurgitation is at least doubtful.

To determine the systolic or diastolic character of a murmur, the pulse at the wrist should be carefully noted during auscultation: if systolic, the bruit must of course be synchronous with the pulse, and if most audible at the apex, is indicative of mitral disease; if diastolic, not synchronous with the pulse, and most audible over the centre of the sternum and along the course of the aorta, it is indicative of aortic disease.

Inorganic or *functional murmurs* generally counterfeit aortic or pulmonic bruits as regards their position. A murmur which is best heard over the base of the heart and the great arteries, which is single and systolic, which is accompanied by an anæmic murmur in the neck, which varies in intensity under different states of the system, and which is not attended by a turgid condition of the vessels,—such may be set down as a functional bruit.

2. The Functional Symptoms.—The following are the chief results of valvular disease :—

a. Palpitation and irregular action of the heart appreciable to the patient. *b.* Congestion of the lungs ; bronchitis ; pneumonia ; and pulmonary hæmorrhage, with or without pulmonary apoplexy. These symptoms are most urgent in mitral disease. *c.* Hæmorrhages from the nose, bronchial tubes, or mucous membrane of the stomach. *d.* Œdema of the lower and sometimes of the upper extremities, and face ; hydrothorax ; and ascites. Dropsy is more common in disease of the right cavities of the heart than in affections of the left. *e.* Cephalalgia, tinnitus aurium, vertigo, syncope, cerebral congestion, and cerebral hæmorrhage. These consequences are most urgent in aortic disease. *f.* Broken rest, with startings during sleep, and frightful dreams : the latter often so bad, that the patient will ask an attendant to keep him awake. *g.* Enlargement of the liver and spleen, with disorder of the digestive organs generally. *h.* A peculiar and almost characteristic appearance of the countenance,—*i.e.* the face is puffed, the cheeks are flushed and of a purple hue, the lips are congested, and the eyes are bright.

While time advances, the heart disease commonly becomes more aggravated. As certain of the functional symptoms are developed, the patient gets weak and nervous. He suffers immediately from over-exertion, mental emotion, improper food, or exposure to wet and cold ; and subsequently death ensues,—either suddenly from syncope, or gradually from exhaustion aggravated by sleeplessness, or from the progress of one or other of the secondary affections. The latter termination is decidedly the most common.

Prognosis.—The danger of structural cardiac disease will be in proportion to the extent to which the change impairs the power of the heart in carrying on the circulation; as well as partly in proportion to the degree to which the blood is deteriorated in quality. So long as the natural sounds are distinct, and the impulse of the apex is not felt beyond its natural limits, there is no present danger (provided there be no great amount of anæmia) however loud or harsh the accompanying murmurs happen to be; while even if the general symptoms be distressing, we may entertain very sanguine expectations of relieving them to such an extent that moderate health may be regained. Whether the improvement will persist for any length of time, must of course depend upon the fact of the valvular lesion becoming stationary or aggravated; for it may so increase, from many causes, as to develope dangerous disorder. But if the history of the case is not that of a sudden or recent attack, and if the physical signs do not grow more marked in the course of a few weeks, a favourable prognosis can be given, and hopes encouraged of some years of comfort.

On the contrary, if the natural sounds are indistinct, or are nearly superseded by abnormal murmurs, then it must be inferred that the heart's power for action is much impaired, and that there exists serious ground for alarm. In such cases, too, the general symptoms usually plainly indicate that the chief organ of the circulation is failing in its work; for there are distressing palpitations with irregular action, frequent attacks of syncope, and congestions of internal organs and tissues. Dropsy is also likely to set in. Those cases are especially dangerous where the valvular lesion is due to some violent exertion; or where the structural change has been aggravated by a second assault of endocarditis, or by the setting in of fatty degeneration and consequent softening. When to the above symptoms there is superadded a thin watery state of the blood, the cause for alarm is proportionately increased; as is also the case when the blood is poisoned by urea, bile, lithic acid, &c.

Treatment.—In the treatment of the valvular diseases of the heart three indications have generally to be followed:—(1) To abate inordinate action of the heart by tonics and sedatives—as digitalis, the American wild cherry, hydrocyanic acid, aconite, belladonna, conium, henbane, hop, and morphia; though these remedies, and especially the last, must be employed with great caution, for where there is a feeble pulse, dyspnœa, and difficult expectoration, a dose of opium may but materially hasten death. (2) To ward off or gradually relieve the results of the cardiac disease,—such as pulmonary congestion, pneumonia, hæmorrhage, congestion of the liver and kidneys, dropsy, &c. This is to be attempted by ordering a nutritious diet, and by maintaining the various secreting organs in a healthy state; saline purgatives and diuretics, repeated at proper intervals, being very valuable. When the dropsical effusion is great in these instances, much benefit may often be derived from mercury; diuretics, which had previously been useless, often causing an astonishing flow of urine directly the gums get touched. The latter effect, however, is frequently obtained with difficulty where the obstruction to the circulation is great. In anasarca of the lower extremities, small incisions along the legs give great relief, by allowing the serum to drain off; the chilly and moist un-comfortable feelings caused by the flow of fluid being best mitigated by wrapping the limbs in soft chamois leather.   And then (3) we must endeavour to give strength and tone to the heart, so as to assist it to do its work.   There will be most hope of accomplishing this by nourishing food, perhaps cod liver oil, a duly regulated supply of stimulants, breathing pure air, warm clothing, early hours, cold or tepid salt-water sponge baths, avoidance of all bodily and mental excitement, and by the administration of tonics—especially one of the various preparations of steel.

XXVIII. HYPERTROPHY OF THE HEART.

The heart is stated roughly to be about the same size as the closed fist.   The average weight of this organ in the adult male may be said to be nine and a half ounces, that of the female being eight and a half.*   After the age of sixty the heart is somewhat heavier, since the thickness of the walls of the left ventricle has then become decidedly increased.   The muscular parietes of one or more of the cavities may become thickened without any diminution in the size of the chamber: this is called *simple hyper-trophy*.   Or, as most frequently happens, the walls will be thickened and the chamber become larger than natural: this is *eccentric hypertrophy*, or *hypertrophy with dilatation*.   On the other hand, the increase in thickness may be accompanied with diminution in the size of the cavity: a condition known as *concentric hypertrophy*.   This last form is now believed only to occur as a congenital mal-formation, and never as the consequence of disease.

The *cause* of the hypertrophy is usually some obstruction either to the flow of blood through the heart, or to the free play of this organ; whence the amplification is frequently a compensatory pro-vision to counterbalance the impediment.   The heart is stimulated to extra exertion; and in consequence it receives an extra supply of nutritive materials, by which its muscular structure is strength-ened.   The left ventricle is more frequently found hypertrophied than the right, and much more so than the auricles.   In a heart which weighed five pounds, the walls of the left ventricle had acquired a thickness of two inches.   Hypertrophy with dilatation of the right ventricle is commonly due to some chronic disease of the lungs obstructing the circulation.   Conversely, it has been thought that hypertrophy of the right ventricle might be an occa-sional cause of the extravasation of blood into the pulmonary

* The weight of the healthy heart in persons from twenty to fifty-five years of age averages, in males 9 oz. 8 dr., and in females 8 oz. 13 dr.   Esti-mates of this description are of course, to a certain extent, arbitrary: for as the heart is found, in some cases, to be considerably above its ordinary weight, without the proportion of its walls and cavities being materially altered, or the organ being otherwise diseased, it is not easy to say at what point it ceases to be healthy.—Dr. Peacock: *Monthly Journal of Medical Science*, vol. xix. p. 211.   Edinburgh, 1854.

structure, possibly by urging the blood onwards with too much force.

The *symptoms* will depend upon the extent of the hypertrophy. Frequently they consist of palpitation, dyspnœa, difficulty of walking quickly, uneasiness and pain in the cardiac region, headache, and repeated attacks of vertigo. If we listen to the heart's movements, the systolic sound will be found less distinct than in health; but we shall also feel that the extent of the pulsation beyond the præcordial region, and especially the degree of impulse against the walls of the chest, are both much increased. Moreover, when there is valvular disease, the morbid sounds indicative of such will be present.

The *treatment* must consist in keeping the patient as free from undue excitement as possible, and in prescribing for his symptoms. If there be much debility, quinine or steel or both (F. 380, 394, 405), bark (F. 371, 376), or the mineral acids (F. 377, 378) had better be given; if the heart's impulse be very great, aconite (F. 330), or digitalis (F. 334), or the American wild cherry (F. 333), can be occasionally but cautiously, tried; while when the dyspnœa is urgent, stimulants, especially ammonia and spirit of ether (F. 361, 367), may be had recourse to. The chief point to be kept in view is this,—that while the effects of the hypertrophy on the circulation are frequently favourable, yet too great force might possibly lead to pulmonary (or even to cerebral) apoplexy.

SIMPLE HYPERTROPHY OF THE LEFT VENTRICLE WITH NO OBSTRUCTION TO THE FLOW OF BLOOD.—This condition is rare. On ausculting the heart the systolic sound is less loud and clear than natural, but no bellows-murmur can be heard. On placing the hand over the præcordial region, the impulse of the heart will be felt increased.

In many cases of chronic Bright's disease, there is found hypertrophy of the heart—especially of the left ventricle—without any disease of the valves or large bloodvessels existing to retard the flow of blood, and thus to explain the increased bulk of the muscular walls. In these cases it is supposed that the blood is impeded in its passage through the minute systemic vessels owing to its contamination by excrementitious materials in consequence of the renal degeneration; and hence the left ventricle has to make extraordinary efforts to propel the blood, and of course acquires increased bulk and strength.

HYPERTROPHY OF LEFT VENTRICLE WITH VALVULAR DISEASE.— This is the most common form of hypertrophy. The chief causes, according to Dr. Markham, are—"Defective aortic valves, permitting regurgitation of the blood into the left ventricle during its diastole; constriction of the aortic orifice, impeding the free passage of the blood from the left ventricle during its systole; deficiency of the aortic valves, associated with constriction of the aortic orifice; defective mitral valves, permitting regurgitation of the blood from the left ventricle into the left auricle;—all these abnormal conditions occasion impediments to the circulation of the blood through the heart, and their immediate effects are, for the most part, communicated directly to the left side, and indirectly to the right side of the heart."*   As the hypertrophy in these cases is an endeavour (so to speak) towards health, the increased power compensating for the obstruction to the flow of blood caused by the valvular disease, we must not unnecessarily interfere with the symptoms.

DILATATION OF THE HEART.—This may occur under three circumstances. First, there may be, as has been just shown, hypertrophy with dilatation; such a condition being known as *active dilatation*, when the expansion predominates over the hypertrophy. Secondly, we have *simple dilatation*, where the thickness of the walls is normal. And thirdly, there is *passive* or *attenuated dilatation*, the walls being thinned. This last is the only state which demands a few words.

Passive dilatation is often combined with malnutrition of the heart, and fatty degeneration of the muscular fibres; both ventricles are usually affected, though the right may be so in a more marked degree than the left; and the attenuation will perhaps be so extreme that the walls are found quite collapsed after death. Passive dilatation may be due to some exhausting disease, or to inflammation of the endocardium, or perhaps to pericardial adhesion. The chief symptoms are a small, weak, and perhaps irregular pulse; coldness and slight lividity of the extremities; with giddiness, and derangement of the digestive organs. There is a tendency to congestion of the liver, to imperfect action of the kidneys, and also to congestion of the lungs. Moreover, the patient is restless at night, gets weak and irritable, and suffers from asthmatic paroxysms (cardiac asthma): palpitation is often distressing, attacks of syncope are not uncommon, and there is anasarca followed by ascites. The physical signs are,—increased præcordial dulness, undue distinctness of the heart's sounds, sometimes irregular action of the heart, sometimes reduplication of the sounds, and generally almost imperceptible cardiac impulse. There will be no murmur if the valves remain healthy; unless the dilatation of the ventricles be so great, that valvular incompetency is necessarily caused by the orifices becoming enlarged. Antispasmodics, ferruginous tonics, and agents to promote the digestion of nourishing food, are the only remedies which afford temporary relief in this serious disease.

XXIX. ATROPHY OF THE HEART.

There are two forms of atrophy of the heart. One, in which the organ simply wastes and dwindles in all its parts; the other, in which the texture of the muscle suffers a sort of conversion into fat—becomes affected with fatty degeneration.

Simple atrophy occurs in connexion with many exhausting dis-

* *Diseases of the Heart, &c.* Second Edition, p. 143. London, 1860.

eases,—to wit cancer, tuberculosis, diabetes, &c. The whole organ diminishes in size; so that after death it may be found to weigh about five ounces instead of nine. Minutely examined, the muscular fibres are detected pale and soft, but otherwise healthy. The treatment must be that which is demanded by the constitutional affection, of which the atrophy is merely one symptom.

Fatty degeneration of the heart is a most interesting disease, which has been already incidentally noticed (p. 176). The student who wishes to study the subject thoroughly may be especially referred to the writings of Dr. Richard Quain, Dr. Ormerod, Mr. Paget, Mr. Barlow, Dr. Wilks, and Prof. Virchow.

This disease occurs under two circumstances; either alone, or in conjunction with fatty disease of other organs, as the kidneys, liver, cornea, &c. Its *diagnosis* is beset with difficulties; so that when existing alone its presence is every now and then unsuspected until after death, and after a microscopic examination of some of the muscular fibres of the heart. Valvular disease very rarely coexists; but where it does, the aortic valves appear to be more generally affected than the mitral. There is no connexion between this process of decay, and the accumulation of adipose tissue around the heart. The most prominent *symptoms* of fatty degeneration are a feeble action of the heart, a remarkably slow pulse—sometimes as low as fifty or forty-five or even thirty-five in a minute, general debility, transient attacks of giddiness or faintness, a tendency to sigh frequently, a pallid and flabby appearance, a feeling of nervous exhaustion, and marked loss of tone, &c. Both sounds of the heart are weak, the first being especially faint; while the impulse of the apex against the chest-walls is feeble or even imperceptible. In advanced cases there are attacks of dyspnœa, produced by even moderate exertion; together with many or all of the symptoms which prevail in angina pectoris. When in addition there is a well-marked arcus senilis (due, as Mr. Canton has shown, to fatty degeneration of the edge of the cornea) the diagnosis may perhaps be facilitated; though I have long been convinced that in many cases of arcus senilis the heart is quite healthy, while the latter is often affected with fatty degeneration without the arcus being present.

Fatty degeneration of the heart seems to occur rather more frequently in men than in women: it may take place at all ages, though it happens principally at advanced periods of life: all classes of society may suffer from it. Moreover, it either exists singly, or with other cardiac diseases; and it is not an uncommon cause of sudden death. "On opening a heart thus affected," says Dr. Ormerod, "the interior of the ventricles appears to be mottled over with buff-coloured spots of a singular zigzag form. The same may be noticed beneath the pericardium also; and in extreme cases the same appearance is found, on section, to pervade the whole thickness of the walls of the ventricle and of the carneæ columnæ." On microscopically examining these spots, their nature is revealed;

they are not deposits, but degenerated muscular fibres. Instead of seeing transverse striæ and nuclei—the evidence of a healthy state, little can be distinguished but a congeries of oil-globules. The muscular fibres are also found to be short and brittle; and Dr. Quain has pointed out that the coronary arteries are often obstructed. Mr. Paget well remarks that "the principal character which all these cases seem to present is, that they who labour under this disease are fit enough for all the ordinary events of calm and quiet life, but are wholly unable to resist the storm of a sickness, an accident, or an operation."—From the foregoing it will appear that the *prognosis* must always be unfavourable. Dilatation, rupture, and aneurism of the heart are the prominent changes most frequently found in connexion with this affection.

Sometimes the fat which is normally deposited upon the heart is increased on and amongst the muscular fibres to a morbid extent; and we then speak of the condition which results as *fatty growth*. This may happen alone, or in conjunction with general obesity; or it will be associated with fatty degeneration. It is possible that the arcus senilis much more frequently accompanies these cases of fatty growth, than those of fatty degeneration. The symptoms of fatty growth, when it exists alone, are those of a heart enlarged and impeded in the performance of its functions. The pulse is permanently quickened above the normal standard, while its force is diminished.

In the present state of our knowledge, the *treatment* of a case of suspected fatty disease of the heart resolves itself chiefly into preventing further degeneration of tissue. The means to adopt therefore are—nourishing animal food, attention to the digestive organs, pure air, early hours, gentle exercise, and the use of ferruginous tonics. Soda water will prove useful as a drink: a little brandy or sherry may be given with it. The patient should daily take a salt-water sponging bath. Everything which can hurry the circulation ought to be avoided; while agents which weaken the power of the heart, such as tobacco, invariably prove mischievous.

Some authors object to the use of fat meats, of milk, and indeed of all oleaginous foods. But it is difficult to understand the ground on which these restrictions are recommended; since the disease is a degeneration of tissue, caused by debility or a wearing-out of the frame, rather than by an excess of power. Hence I believe that cod liver oil, cream and milk, may generally be given with great advantage.

These remarks are not meant to apply to the treatment of fatty growth with general obesity. In such cases, the patient should be dieted according to the directions already (p. 222) given.

XXX. CYANOSIS.

Cyanosis [Κύανος = blue + νόσος = disease], morbus cæruleus, or blue disease, are terms applied to a condition characterized by a blue or purplish discoloration of the skin; arising generally in connexion with some deficiency in the construction of the heart.

The chief malformations are the following :—A permanence of the foramen ovale, allowing the passage of the blood between the two auricles; abnormal apertures in some part of the septum of the auricles or of the ventricles; the origin of the aorta and pulmonary artery from a single ventricle; a transposition of the origins of the large vessels from the heart, the aorta arising from the right and the pulmonary artery from the left ventricle; an extreme contraction of the pulmonary artery; or, lastly, the continued patescence of the ductus arteriosus, permitting a mixture of the bloods of the aorta and the pulmonary artery.

Three explanations have been given as to the immediate cause of the discoloration of the surface in these cases of malformation. Thus, some pathologists refer it solely to general venous congestion; others regard the intermixture of the two currents of blood as the cause; while a third class believes that it is partly due to congestion of the venous system, and partly to the intermingling of the venous with the arterial blood. The truth is probably this,—that the discoloration is owing to systemic venous congestion, but that it may be aggravated by certain malformations. On the other hypothesis it seems impossible to explain the admitted facts, that malformations permitting the free admixture of arterial and venous blood may exist without giving rise to cyanosis; while the latter is sometimes found where no such admixture could have taken place. The cause of the general venous congestion is some obstruction to the flow of blood through the lungs, or from or into the right ventricle; such obstruction frequently consisting in a contraction of the pulmonary artery or its orifice.

In addition to the discoloration of the skin, the patients who survive their birth suffer from coldness of the body (sometimes the temperature, as marked by the thermometer in the mouth, has been as low as 77° Fahr.), palpitation, fits of dyspnœa, syncope on the least excitement, &c. The tips of the fingers, and sometimes of the toes, become bulbous after a time, and the nails are often incurvated. The generative organs are frequently imperfectly formed —there is evidence of early arrest of development. Bronchial hæmorrhage and bronchorrhœa seem to have occurred in many instances. Moreover, in cases about to terminate fatally we have congestion of internal organs, and dropsical effusions. The cutaneous discoloration is generally increased by aught which excites the circulation; while if there is no valvular lesion the sounds of the heart will be found normal. With some few cases the symptoms of cyanosis are not manifested until many months after birth. Infants affected with the disease generally die at a very early age; but occasionally, they live on even to the adult period. Males are notably more prone to cyanosis than females: a satisfactory explanation of this fact remains to be discovered.

The physical signs are diversified, just as the malformations are multifarious.   Whatever the defect may be, however. there is frequently hypertrophy with dilatation of the right ventricle.   Murmurs will of course be detected if there be valvular incompetency, or constriction of the orifices.

Under exceptional circumstances cyanosis may not come on until somewhat late in life.   Cases like the following are related :—A lady, aged 38, under the care of Dr. Theophilus Thompson, was always well until she had an attack of cholera, which impaired her health : two years prior to her death, she suffered from fever, and from this time was cyanotic.—Bouillaud quotes an instance, where cyanosis followed a difficult labour at the age of twenty-six.—Dr. Harrison has recorded the case of a baker, who became cyanotic at 15, after using great exertion in carrying wood.—Dr. Speer has published the history of a girl, thirteen years old, who had to fill a situation needing great exertion, and she was thenceforth cyanotic.—Dr. Reisch of Vienna has given an account of a woman, 49 years old, who always had good health until an attack of rheumatic fever with endo-pericarditis, after which cyanosis and dropsy set in.   Auscultation detected a loud systolic bruit, which had its maximum intensity at the apex of the heart; the second sound being weak and indistinct.   There was intense cyanosis of the face; with considerable swelling of the jugular veins, and evident regurgitation in them.   At the autopsy, in addition to other morbid appearances, the valve of the foramen ovale was found imperfect, there being a crescentic opening which admitted the first joint of the little finger.   Dr. Reisch explains the symptoms in the following way :—The congenital insufficiency of the valve of the foramen ovale had given rise to no cyanosis previous to the rheumatic attack, and accordingly, no communication between the blood in the auricles could have taken place; for, so long as the valves were healthy, the pressure in the two auricles remained equal, so that the passage of blood from one side to the other was impossible.   But when as the result of endocarditis, incompetency of the mitral valve became established, an increased tension was exerted on the blood in the left auricle, whereby not only a congestion of the pulmonary circulation was occasioned, but simultaneously a quantity of blood was pressed into the right auricle.   Thus there was laid the foundation for a high degree of cyanosis, and the bad effects of mitral insufficiency upon the circulation acquired an enormously increased potency.   The passage of blood from one side to the other must have taken place at the moment of ventricular systole, for this was manifestly the time when the difference of tension in the auricles had reached its maximum.   The blood flowing from the left into the right auricle must have presented an obstacle to that entering by the venæ cavæ, and by imparting to it an impulse in the centrifugal direction, have given rise to the systolic venous impulse.

The *treatment* should be simply palliative, the organic cause being irremediable. A very nourishing diet, warm clothing, the avoidance of fatigue or undue mental excitement, and residence in a pure mild air, will give the sufferers from cyanosis every chance of life which can be afforded them.

XXXI. RUPTURE OF THE HEART.

Rupture of the heart may occur spontaneously from previous disease, or it may be caused by external violence. Rupture from disease is much more frequent on the left than on the right side of the organ; whereas when it occurs from external violence we find just the reverse. The laceration most commonly has its seat in the ventricles, and in that of the left side when disease is its source. Out of fifty-two cases collected by Gluge, the left ventricle was the seat of the lesion in thirty-seven, the right ventricle in eight, the left auricle in three, and the right auricle in two cases. Rupture of the valves or their tendons is generally the consequence of a prior attack of endocarditis; whereas laceration of the muscular wall of the heart most frequently is symptomatic of fatty degeneration. Probably there are six ruptures from fatty degeneration, to one from any other cause. Laceration may also be due to an aneurism in the ventricular wall; to malignant degeneration; and perhaps hydatids, by causing atrophy of the muscular fibres, might lead to it. The rupture takes place as frequently at the apex as at the base. The immediate cause is usually some sudden strain or emotion. This accident happens more frequently in males than females; while its occurrence is rare until after the fiftieth or sixtieth year.

I have seen a case of sudden death from ulceration of the wall of the left ventricle ending in rupture, where there had been no previous symptoms of heart disease. And yet the ulcer was nearly if not quite the size of a florin; was in my opinion of a cancerous nature; and had fairly eaten its way through the tissues, the rent being one inch in length. The gentleman who was the subject of this disease was 68 years old. He had gone to bed apparently quite well; must have got up in the night; and was found dead in his chair the next morning. There could scarcely have been any suffering, for his features were calm; while a book he had been reading remained open on his lap.

Supposing that death is not the immediate result of this accident, the symptoms which indicate the occurrence of rupture are great orthopnœa, intense prostration, syncope, and convulsions. In laceration of the valves, of the chordæ tendineæ, or of the musculi papillares, there is sudden great oppression about the præcordia, together with a loud endocardial bruit.

As regards the majority of cases, rupture of the heart kills instantaneously; not so much, however, as a rule, by the loss of blood, as by the embarrassment to the play of the heart or lungs which arises from the extravasation. In more than one instance, however, the patient has been known to survive some hours, or even days; the wound having become plugged by coagula, so that the extravasation of blood into the pericardium has taken place slowly and gradually.

XXXII. ANGINA PECTORIS.

This is a paroxysmal disease, first described by Dr. Heberden in 1768, who called it a *disorder of the breast;* remarking that " the seat of it and the sense of strangling and anxiety with which it is attended, may make it not improperly be called *angina pectoris.*" It is of not very frequent occurrence.

The *symptoms* of " suffocative breast-pang" consist of paroxysms of intense pain about the præcordial region, accompanied with a feeling of suffocation and a fearful sense of impending death. The pain in the breast is variously described by sufferers as lancinating, burning, or constrictive; and it often seems to radiate from the centre of the sternum to the neck, or to the back, or to the left shoulder and arm. If the paroxysm come on while the patient is walking, immediate rest is necessary; the anguish being most extreme for the time. During the attack the pulse is slow and feeble, the breathing short and hurried, the countenance pale and anxious, the surface of the body cold and perhaps covered with a clammy sweat, while the consciousness is unimpaired. As the struggle passes off, the patient regains his usual health, and perhaps appears perfectly well.

The duration of the seizure rarely exceeds two or three minutes; though it may last for half an hour, or an hour, or even longer. The attacks occur at uncertain intervals of weeks or months; but in confirmed cases the periods of recurrence approximate more and more with each successive paroxysm. The seizure may come on at any time: not only when the patient is walking, but even when in bed. The pain is most severe, and is attended with a feeling as if life were about to cease; while in several cases the paroxysm has at once proved fatal.

It necessarily follows from the foregoing, that the *prognosis* is unfavourable to a marked degree; for if death do not ensue in an early seizure, it generally does so in some subsequent attack. The disease occurs most frequently in advanced life, and is much more common in men than in women. In some few instances it has seemed to have an obscure connexion with gout; and I have read of gout and angina pectoris alternating with each other in the same individual. But I apprehend this only happens in gouty subjects who have a weakened heart, either from attenuation or from fatty degeneration.

With regard to the *pathology* of angina pectoris, it may be said that our improved means of observation have rendered it almost certain that this most distressing disorder is always associated with some important organic cardiac affection; although, in all probability, it is not connected with one form of heart disease only. In many instances fatty degeneration of the muscular fibres of the heart has been detected; a condition which, occasionally at least, seems to be connected with partial obstruction of the coronary arteries. Sometimes possibly, atheromatous deposit, or a syphiloma, about the root of the aorta and aortic valves will be found to have obstructed the coronary arteries by encroaching upon their openings.

Sir John Forbes, in an essay published in 1833, before the value of the microscope was appreciated, collected the histories of forty-five examples of angina pectoris, in which the body had been examined after death. In two of the cases there was disease of the liver only; in four, there was nothing morbid except an excessive coating of fat about the heart; while in the remaining thirty-nine there was found organic disease of the heart or great vessels. Of these latter cases, in ten there was organic disease of the heart alone; in three of the aorta alone; in one of the coronary arteries alone. But there was ossification, or cartilaginous thickening of the coronary arteries, combined with other disease, in sixteen instances; and there was a morbid condition of the cardiac valves in sixteen cases likewise. The aorta was diseased in twenty-four cases, and in twelve there was preternatural softness of the heart.

The *treatment* during a paroxysm consists in the administration of stimulants, such as ammonia, wine, and brandy; and of antispasmodics,—as ether, opium, chloroform, hydrocyanic acid, &c. I have found a mixture of ammonia, spirit of chloroform and of ether, a little belladonna, and tincture of cantharides (F. 85), exceedingly valuable in giving speedy relief. The patient should always carry a dose of this medicine about with him, in order that it may be taken on the least threatening of an attack. Sinapisms, turpentine stupes, hot fomentations, and liniments containing belladonna and chloroform will help to relieve the suffering.

The return of the seizure is to be guarded against by improving the general health; by constant attention to diet; by the occasional use of well-selected tonics; and by the avoidance of stimulants, strong exercise, walking soon after meals, and all mental excitement. A belladonna plaster worn constantly over the præcordial region may do good.

XXXIII. CARDIAC ANEURISM.

Aneurism of the heart was formerly said to occur in two forms:—either as a simple dilatation of the wall of a ventricle, forming the improperly called *passive aneurism* of Corvisart; or as a pouched fulness arising abruptly from the ventricle, constituting a tumour on the heart's surface. The latter is the only disease to which the designation of cardiac aneurism (or partial dilatation) should be applied. In it the tumour may vary in size from that of a small filbert to a growth as large as the fist; the sac is found to contain layers of fibrin or laminated coagula of blood, especially when its mouth is constricted, like arterial aneurisms; while it generally has its seat in the left ventricle, much more rarely in the left or right auricle, but never in the right ventricle.

According to Rokitansky there are two distinct kinds of cardiac aneurism. The first or acute variety depends upon a laceration of the endocardium and muscular tissue, through which the blood passes and gradually makes a pouch; while in this pouch fibrin is deposited, its entrance presenting a fringed margin of endocardium with vegetations attached. The second or chronic form is the result of some inflammatory condition of the muscular fibre, or of the investing or lining membrane of the heart. The walls of the sac consist of the endocardial and pericardial membranes unbroken, while the muscular fibre seems to be replaced by a fibroid tissue. Either kind gives rise to symptoms which are uncertain and obscure. Often the passage of the blood into the sac has caused a murmur, but this has been mistaken and thought to be due to some valvular lesion. Death occurs in consequence of the supervention of extraneous disease unconnected with the aneurism; or it will happen suddenly from the wall of the latter giving way, the blood being poured into the pericardium, or into the pleura—if the free surfaces of the pericardium be adherent, as they often are in these cases.

The *coronary arteries* are now and then diseased. Fatty degeneration and ossification of their coats, obstruction of their canals, and small aneurismal dilatations of their walls are not frequent events. There may be only one aneurism; or several branches of both the right and left coronary artery, or one or both main trunks will perhaps be found dilated into a set of sacculated little tumours. With this condition, all the other vessels in the body need not necessarily be otherwise than healthy. In the instances which have been recorded there have been no symptoms during life to allow of a correct diagnosis, or sometimes even of a suspicion of heart disease; while death has occurred gradually from a progressive loss of strength and exhaustion, or suddenly from rupture of the aneurism—the pericardium being afterwards found filled with blood.

XXXIV. TUMOURS OF THE HEART.

Morbid growths of a benignant or malignant character in the interior of the heart are of rare occurrence, and consequently very little is known of the clinical history of these cases. The chief features which have been noticed seem to have consisted of progressive weakness, with paroxysms of dyspnœa; the latter gradually increasing, until the breathing has become permanently laborious and panting. With this breathlessness, there has been an incessant dry cough; as well as a frequent small pulse, an occasional paroxysm of substernal pain, disturbed rest from fearful dreams, and nausea with disgust for food.

Examples of true *polypus of the heart* are infrequent even amongst the exceptional cases of disease. An instance has been reported by Dr. Douglas, who gives the following summary of the signs which were presented :*—The patient was a gentleman, aged 35, of large frame and development. There was a rapid development of the symptoms. A previously robust state of health. Dyspnœa, with an absence of signs of pulmonary obstruction. Persistent hurry of the circulation, with regularity. Reflex nervous irritation, with a kind of hysteric breathing; paroxysmal cough without expectoration; retching, semi-convulsive attacks, and tearing substernal pain. Delayed obstruction of the circulation through the lungs, the kidneys, and the liver. Anasarca delayed, but rapidly developed. Pulse small and regular. Contrast of a more marked cardiac impulse than radial pulse. Absence of cardiac murmur. Assimilation in the "clang" of the heart's sounds. *Death* occurred after one of those semi-convulsive attacks which usually ended in syncope. At the *necroscopy*, on opening the left ventricle, the rounded nodulated extremity of a tumour was seen projecting through the mitral orifice. On opening the left auricle, this tumour was found growing from its posterior wall; of such bulk as seemed nearly to fill the cavity of the auricle, and hanging downwards, its point projecting into the left ventricle. The tumour was $4\frac{1}{4}$ inches long, $2\frac{1}{2}$ broad, and $1\frac{1}{4}$ deep at its deepest part. Its superficial and dependent part was coated with some layers of coagulated fibrin, and it presented nodules of a translucent appearance; but its base was organically connected with the auricular wall, and was dense in structure. On the outer side of the auricle, opposite the point where the tumour had its attachment, there were small outgrowths of a structure identical with that of the tumour itself; this structure being afterwards found rich in cells, many of them resembling connective tissue bodies, but none having the appearance of typical cancer cells. There was no coagulum in the auricular appendage, nor between the bands of the columnæ carneæ. The right side of the heart presented no abnormality. The pulmonary veins were open; and the valves of the heart were healthy. The aorta was slightly dilated in its ascending portion, and just above it presented an insignificant narrowing, with a small cicatrix at the part.

* *Edinburgh Medical Journal*, p. 908. No. 154, April 1868.

Dr. Morgan exhibited at the Manchester Medical Society, in March 1868, a preparation which he believed to be unique. The patient, 28 years of age, had suffered from one or two attacks of rheumatic fever. He had a complicated cardiac murmur, partly exocardial and partly double mitral. Death took place very gradually. At the subsequent examination it was found that the right auricle contained a *loose tumour*, about as large as a pigeon's egg, composed of phosphate of lime and fibrous stroma. This tumour had evidently grown from the wall of the auricle, had become detached, and had then rolled about in the current of blood ; for both on its surface and on the inside of the wall were to be seen the remains of a pedicle. Another tumour, still small, was also in process of formation. The auriculo-ventricular valve was worn away at one part by the attrition of the substance.

In a case of rupture of the heart shown to the Pathological Society by Dr. Moxon in February 1866, there was seen, on cutting into the substance of the septum of the left ventricle, a pale cheese-coloured *fibrinous mass*, resembling decolorised blood-clot. Dr. Moxon expressed his belief that deposits such as this, which are nearly always in the septum, are none other than clots formed in the substance of the ventricular wall by injury to the vessels, occurring in ruptures that are not sufficiently extensive to reach either surface of the wall.

According to Dr. Oppert, up to the year 1867, eight cases of *syphilomata* of the heart had been recorded in medical literature. The little tumours appear to have given rise to pain, irregular action of the heart, palpitations, dyspnœa, &c. ; while sometimes a slight systolic murmur was noticed. The histories show that these growths are liable to soften, and that they may produce ulceration of the heart and embolism. Their diagnosis must be made through the presence of syphilitic affections of other organs.

Occasionally a cure can be hoped for from the use of specific remedies, provided they are employed at an early period before degeneration of the muscular tissue has set in.

Where the syphilitic deposit on the walls of the heart has taken place slowly, there has been found hypertrophy of the organ. In an instance related by Ricord, the constitutional infection was of long standing ; the first sore being contracted in 1824, while death from syphilitic degeneration of the muscular fibres of the heart did not happen until 1845. Mr. Morgan, of Dublin, has published the medical history of a prostitute who had sores on the genitals eighteen years before death took place, in July 1868, from the formation of gummata in the walls of the ventricles.

Cases of primary *cancer* of the heart are very seldom met with. Less uncommon, are instances where the malignant disease has spread to the heart from adjacent organs,—from the glands in the neck, the bronchial glands, or the lungs. But most frequently where the heart is invaded by cancer, this affection has occurred secondarily : there either is or there has been malignant disease in some other organ of the body.

Cancer of the heart, whether primary or secondary, has rarely given rise to such symptoms that its existence has been diagnosed during life. In a case of this disease which was under the care of Dr. Peacock at the Victoria Park Hospital, and in which particular attention was paid to the heart because it appeared clear that there was a tumour in the chest, and the patient stated that his father died of cancer of the heart, yet no symptoms specially indicating that the heart was involved could be detected.

The cancerous deposit, which is most frequently of the medullary kind, may be found about the pericardium, or in the muscular substance of the heart. In an instance reported by Dr. Bright, a thick layer of yellow malignant disease covered the whole of the visceral and parietal portions of the pericardium : so that this fibro-serous membrane was glued to the heart. The external wall of the right ventricle has been found occupied by a large knotted tumour, looking like a supernumerary heart and formed of medullary cancer. In addition to masses of cancer involving the walls of the heart, the columnæ carneæ, and the musculi pectinati, we find that the surfaces of one or more of the valves may have cancerous vegetations impeding the proper closure of the openings.

XXXV. FUNCTIONAL DERANGEMENT OF THE HEART.

The disorder now to be considered is of special importance on account of the mental distress to which it gives rise. For it is a curious feature in medical practice, that whereas patients with grave structural disease of the heart (prior to the occurrence of the secondary evils) seldom consider that there is anything radically wrong, individuals with mere deranged action can scarcely be persuaded that they are not doomed to an early and sudden death. The latter are unable to understand how indigestion, fast living, the abuse of tobacco and tea, or severe mental labour with insufficient bodily exercise, can produce palpitation with an intermittent pulse ; while the physician who assures them that there is no cardiac disease, is either regarded as one ignorant of his business, or as a good-natured fellow afraid to tell an unwelcome truth.

Functional disorder can closely simulate organic disease of the heart. There may be an irregular feeble pulse, palpitation, and fluttering ; with a cardiac murmur and subcutaneous œdema in anæmic subjects. A systolic murmur, sometimes audible at the base and apex, may even be heard in a few healthy individuals under the influence of great nervous excitement. The local suffering is usually greater than in organic disease; the patient complaining either of a dull wearying ache in the præcordial region, or of occasional lancinating pains. Frequently there is inability to lie on the left side, owing to tenderness. There is always great depression of spirits; the digestive organs are deranged, flatulence and acid eructations being especially common; a sense of choking, or of the rising of a ball in the throat, is complained of; and there may be occasional attacks of giddiness, faintness, headache, noises in the ears, flushing of the face, violent pulsation in the aorta and other arteries, &c. There is rarely any dyspnœa, if the blood be healthy; and even when the breathing is hurried the patient hardly refers to it, all his thoughts being fixed on the palpitation or thumping of his heart, and the pain.

Some remarkable examples of unusually rapid action of the heart are to be found recorded in the medical periodicals. In one instance, a patient who consulted Dr. Cotton, had a pulse too rapid to be counted; the respirations were forty; while the pulsations of the heart were 230 in a minute. Three weeks after the commencement of the attack, the action of the heart suddenly became natural in every respect, and the pulse fell to 80. Four or five similar attacks took place; most of these ending in recovery while the patient was taking digitalis. Dr. Cotton believes that such rapid action of the heart, when unconnected with organic mischief or inflammatory disease or displacement, must be due either to the heart being so extremely sensitive that it contracts upon the healthy blood before the cavities have got filled; or else the blood is of such an abnormal and irritating character, that it excites premature contraction. One symptom remained after recovery from the last attack, viz. pulsation of the right jugular vein; this being probably due to the tricuspid valve allowing of regurgitation. Why the valve should continue incompetent, and should not give rise to a regurgitant murmur, are questions difficult to answer.*— A second case is reported by Dr. Edmunds. It ended in recovery.— A similar instance happened in the practice of Sir Thomas Watson; where the beatings, "or rather the waggings," of the heart were found to number 216 in the minute. There was no murmur. In a day or two, the inordinate action suddenly ceased, and the pulse numbered 72. During a third seizure, the attack suddenly passed off while Sir Thomas Watson was present. A fourth attack proved fatal. At the autopsy the heart was found large, as if it had been distended; while the muscular walls were very thin and soft. No other morbid state could be detected.

To prevent any error in the diagnosis of functional from organic

---

* *British Medical Journal*, p. 630. London, 1 June 1867. The case by Dr. Edmunds will be found in the same journal, p. 721, for the 15 June; while that mentioned by Sir Thomas Watson is at p. 752, 22 June 1867.

affections of the heart, the physical signs of valvular disease (as already described) must be borne in mind.   Moreover, the patient ought to be examined with the greatest care; and the practitioner if in doubt, should reserve his opinion until he can make a second investigation.   The disease perhaps most likely to be overlooked is fatty degeneration, especially if the pulse be temporarily hurried and the corneæ appear healthy.

Functional disturbance of the heart often occurs in cases of hysteria, ovarian or uterine irritation, neuralgia, and anæmia; it is frequently complained of by women at " the change of life;" it may be associated with the derangements due to nervous exhaustion, —such as over study, mental anxiety, sexual excesses, &c.; morbid states of the blood, gout, rheumatism, or chronic disease of the liver can produce it; the use of tobacco or strong tea not uncommonly originates it; and lastly it is a frequent result of all forms of dyspepsia.

The object of our treatment must be to allay the symptoms, while we also endeavour to remove their source.   The cause of the suffering ought to be fully explained to the patient, and he must be led to feel confidence in our ability to cure him.   To quiet the circulation, antispasmodics and sedatives and special tonics will be needed.   Perhaps few remedies of this description answer better than ammonia, ether, sumbul, henbane, belladonna, hop, opium, &c. (according to F. 86, 93, 95, 326, 337, 361).   The officinal belladonna or opium plaster, applied over the præcordia, gives relief. Where the patient can bear digitalis, which most probably acts as a cardiac tonic, this drug (F. 334) will prove very useful.   Supposing it be desirable to effect a compromise in the treatment,—to feel one's way, the American wild cherry (F. 333) can be prescribed instead of digitalis.   If there be constipation with unhealthy secretions, a warm aperient (F. 146, 149, 162) should be ordered. Then, if the deranged cardiac action appear to have any connexion with gout, saline effervescing draughts with colchicum (F. 46, 348, 352) ought to be administered.   Where there are acid eructations with dyspepsia, bismuth, soda or potash, hydrocyanic acid, laurel water, &c. (F. 65, 67, 70), will be necessary; followed at the end of a few days by the nitro-hydrochloric acid in some bitter infusion (F. 378).   Pepsine (F. 420) frequently does good in these cases of dyspeptic misery, although it will be useless without particular attention to the diet.   The patient who cannot afford time to eat his meals quietly, and to masticate his food thoroughly, must bear his troubles.   The practitioner will have to see that the teeth and gums are in a proper condition.   It is astonishing that people should expect to enjoy good health, while their gums are sodden and filled only with decayed teeth and useless stumps.   In these days of painless dentistry and the skilful adaptation of artificial teeth, every mouth ought to be clean and sound.   Supplementary to the foregoing, the use of tobacco and tea should be forbidden; while it must be remembered that malt liquors more frequently than not disagree.   A small quantity of brandy in iced soda water is generally most suitable.   And lastly, if there be symptoms of nervous exhaustion, or if the patient be anæmic, steel will be required.   The best preparations in these cases, as a rule, are the citrate of iron and ammonia (F. 401, 403), the reduced iron (F. 394, 404), the citrate of iron and strychnia (F. 408), or quinine and iron (F. 380).

XXXVI. INTRA-THORACIC TUMOURS.

An intra-thoracic tumour either consists of an aneurism ; or it may be composed of cancer, of simple exudation matter, of fibrous tissue, or of masses of fatty or steatomatous matter.   Putting aside the cases of aneurism, we find that the other tumours, whatever be their nature, commonly have their origin in the connective tissue and glandular structures, and are developed in the mediastina. The symptoms they produce are chiefly due to the pressure exerted on the heart or lungs, or on the nerves or vessels ; and consequently there may be no indications of disease for a time, as a tumour oftens attains some size before it interferes with the circulation or the respiration.

The symptoms of mediastinal tumour are exceedingly variable. Speaking generally, we find more or less pain, restlessness, cough, dyspnœa or even orthopnœa, frothy or viscid expectoration, palpitation, hoarseness, frequently dysphagia, and every now and again hæmoptysis.   By its irritating effects the tumour may produce pleurisy, bronchitis, pneumonia, and inflammation of the larynx or trachea.   By the pressure exerted it is not unlikely to cause pulmonary collapse, if a main bronchus be obstructed ; or a bulging or even perforation of the ribs and sternum; or displacement of the heart ; or it will perhaps impede the circulation through the aorta, or through the superior or inferior vena cava.   The dulness on percussion becomes more marked as the growth protrudes into the anterior mediastinum ; while the auscultatory signs will vary according to the nature of the secondary phenomena.

Primary hydatid disease of the lung, or of the mediastinal structures, is hardly ever met with.   In cases where hydatids, or portions of their cystic membranes, are expectorated, the original seat of the parasitic growth has been the liver.   At least, this has been the case with the great majority of instances.

With regard to cases of primary cancer involving the root of the lung, it is remarkable that inflammatory condensation of the pulmonary tissue, with disorganization and abscess, may result comparatively early.   In the only three examples of this rare and obscure disease which fell under Dr. George Budd's observation at King's College Hospital, during nearly twenty years, the tumour implicated the root of the right lung.* The extent of change in the lung in these three cases was greater as the tumour was larger, and involved more completely the root of the lung; while in all, the left lung was free from adhesions, and presented only those appearances which result from recent congestion. As to the way in which these changes arose, Dr. Budd suggests that they resulted from the tumour involving and destroying all or a greater part of the pulmonary nerves; and consequently the inflammatory affections of the tissues of the lung in these instances are analogous to that destructive inflammation of the eyeball which results from disease involving the fifth nerve within the orbit. The lung resembles the eyeball in this respect, that all the nerves which supply it are comprised at its root in a very small space, so that they can there be destroyed or paralysed (and the organ, in consequence, be deprived entirely of nervous influence) by disease of no very great extent.

Mediastinal cancer is seldom primary. It may occur secondarily to disease of distant organs, or it can possibly spread from the lungs. The fatal termination in mediastinal tumour, whether this be cancerous or not, often takes place slowly; the patient's sufferings from impeded respiration, want of sleep and appetite, debility, and anæmia, gradually increasing until he dies anasarcous and exhausted. Sometimes, however, death takes place almost suddenly from hæmorrhage, from thrombosis, or from spasm of the glottis. All that art can do in these very distressing cases is to palliate the prominent symptoms. Great temporary relief may, however, be often given by the cautious use of diuretics or of aperients; by dry cupping; by inunction with the ointment of red iodide of mercury (one part of the officinal ointment to three of lard), or by freely rubbing in the compound iodine ointment (equal parts of the ointment and cod liver oil); by venesection, to the extent of six or eight ounces, if symptoms of pulmonary or cardiac congestion predominate; and by employing antispasmodics,—such as ether, spirit of chloroform, ammonia, opium, belladonna, stramonium, &c.

* *Medico-Chirurgical Transactions*, vol. xlii. p. 215. London, 1859.

PART VI.

DISEASES OF THE THORACIC WALLS.

I. PLEURODYNIA.

PLEURODYNIA [from Πλευρὰ = the side + ὀδύνη = pain], or chronic rheumatism of the walls of the chest, is a disorder of almost every day occurrence. It is of importance on account of the long-continued pain to which it often gives rise; and partly because it is always believed by the patient to be an inflammation of the side, while every now and then it is mistaken by the practitioner for pleurisy or pericarditis, or even for peritonitis.

This affection is sometimes associated with rheumatism of the joints, but in by far the greater number of cases there is no such combination. In nineteen cases out of twenty, the muscular and fibrous textures of the left side of the chest are alone affected. The pain may be acute, and it often comes on suddenly; being referred to the infra-mammary region (though sometimes it extends rather lower), and being increased by a deep inspiration or by any stretching movement of the trunk.

The *diagnosis* is easy with moderate care; for although there is often tenderness on pressure, with slightly impaired thoracic movement, yet there are none of the physical signs of pleurisy, &c. The pulse also does not betoken inflammation; while the tongue is clean, the skin inclined to be cool rather than unduly hot, and there is no real dyspnœa. Out of the large number of cases which I have seen, I can recollect none where the general symptoms have not been those of impaired health, with debility; there usually being found, moreover, more or less constipation, loss of appetite, mental depression, and the secretion of urine containing an excess of phosphates or urates. One of the worst examples of pleurodynia which I have met with occurred in a medical man who was suffering from acute rheumatism affecting the knees and ankles; and I well remember the incredulity with which he received my opinion that his pericardium was healthy, as well as the difficulty that was experienced in preventing him from taking calomel and having a vein opened. The success which followed the use of simple treatment, however, quite reassured him.—In tertiary syphilis there is often pain about the middle of the sternum, and sometimes costal periostitis; but a consideration of the general symptoms, together with a local examination, will prevent this disease from being mistaken for pleurodynia.—In herpes zoster or the shingles, sharp pain often precedes the appearance of the vesicles; but the suffering is usually of a burning character, is not increased by movement, and in the great majority of cases is on the right side of the body.

Pleurodynia affects men rather more frequently than women, probably because of the greater exposure of the former to the sources of rheumatism. The residents of marshy districts, the inhabitants of damp houses, coal porters and other labouring men who drink large quantities of beer, as well as policemen or soldiers on night duty, are very liable to this affection.

In the *treatment* of these cases, over-active remedies ought decidedly to be avoided. Cupping, leeching, severe purging or sweating, and blistering will only render the disorder more intractable. If the pain come on in the course of rheumatic fever, it may merely be necessary to order fomentations or hot poultices in addition to the remedies which are being employed. But in ordinary cases, where the pleurodynia is the sole manifestation of any disease, a cure may generally be effected in from three or four days to a fortnight, by a mixture of ammonia, tincture of aconite, and bark (F. 371); by one or two warm water or Turkish baths (F. 130); by friction night and morning with a belladonna and opium liniment (F. 281); and by plain nourishing food. Stimulants can be given, if necessary; but all kinds of beer and port wine should generally be avoided. In obstinate cases, iodide of potassium (F. 31) may be required; while cod liver oil will often prove extremely useful.

II. INTERCOSTAL NEURALGIA.

Neuralgia [from Νεῦρον = a nerve + ἄλγος = pain] may affect the intercostal, as it does the other nerves of the body. The pain is either of a dull and continued aching character, or it comes on in sharp paroxysms; while it is most frequently situated in the sixth, seventh, eighth, or ninth nerves of the left side. These nervous trunks (anterior primary branches of the dorsal nerves) pass forwards in the intercostal spaces with the vessels, and are distributed to the parietes of the thorax and abdomen. The pains, whether dull or severe, follow the course of the nerves, and extend from the thoracic wall directly backwards to the vertebræ. One or two particularly painful spots can often be detected by pressure, while sometimes there is cutaneous hyperæsthesia of the whole mammary or infra-mammary region. There are no febrile symptoms; the pleuræ, lungs, and heart are found healthy; but there are often indications of debility. The catamenia are sometimes irregular, or the flow may be supplemented by an abundant leucorrhœal discharge.   Oftentimes there is some uterine or ovarian disorder present ; particularly such as retroflexion, excoriation of the labia, or chronic ovaritis.

Chlorotic and hysterical women suffer most frequently from this species of neuralgia.   I have met with it during the progress of Bright's disease.   It may form a subsidiary phenomenon in phthisis.   The pain sometimes lasts for weeks ; being got rid of with the greatest difficulty in those cases where there is no obvious condition of the general health, or no local affection, to account for it.   Intercostal neuritis is the only disease with which it can be really confounded, and this is of very rare occurrence.   A dull tensive aching, referred to the left hypochondrium, is not unfrequently complained of in affections of the spleen ; but the pain is seldom troublesome until the gland has become so much enlarged that it can be readily felt.

The remedies which are usually the most beneficial, consist of quinine, iron, cinchona, cod liver oil, and a nutritious diet. Friction with liniments containing belladonna and aconite gives relief. Sometimes, pressure by means of strips of belladonna plaster applied all round the thorax is a source of great comfort.   Where there are one or more obstinately tender points, the subcutaneous injection of the sixth of a grain of morphia (F. 314) will effect a cure, if employed in conjunction with remedies that improve the general health.

III. THORACIC MYALGIA.

The tendinous insertions of the fleshy bodies of the pectoral muscles, and sometimes of the intercostal muscles, every now and then become the seats of a hot wearying pain, which is often mistaken for pleurodynia and even for more serious diseases.   It is probable also that the diaphragm, like the other muscles of respiration, occasionally suffers from myalgia; especially where the ceaseless action of this septum gets exaggerated by affections attended with dyspnœa.

Myalgia [Μῦς = a muscle + ἄλγος = pain] is generally due to over-work of the affected muscles.   It is a disorder common to both sexes, though probably arising most frequently in males. The pain is seldom complained of in the morning, especially after a good night's rest ; but it follows upon a few hours' exertion, and gradually increases towards the evening. Patients give various accounts of the amount of suffering, and frequently the descriptions appear to be exaggerated.   No doubt some individuals feel pain much more acutely than others ; so that what is regarded as almost torture by one would be looked upon as trifling by another. The physical suffering, however, is not on these grounds to be lightly thought of; and especially should the practitioner avoid the habit easily acquired, of looking upon a reputed pain as imaginary, because it is spoken of in more extravagant terms than he may think warrantable.

In all cases of persistent myalgia the blood is more or less impoverished, and consequently the general health will be found depressed. Sometimes the appetite is bad, and the digestion impaired; the bowels are constipated; attacks of palpitation are common; the sexual functions are disordered; and there is a disinclination for work of any kind. The patient also is irritable or low-spirited. From this it follows that the treatment should consist in diminishing for a time those exertions or movements which have been the partial cause of the disorder; while a certain amount of rest is to be especially ensured to the affected muscles by the application of a flannel bandage round the thorax. Friction with anodyne liniments will also be of service; but above all the general health ought to be improved by remedies to promote digestion, quinine with ferruginous tonics, and nourishing food. The use of strips of opium or belladonna plaster around the painful part of the chest often does good; the favourable result being partly due to the support afforded to the muscles, and partly to the soothing of their excessive irritability.

IV. ABNORMAL CONDITIONS OF THE DIAPHRAGM.

Considering the very important parts with which the diaphragm is in relation, it cannot appear surprising that this thin musculo-fibrous septum often gets involved in the diseases of adjoining organs and tissues. Independently of its position as a barrier between the thorax and abdomen, the diaphragm is the most important inspiratory muscle. Then its upper or thoracic surface is in relation with three serous membranes—the pleura on either side, and the pericardium covering the tendinous centre; while its under or abdominal surface is closely connected with the peritoneum. Moreover, through three large openings in its coats are transmitted the aorta and thoracic duct and right azygos vein, the œsophagus and pneumogastric nerves, and the inferior vena cava. Being thus placed in such close approximation with the pleuræ, lungs, and heart by its upper convex surface, it cannot but often become involved when morbid action is set up in these vital organs. So the connection of its under concave surface with the liver, the spleen, and the left or greater extremity of the stomach; and less intimately with the kidneys, pancreas, transverse portion of the duodenum, and solar plexus must materially tend not only to influence its action, but also to make it a frequent secondary seat of disease.

Inflammation of the diaphragm, or diaphragmitis [Διάφραγμα = a separation between two parts, from διαφράγνυμι, with the terminal -*itis*], is probably only met with by the physician when it sets in consecutively to disease in adjoining organs. The morbid action may possibly, however, have its starting point in a rheumatic state of the system; none of the thoracic or abdominal viscera being at the same time affected. As a consequence of punctured wounds, fractured ribs, and other mechanical injuries, diaphragmitis is every now and then observed in hospital practice.

The chief symptoms of this disease are those presented in other important inflammations; supplemented by the occurrence of severe tenderness with a sense of constriction around the upper part of the abdomen and back, great pain about the sternum and lower ribs on coughing or sneezing or making a deep inspiration, more or less dyspnœa, the performance of the respiratory movements almost wholly by the intercostal muscles, painful deglutition, anxiety of countenance, frequent hiccup and sobbing, spasms or cramps of all the abdominal muscles, and perhaps a sense of suffocation with delirium. Where, in fatal cases, an opportunity has been afforded of ascertaining the effects of the inflammatory action the results which have for the most part been observed have consisted of effusions of coagulable lymph or of a sero-albuminous fluid, or of patches of ulceration, or of small collections of pus. When recovery has happened and examinations have been made after the lapse of years, the diaphragm has been seen to have become abnormally adherent to neighbouring viscera; while it has also perhaps been found considerably thickened, with its tissue rendered almost as dense as cartilage.

The treatment should be of the same character as that required in inflammations of the organs connected with this muscle. Belts of linseed poultice, made very hot and moist, and medicated with the extracts of belladonna and poppies (F. 297) are especially serviceable. Vomiting is to be allayed by the use of ice. The inhalation of chloroform and ether (F. 313) will often relieve the hiccup when all other remedies fail. The persistence of pain at any one point can be stopped by the use of the ether spray, or by subcutaneous injections of morphia and atropine (F. 314). The importance of milk as an article of nourishment is not to be overlooked.

Fatty degeneration of the diaphragm is a morbid state which is probably more common than at first sight the practitioner will feel inclined to believe. The affection, however, has been overlooked; and chiefly for the reason that in a large number of post mortem examinations the condition of this septum still escapes investigation. So far as I can call to mind, Mr. G. W. Callender has been the first to notice this disease.* Here and there cases have been reported where the diaphragm has been discovered wasted in connection with a similar affection of the other muscles of the body. But in the widely different instances published by Mr. Callender, the tissue of the diaphragm has been found to have undergone conversion into fat; the granules of which have destroyed and taken the place of the muscular fibres. For the most part, this degeneration has been met with in connection with a similar change in the muscular structure of the heart; so that sometimes death has occurred from a failure of the action of this organ, sometimes from severe disturbance and embarrassment of the breathing owing to the inability of the spoiled and fatty diaphragm to contract properly and to allow of normal inspiration. Now and then not only the structure of the heart and diaphragm is more or less destroyed by fatty degeneration, but other muscles, with the liver, and coats of the bloodvessels, are injured in a similar way. In such, death may of course happen in one of several ways,—from exhaustion, from syncope, from rupture of the heart, from cerebral hæmorrhage owing to the coats of a vessel giving way, or from the breathing becoming laboured to a degree incompatible with life. The question as to which organ shall first give way, will probably be determined by accident; that which becomes over-strained or excited being the one to yield.

Cancer of the diaphragm as a primary disease is unknown. Cancerous infiltration or deposit, the consequence of the extension of malignant disease from the liver or œsophagus or other adjoining organs, is not very uncommon. Under these circumstances, one or more large masses of cancer will perhaps be found, on the under or upper surface of the diaphragm; or there may be merely a number of papulæ, with small patches or laminæ formed by the coalescence of several of these pimples. Moreover, isolated cancers have been observed in this structure; that is to say, cancer of the diaphragm may be the only disease detected at the necroscopy, the original mischief having been removed some time previously by operation. This appears to have been so in a case related by Sir Robert Carswell; in which several nodules varying in diameter from a pea to half-a-crown, and formed of a scirrhous stroma with a milky-looking infiltration, were discovered in the diaphragm of a woman who had previously had her breast amputated.

Syphilitic gummous tumours have been found in the diaphragm; these growths oft-times extending upwards into the lung, in other instances downwards into the liver. Now and then, both the lung and liver are firmly adherent to the gummous mass. In a woman who died at the Middlesex Hospital, in November 1861, of syphilitic disease of the dura mater and liver, there was found a firm and pale-yellow tumour with white septa running through it, the

* *The Lancet*, p. 39. London, 12 January 1867.

size of half a large orange, embedded in the substance of the diaphragm. The growth projected downwards, and was inseparably connected with the left lobe of the liver, as well as with the spleen. I know of no means by which such a morbid condition could be detected during life.

Laceration or perforation of the diaphragm has occurred from falls and other accidents; from attempts to suppress the pains of parturition; and from violent vomiting. It has also taken place in consequence of the extension of suppuration and ulceration from the liver, spleen, or even stomach; from the rupture of an aortic aneurism which had encroached on its texture; from malignant degeneration; from the extension of hydatid cysts upwards from the liver, or downwards from the lungs; as well as from some congenital malformation or cleft becoming unusually strained and so giving way at its border.

Finally, *convulsive action of the diaphragm,* or spasms of the midriff, may prove troublesome as a mild idiopathic affection, or as a consequence of irritation from morbid action going on in adjoining tissues, or as a result of general exhaustion from disease in distant organs. Hiccup is a curious effect of the sudden and involuntary and momentary contraction of the diaphragm, the glottis being simultaneously narrowed. In vomiting, crying, sobbing, sneezing, &c., there is convulsive action of the midriff; the other muscles of respiration being likewise affected. Moreover, in weakly subjects long-continued attacks of hiccup or vomiting, of chronic cough, of dyspnœa, &c. may lead to diaphragmatic myalgia; a painful affection which has been referred to in the preceding section.

END OF THE FIRST VOLUME.

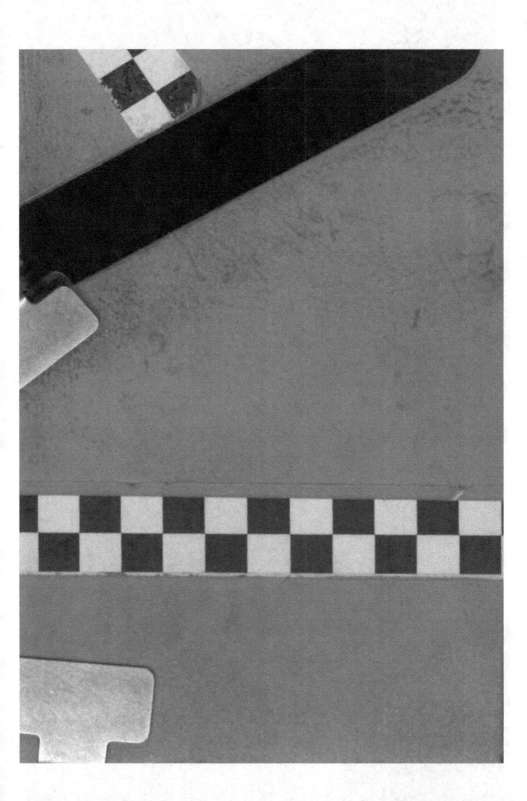

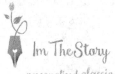
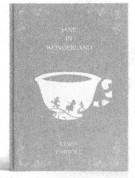